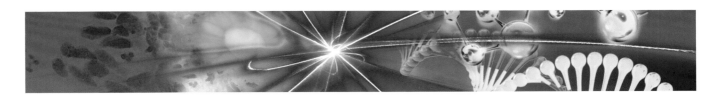

Cytopathology Review Guide
4e

Dedication

I'd like to express my extreme thanks to my family for supporting me throughout the past 30 years of my career—it may come as no surprise to you that I intend to have 30 years more. I know it's difficult that I spend 200 days in the air working throughout around the world, either giving speeches or building bridges for our profession by helping to providing access to appropriate, fair and equitable healthcare for all people. I firmly believe that access to appropriate and affordable healthcare is a fundamental right. It is because of your support that I have been able to make an impact, hopefully advance our profession, and play a small role in the revolution of medicine. To my late mother, who always loved to watch me in action—whether it was interviewing or working with former or future presidents, and who consistently bestowed her admiration upon my professional pursuits, I dedicate this book to you. Thanks also to my dear father, whose ceaseless, inquisitive mind continues to probe my professional endeavors. My father has faced his share of benign and malignant diseases—including a recent bout where I had the rare privilege to help overturn an established diagnosis of an inoperable glioblastoma to that of an operable meningioma. I'm pleased to report he's still with us 2 years later and disease free. Dad, your investment in me paid off.

Lastly, to Liesl and the kids (Caleb, Noah, and Frances), who understand the reason why I spend most of my time away. Thank you for the latitude in letting me pursue my dreams and help patients worldwide have access to the right test, at the right time, at the right cost. There's nothing more powerful than being given the opportunity to pursue one's own dreams, and nothing more rewarding than seeing them come true. I thank you with all my heart.

EBH

ISBN 978-089189-6357 ©ASCP 2015

E Blair Holladay, PhD, SCT(ASCP)^{CM}
CEO
American Society for Clinical Pathology
Chicago, IL

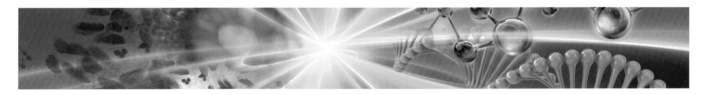

Cytopathology Review Guide
4th edition

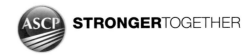

Erik N Tanck (production)
Martin Tyminski (cover & chapter opener art)
Joshua Weikersheimer (publishing direction)

Notice

Trade names for equipment and supplies described are included as suggestions only. In no way does their inclusion constitute an endorsement of preference by the Author or the ASCP. The Author and ASCP urge all readers to read and follow all manufacturers' instructions and package insert warnings concerning the proper and safe use of products. The American Society for Clinical Pathology, having exercised appropriate and reasonable effort to research material current as of publication date, does not assume any liability for any loss or damage caused by errors and omissions in this publication. Readers must assume responsibility for complete and thorough research of any hazardous conditions they encounter, as this publication is not intended to be all inclusive, and recommendations and regulations change over time.

PRESS

Printed in Singapore

19 18 17 16 15

Contents

©ASCP 2015 ISBN 978-089189-6357

Acknowledgments

Since the first edition of the textbook, I have joined the ASCP in Chicago, Illinois, originally in 2005 as the Executive Director for the Board of Certification and Vice President for Scientific Activities, and since 2010, as the Chief Executive Officer (CEO). It has been and continues to be a pleasure to work with so many wonderfully talented individuals on a day to day basis–both volunteers and staff alike. Together, we have built an organization that is second to none and serves as the largest pathology association in the world with over 120,000 members.

Since the first edition of this book in 1998, I've had the pleasure of collaborating with many friends and colleagues, including the visionary Karen Allen Linder, SCT(ASCP), Mac DeMay, MD, FASCP–author of the gold standard cytopathology textbook (published by ASCP Press), Laurie Charles, MT(ASCP)–an expert in Clinical Laboratory Management, and Dr Joshua Weikersheimer, an impeccable editor, publisher, and acclaimed microbiologist.

In this latest edition, I have many more to thank for their support and contributions to the overall content. First, a special thanks to our esteemed colleagues and scientists who have served on the ASCP GYN and non-GYN Cytopathology Committees. I requested and received permission from the chairs/cochairs of these committees to repurpose some of the out of print content in order for it to be distributed throughout various sections of this book. As such, I would like to personally acknowledge them: Bob Goulart, MD, FASCP, Stan Eilers, MD, FASCP, Eva Wojcik, MD, FASCP and Mike Facik, SCT(ASCP). These committee Chairs and their respective committee members have assisted the ASCP by donating their time and talents, and we are ever indebted to each of you for your dedication to the profession and to the advancement of diagnostic pathology worldwide.

To Amy Wendel Spiczka, SCT(ASCP)[CM], HTL[CM], MB[CM], Manager of Anatomic Pathology at Mayo Clinic Arizona, for her visionary insight and exceptional skills in both cytopathology and molecular biology. Amy served as the principal editor for the new theranostics chapter of the text, which significantly differentiates this text from previous editions. Amy continues to enhance the profession by embracing change and helping diagnostic cytologists evolve their molecular diagnostic skills. We are indebted to her tireless vision and forthright positivity.

Lastly, and most importantly, I'd like to especially thank Jennifer Clark, SCT(ASCP)[CM], MB[CM], who served as my chief editor. In particular, Jennifer assisted me with editing the chapter on molecular theranostics as well as serving as editor for many of the new questions, images, and references throughout the text. In addition to her superb editing skills, Jennifer was a significant contributor of content in the areas of the Bethesda System, ASCCP-NIH-ASCP guidelines, the Bethesda thyroid, and the Paris urine. Her painstaking perfection and can do/will do attitude made collaboration truly a pleasure. Without Jennifer, this new edition would not have been completed. It has been an honor to work with you over the past 20 years, and I thank you for all you do on behalf of ASCP and the profession.

Preface

This book is dedicated to those cytology students, pathology residents, pathology fellows in training, and pathologists who have chosen to advance their careers in the subspecialty area of cytopathology and, more recently, in its relationship to genomic medicine. Since its original publication in 1998, this text has prepared thousands of individuals throughout the world to successfully pass the national board examinations. I'm often humbled by their testimony and the candid remarks they have shared with me regarding how this text had a positive influence on their lives as they prepared to practice the profession.

The field of cancer diagnostics has rapidly evolved since the advent of genetic cloning and the completion of the mapping of the human genome. Because of this, the specificity of molecular testing continues to play an increasingly important role in aiding cellular morphology for the diagnosis of cancer. I've spent my career as a proponent of genomic testing, being supportive of the molecular revolution, and as such, am elated that these professions are finally merging as a better alternative to conventional cancer diagnostics. That being said, it's critical that educators embrace the complementary nature of both of these modes of diagnostic medicine in order to ensure that the future practitioners they educate are equipped with the complete set of skills that ensure their patients will have access to the personalized therapeutic interventions that are now available to save their lives. Our patients depend on us, and we have obligation to teach future legions of practitioners, the significant relationship between cytopathology and molecular diagnostics. I've been preaching this since 1985–and yes, there have been many skeptics throughout the years–but I'm pleased to see this dream has finally come to fruition.

I have expanded this book significantly in each of the areas of diagnostic cytopathology, thanks to the contributions of many individuals that have been aforementioned in the Acknowledgments section. As such, the book has increased almost 25%, and I have modernized the content to reflect the current state of practice. New and enhanced questions and images will allow the reader to use this text as the quintessential preparation tool for successfully passing the board examinations. In addition, I have added a new cutting edge chapter on theranostics. It is critically important that, as new FDA approved therapeutic modalities continue to emerge within the market, we complement our diagnostic toolkit with these companion diagnostics, thus allowing the patient to receive personalized therapy. This new chapter showcases those diagnostic tools that are currently FDA approved. As new drugs are approved, I will add additional content to the virtual edition of this text. I strongly believe that molecular diagnostics and subsequent theranostics are the future of the profession. These personalized diagnostic markers and their subsequent therapeutic implications will help make the profession more vibrant, exciting and showcase that cytologists are the lynchpin to the future of diagnostic medicine. Clinicians are relying on us. We must help them choose the right test and consult with them on the appropriate clinical follow-up. That's the future.

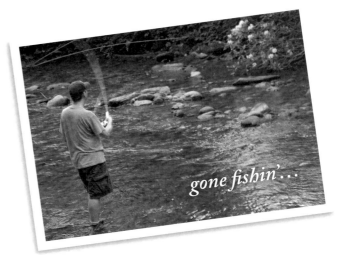

gone fishin'…

E Blair Holladay, PhD, SCT(ASCP)ᶜᴹ

CEO, American Society for Clinical Pathology
Chicago, IL April 2015

Bibliography

Carson F, Cappellano CH [2014] *Histotechnology: A Self-Instructional Text*, 4e. Chicago: ASCP Press [ISBN 978-089189-6319]

Chowdhury S [2001] *The Power of Six Sigma: An Inspiring Tale of How Six Sigma Is Transforming the Way we Work*. Chicago: Dearborn Trade [ISBN 978-079314-4341]

Cibas ES, Ducatman BS, eds [2009] *Cytology: Diagnostic Principles and Clinical Correlates*, 3e. Philadelphia: Saunders Elsevier [ISBN 978-141605-3293]

Davis D [2008] *Laboratory Safety: A Self Assessment Workbook*. Chicago: ASCP Press [ISBN 978-089189-5701]

DeMay, RM [2012] *The Art & Science of Cytopathology*, 2e. Chicago: ASCP Press [ISBN 978-089189-6449]

Keebler CM, Somrak TM [1993] *The Manual of Cytotechnology*, 7e. Chicago: ASCP Press [ISBN 978-089189-3520]

Nayar R, Wilbur D, eds [2015] *The Bethesda System for Reporting Cervical Cytology* [in press]

Perney S [2002] *HIPAA Training Handbook for the Healthcare Staff: An Introduction to Confidentiality and Privacy Under HIPAA*. USA: Opus Communications [ISBN 978-157839-1516]

Snyder JR, Wilkinson DS, eds [1998] *Management in Laboratory Medicine*, 3e. Philadelphia: Lippincott [ISBN 978-039755-1491]

A full list of all references including journal articles may be found at www.ascp.org

ISBN 978-089189-6357 ©ASCP 2015

Chapter 1

Female Reproductive Tract

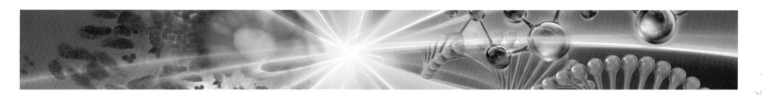

syncytiotrophoblasts

1 The portion of the menstrual cycle that is constant is:
   a follicular phase
   b secretory
   c ovulation
   d proliferative

2 Which of the following is considered a pituitary gonadotropin?
   a luteinizing hormone
   b estrogen
   c androgen
   d glucocorticoid

3 Cells normally found in the endocervical canal that resemble histiocytes, possess uniform nuclei with fine, regular chromatin distribution, and have discretely vacuolated but poorly defined cytoplasm are:
   a reserve cells
   b cells from microglandular hyperplasia
   c metaplastic cells
   d oxyphilic cells

4 LH peaks at which day of the menstrual cycle?
   a 28
   b 5
   c 14
   d 1

5 The presence of mitotic figures indicates:
   a the possibility of neoplasia
   b reparative/regenerative processes
   c a current HPV infection
   d no pathologic information

6 An example of a protective reaction of the uterine cervix is:
   a hyperkeratosis
   b pemphigus
   c folic acid deficiency
   d chronic lymphocytic cervicitis

7 Which of the following may be associated with a threatened abortion?
   a increase in desquamation and cytolysis
   b boat shaped intermediate cells
   c large cells with multiple, tightly clustered nuclei
   d intermediate cell maturation

8 A vaginal smear from a 23-year-old female contains ciliated glandular cells, metaplastic epithelial cells, and mixed mature squamous cells in the presence of a moderate inflammatory exudate. The appropriate diagnosis is:
   a negative for squamous intraepithelial lesion
   b negative for squamous intraepithelial lesion, limited by inflammation
   c vaginal adenosis
   d a diagnosis cannot be rendered based on the above cytologic findings

9 Estrogen reaches its greatest concentration in the bloodstream at which day of the menstrual cycle?
   a 1
   b 14
   c 21
   d 28

10 A masculinizing tumor of the ovary is:
   a Sertoli-Leydig cell tumors
   b Brenner tumor
   c gynandroblastoma
   d endodermal sinus

   ↑ serum androgens → atrophic vaginal smears

11 In order for menses to occur, which structure in the ovary must degenerate?
   a corpus luteum
   b tunica albuginea
   c Call-Exner bodies
   d medulla

12 The ratio of estrogen to follicle stimulating hormone in the bloodstream is:
   a proportional
   b inverse
   c unrelated
   d these 2 hormones are never found together

   estrogen is negative feedback to FSH secretion

13 Microglandular hyperplasia is most often associated with:
   a squamous dysplasia
   b broad spectrum antibiotics
   c oral contraceptives
   d chronic lymphocytic cervicitis

14 Which phase of the menstrual cycle directly follows a degenerated corpus albicans?
   a menses
   b follicular
   c secretory
   d ovulation

15 Which pituitary hormone stimulates the primordial follicles of the ovary to grow?
   a LH
   b FSH
   c estrogen
   d progesterone

16 A 22-year-old female presents with primary amenorrhea. Upon clinical investigation, she was found to have a low hairline, large numbers of pigmented nevi, polydactyly, and a short webbing of the neck. A smear from the lateral vaginal wall was collected for hormonal analysis. What maturation index is compatible?
   a 0/0/100
   b 0/50/50
   c 0/100/0
   d 100/0/0

17 What may explain why some postmenopausal women have an intermediate cell maturation while others will have deep atrophy?
   a increased vascularization near the basal lamina in women with intermediate cell atrophy
   b women with deep atrophy are most likely to have undergone castration early in their reproductive years
   c weak adrenal hormonal production in those patients with intermediate cell maturation
   d weak ovarian stromal hormonal production in those patients with intermediate cell maturation

18 A 64-year-old asymptomatic woman presents for a routine Pap smear. A vaginal smear is performed for hormonal analysis. Which of the following maturation indices are feasible given this patient's age?
   a 0/0/100
   b 75/25/0
   c 0/25/75
   d 0/10/90

19 Which of the following are contraindications for performing hormonal analyses?
   a mature cycling female
   b correlation of follicular persistency
   c Trichomonas vaginalis infection
   d correlation of Turner syndrome

20 A 52-year-old female with advanced cirrhosis of the liver is likely to show:
   a increased estrogenic effect
   b decreased estrogenic effect
   c increased progesterone effect
   d decreased progesterone effect

21 A patient with secondary amenorrhea would have a maturation index of:
   a 100/0/0
   b 0/100/0
   c 0/0/100
   d cannot be determined based on the above clinical information

22 The significance of hyperkeratosis and/or parakeratosis is that they:
   a may overlie and/or be associated with a possible lesion
   b are usually associated with a high grade squamous intraepithelial lesion
   c are predictive of reparative/regenerative processes
   d are of no significance

23 Severe hypothyroidism may be represented by which of the following maturation indices?
   a 0/100/0
   b 0/0/100
   c 0/50/50
   d 75/25/0

24 The administration of tamoxifen citrate in postmenopausal breast cancer patients:
   a increases cellular maturation
   b has no effect on cellular maturation
   c promotes formation of navicularlike cells
   d decreases cellular maturation

25 Cells with spinelike processes protruding from the cytoplasmic membrane (spider cells), occurring singularly and rarely in sheets, with smooth nuclear margins found proximal to the endocervical canal are diagnostic of:
   a adenocarcinoma in situ, endocervix
   b endocervical columnar cells
   c immature metaplastic cells
   d mature metaplastic cells

26 Torulopsis glabrata is similar in morphologic appearance to Candida albicans with the exception that:
   a Torulopsis glabrata lacks hyphae
   b Candida albicans has true mycelium
   c Torulopsis glabrata contains sulfur granules
   d Torulopsis glabrata reproduces by binary fission

27 An abortive attempt at keratinization is termed:
   a hyperkeratosis
   b reserve cell hyperplasia
   c parakeratosis
   d Arias-Stella reaction

ISBN 978-089189-6357 ©ASCP 2015

28 What is the effect of progesterone therapy upon an estrogen primed epithelium?
   a no change
   b decreased maturation to the intermediate cell level
   c decreased maturation to the deep parabasal cell level
   d increased maturation to a thick superficial cell level

29 A 42-year-old female suffers from menometrorrhagia of 3 months' duration following an automobile accident involving head injury. What might explain her condition?
   a pituitary hypogonadism
   b glioblastoma multiforme
   c pseudocyesis
   d Sertoli-Leydig cell tumors

30 Useful criteria to employ in the differential diagnosis between "atypical" reparative processes and nonkeratinizing squamous cell carcinoma include:
   a presence of single cells in repair
   b presence of nucleoli in carcinoma
   c coarse, irregular chromatin in carcinoma
   d nuclear polarity in carcinoma

31 A Pap smear reveals pools of mature and immature lymphocytes found in the company of tingible body macrophages. The diagnosis is consistent with:
   a lymphocytic leukemia
   b lymphoblastic lymphoma
   c follicular cervicitis
   d subacute inflammation

32 The smear pattern for a patient with Stein-Leventhal syndrome would reveal:
   a superficial predominance, intermediate cells without folding or clustering
   b parabasal cells
   c mixed parabasal and intermediate cells
   d intermediate cell predominance with excessive Döderlein cytolysis

33 A 32-year-old patient presents with severe bullous dermatitis and vulvar itching. A vulval smear revealed numerous parabasal squamous cells in sheets with large oval nuclei, perinuclear halos, regular to coarse chromatin, and prominent nucleoli. The most likely diagnosis is:
   a well differentiated squamous cell carcinoma
   b poorly differentiated squamous cell carcinoma
   c Haemophilus ducreyi
   d pemphigus vulgaris

34 Which pregnancy related deficiency produces multinucleated giant cells with relatively normal N:C ratios?
   a folic acid
   b benzopyrene
   c birth control pills
   d podophyllin

35 Cells resembling metaplastic cells arranged in sheets, exhibiting cytoplasmic streaming, moderate anisocytosis, fine to coarse chromatin, and prominent macronucleoli are haphazardly scattered throughout a cervical/endocervical smear. The diagnosis is consistent with:
   a poorly differentiated squamous cell carcinoma
   b high grade squamous intraepithelial neoplasia
   c koilocytic changes associated with HPV infection
   d reparative/regenerative process

36 The cellular effects of radiation include:
   a hyperchromasia, high N:C ratio
   b macrocytic changes, polychromasia
   c intranuclear cytoplasmic inclusions
   d eosinophilic intranuclear inclusions and polymorphonuclear neutrophils

37 Which of the ovarian tumors frequently present with bilateral involvement?
   a serous
   b mucinous
   c endometrioid
   d Sertoli-Leydig cell

38 The Schiller test is performed to identify:
   a glycogenated areas that stain with iodine
   b nonglycogenated areas that stain with methylene blue
   c glycogenated areas that do not stain with methylene blue
   d nonglycogenated areas that do not stain with iodine

39 What microorganism maintains the vaginal pH?
   a Lactobacillus acidophilus
   b Leptothrix
   c Bacterionema species
   d staphylococci

40 It has been determined that squamous cell carcinoma of the uterine cervix is associated with:
   a expression of HPV6, 11 viral DNA
   b expression of HPV6, 16 viral DNA
   c expression of HPV16, 18 viral DNA
   d antibody titer against episomal viral DNA

41 The most common clinical term that describes a benign ovarian tumor is:
   a embryonal teratoma
   b mature cystic teratoma
   c Krukenberg tumor
   d gynandroblastoma

42 The Clinical Laboratory Improvement Amendments of 1988 (CLIA '88) implement all of the following conditions except:
a all cases of atypical squamous cells of undetermined significance (ASCUS) are considered part of the 5 year retrospective review process
b a diagnosis of a high grade squamous intraepithelial lesion mandates follow-up of the patient
c daily records of the number of slides reviewed as well as the amount of time spent reviewing the slides must be kept on each cytotechnologist
d board certified pathologists may not perform primary review of >100 slides in any 24 hour period

43 Which of these diagnostic entities is associated with hyperestrinism and endometrial adenocarcinoma?
a endometrial polyps
b HPV
c endometrial hyperplasia
d atypical squamous metaplasia

44 Abnormal cells originating from endocervical adenocarcinoma may be distinguished from cells originating from endometrial adenocarcinoma by:
a presence of granular cytoplasm and columnar cellular shape
b frothy, delicate cytoplasm and round cellular shapes
c nucleoli and polymorphonuclear neutrophilic cannibalism
d diathesis background with 3D hyperchromatic cell groupings

45 If a uterine cancer were described as a heterologous mixed Müllerian tumor it could be:
a endometrial carcinoma only
b endometrial carcinoma + osteosarcoma
c endometrial sarcoma only
d endometrial carcinoma + leiomyosarcoma

46 The clinical utility of performing molecular HPV testing and the use of cervicography are considered:
a specific for determining the likelihood of progression of any one lesion
b adjunctive methods that currently lack the specificity needed to determine the progression rate of any one lesion
c important in determining the progression rate for patients with HPV
d basically equal in comparison

47 The vagina, uterus, and ovaries are formed embryologically from which germ cell layer(s)?
a ectoderm
b mesoderm
c endoderm
d ectoderm and mesoderm

48 Large numbers of small to medium, round, single cells exhibiting hyperchromasia and finely granular, evenly distributed nucleus comprising most of the cellular area is most suggestive of:
a spider cells
b nonkeratinizing dysplasia, severe (high grade squamous intraepithelial lesion)
c atypical squamous cells of undetermined significance
d nonkeratinizing dysplasia, mild (low grade squamous intraepithelial lesion)

49 Which of the following variants of endometrial adenocarcinoma are aggressive, arise in atrophic endometrium of older postmenopausal women, and are unrelated to hyperplastic precursor lesions?
a well differentiated type
b poorly differentiated type
c secretory type
d mucinous type

50 Which characteristic serves as the most important hallmark of ectocervical squamous lesions?
a opaque nuclei
b pleomorphism
c orangeophilic/amphophilic staining
d sheets of cells

51 An in situ carcinoma of the vulva is termed:
a Nabothian cyst
b Paget disease
c Gartner disease
d Bowen disease

52 A benign proliferation of undifferentiated cells under endocervical type glandular epithelium is termed:
a reserve cell hyperplasia
b cervical hypertrophy
c atrophy
d neoplasia

53 The histologic presentation of condyloma of the cervix includes:
a abnormal cells comprising 90% of the epithelial thickness
b submucosal dyskeratosis
c smudged nuclear features and cavelike perinuclear vacuoles
d mononuclear hypochromatic cells

54 Remnants of the mesonephric system found in the lateral vaginal wall are termed:
a Gartner cysts
b cloacal fold
c Bartholin ducts
d Skene glands

55 The correct order for chromatin degeneration associated with cell death is:
a karyolysis, pyknosis, karyorrhexis
b karyorrhexis, cytolysis, pyknosis
c pyknosis, karyorrhexis, karyolysis
d karyorrhexis, pyknosis, karyolysis

ISBN 978-089189-6357 ©ASCP 2015

56 Which of the human papillomavirus (HPV) types have episomal replication and are considered "low risk"?
   a HPV6, HPV16
   b HPV6, HPV11
   c HPV11, HPV16
   d HPV16, HPV18

57 Which cytomorphologic criteria are essential when establishing a diagnosis of a reparative process over a malignant one?
   a anisonucleosis, hyperchromasia
   b hyperchromasia, single cells
   c anisonucleosis, syncytial fragments
   d normochromasia, cytoplasmic streaming

58 Which clinical finding would place the patient at risk for infection by *Candida* species?
   a follicular phase of the menstrual cycle
   b diabetes mellitus
   c intrauterine devices
   d antibodies against cytomegalovirus

59 During the embryological development of a female, if the Müllerian ducts fail to fuse, the end result may be a(n):
   a pseudohermaphroditic female
   b bicornuate uterus
   c improper ovarian ligament support
   d Wolffian duct continuation

60 A 24-year-old female presented to the clinician with hyperemic, petechial hemorrhages of the vaginal walls and fornices. Which of the following may be responsible for the clinical findings?
   a a yeast infection
   b *Trichomonas vaginalis* infection
   c Bowen disease
   d condyloma acuminata

61 Puerperal endometritis may present cytologically as:
   a reactive trophoblasts
   b psammoma bodies
   c Curschmann spirals
   d folate changes

62 Cervical smears containing irregular spherical structures that take on a radiated appearance and are associated with hemorrhagic infarcts are:
   a cockleburs
   b brown artifact ("cornflaking")
   c impossible to identify without special stains
   d hematoidin crystals

63 Which of the following occurs due to the estrogenic effect upon normal squamous epithelium during the follicular phase of the menstrual cycle?
   a increased deposition of glycogen in the cytoplasm
   b folding and clustering of intermediate cells
   c desquamation of squamous cells
   d increased Döderlein cytolysis

64 A morphologic change seen in late secretory phase and pregnancy is:
   a an increase in the N:C ratio
   b glycogenated navicular cells
   c an increase in cellular eosinophilia
   d the presence of syncytiotrophoblasts

65 A 42-year-old nulliparous woman complaining of irregular menses frequently sheds fragments of normal endometrium in the midluteal phase of her menstrual cycle. Further clinical evaluation might suggest:
   a dilation and curettage to rule out hyperplasia of the endometrium
   b conization for endometriosis
   c hysterectomy
   d further evaluation not necessary; endometrial cells are normally found in midluteal phase

66 Radiated crystalline arrays lacking central filaments, found in late pregnancy, formed from stagnating products of degenerated cells, and composed of nonimmune glycoprotein, lipid, and calcium are diagnostic of:
   a *Actinomyces* species
   b hematoidin crystals
   c cockleburs
   d corpora amylacea

67 Which clinical feature is associated with an increased risk for well differentiated endometrial cancer?
   a a history of opposed estrogen
   b nulliparous
   c early menopause
   d increased number of sexual partners

68 What has been hypothesized to promote squamous cell carcinoma of the uterine cervix?
   a oncogene activation secondary to HPV
   b increased progesterone stimulation
   c episomal viral types
   d HPV induced exophytic lesions

69 Human chorionic gonadotropin is:
   a produced by the corpus luteum in early pregnancy
   b found during the third trimester of pregnancy only
   c considered important in menstruation
   d produced by the Graafian follicle in early pregnancy

70 Which embryological duct system develops internal genitalia in the female?
   a Wolffian
   b mesonephric
   c paramesonephric
   d mesentery

71 Multinucleated cells with cytoplasmic tails and tightly packed centrally located small hyperchromatic nuclei found in pregnancy are diagnostic of:
   a cytotrophoblasts
   b endometrial adenocarcinoma
   c syncytiotrophoblasts
   d choriocarcinoma

72. Of the following tissues, which is considered the most radiosensitive?
    a muscle
    b brain
    c uterus
    d gastrointestinal epithelium

73. Which finding is associated with the diagnosis of well differentiated endometrial adenocarcinoma?
    a basophilic watery diathesis
    b coarsely granular necrotic diathesis
    c sheets of neoplastic cells
    d papillary groups with associated psammoma bodies

74. Which condition is associated with the development of endometrial adenocarcinoma?
    a multiparity
    b exposure to the human papillomavirus
    c granulosa-theca cell tumor
    d exposure to cytomegalovirus

75. The most common metastatic tumor found in Pap smears is:
    a ovarian
    b fallopian tube
    c breast
    d colon

76. A 51-year-old patient with a history of normal Pap smears has a large population of malignant cells with hyperchromatic fine, irregular chromatin patterns, seen in sheets and single cells. Cytoplasmic configurations resemble a columnar formation. Endocervical curettings revealed no pathologic abnormality. In determining the origin of these cells, you might consider:
    a colon for malignancy
    b vagina for malignancy
    c breast for malignancy
    d lung for malignancy

77. A cervical/endocervical sample from a 38-year-old patient reveals large groups of cells in columnar formation with hyperchromatic nuclei and irregular chromatin. The cells have anisocytosis with intact cilia. These cells represent:
    a adenocarcinoma in situ, endocervix
    b well differentiated adenocarcinoma, endocervix
    c well differentiated adenocarcinoma, colon
    d tubal metaplasia

78. Which malignancy is often associated with psammoma bodies?
    a mucinous cystadenocarcinoma, ovarian primary
    b serous adenocarcinoma, ovarian
    c adenocarcinoma, colon
    d endocervical adenocarcinoma

79. Cells exhibiting multiple frondlike projections arranged in a papillary group with hyperchromatic, fine, irregular chromatin patterns and "bird's eye" macronucleoli were observed in a cervical/endocervical smear from a 40-year-old patient. The background was clean with a mild inflammatory component. Endocervical curetting was negative. The origin of the cells suggests:
    a vagina
    b fallopian tube
    c ovary
    d colon

80. The cytoplasm of cells from vulvar intraepithelial neoplasia grade 3 (VIN III) is:
    a pleomorphic
    b polygonal
    c round to oval
    d frothy, lacy, delicate

81. Which of the following statements is true regarding discrimination of endocervical adenocarcinoma from endometrial adenocarcinoma?
    a morula configuration and frothy cytoplasm are observed in endocervical adenocarcinoma
    b columnar configuration and granular cytoplasm are observed in endometrial adenocarcinoma
    c columnar configuration and granular cytoplasm are observed in endocervical adenocarcinoma
    d micronucleoli are observed in endocervical adenocarcinoma, while macronucleoli are observed in endometrial adenocarcinoma

82. Which vulvar infection clinically presents as a vesiculopustule and requires the identification of Gram– bacilli arranged in pairs or clusters?
    a *Neisseria gonorrhoeae*
    b *Torulopsis glabrata*
    c molluscum contagiosum
    d *Haemophilus ducreyi*

83. The most common sarcomatous element associated with a homologous mixed Müllerian tumor of the uterus is:
    a rhabdomyosarcoma
    b endometrial stromal sarcoma
    c leiomyosarcoma
    d osteosarcoma

84. A differential diagnosis for keratinizing dysplasia is:
    a dyskeratosis
    b koilocytosis
    c reactive/reparative cells
    d superficial stromal cells

85. A differential diagnosis for the bare nuclei of normal endocervical cells found in postmenopausal patients is:
    a atypia of atrophy and maturity
    b parakeratosis
    c pemphigus vulgaris
    d chronic follicular cervicitis

ISBN 978-089189-6357 ©ASCP 2015

86 A 41-year-old female with a history of diabetes presents for an annual Pap smear. Her last menstrual period, regularly 28 days in length, was 3 weeks prior to the current date. Cytology reveals large numbers of 3D glandular cells in tight clusters with indistinct cellular outlines, surrounded by a clean background. What clinical follow-up may help determine the origin of these cells?
  a cervical biopsy to rule out endocervical adenocarcinoma
  b cervical biopsy to rule out infiltrating squamous cell carcinoma
  c endometrial biopsy to rule out cystic hyperplasia
  d ovarian biopsy to rule out endometriosis

87 A 72-year-old female presents with pruritus and vaginal dryness. Cytologic examination reveals large numbers of deep parabasal cells masked by severe acute inflammation. A small population of round cells displaying an eosinophilic to orangeophilic appearance with India ink nuclei are diagnostic of:
  a low grade squamous intraepithelial lesion, mild keratinizing dysplasia
  b high grade squamous intraepithelial lesion, severe keratinizing dysplasia
  c degenerated parabasal cells of atrophy
  d keratinizing pearls

88 Which of the following may mimic follicular cervicitis?
  a metaplastic cells
  b well preserved neutrophils
  c nonkeratinizing dysplasia
  d malignant lymphoma

89 When differentiating a reparative process from a malignant one, which of the following criteria is important?
  a single cells in repair
  b sheets of cells without single cells in repair
  c nucleoli in repair
  d nucleoli in malignancy

90 Cells from a 62-year-old female that possess scalloping borders, finely vacuolated cytoplasm often containing polymorphonuclear neutrophils, anisonucleosis, and nuclei with irregular chromatin distribution and slight hyperchromasia are found in concert with mucicarmine+ signet ring cells among a dense, wispy background demonstrated with the Diff-Quik stain. The diagnosis is consistent with:
  a adenoacanthoma
  b clear cell endometrial adenocarcinoma
  c papillary serous endometrial adenocarcinoma
  d mucinous endometrial adenocarcinoma

91 Adenoacanthoma is identified cytologically by the presence of:
  a lipophages
  b superficial stromal cells
  c a squamous metaplastic component
  d deep stromal cells

92 A cervical/endocervical smear from a 41-year-old patient reveals cells possessing hyperchromatic nuclei with smooth chromatin patterns. A slight degree of anisonucleosis with a loss of polarity is also found in cells exhibiting a "feathering" effect. In addition, a hyperchromatic population of well preserved, round to oval, bare nuclei are seen. The diagnosis is:
  a endocervical adenocarcinoma
  b endometrial adenocarcinoma
  c AGUS/endocervical dysplasia
  d adenoid basal carcinoma

93 A cervical/endocervical smear reveals cells in sheets, and microbiopsies reveal columnar formation, pseudostratification, granular cytoplasm, fine irregular chromatin, and micronucleoli. Red blood cells and fibrin are also identified. The cytology is diagnostic of:
  a endometrial adenocarcinoma
  b endocervical adenocarcinoma
  c endometrial reparative/regenerative processes
  d endocervical reparative/regenerative processes

94 What cytologic feature found in endometrial cells is associated with patients who have an intrauterine device?
  a macronucleoli
  b coarse, irregular chromatin
  c large, distended vacuoles
  d diathesis

95 Which of the following is not considered a precursor lesion for adenocarcinoma of the endometrium?
  a cystic hyperplasia
  b atypical hyperplasia
  c endometrial CIS
  d endometrial polyps

96 Cells exhibiting coarse, irregular chromatin, irregularly defined cytoplasmic borders, and large distended vacuoles were identified in a cervical/endocervical smear from a 41-year-old patient. Endocervical and endometrial curettings revealed no pathologic abnormality. The diagnosis/origin of these cells is:
  a medullary carcinoma/breast
  b papillary carcinoma/thyroid
  c serous cystadenocarcinoma/ovary
  d mucinous cystadenocarcinoma/ovary

97 The cytologic diagnosis of lichen sclerosus is based on the presence of:
  a hyperkeratosis, plasma cells
  b koilocytosis, polymorphonuclear neutrophils
  c squamous cell carcinoma
  d pseudoepitheliomatous hyperplasia

98 An example of solid primary tumor of the vulva is:
  a granular cell tumor (myoblastoma)
  b minimal deviation adenocarcinoma
  c clear cell adenocarcinoma
  d adenocarcinoma, Skene duct origin

99 Poorly differentiated endometrial adenocarcinomas possess which of the following cytologic features?
  a an increase in sheets over gland formation
  b an increase in gland over sheet formation
  c an increase in the number of oxyphilic cells present
  d a decrease in nucleoli

100 A 42-year-old patient presents with pelvic ascites for a pelvic examination. A Pap smear was performed and the cytologic evaluation revealed a large population of 3D cells exhibiting anisocytosis, polymorphic nuclear features, and hyperchromatic nuclei with fine irregular chromatin patterns. Macronucleoli and psammoma bodies are seen. The background is clean or free of diathesis. The diagnosis is:
  a cervical polyp
  b well differentiated endometrial adenocarcinoma
  c serous adenocarcinoma of the ovary
  d endocervical adenocarcinoma

101 As the differentiation of an endometrial adenocarcinoma decreases, the size and number of nucleoli:
  a increase
  b decrease
  c stay the same
  d are not predictable

102 Multinucleation is commonly associated with:
  a folic acid deficiency
  b squamous cell carcinoma
  c cytotrophoblasts
  d lymphocytes

103 Bean shaped Gram– bacilli with a "safety pin" appearance found within the cytoplasm of histiocytes are diagnostic of:
  a Donovan bodies, *Calymmatobacterium granulomatis*
  b *Haemophilus ducreyi*
  c *Neisseria gonorrhoeae*
  d *Gardnerella vaginalis*

104 A 22-year-old patient with a history of birth control pill usage (6 years) recently terminated usage. The patient currently suffers from galactorrhea (3 weeks). What condition is associated with the clinical findings?
  a Sheehan syndrome
  b del Castillo syndrome
  c Forbes-Albright syndrome
  d Stein-Leventhal syndrome

105 On colposcopic examination, HPV related cervical abnormalities may be represented by:
  a mosaic patterns
  b decrease in vascularity
  c uterine prolapse
  d atrophic uterine cervix

106 The pathognomonic indication for HPV infection in cytology is:
  a the presence of chromatin smudging
  b koilocytosis
  c nuclear wrinkling
  d parakeratosis

107 What significant postirradiation finding might raise suspicion of a possible recurrent squamous cell carcinoma?
  a macrocytosis
  b amphophilic staining
  c an abrupt increase in squamous cell maturation
  d intermediate cells with concentric cytoplasmic fibrils

108 Which of the following is (are) a possible treatment regimen for high grade intraepithelial lesions?
  a LEEP/LLETZ
  b DNA ploidy analysis
  c vitamin D therapy
  d methotrexate

109 What diagnosis might be confused with an HPV infection?
  a changes associated with *Trichomonas* infections
  b repair
  c microglandular hyperplasia
  d squamous cell carcinoma

110 The smear pattern taken from a patient suffering from extreme anorexia nervosa will show:
  a parabasal cell predominance
  b intermediate and superficial cells
  c superficial cell predominance
  d normal cyclic pattern dependent upon the last menstrual period

111 All of the following are possible carcinogenic mechanisms for the initiation and promotion of squamous cell carcinoma except:
  a uncontrolled transcription of E6 and E7
  b HPV integration disrupting the E1-E2 region
  c double point mutations of oncogene p53
  d high risk HPV types inducing exophytic lesions

112 The presence of malignant cells postirradiation may be considered persistent or recurrent after what length of time?
  a 1 week postirradiation
  b 2 weeks postirradiation
  c 4 weeks postirradiation
  d 8 weeks postirradiation

ISBN 978-089189-6357 ©ASCP 2015

113 The stem cell from which large cell nonkeratinizing carcinoma arises is:
a endocervical reserve cell
b immature squamous metaplasia
c mature nonkeratinizing squamous epithelium
d mature keratinizing squamous epithelium

114 Minor (nonspecific) criteria suggestive of condyloma infection include:
a macrocytes, kite, polka dot, and balloon cells
b abundant reparative epithelial cells
c immature squamous metaplastic cells
d cytoplasmic vacuolization

115 Which of the following is (are) not considered a morphologic variant of carcinoma in situ?
a immature round dysplastic cell
b syncytial-like arrangement
c hyperchromatic crowded groups
d intermediatelike cells in cobblestone pattern

116 An indication of recurrent postirradiation adenocarcinoma is:
a large, round to oval stripped nuclei
b cytoplasmic vacuolization
c polymorphic cells with orangeophilic cytoplasm
d opaque nuclear features

117 The most common histologic appearance associated with the "high risk" HPV viral types is:
a flat
b spiked
c exophytic
d inverted

118 A 65-year-old female on long term, low dose estrogen therapy will most likely show:
a parabasal cell predominance
b intermediate cell predominance
c superficial cell predominance
d cannot be predicted

119 Which process mimics a dyskeratotic process but is not considered part of the cytologic spectrum of HPV infection?
a dyskeratocyte
b koilocyte
c parabasal-like cells
d pseudokeratosis

120 Recurrent carcinoma cells found in patients who have previously received radiation therapy are:
a smaller than the original tumor cells
b larger than the original tumor cells
c the same size as the original tumor cells
d size cannot be predicted

121 Which of the following histologic criteria are helpful in diagnosing carcinoma in situ instead of dysplasia?
a abnormal cells throughout the full thickness; differentiated at the surface
b abnormal cells replacing the full thickness of the squamous mucosa; no differentiation at the surface
c abnormal cells are present in only 1/3 of the epithelial thickness; normal mature differentiation is present in the upper 2/3
d abnormal cells are present in only 1/2 of the epithelial thickness; normal mature differentiation is present in the upper 1/2

122 Orangeophilic small parakeratotic cells with enlarged, smudged, and opaque nuclei, exhibiting slight pleomorphism, are:
a severe keratinizing dysplasia
b reserve cell hyperplasia
c dyskeratocytes
d microglandular hyperplasia

123 What is a useful criterion in distinguishing low grade squamous intraepithelial lesions from high grade lesions?
a cytoplasmic inclusions in low grade lesions
b co-infection with HPV in high grade lesions
c increased nuclear to cytoplasmic area in high grade lesions
d larger nuclear size in high grade lesions

124 Cells found in 3D syncytial-like arrangements with chaotic architecture, coarse regular chromatin, and hyperchromatic crowded groups are found in a clean background. The diagnosis is:
a low grade squamous intraepithelial neoplasia, mild dysplasia
b high grade squamous intraepithelial neoplasia, moderate dysplasia
c high grade squamous intraepithelial neoplasia, severe dysplasia
d high grade squamous intraepithelial neoplasia, carcinoma in situ

125 Which of the following is considered a synonym for carcinoma in situ?
a Paget disease
b CIN3
c infiltrating epithelioma
d low grade squamous intraepithelial carcinoma

126 A mechanism that might prove useful to differentiate severe keratinizing dysplasia from invasive keratinizing carcinoma is:
a diathesis, increased cellular pleomorphism in carcinoma
b nucleoli in dysplasia
c increased mitotic activity in dysplasia
d presence of pearl formation in carcinoma

127 What sexually transmitted condition, related to pelvic inflammatory disease, is the most prevalent in the United States?
a *Chlamydia trachomatis*
b gonorrhea
c human papillomavirus
d herpes

128 Benign cellular changes related to irradiation include:
a karyomegaly and macrocytosis
b viable cells with increased mitosis
c aneuploidy
d coarse, irregular chromatin with macronucleoli

129 What benign cellular change mimics dysplasia?
a irradiation
b severe inflammation
c nuclear vacuolation
d decreased N:C ratios

130 Cytology reveals single cells and syncytial-like aggregates, extreme pleomorphic cytoplasmic features, opaque nuclei, and occasional cells with irregular chromatin distribution. Background material is granular with eosinophilic fibrinous material. The diagnosis is:
a high grade intraepithelial neoplasia, moderate dysplasia
b squamous cell carcinoma, keratinizing type
c atypical reparative/regenerative process
d pleomorphic parakeratosis

131 The morphogenesis of small cell squamous carcinoma of the uterine cervix is related to the development of:
a atypical squamous metaplasia
b mature squamous metaplasia
c native squamous epithelium
d atypical reserve cell hyperplasia

132 In a subclinical HPV infection, the virus is most likely harbored in:
a dysplastic epithelium
b reserve cells
c ectocervical cells
d the underlying stroma

133 The most common malignancy that involves the uterine cervix is:
a keratinizing squamous cell carcinoma
b nonkeratinizing squamous cell carcinoma
c small cell squamous carcinoma
d adenocarcinoma, endocervical type

134 Which viral genomic segment is responsible for host cellular transformation in vivo?
a late region 1,2
b early region 1,2
c upstream regulatory region
d early region 6,7

135 What is a pitfall in the diagnosis of benign radiation changes?
a vitamin C deficiency
b folic acid deficiency
c chronic follicular cervicitis
d vitamin A deficiency

136 The presence of keratin pearls in a cervical smear is associated with:
a keratinizing squamous cell carcinoma
b keratinizing dysplasia, not otherwise specified
c keratinizing processes, nonspecific
d no relation to any process

137 Small cells exhibiting cell to cell compression, high N:C ratios, and coarse, irregular chromatin distribution in a "dirty" necrotic background represent:
a small cell neuroendocrine carcinoma, cervix
b squamous cell carcinoma, cervix
c high grade intraepithelial neoplasia, carcinoma in situ
d serous cystadenocarcinoma, metastatic from ovary

138 The most sensitive technique to identify a specific HPV virotype is:
a immunohistochemistry
b cytologic morphology
c histomorphology
d nucleic acid analysis

139 Which of the following special stains will help verify the neuroendocrine differentiation (ND) found in small cell neuroendocrine carcinoma of the cervix from nonneuroendocrine in poorly differentiated small cell squamous carcinoma?
a synaptophysin
b HMB45
c PAS
d alcian blue

140 Which technique might be useful in determining the primary site of a carcinoma metastatic to the vaginal/cervical area?
a ploidy analysis
b DNA analysis for human papillomavirus
c immunohistochemistry
d flow cytometry

141 The progression rate of immature metaplastic dysplasia compared with the most common dysplasia variant is:
a greater
b less
c the same
d dependant upon coexisting infections

142 The cytologic features of mucinous/intestinal endometrial adenocarcinoma are which grade?
a 1
b 3
c 4
d cannot be determined with available information

ISBN 978-089189-6357 ©ASCP 2015

143 Extrauterine tumors that spread to the vagina via direct extension may be cytologically distinguished from those metastasizing from distant locations (nonimplanting) by:
a diathesis related changes with malignancies involving direct extension
b signet ring cells in malignancies involving distant metastasis
c nuclear chromatin patterns providing delineation
d pools of mucin, which are more common in malignancies involving direct extension

144 The most helpful cytologic criteria for verifying the "atypical" features associated with cone biopsy artifact as merely benign degenerative changes are:
a increased crowding resembling neoplasia, large nucleoli
b increased crowding resembling neoplasia, abundant mitotic figures
c few "atypical" cells, associated benign epithelial elements
d increased numbers of hyperchromatic crowded groups, increased crowding resembling neoplasia

145 Hyperchromatic crowded groups and syncytial-like formation as identified by low power analysis are helpful features for the cytologic identification of:
a LSIL
b endometrial adenocarcinoma
c Arias-Stella reaction
d carcinoma in situ

146 The risk for development of vaginal adenosis is greatest if exposure to DES is during the:
a 2nd week of embryonic development
b 8th week of gestation
c 12th week following conception
d 3rd trimester

147 Which is considered an uncommon protozoan found in the female genital tract?
a *Vorticella* species
b *Hormodendrum* species
c *Gaffkya* species
d *Aspergillus* species

148 Single basophilic cells with variable sizes with scarce, wispy, trailing cytoplasm resembling "rootlets," oval nuclei, and finely granular, evenly distributed chromatin with prominent nucleoli, found in patients with a history of radiotherapy for squamous cell carcinoma, are representative of:
a recurrent squamous cell carcinoma
b myofibroblasts
c leiomyosarcoma
d postirradiation dysplasia

149 The most frequent heterologous constituent of a mixed Müllerian uterine tumor is:
a leiomyosarcoma
b rhabdomyosarcoma
c osteosarcoma
d chondrosarcoma

150 Clear cell adenocarcinomas of the endometrium cytologically present as:
a well differentiated cells
b poorly differentiated, delicate cytoplasm, prominent nucleoli
c well differentiated, mucin+ with signet ring cells
d poorly differentiated, papillary, psammoma bodies

151 A neuroendocrine malignancy arising in the cervix is:
a clear cell adenocarcinoma
b small cell carcinoma
c nonkeratinizing (large) cell carcinoma
d adenosquamous carcinoma

152 Difficulties in distinguishing squamous carcinoma in situ (CIS) from endocervical adenocarcinoma in situ (AIS) may arise when:
a CIS involves the underlying glandlike spaces
b AIS involves the transformation zone
c CIS is derived from ectocervical mucosa
d AIS stains eosinophilic

153 An endometrial adenocarcinoma that cytologically possesses uniform nuclear features and stains positive with periodic acid-Schiff is diagnostic of:
a secretory adenocarcinoma
b adenoacanthoma
c papillary serous adenocarcinoma
d clear cell adenocarcinoma

154 The possibility of microinvasive squamous carcinoma is suggested when what feature is present?
a syncytial formation, pronounced chromocenters
b fine regular chromatin patterns
c micronucleoli, diathesis
d macronucleoli

155 Granulomatous cervicitis may be associated with:
a radiation
b Arias-Stella reaction
c psammoma bodies
d *Candida* species. infections

156 A normal cell type commonly found in smears from postmenopausal patients is the:
a superficial squamous cell
b multinucleated giant histiocyte
c dyskeratocyte
d anucleate squame

157 In addition to the human papillomavirus, possible cofactors associated with cervical carcinogenesis may include:
   a the use of progesterone based birth control pills
   b vitamins A, B, and C deficiency
   c the use of an intrauterine device (IUD)
   d a history of endometritis

158 The most common primary carcinoma of the vulva is:
   a basal cell carcinoma
   b malignant melanoma
   c verrucous carcinoma
   d squamous cell carcinoma, keratinizing type

159 A vulvar smear from a 43-year-old patient shows a large group of columnar cells with anisocytosis, large hyperchromatic nuclei, fine irregular chromatin, macronucleoli, and signet ring formation. A mucinous background was identified. Subsequent endocervical and endometrial biopsies were normal. Which of the following may represent the possible origin of these cells?
   a transitional cell carcinoma, bladder
   b vulvar adenosis
   c Bartholin gland adenocarcinoma
   d ductal carcinoma, breast

160 Which ovarian tumor presents bilaterally and has cells that are positive with the CA125 monoclonal antibody?
   a serous cystadenocarcinoma
   b mucinous cystadenocarcinoma
   c endometrioid tumor
   d malignant teratoma

161 A pure uterine sarcoma presenting with small, round, and uniform cells with high nuclear to cytoplasm ratios, coarse chromatin, and frequent micronucleoli is considered:
   a leiomyosarcoma
   b endometrial stromal sarcoma
   c rhabdomyosarcoma
   d osteosarcoma

162 Psammoma bodies may be seen with all of the following except:
   a endometrial adenocarcinoma
   b fallopian tube adenocarcinoma
   c patients with an IUD
   d Sertoli-Leydig cell tumor

163 The nuclei of adenocarcinoma in situ of the endocervix present with:
   a great pleomorphism
   b little pleomorphism
   c macronucleoli
   d spindle shapes

164 When should one analyze smears taken from patients who have received radiation therapy?
   a within 3-6 days postadministration
   b not before 6-8 weeks postadministration
   c in patients receiving external beam instead of radium application
   d in patients receiving polonium induced radiation

165 Which statement is true?
   a atypical glandular cells (AGUS) often accompany squamous dysplasia
   b atypical endocervical repair is associated with Döderlein bacillus metaplasia
   c endometrial adenocarcinoma presents in strips or a "feathering" cellular pattern
   d cells associated with Arias-Stella reaction may be distinguished from squamous carcinoma in situ because of their small cell size

166 Stratified strips, rosettes, and columnar shaped cells presenting with palisading, enlarged, (crowded and overlapping), hyperchromatic nuclei possessing coarse chromatin and micronucleoli are diagnostic of:
   a high grade intraepithelial neoplasia, carcinoma in situ
   b squamous cell carcinoma
   c atypical glandular cells of undetermined significance, favor neoplastic
   d adenocarcinoma, endometrial

167 The cytoplasm of endocervical adenocarcinoma is:
   a diffusely vacuolated
   b generally cyanophilic
   c granular
   d amphophilic

168 Cervical smears containing pleomorphic cells with enlarged, eccentrically located, fine to granular hyperchromatic nuclei, prominent nucleoli, PAS+ vacuolated cytoplasm, and occasional giant cells with low N:C ratios resembling chemotherapeutic changes found in a late stage pregnancy are diagnostic of:
   a choriocarcinoma
   b endometrial adenocarcinoma
   c endocervical repair/regeneration
   d Arias-Stella reaction

169 Which cytologic criteria are helpful in distinguishing endocervical adenocarcinoma from endometrial adenocarcinoma?
   a cells with columnar morphology arranged into rosettes and crowded sheets with holes for endocervical adenocarcinoma compared with round, plump cells arranged into balls and molded groups for endometrial adenocarcinoma
   b granular cytoplasm, coarse chromatin in endometrial adenocarcinoma
   c diffusely vacuolated cytoplasm, limited hyperchromasia in endocervical adenocarcinoma
   d cells in sheets, larger cell size, and cyanophilia in endometrial adenocarcinoma

ISBN 978-089189-6357 ©ASCP 2015

170 Arias-Stella reaction may be normally seen with which of the following?
 a prolonged progesterone stimulation
 b vaginal cuff smears from hysterectomy patients
 c scraping the lower 1/3 of the vaginal wall
 d vulval scrapes

171 A 70-year-old female complains of vulvar pruritus and bleeding. Cytology reveals a large population of loosely arranged pleomorphic cells with oval nuclei, often binucleate. Nucleoli, often representing 1/3 of the nuclear diameter, are found, as well as intranuclear vacuolization. Intracytoplasmic deposits are seen in many of the cells. The diagnosis is most consistent with:
 a pseudoepitheliomatous hyperplasia
 b basal cell carcinoma
 c bowenoid papulosis
 d malignant melanoma

172 Endocervical adenocarcinoma in situ (AIS) may be distinguished from invasive adenocarcinoma of the endocervix using which criteria?
 a increase in single cells, loosely arranged cell groups, macronucleoli, diathesis present in endocervical adenocarcinoma
 b increase in single cells, loosely arranged cell groups, macronucleoli, diathesis present in endocervical adenocarcinoma in situ
 c 3 dimensionality (morula or cell ball formation) of endocervical AIS vs feathering in endocervical adenocarcinoma
 d eosinophilic cytoplasm is found in endocervical AIS, whereas cyanophilia is associated with endocervical adenocarcinoma

173 When discriminating minor endocervical atypia from that of endocervical adenocarcinoma in situ (AIS), which of the following is helpful?
 a chromatin is fine to moderately granular, and cells present with minimal anisocytosis and lack pseudostratification in endocervical glandular dysplasia
 b chromatin is fine to moderately granular, and cells present without pseudostratification in endocervical adenocarcinoma in situ
 c apoptosis is present in endocervical glandular dysplasia while absent in adenocarcinoma in situ
 d chromatin is moderate to coarse with prominent pseudostratification in endocervical glandular dysplasia, while less pronounced chromatin and pseudostratification are associated with endocervical adenocarcinoma in situ

174 The cytologic criteria most helpful in establishing a diagnosis of large cell squamous carcinoma from poorly differentiated endometrial adenocarcinoma are:
 a vacuolated cytoplasm, finely granular chromatin with macronucleoli in large cells in squamous carcinoma
 b vacuolated cytoplasm, finely granular chromatin with macronucleoli in endometrial adenocarcinoma
 c syncytial aggregates, micronucleoli in endometrial adenocarcinoma
 d eosinophilic staining cytoplasmic features in endometrial adenocarcinoma vs cyanophilic staining in large cell squamous carcinoma

175 The mean age of detection of clear cell adenocarcinoma of the vagina is:
 a 10
 b 20
 c 30
 d 50

176 A poorly differentiated uterine glandular tumor presenting as papillary structures lined with stratified cuboidal to columnar cells and accompanying psammoma bodies is a(n):
 a adenoacanthoma
 b clear cell adenocarcinoma, endometrium
 c "hobnail" serous adenocarcinoma, endometrium
 d leiomyosarcoma

177 A differential diagnosis for an endometrial adenocarcinoma that extends into the endocervical canal is:
 a endocervical glandular repair/regeneration
 b grade 1 endocervical adenocarcinoma
 c endocervical glandular dysplasia
 d primary endometrioid endocervical adenocarcinoma

178 A 22-year-old female presents with multiple papules on the vulva, resembling dysplastic nevi. Polymerase chain reaction revealed HPV+. The cells have anisocytosis, syncytial formation, and large nuclei with coarse, regular chromatin features. The diagnosis is consistent with:
 a squamous cell carcinoma
 b vulvar intraepithelial neoplasia, grade 1 (VIN I)
 c verrucous carcinoma
 d bowenoid papulosis

179 Compared with conventional smears, the nuclear borders of HSIL in liquid based Paps are:
 a not evident
 b identical
 c more rounded
 d more irregular

180 Compared with conventional smears, the nuclear chromatin of liquid based Paps shows:
   a more detail
   b less detail
   c more smudging
   d more opacity

181 Compared with conventional smears, tumor diathesis seen in liquid based Paps is often:
   a absent
   b clinging to cells
   c found at the periphery of the preparation
   d obscuring cellular material

182 Compared with liquid based Paps, metaplastic cells in conventional smears appear to have:
   a thicker cytoplasm
   b more cytoplasm
   c increased cyanophilia
   d increased eosinophilia

183 Compared with conventional smears, endocervical cells in liquid based Paps may appear:
   a more flattened
   b more elongated
   c more hypochromatic
   d more hyperchromatic

184 Endocervical component, as seen in liquid based preparations, is composed of:
   a mature superficial squamous cells
   b endometrial cells
   c endocervical and/or squamous metaplastic cells
   d cervical mucus

185 Compared with conventional smears, cells in liquid based Paps demonstrate:
   a larger nuclear diameter
   b smaller nuclear diameter
   c paler staining
   d more atypia

186 An important feature in distinguishing cells of HSIL from small metaplastic cells in liquid based Paps is the presence of:
   a hyperchromasia
   b higher N:C ratios
   c irregular nuclear borders
   d homogeneous chromatin distribution

187 The greatest cause of false negative Paps, both conventional and liquid based, is attributed to:
   a screening locator error
   b screening interpretation error
   c slide preparation error
   d sampling error

188 Compared with conventional smears, liquid based Paps statistically report fewer interpretations of:
   a limited cellularity
   b LSIL and HSIL
   c endocervical adenocarcinoma
   d *Trichomonas* infection

189 Following an interpretation of atypical glandular cells of undetermined significance (AGUS) in a liquid based Pap, compared with AGUS in a conventional smear, the follow-up diagnosis of the cervical biopsy is more often:
   a carcinoma in situ
   b reactive endocervical epithelium
   c glandular pathology
   d normal

190 Compared with conventional smears, red blood cells seen in liquid based Paps are usually:
   a better preserved
   b lysed
   c absent
   d nucleated

191 Compared with conventional smears, the cell groups of adenocarcinoma as seen in liquid based Paps show:
   a greater depth of focus
   b flattening of cell sheets
   c larger clusters
   d less nuclear overlap

192 Compared with conventional smears, the cells of squamous cell carcinoma as seen in liquid based Paps may:
   a show increased orangeophilia and keratinization
   b lack orangeophilia and keratinization
   c exhibit more tadpole forms
   d be larger in size

193 The incidence of infectious organisms in liquid based Paps, compared with conventional smears, is:
   a higher
   b lower
   c identical
   d infectious organisms cannot be diagnosed with liquid based Paps

194 When atypical glandular cells of endocervical origin are reported in Pap tests, they are:
   a of limited diagnostic significance for patient care
   b rarely associated with polyps
   c best evaluated by colposcopy
   d often seen concurrent with squamous atypia or intraepithelial lesions

195 Chlamydia trachomatis as seen in Pap tests is characterized by the presence of:
   a clue cells
   b granular intracytoplasmic inclusions
   c sulfur granules
   d large intranuclear inclusions

ISBN 978-089189-6357 ©ASCP 2015

196 Hematoidin cocklebur crystals have been described most often in cervical smears of patients who:
  a have endometrial adenocarcinoma
  b have low grade squamous intraepithelial lesions
  c have an endometrial polyp
  d are pregnant

197 The most common cancer metastatic to the uterine cervix is:
  a malignant melanoma
  b lung adenocarcinoma
  c ovarian carcinoma
  d malignant lymphoma

198 The most useful cytologic criteria for the differentiation between high grade squamous intraepithelial lesion and endocervical adenocarcinoma in situ are:
  a nuclear size and shape
  b nuclear chromatin patterns
  c cell arrangements and architecture
  d slide background characteristics

199 Cytomegalovirus effects as seen in Pap tests are characterized by:
  a frequent multinucleated giant cells
  b intranuclear and intracytoplasmic inclusions
  c perinuclear cavities
  d hyperdistended cytoplasmic vacuoles

200 Bacterial vaginosis as seen in Pap tests is characterized by the presence of:
  a abundant lactobacilli
  b marked inflammatory background
  c clue cells
  d sulfur granules

201 Approximately what percentage of women with a diagnosis of high grade squamous intraepithelial lesion Pap test result will test positive for high risk human papillomavirus (HPV) cytopathic effect?
  a 17%
  b 47%
  c 67%
  d 97%

202 Which of the following principle diagnostic features can aid in distinguishing invasive squamous cell carcinoma from a high grade squamous intraepithelial lesion:
  a tumor diathesis and prominent nucleoli
  b coarse chromatin pattern and irregular nuclear contours
  c syncytial aggregates and coarse chromatin pattern
  d syncytial aggregates and inconspicuous nucleoli

203 Which of the following HPV types is associated with endocervical adenocarcinoma in situ?
  a type 6
  b type 11
  c type 18
  d type 42

204 Single cells from which of the following lesions are most commonly missed on initial cytologic interpretation (false negative)?
  a endocervical adenocarcinoma
  b squamous cell carcinoma
  c low grade squamous intraepithelial lesion
  d high grade squamous intraepithelial lesion

205 A 25-year-old female has her first Pap test, and many cells with this morphology are identified. Which of the following statements are true?

   a her risk of having biopsy proven CIN2/3 identified in the next 2 years approaches 25%

   b she is most likely infected with a low risk HPV serotype

   c if her colposcopy and biopsy are negative, she is not really infected with HPV

   d her risk of having biopsy proven CIN2/3 identified in the next 2 years is <10%

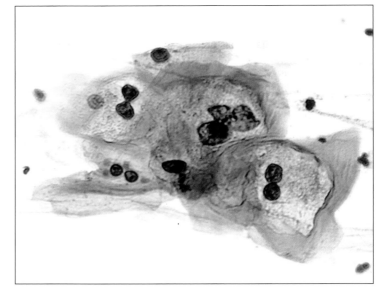

206 A 26-year-old postpartum (post 8 weeks) female presents to the clinician for a repeat ThinPrep Pap test after a previous ASCUS diagnosis during the first trimester. The HPV test was negative. The diagnosis is:

   a atypical atrophy

   b HSIL

   c NILM

   d AGUS, favor neoplastic

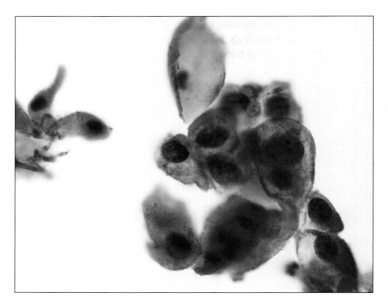

207 A 58-year-old postmenopausal female with complaints of vaginal bleeding presents to the clinician for a pelvic examination. At the time of visual inspection, a vaginal cuff specimen was taken and processed with the ThinPrep 3000. The cells are diagnostic of:

   a adenocarcinoma, ovarian primary

   b vaginal adenosis

   c adenocarcinoma, endometrial origin

   d benign endometrial cells

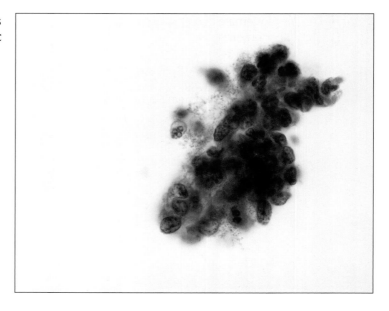

ISBN 978-089189-6357 ©ASCP 2015

208 An 18-year-old female, LMP 3 weeks prior, presents
for annual Pap test. Based on the cells shown,
what is the diagnosis and the appropriate clinical
management?
  a ASCUS, repeat Pap test in 6 months
  b ASCUS, recommend colposcopy
  c LSIL, recommend colposcopy
  d LSIL, repeat Pap test in 12 months

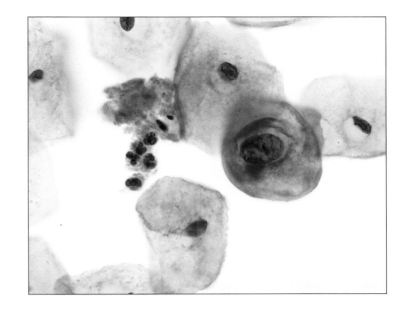

209 A 45-year-old female presents to the clinician with
postcoital bleeding. Her last Pap test was 10 years
prior, in her first trimester or pregnancy. The cells are
diagnostic of:
  a HSIL
  b squamous cell carcinoma, nonkeratinizing type
  c AGUS, endometrial origin
  d ASCUS

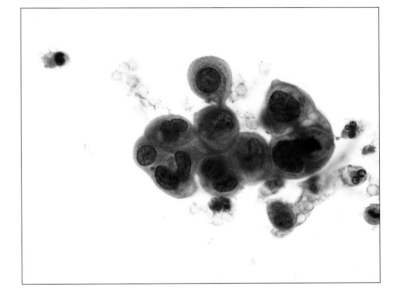

210 A 62-year-old female presents with intermittent
bleeding. Endometrial curettings are negative.
The following cells from a ThinPrep Pap test were
subsequently stained for p16 immunomarkers.
The diagnosis is:
  a adenocarcinoma, endometrial type
  b small cell squamous carcinoma
  c adenocarcinoma, endocervical type
  d adenocarcinoma in situ; endocervix

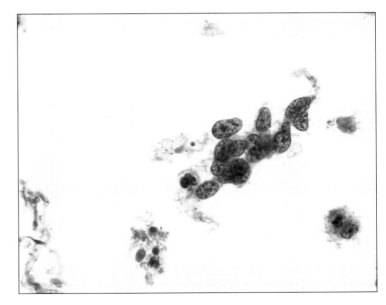

211 A 41-year-old female with a 2 year history of atypical Pap tests presents for a follow-up Pap after 6 months. High risk HPV testing was positive. The cells are from a ThinPrep Pap test. The diagnosis is:

a AGUS, endometrial
b NILM, reactive endocervical cells
c small cell carcinoma
d adenocarcinoma in situ, endocervical type

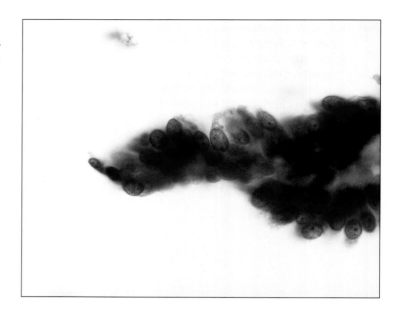

212 The following cells represent a routine Pap test from a 28-year-old female, day 18. The diagnosis is:

a small cell carcinoma
b HSIL
c NILM; inflammatory cells
d endometrial hyperplasia

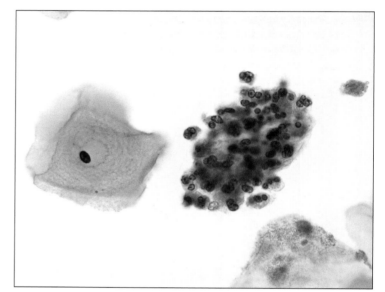

213 These cells are from a cervical scrape and an endocervical brushing from a 23-year-old female, months pregnant. The clinical management should be:

a colposcopy
b repeat Pap in 12 months
c perform HPV testing
d vaginal delivery should be avoided

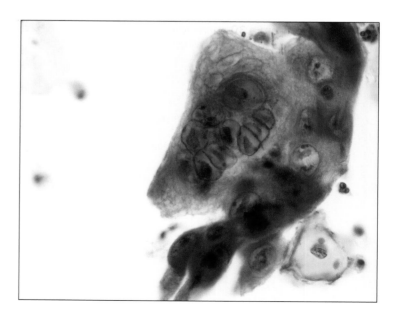

ISBN 978-089189-6357 ©ASCP 2015

214 A 66-year-old obese nulliparous female with a previous history of a gynecologic malignancy 2 years ago (treated with hysterectomy, radiation and chemotherapy) presents to the clinician with vaginal bleeding. Visual inspection of the vagina reveals a 3 cm mass in the cul de sac. A direct scraping of the lesion was immersed into ThinPrep vial containing 20 mL of fluid. The diagnosis is:

    a reactive endocervical cells
    b primary adenocarcinoma of the vagina
    c metastatic endometrial stromal sarcoma
    d HSIL

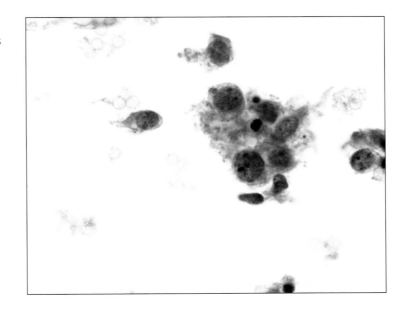

215 These cells were found in a 48-year-old female with a rectal vaginal fistula of previous unknown etiology. A ThinPrep Pap of the vagina/cervix was performed. The cells are diagnostic of:

    a metastatic colon cancer
    b reactive endocervical cells
    c AGUS; endocervical
    d primary adenocarcinoma, endocervix

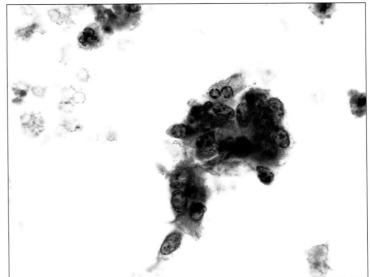

216 A Pap test from a 30-year-old female reveals aggregates of long filamentous organisms accompanied by masses of bacteria. This finding is associated with:

    a infection due to *Gardnerella vaginalis* with resultant bacterial vaginosis
    b use of an intrauterine device (IUD)
    c overgrowth of lactobacilli
    d use of oral birth control with associated estrogen related changes

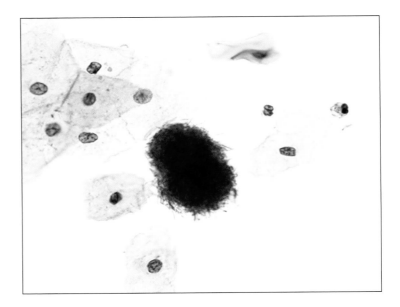

217 The cytologic identification of this organism is described best by which of these statements?

  a a spore form predominates in this species
  b this is a true mycelial form lacking the pseudohyphae form of other *Candida* species
  c sulfur granules are present in its mature form
  d the mature form is usually peripherally aggregated on an intermediate cell membrane

Torulopsis

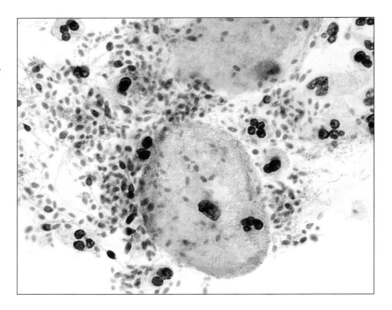

218 The identifiable components within the cytoplasm of these cells are:

  a elementary bodies
  b molluscum bodies
  c Type A inclusions of Cowdry
  d nucleoli

chlamydia

Nebular bodies

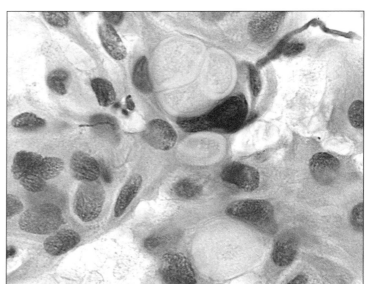

219 The broad alterations in the background (milieu) seen in this specimen are consistent with:

  a coccoid bacteria
  b a mild inflammatory exudate
  c changes secondary to *Trichomonas vaginalis* infection
  d diathesis changes associated with an invasive primary malignancy

RBCs

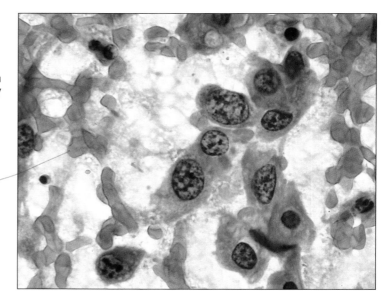

ISBN 978-089189-6357   ©ASCP 2015

220 What clinical finding is associated with these cytologic findings?

   a increased risk of fetal infection, possibly resulting in death in utero
   b vesicles, erythematous papules
   c *Trichomonas vaginalis* infection
   d *Candida* species infections

CMV

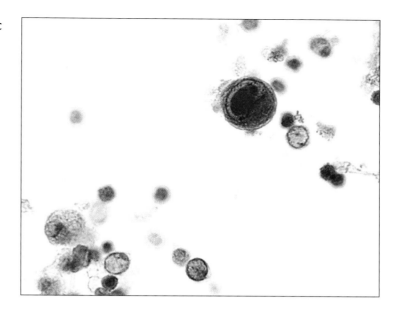

221 These organisms are commonly accompanied by:

   a herpesvirus
   b Döderlein bacillus
   c human papillomavirus
   d *Trichomonas vaginalis*

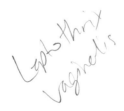

Leptothrix vaginalis

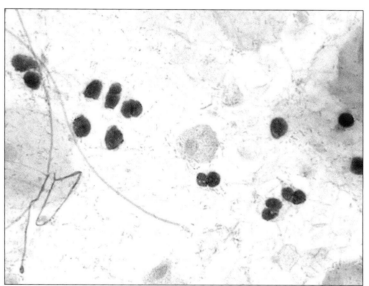

222 These cells are from a vaginal scrape from a 22-year-old female. The diagnosis is most consistent with:

   a normal endocervical cells
   b normal endometrial glandular cells
   c normal endometrial stromal cells
   d adenosis

DES associated

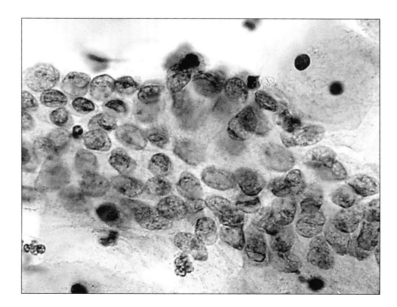

223 Which of the following statements does not correlate with the cytologic findings?

   a these cells are indicative of infection by human papillomavirus

   b the presence of these cells is often associated with keratinizing lesions

   c the cells may be associated with an underlying dysplasia

   d hyperkeratosis may accompany these cells

Parakeratosis →

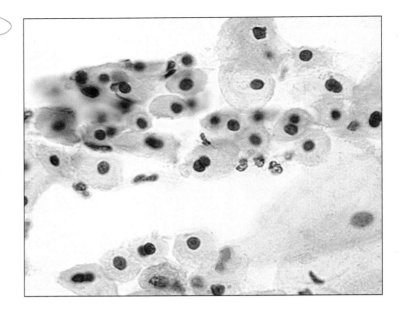

224 These cells are from a cervical scrape and an endocervical brushing from a 23-year-old female, 4 months pregnant. The diagnosis is consistent with:

   a human papillomavirus

   b cytomegalovirus ✓

   c herpesvirus

   d vaccinia virus

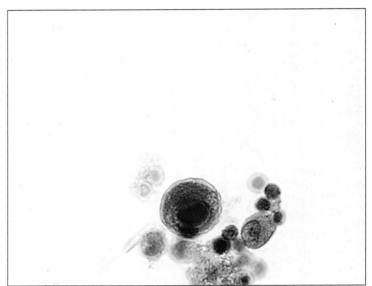

225 What clinical description is associated with these cytologic findings?

   a mature cycling woman

   b use of birth control pills

   c creates a green-yellowish discharge

   d use of an intrauterine device

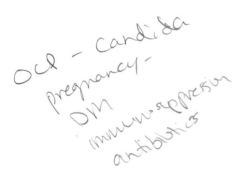

OCP — Candida
Pregnancy
DM
immunosuppression
antibiotics

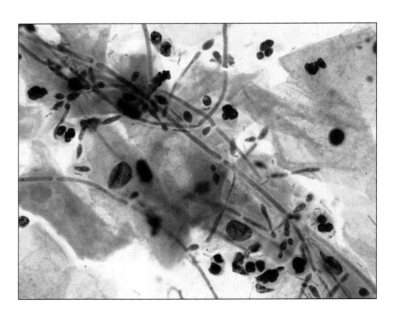

ISBN 978-089189-6357 ©ASCP 2015

226 Which of the following applies to these cells observed in a cervical smear?
  a hyperkeratosis
  b hypodifferentiation
  c an abortive attempt at keratinization
  d histologic differentiation to the stratum spinosum

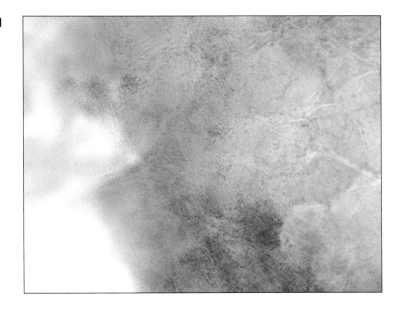

227 The entities depicted are diagnostic of:
  a *Candida albicans*
  b *Candida glabrata*
  c *Geotrichum candidum*
  d *Mucor* species

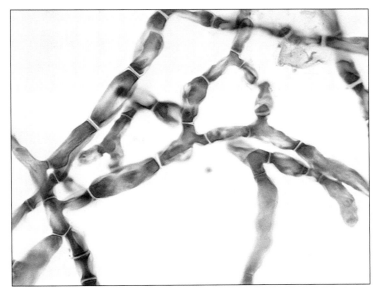

228 Which of the following clinical histories is compatible with the cytologic findings?
  a postmenopausal patient on high dose, short term estrogen therapy
  b postmenopausal patient with adrenal hyperplasia
  c postmenopausal patient with senile atrophy
  d postmenopausal patient with deep atrophy

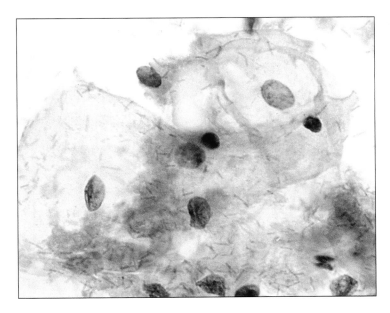

229 These structures found in Pap smears are:
   a of pathologic significance
   b suggestive of systemic *Cryptococcus* species infection
   c suggestive of mites
   d suggestive of pollen

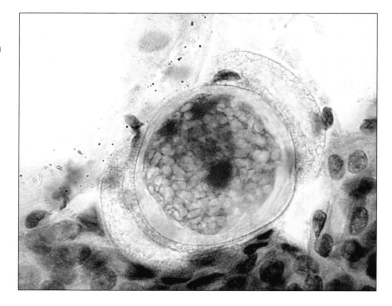

230 What is the significance of these cellular findings?
   a may mask an underlying pathologic condition
   b diagnostic of severe dysplasia and must be treated
       aggressively
   c suggestive of an invasive lesion
   d associated with progesterone based birth control pill
       usage

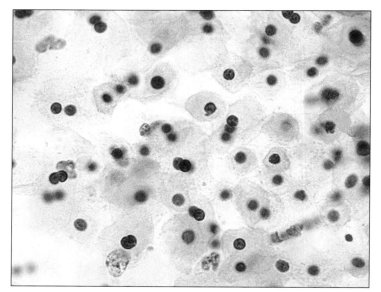

231 These cells are consistent with a:
   a benign protective reaction
   b destructive reaction
   c reparative reaction
   d dysplastic reaction

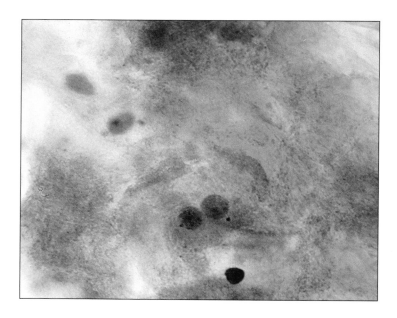

ISBN 978-089189-6357   ©ASCP 2015

232 These organisms may be associated with which clinical condition?

   a endometrial hyperplasia
   b endocervical stenosis
   c vaginal acidity
   d vaginal alkalinity

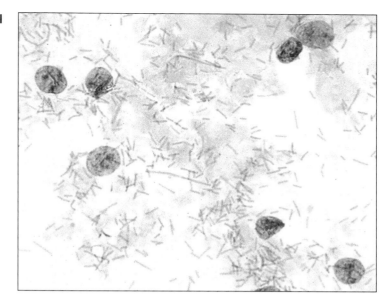

233 What clinical finding is associated with this organism?

   a curdlike yeast discharge
   b use of intrauterine devices
   c ulceration of vaginal mucosa
   d vesicles, erythematous papules

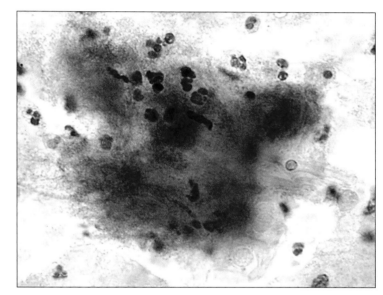

234 This cytologic sample was taken from a patient with:

   a atrophy
   b endocervical adenocarcinoma in situ
   c severe parakeratosis
   d small cell carcinoma

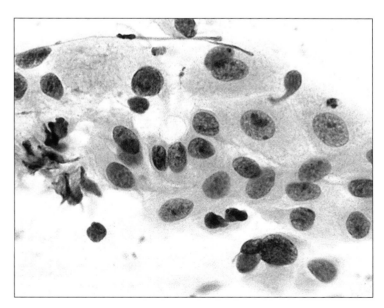

235 The material covering these cells is:
  a hematoxylin sheen
  b endocervical mucus
  c lubricant jelly
  d drying artifact

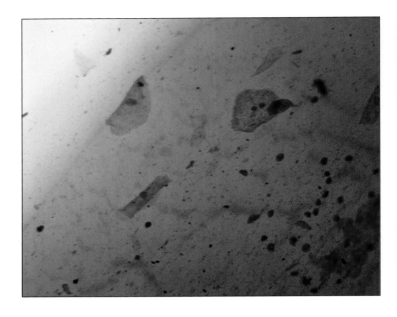

236 What hormonal state is consistent with these cytologic findings?
  a early proliferative
  b ovulation
  c late secretory
  d postpartum with galactorrhea

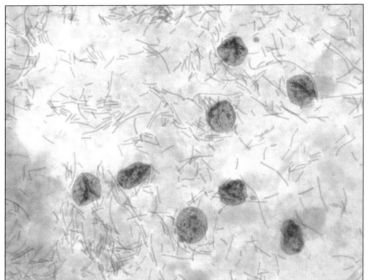

237 These cells are from a cervical scrape and an endocervical brushing from a 18-year-old female, last menstrual period 3 weeks prior. The findings are consistent with:
  a human papillomavirus
  b multinucleated histiocyte
  c syncytiotrophoblast
  d herpesvirus

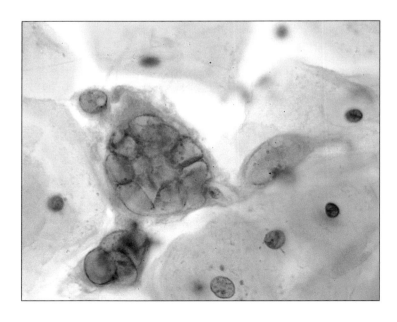

ISBN 978-089189-6357 ©ASCP 2015

238 Based on these cytologic findings, which clinical statement applies?

a prediction of disease progression is possible
b it is impossible to predict the progression rate of the lesion
c increased risk for the development of endometrial cancer
d high risk of transplacental infection

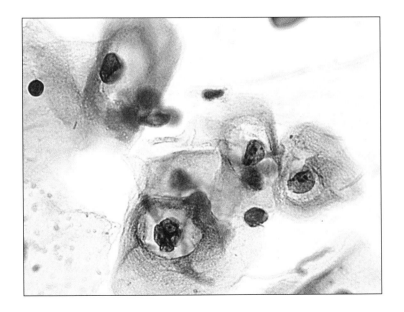

239 Which of the following is a compatible clinical condition for these cytologic findings?

a diabetes mellitus
b Stein-Leventhal syndrome
c vaginal adenosis
d marked estrogen effect

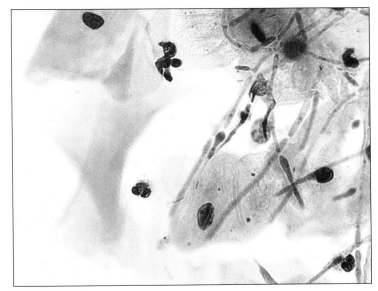

240 Which of the following is responsible for the nature of this smear taken from the vaginal/cervical area?

a improper fixation
b water in the xylene
c hardening of the mounting medium
d too long between application of mounting medium and coverslipping

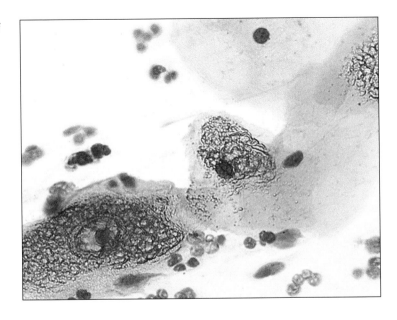

241 Which of the following is a compatible clinical setting for these cytologic findings?

   a perimenarche
   b proliferative phase of the menstrual cycle
   c secretory phase of the menstrual cycle
   d postmenopausal, postcastration (20 years)

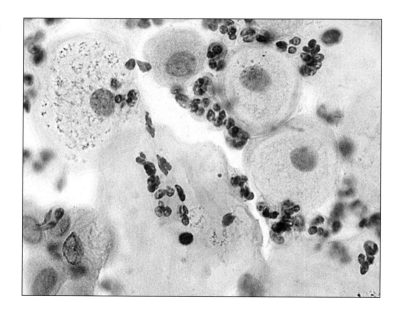

242 The maturation index in the cytologic presentation is:

   a 0/50/50
   b 50/50/0
   c 50/0/50
   d cannot be determined

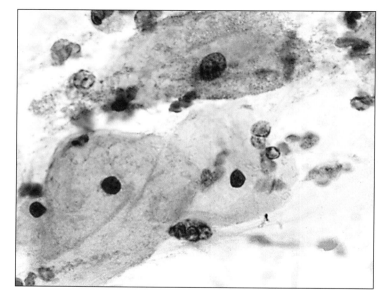

243 These cells may be associated with which hormonal condition?

   a menopausal patient on androgenic therapy
   b menopausal patient on high dose, short term estrogen therapy
   c menopausal patient on low dose, long term estrogen therapy
   d menopausal patient on corticosteroid therapy

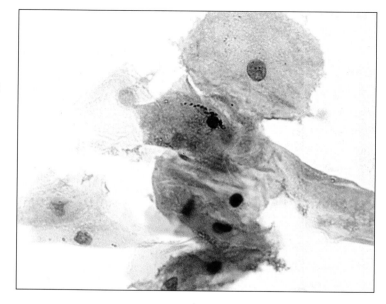

ISBN 978-089189-6357 ©ASCP 2015

244 These cells are from a vaginal smear of an 18-year-old female who is currently requesting birth control pills. Which of the following applies?
  a findings consistent with normal metaplastic epithelium found within the transformational zone
  b vaginal adenosis
  c atypical squamous cells of undetermined significance
  d metaplastic dysplasia

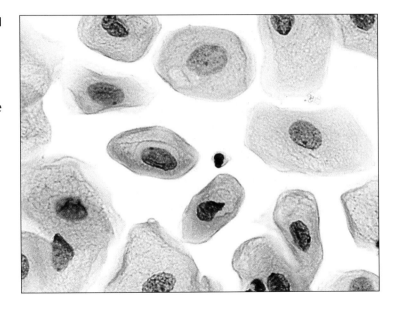

245 What clinical setting could be associated with these cytologic findings?
  a 18-year-old female with primary amenorrhea
  b 28-year-old female in the early secretory phase
  c 22-year-old female in late pregnancy
  d 35-year-old female, last menstrual period 3 days ago

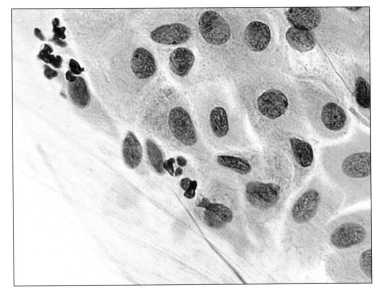

246 Represented is a vaginal smear from a 32-year-old female in her 3rd trimester. The presence of this entity is associated with preexisting vaginal:
  a acidity
  b lesion
  c alkalinity
  d infection

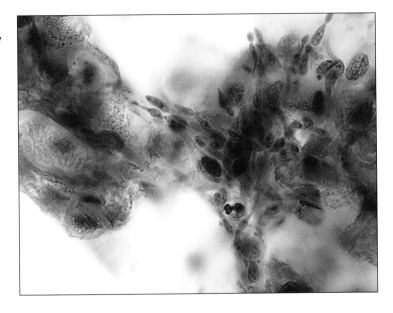

247 These cellular findings represent a sample from a 40-year-old female with small papillomatous vulval lesions. The most likely diagnosis is:
    a human papillomavirus
    b molluscum contagiosum
    c herpes simplex virus
    d pemphigus vulgaris

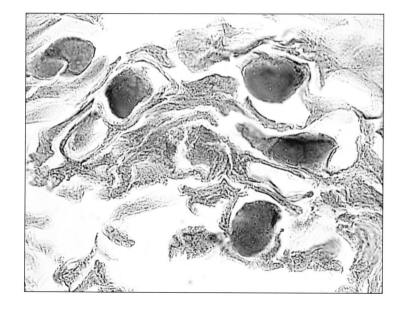

248 These cells are from a 32-year-old female, 3 months pregnant. Because the patient had previously suffered several spontaneous abortions, the clinician administered estrogen therapy. The cytologic studies are performed 6 weeks post therapy. Based on the cytologic findings, which of the following applies?
    a poor prognostic information
    b good prognostic information
    c a progesterone test should be performed to confirm a threatened pregnancy
    d prognostic information cannot be determined

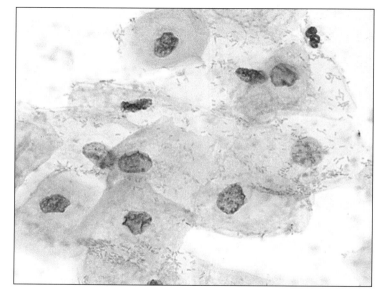

249 These cells represent a vaginal smear from a 50-year-old perimenopausal woman. A hormonal analysis was requested. Which of the following applies?
    a progesterone effect
    b decreased estrogenic effect
    c treat and repeat due to presence of microbiologic agent
    d atrophy

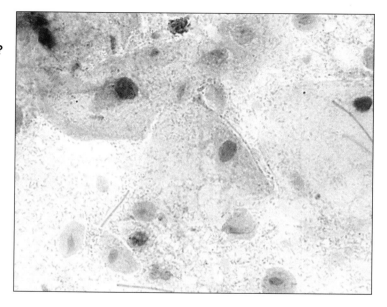

ISBN 978-089189-6357 ©ASCP 2015

250 Which of the following clinical settings would not typically support these cytologic findings?
   a long term estrogen therapy
   b late secretory phase of the menstrual cycle
   c pregnancy
   d late proliferative phase of the menstrual cycle

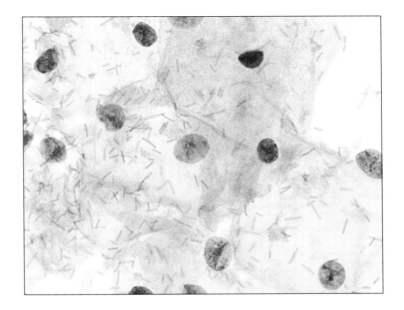

251 Based on this histologic section, which cytomorphologic features would be seen?
   a pleomorphism/caudate shape/opaque, irregular chromatin distribution
   b back to back glands/increased nuclear size/irregular chromatin distribution
   c spiderlike/attenuated processes/regular chromatin distribution
   d cytoplasmic streaming/polygonal shape/regular chromatin distribution

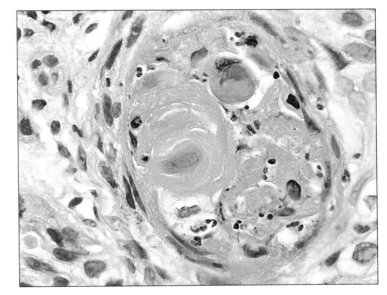

252 Based on these cells, the differential diagnosis is:
   a repair/squamous cell carcinoma
   b metaplastic dysplasia/immature metaplastic cells
   c adenocarcinoma in situ/carcinoma in situ
   d deep stromal cells/superficial stromal cells

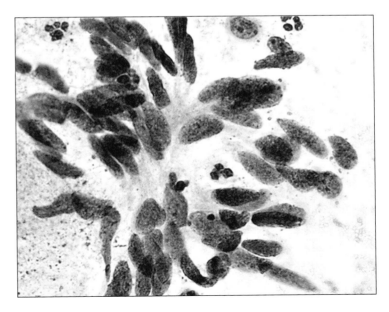

253 These cells are from a 42-year-old female who has a lesion on the anterior lip of the cervix. The cytologic pattern is most consistent with a diagnosis of:
  a atypical repair
  b low grade squamous intraepithelial lesion (LSIL)
  c endocervical adenocarcinoma
  d squamous cell carcinoma, keratinizing type

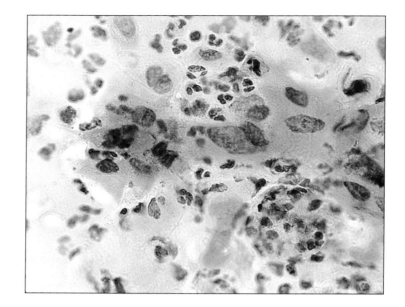

254 These cells, found in a vaginal pool sample from a 58-year-old female with a history of Stein-Leventhal syndrome of 20 years' duration, are diagnostic of:
  a polycystic ovaries
  b endocervical repair
  c endometrial adenocarcinoma
  d deep atrophy

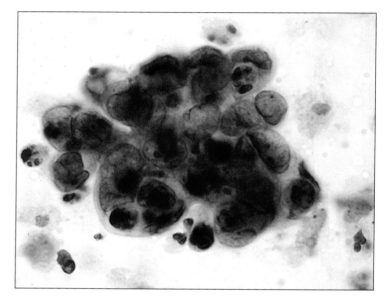

255 These cells are identified in a cervical smear from a 39-year-old female on day 9 of her menstrual cycle. They are most consistent with a diagnosis of:
  a carcinoma in situ, intermediate cell type
  b carcinoma in situ, small cell type
  c small cell carcinoma
  d chronic lymphocytic cervicitis

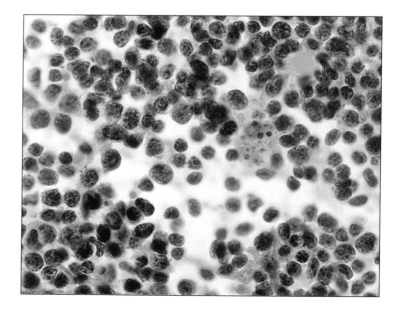

ISBN 978-089189-6357 ©ASCP 2015

256 Using the Bethesda System, this specimen would be classified as:
   a satisfactory for evaluation but limited by contaminant
   b unsatisfactory for evaluation because of obscuring inflammation
   c unsatisfactory for evaluation because of poor fixation
   d unsatisfactory for evaluation because of drying artifact

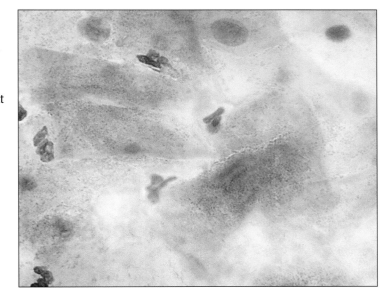

257 These cells may represent an aspirate from the:
   a Bartholin glands
   b pouch of Douglas
   c vulval apocrine glands
   d endometrial stroma

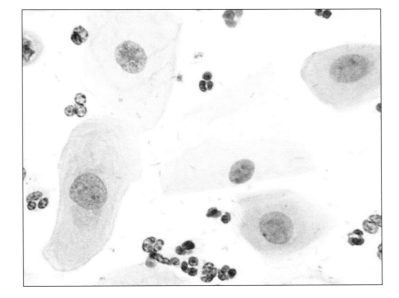

258 These cells are from a 57-year-old female with a history of irradiation for squamous cell carcinoma of the uterine cervix. The diagnosis is most consistent with:
   a radiation changes
   b recurrent carcinoma
   c changes secondary to infection with human papillomavirus
   d carcinoma in situ

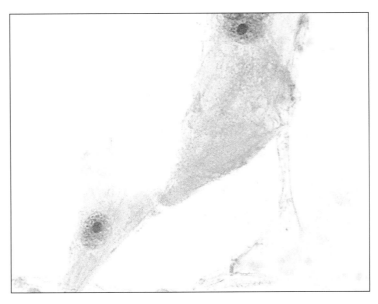

259 These cells represent a process that generally originates from the:

a native squamous epithelium
b transformation zone
c endocervical area
d endometrial area

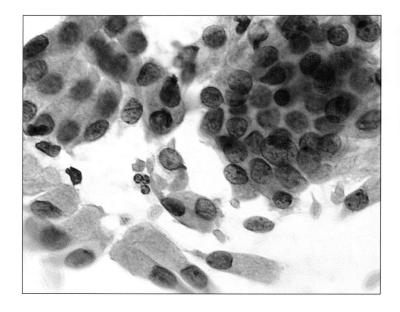

260 These cells represent normal cellular findings from the:

a endocervix
b cervical os
c endometrium
d fallopian tube

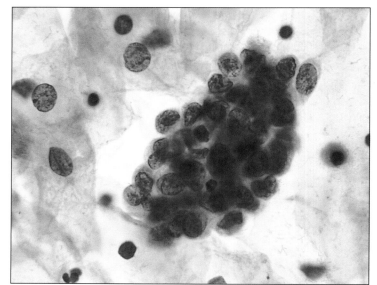

261 A 44-year-old female presents with an enlarged abdominal girth. A complete workup, including paracentesis, is performed. These cells, obtained from a cervical scrape and an endocervical brushing, suggest:

a hepatocellular carcinoma
b papillary serous cystadenocarcinoma, ovarian primary
c mucinous cystadenocarcinoma, ovarian primary
d renal cell carcinoma

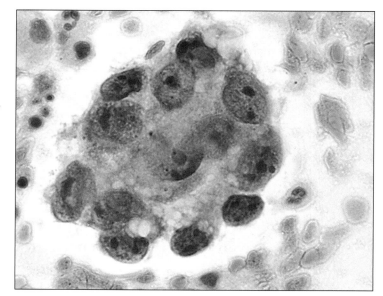

ISBN 978-089189-6357 ©ASCP 2015

262 The clinical condition depicted in this ectocervical scraping from a 12-year-old female is:

   a erosion
   b endometritis
   c retroflexion
   d cervicitis

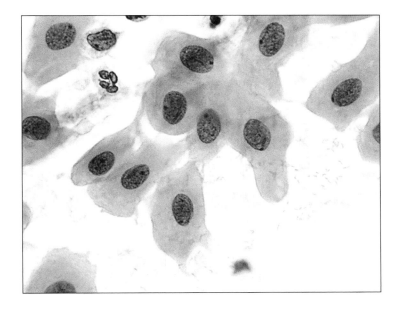

263 A 61-year-old postmenopausal woman presents with a profuse, watery discharge of 4 weeks' duration and lower abdominal cramps. Colposcopic evaluation, endocervical biopsy, and dilation and curettage of the endometrium are nonconfirmatory. The patient has no history of malignant disease. Based on these clinical and cytologic findings, the diagnosis suggests:

   a endometrial adenocarcinoma
   b adenocarcinoma, fallopian tube
   c dysgerminoma
   d endocervical adenocarcinoma

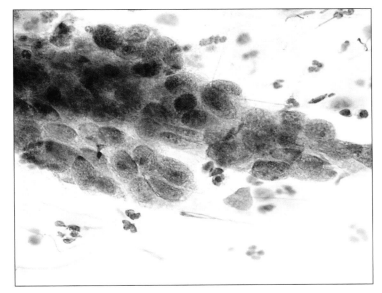

264 These cells are taken from a 43-year-old female with a history of abnormal cytologic findings. What diagnosis and patient management guidelines apply?

   a HSIL; women with this diagnosis should undergo colposcopy and directed biopsy
   b ASCUS; ablation without histologic confirmation is considered unacceptable
   c LSIL; ablation without histologic confirmation is considered unacceptable
   d negative for squamous intraepithelial lesion; no management is necessary

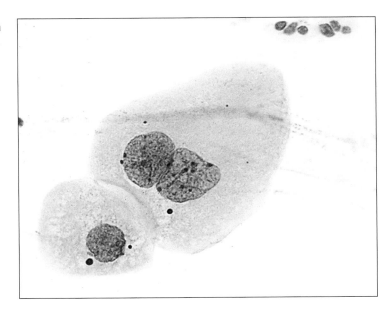

265 These cells are identified in a cellular sample obtained by an ectocervical scrape and an endocervical brushing from a 49-year-old patient complaining of a watery discharge outside of menses. The findings are most consistent with:

  a endocervical adenocarcinoma, grade III
  b metastatic colonic adenocarcinoma
  c endometrial adenocarcinoma, grade I
  d metastatic serous cystadenocarcinoma of the ovary

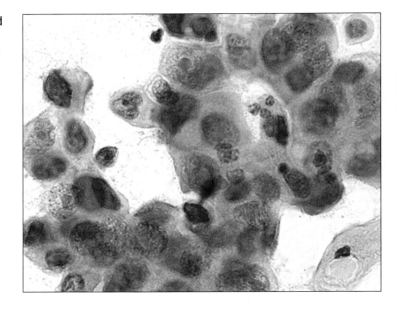

266 These cells are taken from a 22-year-old female on day 18 of her menstrual cycle. The cytologic picture represents:

  a koilocytosis
  b degenerated squamous cells
  c navicular cells
  d changes secondary to *Trichomonas* infection

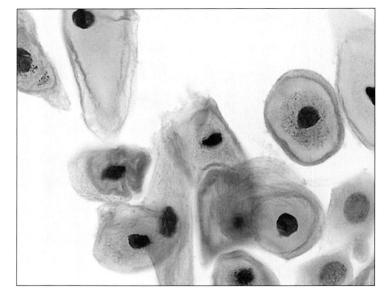

267 The cellular findings represent a vaginal/cervical/endocervical (VCE) sample taken from a 65-year-old female with a recent onset of vaginal bleeding. The findings are most consistent with:

  a normal endometrial cells
  b endometrial hyperplasia
  c atypical endometrial hyperplasia
  d endometrial adenocarcinoma

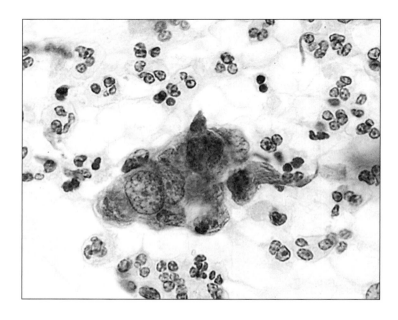

ISBN 978-089189-6357   ©ASCP 2015

268 The cells depicted are derived from what type of squamous epithelium?

   a native squamous
   b mature metaplastic
   c endocervical glandular
   d immature metaplastic

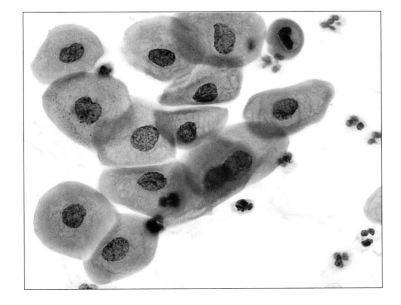

269 The presence of these cells in a vaginal smear suggests:

   a congenital abnormality; maldescension of the paramesonephric ducts
   b congenital abnormality; maldescension of the mesonephric ducts
   c possible exposure to diethylstilbestrol (DES) in utero
   d normal findings

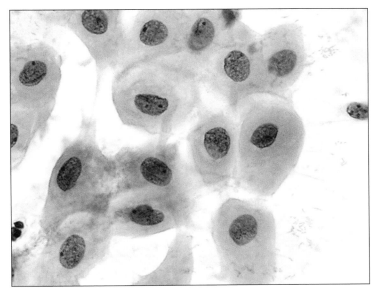

270 These cells were taken from a 40-year-old patient on day 6 of her menstrual cycle. They represent:

   a endometrial stromal cells, in cycle
   b endometrial stromal cells, out of cycle
   c endometrial glandular cells, in cycle
   d endometrial leiomyosarcoma

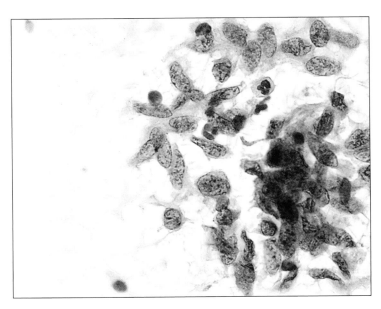

271 Using the 2002 Bethesda System, these cells would be classified as:

a within normal limits, negative for squamous intraepithelial lesion

b negative for squamous intraepithelial lesion, reactive cell changes seen

c epithelial cell abnormality, atypical squamous cells of undetermined significance (ASCUS)

d epithelial cell abnormality, LSIL

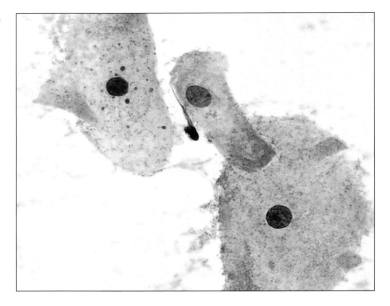

272 A 44-year-old female, on day 18 of her menstrual cycle, presents for an annual Pap smear. Cytology suggests:

a normal findings for clinical history

b endometrial hyperplasia

c endometrial adenocarcinoma

d reparative/regenerative endocervical cells

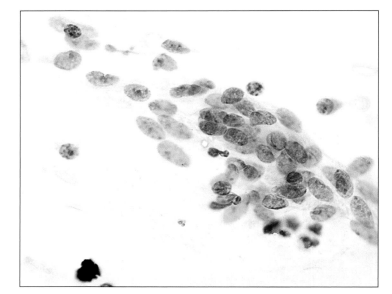

273 These cells are observed from a 65-year-old female with recent onset of bleeding. The most appropriate diagnosis is:

a endometrial adenocarcinoma, grade I

b endometrial adenocarcinoma, grade III

c mixed Müllerian tumor, homologous type

d mixed Müllerian tumor, heterologous type

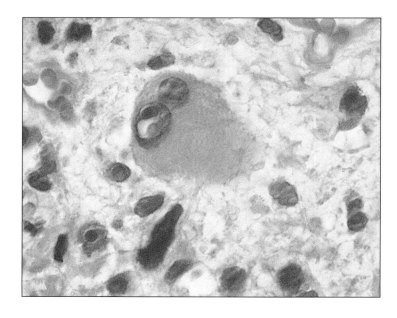

ISBN 978-089189-6357   ©ASCP 2015

274 Which of the following is associated with these cytologic findings?
   a production of lactic acid
   b *Trichomonas vaginalis*
   c intracellular diplococcus
   d alkaline pH

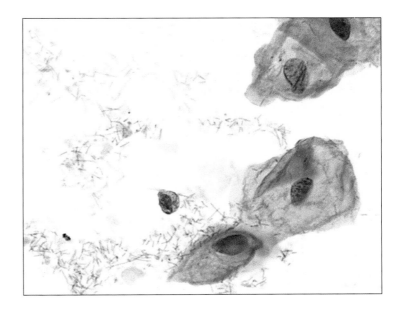

275 These cells are from a 62-year-old female with recent complaints of vaginal bleeding. The diagnosis that correlates best with her clinical history is:
   a normal endocervical cells
   b endometrial adenocarcinoma, grade I
   c metastatic serous cystadenocarcinoma of the ovary
   d endometrial hyperplasia, suggest further evaluation

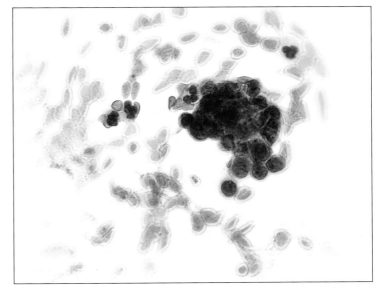

276 Which of the following terms best describes the depicted cellular findings?
   a air dried
   b karyolytic
   c karyorrhectic
   d karyopyknotic

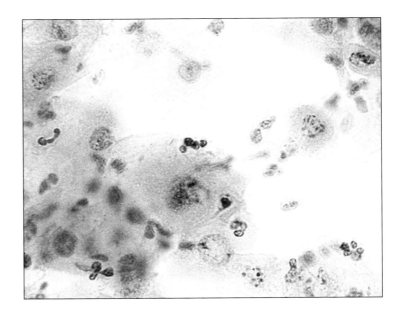

277 This cellular smear represents a cervical scrape and an endocervical brushing from a 33-year-old female on day 12 of her menstrual cycle. This is diagnostic of infection with:

   a *Lactobacillus acidophilus*
   b *Chlamydia trachomatis*
   c *Gardnerella vaginalis*
   d *Actinomyces* species

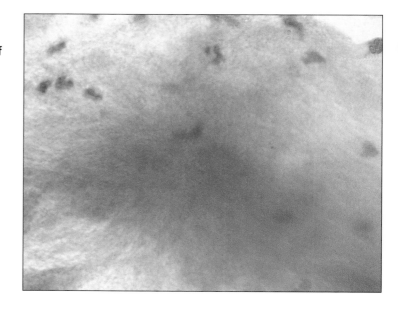

278 These cells are observed in a 44-year-old patient with dyschezia and dyspareunia. A CAT scan reveals a 3 cm lesion in the smooth muscular area of the uterus. A fine needle aspiration (FNA) was performed. The diagnosis is:

   a adenomyosis
   b metastatic cervical carcinoma
   c leiomyoma
   d leiomyosarcoma

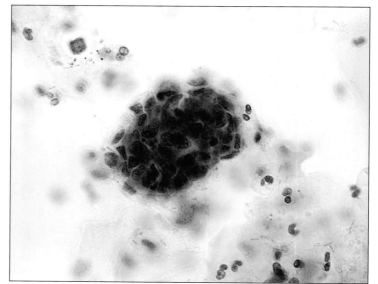

279 These cytologic findings are from a 34-year-old female in her third trimester. What is the most appropriate clinical recommendation?

   a check placenta at delivery to rule out choriocarcinoma
   b deliver via cesarean
   c treat patient with penicillin
   d advise patient of the possibility of endometrial adenocarcinoma

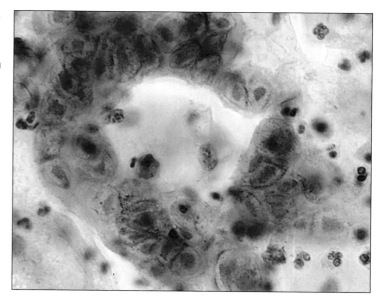

ISBN 978-089189-6357 ©ASCP 2015

280 Which clinical profile is associated with these cellular findings?

   a endometritis
   b infection by a high risk human papillomavirus viral subtype
   c unopposed estrogen stimulation
   d increased number of sexual partners

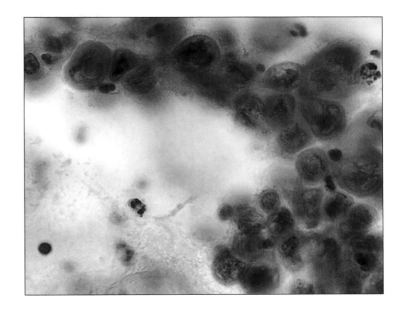

281 A 36-year-old female presents with infertility, menorrhagia, and recent onset of incontinence. A pelvic CT scan reveals a 2 cm mass involving the uterine wall with direct extension into the left ureter. Represented is an endometrial aspirate. The diagnosis is:

   a endometrial stromal sarcoma
   b endometrial adenocarcinoma, grade III
   c mixed Müllerian tumor, heterologous type
   d leiomyosarcoma

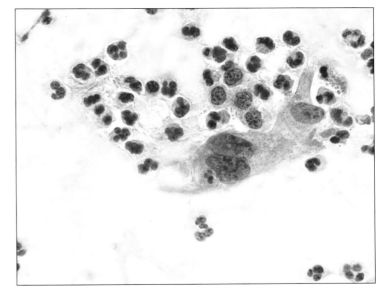

282 The clinical findings associated with this vaginal/cervical scrape specimen are:

   a frothy, yellow-green discharge/strawberry cervix
   b white, curdlike discharge/normal cervix
   c absence of discharge/leukoplakia on cervix
   d menorrhagia/exophytic mass

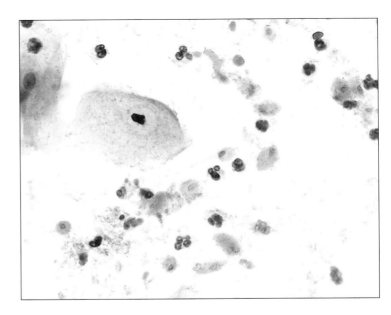

283 The cells of this lateral vaginal wall scraping are compatible with which of the following conditions?

   a Stein-Leventhal syndrome
   b granulosa-theca cell tumor
   c hepatic insufficiency
   d Turner syndrome

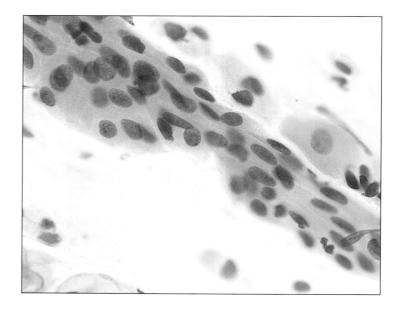

284 The diagnostic criteria that differentiate these cells from those of carcinoma in situ are:

   a finely granular, evenly distributed chromatin
   b nucleoli, diathesis, irregular chromatin distribution
   c hyperchromasia, regular chromatin distribution
   d koilocytic changes, parakeratosis

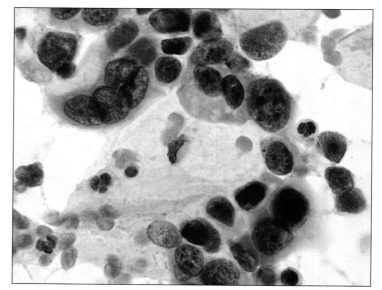

285 These cells are from a 34-year-old female. Based on the morphologic findings, what is their likely source?

   a endometrium
   b internal cervical os
   c endocervical canal
   d vagina

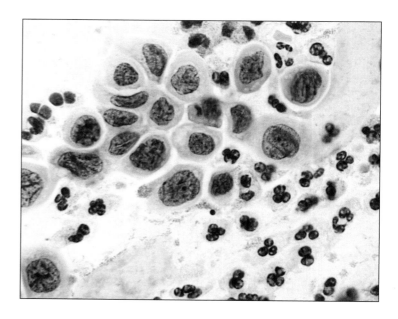

ISBN 978-089189-6357 ©ASCP 2015

286 These cells are observed in a vaginal/cervical/endocervical sample taken from an 18-year-old female. The findings are most consistent with:
  a LSIL, mild nonkeratinizing dysplasia
  b atypical glandular cells of undetermined significance (AGUS)
  c LSIL, mild metaplastic dysplasia
  d squamous atypia/mature metaplastic ASCUS (mimicking mature native squames)

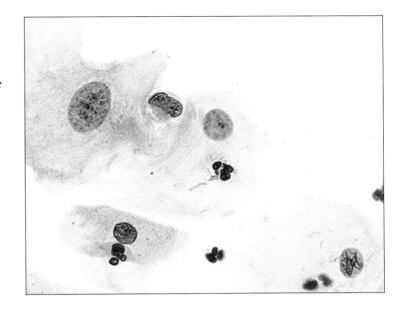

287 Compared with cells of other lesions arising within the cervix, the mitotic rate of this cell type is considered:
  a high
  b low
  c variable
  d equal

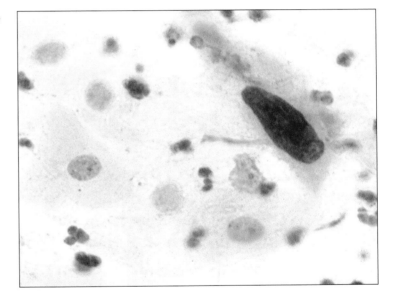

288 A 26-year-old female was treated with electrocautery for a cervical intraepithelial neoplasia 2 (CIN2) 6 months before collection of these cells. The cells were collected on day 16 of a normal 30 day estrous cycle. The cellular changes are suggestive of:
  a residual dysplasia, not otherwise specified
  b invasive squamous cell carcinoma
  c CIN2
  d reparative/regenerative changes secondary to therapy

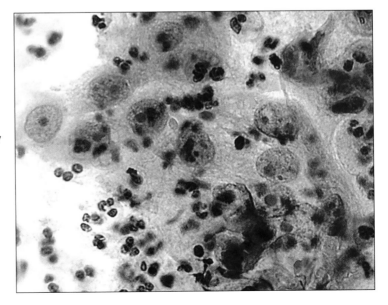

289 These cellular findings are representative of:
  a HSIL
  b radiation induced cell changes
  c squamous cell carcinoma
  d parakeratosis

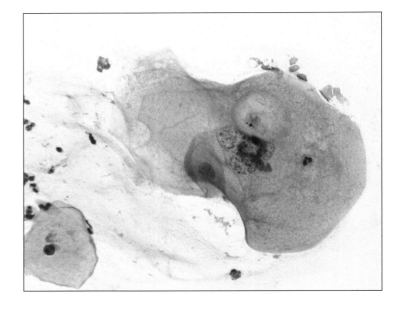

290 A 33-year-old female presents with dysfunctional uterine bleeding. These cells were collected with conventional cervical/endocervical brushings. The findings are most consistent with:
  a endometrial adenocarcinoma, grade I
  b endometrial polyp
  c normal endometrial cells, possibly associated with endometrial hyperplasia
  d endometrial adenocarcinoma, grade IV

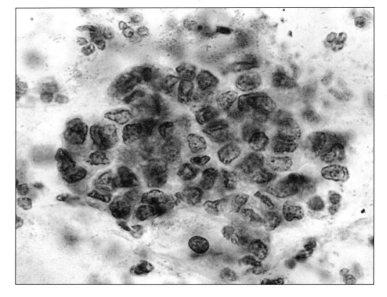

291 What percentage of the epithelial thickness is replaced in situ given these cytologic findings?
  a 25%
  b 50%
  c 75%
  d 100%

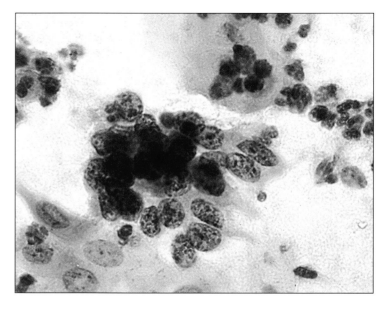

ISBN 978-089189-6357 ©ASCP 2015

292 These cells represent a cervical/endocervical smear from a 66-year-old female. The cytology represents:

   a atypia of atrophy
   b *Chlamydia trachomatis* infection
   c LSIL, koilocytosis associated with HPV
   d navicular cells

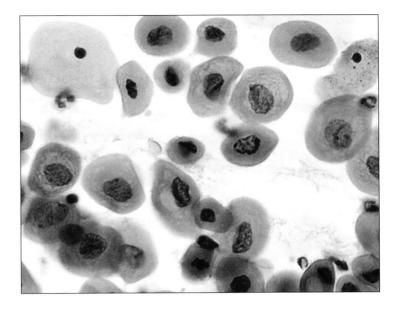

293 These cells are from a 40-year-old female, gravida 8, para 4, abortus 4, last menstrual period 9 days ago. The findings are consistent with:

   a normal endometrial cells
   b atypical endometrial hyperplasia
   c reactive/reparative endocervical cells
   d endometrial adenocarcinoma

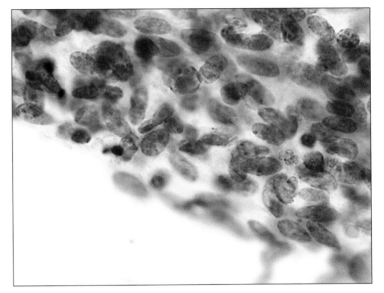

294 These cells are derived from a vaginal/cervical/endocervical scraping taken from a 31-year-old female, last menstrual period 12 days ago. The findings are most consistent with:

   a HSIL, moderate nonkeratinizing dysplasia
   b LSIL, mild nonkeratinizing dysplasia
   c HSIL, moderate metaplastic dysplasia
   d LSIL, mild metaplastic dysplasia

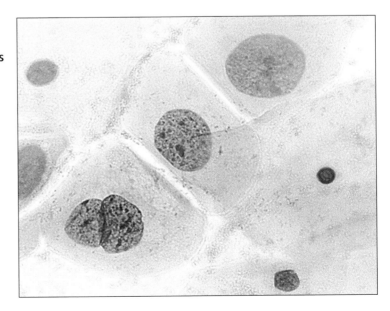

295 These cells would most likely originate from the:
  a ectocervix
  b mature metaplastic transformational zone
  c immature metaplastic transformational zone
  d endocervical glandular epithelium

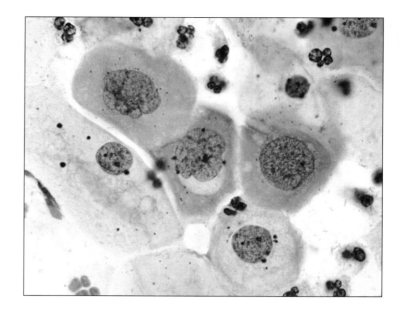

296 The hallmark for diagnosing the lesion represented is the presence of:
  a fine chromatin
  b hyperchromasia
  c irregular chromatin
  d cytoplasmic streaming

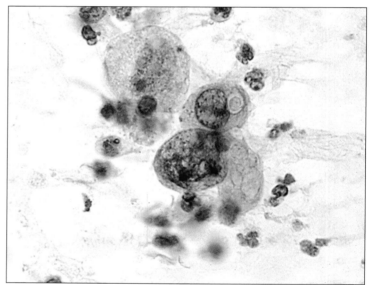

297 These cells represent a cervical specimen from a 48-year-old female with an anterior lip cervical lesion. The findings are most consistent with:
  a squamous cell carcinoma, keratinizing type
  b HSIL, moderate dysplasia, keratinizing type
  c dyskeratosis associated with HPV
  d poorly differentiated squamous cell carcinoma

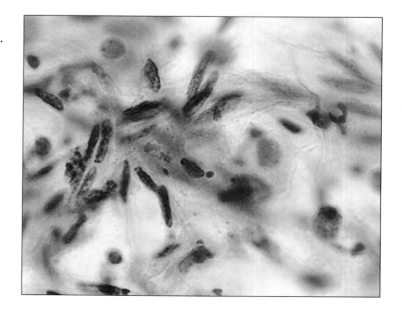

ISBN 978-089189-6357 ©ASCP 2015

298 What feature becomes less predictable as the depicted lesion becomes poorly differentiated?

a pleomorphism
b anisocytosis
c anisonucleosis
d macronucleoli

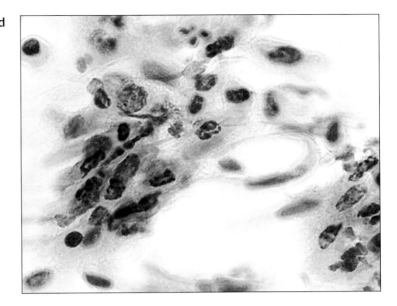

299 These cells are found 6 months after irradiation therapy for stage IB squamous cell carcinoma of the uterine cervix. Their presence indicates:

a hyperkeratosis, a benign cellular change related to the irradiation therapy
b a hyperdifferentiation that places the patient at a higher risk for postirradiation dysplasia
c normal findings
d unrelated to the history

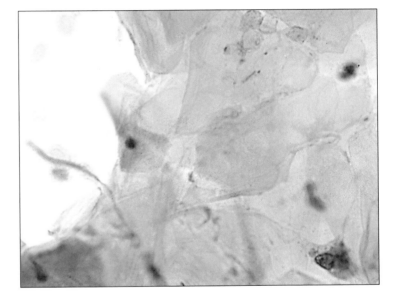

300 These cells are best differentiated from an intraepithelial squamous lesion by:

a strips of pseudostratified or "feathering" epithelium in glandular lesions
b elevated nuclear to cytoplasmic (N:C) ratios in squamous lesions
c increased hyperchromasia in squamous lesions
d the presence of nucleoli in squamous lesions

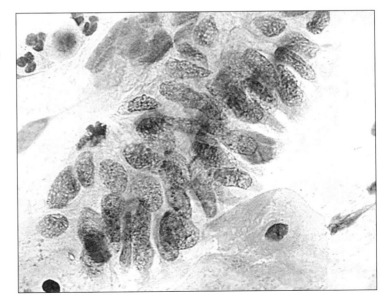

301 One of the best criteria for distinguishing these cells from their immediate precursor is:

   a coarse chromatin
   b diathesis
   c nucleoli
   d hyperchromasia

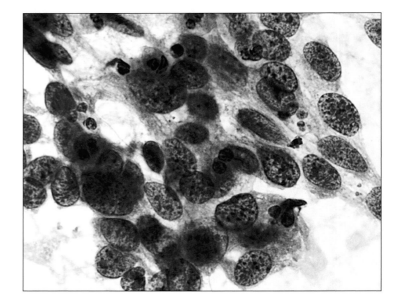

302 How common is the lesion shown relative to a nonkeratinizing squamous lesion?

   a it is more common
   b it is less common
   c they have about the same frequency
   d it cannot be determined with the information provided

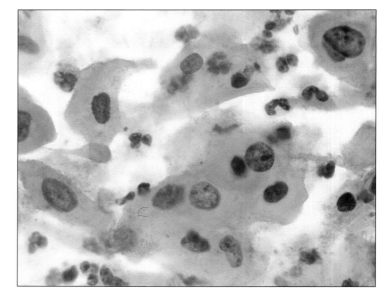

303 Which of the following criteria are helpful in establishing the diagnosis in this photomicrograph?

   a predominantly single cells
   b low nuclear to cytoplasmic (N:C) ratio
   c hyperchromatic crowded groups
   d rosettes, acinar morphology, feathering cytoplasmic borders

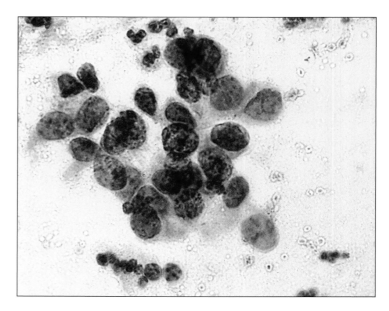

ISBN 978-089189-6357   ©ASCP 2015

304 These cells are from a 35-year-old patient with a history of normal Pap smears. The cellular findings are suggestive of:
  a reserve cell hyperplasia
  b small cell carcinoma in situ
  c reactive endocervical cells
  d endocervical adenocarcinoma in situ

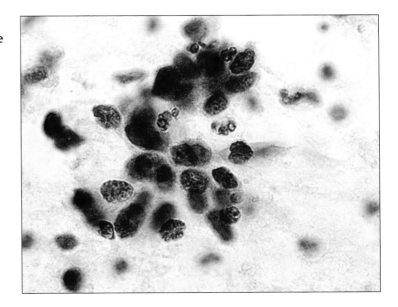

305 These cells are observed in a 32-year-old female, 6 months postpartum, with a history of HPV infection. The findings are most consistent with:
  a LSIL, mild dysplasia with associated HPV infection
  b parakeratosis
  c dyskeratotic cells related to HPV infection
  d atrophic vaginitis

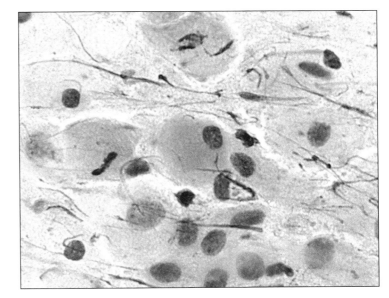

306 The origin of these cells in a cervical/vaginal smear taken from a 44-year-old patient is most likely:
  a vaginal, immature metaplastic
  b vaginal, endocervical
  c ectocervical, immature metaplastic
  d ectocervical, mature metaplastic

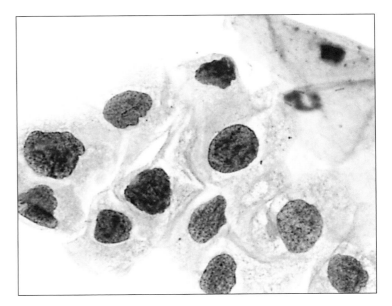

307 Cytologically, this tissue section is best characterized as:

    a possessing macronucleoli
    b pleomorphic, caudate, spindled
    c possessing large, round to oval cells with anisocytosis
    d isodiametric

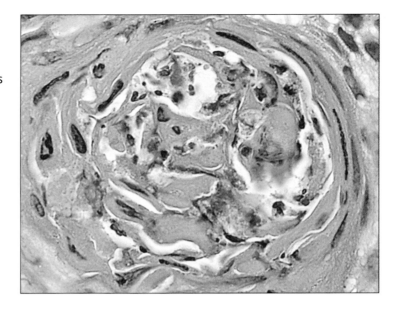

308 What histologic growth pattern may be associated with these cellular findings?

    a endophytic
    b verrucous
    c flat
    d inverted

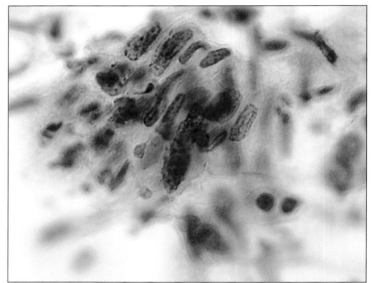

309 Based on these cytologic findings, is it possible to predict the histologic growth pattern of the lesion?

    a yes
    b no
    c not sure based on these cellular changes

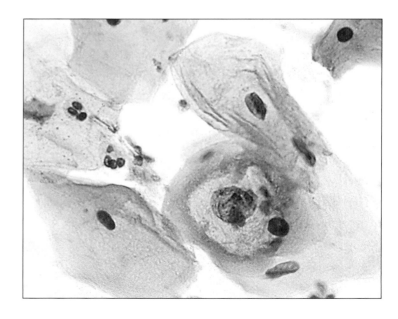

ISBN 978-089189-6357 ©ASCP 2015

310 These cells, representative of a cervical scraping and an endocervical brushing, are diagnostic of:
a cervical intraepithelial lesion, grade III
b small cell squamous cell carcinoma
c nonkeratinizing squamous carcinoma, moderately differentiated
d mixed mesodermal tumor, homologous variety

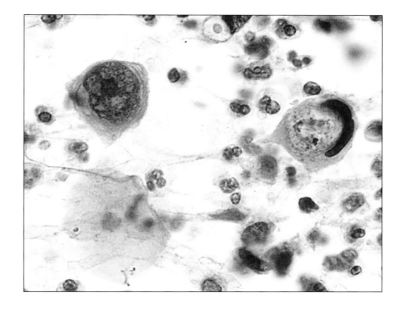

311 These cells are found in a 26-year-old patient, last menstrual period 8 days ago. The findings are consistent with:
a follicular cervicitis
b pseudoparakeratosis/microglandular hyperplasia
c degenerated neutrophils
d small cell histiocytes

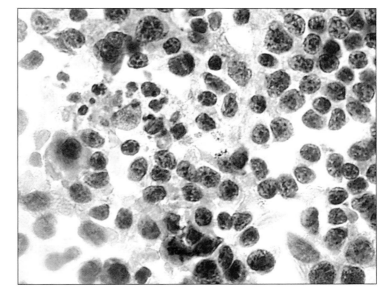

312 These cells represent a cervical scraping from a 33-year-old female with a friable lesion within the endocervical canal. The findings are consistent with:
a reactive/reparative reaction
b carcinoma in situ, large cell type
c sarcoma, NOS
d squamous cell carcinoma, nonkeratinizing type

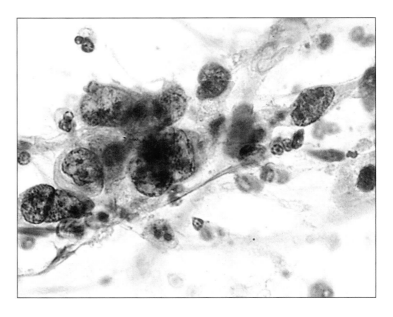

313 These cells are from a patient, after radiation therapy for squamous cell carcinoma, grade I. She recently underwent hormonal therapy for vaginal atrophy. The diagnosis is most consistent with:
   a folic acid deficiency
   b atrophic vaginitis
   c benign radiation induced cellular changes
   d postirradiation dysplasia

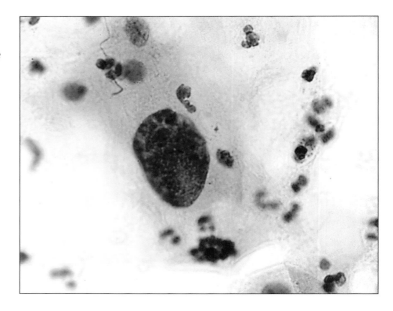

314 These cells represent an endocervical aspirate from a 52-year-old female with a recent history of vaginal bleeding. The cells are consistent with a diagnosis of:
   a degenerated endocervical cells
   b endometrial hyperplasia
   c nonkeratinizing squamous cell carcinoma
   d small cell neuroendocrine carcinoma

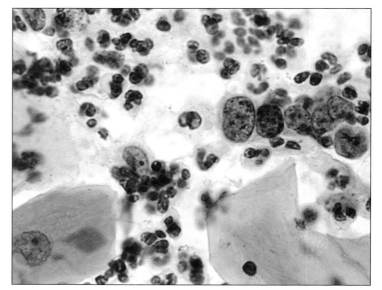

315 These cellular changes are diagnostic of:
   a benign radiation cellular changes
   b autolysis
   c cellular degeneration, secondary to inflammation
   d postirradiation dysplasia

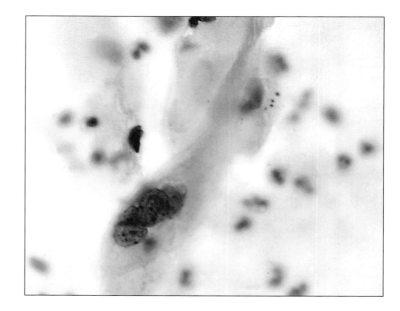

ISBN 978-089189-6357 ©ASCP 2015

316 A 55-year-old patient, status post total abdominal hysterectomy and bilateral tubal ligation and 6 weeks postirradiation for stage IIB squamous cell carcinoma of the uterine cervix, presents for a follow-up Pap smear. These cells are suggestive of:

a residual carcinoma
b negative for squamous intraepithelial lesion with radiation induced cellular changes
c postirradiation dysplasia
d ASCUS

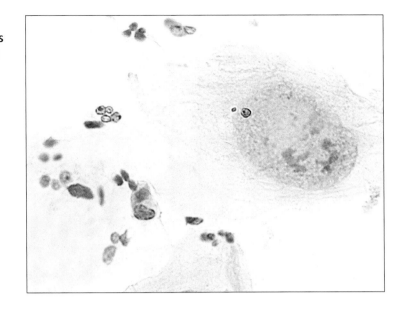

317 These cells are found in a vaginal cuff sample taken from a patient who had undergone irradiation therapy for squamous cell carcinoma of the cervix. The cellular findings suggest a diagnosis of:

a postirradiation dysplasia
b residual carcinoma
c reparative/regenerative changes
d parakeratosis

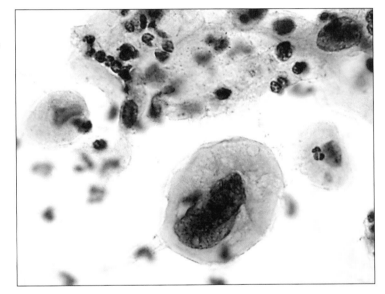

318 The cellular aggregate shown is most commonly described as:

a a sheet
b syncytial-like
c a cluster
d a rosette

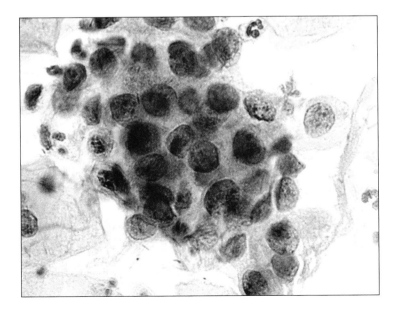

319 These cells are normally located:
  a in a prepubescent female
  b at the internal cervical os
  c within the vagina
  d in the transformation zone

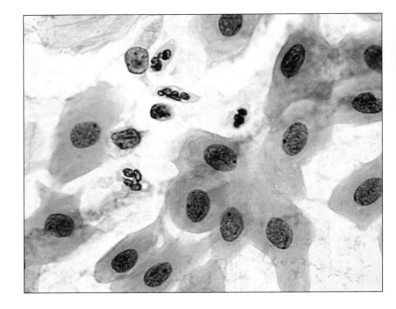

320 These cells are from an ectocervical scrape and endocervical brushing. The findings depicted represent:
  a malignant lymphoma
  b toxoplasmosis
  c chronic follicular cervicitis
  d acute inflammatory process

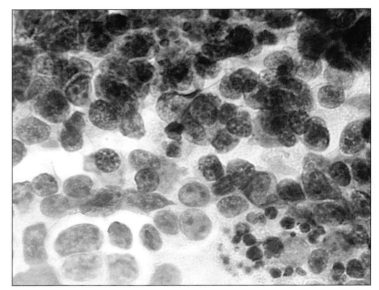

321 Which of the following may be associated with these cells obtained from a vaginal/cervical scrape of a 42-year-old female?
  a invasive squamous cell carcinoma
  b endocervical dysplasia
  c severe cervicitis
  d pemphigus vulgaris

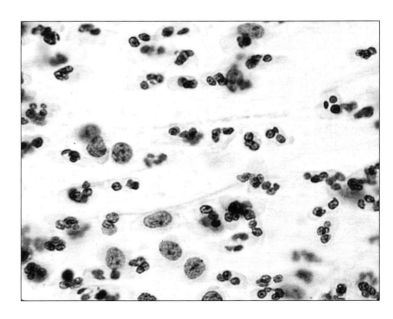

ISBN 978-089189-6357   ©ASCP 2015

322 A 35-year-old diabetic woman presents in the second trimester of pregnancy. Which of the following correlates with the cytologic findings represented in this vaginal smear?

a normal cytologic pattern for pregnancy
b possible fetal death in utero
c vaginal infection
d folic acid deficiency

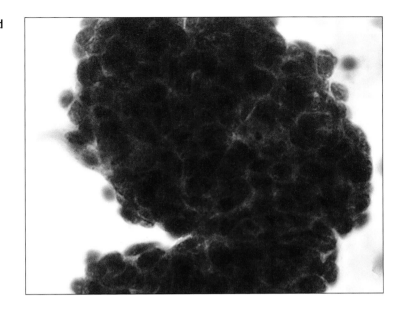

323 The background in the depicted cellular process may be described as:

a a tumor diathesis
b clean—no tumor diathesis
c severe acute inflammation
d cytolysis

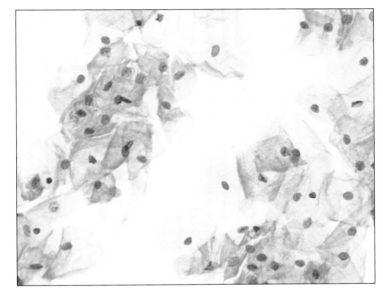

324 These cells are diagnostic of:

a microglandular hyperplasia
b parakeratosis
c dyskeratosis
d low grade squamous intraepithelial lesion (LSIL)

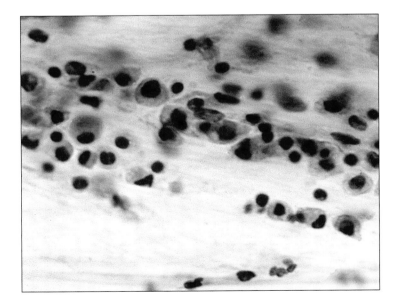

325 This vaginal smear is from a 42-year-old infertile patient. A diagnostic tool useful in evaluating the hormonal status of infertile patients is:

  a lateral vaginal wall smear (taken from the upper third)
  b lateral vaginal wall smear (taken from the lower third)
  c serum levels
  d cervical smear

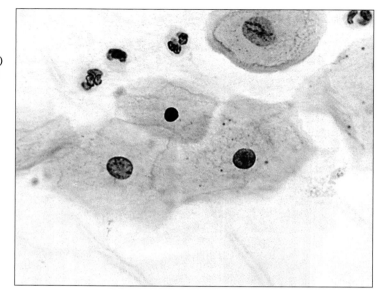

326 Which clinical condition may be associated with these cytologic findings from a vaginal smear from a 35-year-old female?

  a Cushing syndrome
  b Stein-Leventhal syndrome
  c follicular persistency
  d hepatic insufficiency

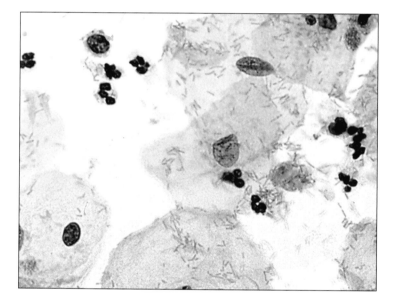

327 These cells are found in a cervical scrape and endocervical brushing from a 26-year-old female with a history of cauterization for an abnormal Pap smear. The diagnosis is consistent with:

  a reparative/regenerative process
  b low grade squamous intraepithelial lesion (LSIL)
  c high grade squamous intraepithelial lesion (HSIL)
  d invasive squamous cell carcinoma

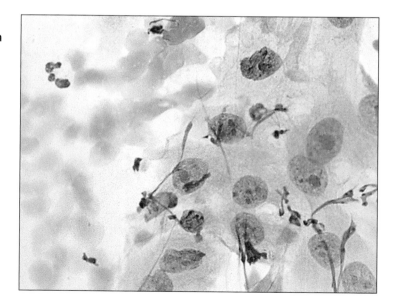

ISBN 978-089189-6357   ©ASCP 2015

328 These cells are from a cervical scrape and endocervical brushing specimen from a 28-year-old female suffering from a chronic skin disease. The diagnosis is:

a pilomatrixoma
b amelanotic melanoma
c pemphigus vulgaris
d basal cell carcinoma

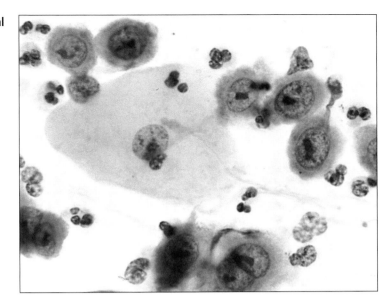

329 A 22-year-old female presents with secondary amenorrhea. Clinical findings reveal that the patient suffers from Stein-Leventhal syndrome. Based on these cellular findings, the hormonal analysis:

a correlates with history
b does not correlate with history

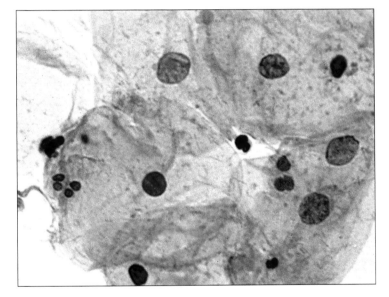

330 These cells represent a cervical/endocervical smear from a 43-year-old female. The diagnosis is:

a squamous cell carcinoma, keratinizing variety
b LSIL, keratinizing variety
c HSIL, keratinizing variety
d parakeratosis

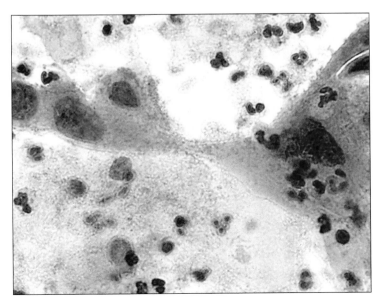

331 These cytologic findings represent a vaginal/cervical smear from a 28-year-old asymptomatic woman. The diagnosis is consistent with:

a glycogenated cells
b ASCUS
c LSIL, HPV
d HSIL

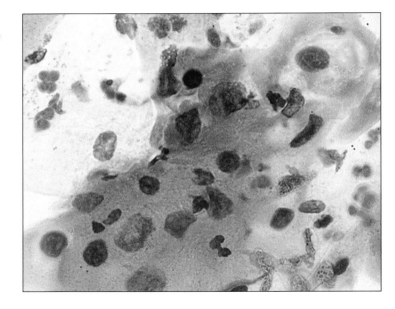

332 Which clinical condition may be associated with this vaginal smear pattern?

a del Castillo syndrome
b precocious puberty
c granulosa-theca cell tumor
d advanced cirrhosis of the liver

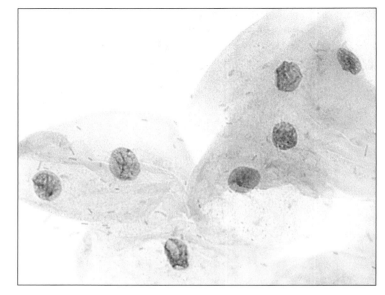

333 A 16-year-old patient presents with primary amenorrhea. Primary clinical findings suggest feminizing testicular syndrome. A smear is performed for hormonal analysis. Based on the cellular findings, one would conclude:

a the hormonal analysis is compatible with history
b the hormonal analysis is not compatible with history

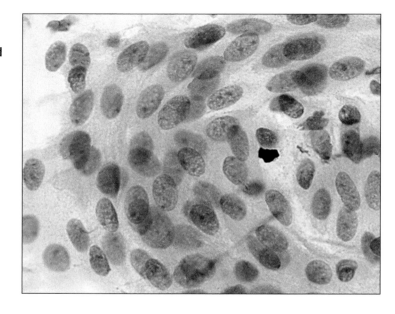

ISBN 978-089189-6357　©ASCP 2015

334 Which of the following might subsequently develop
based on these cytologic findings?
a keratinizing dysplasia
b high grade intraepithelial lesion, metaplastic dysplasia
c atypical reserve cell hyperplasia
d small cell carcinoma in situ

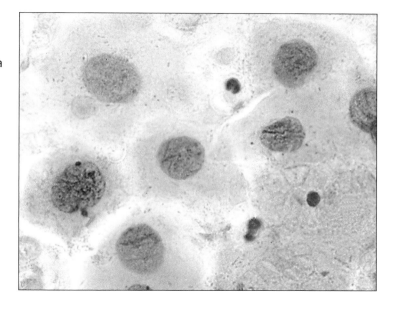

335 These cytologic findings from a vaginal smear are
compatible with:
a masculinizing ovarian tumor
b patient with amenorrhea with galactorrhea
c Chiari-Frommel syndrome
d granulosa-theca cell tumor

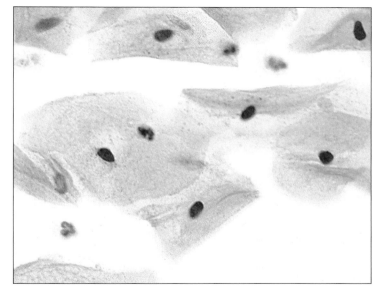

336 A 22-year-old postpartum (1 week) patient presents
to her physician with vaginal bleeding. A Pap test is
performed. The findings are consistent with:
a HPV associated dyskeratosis
b reparative/regenerative process
c endometrial stromal cells
d syncytiotrophoblasts

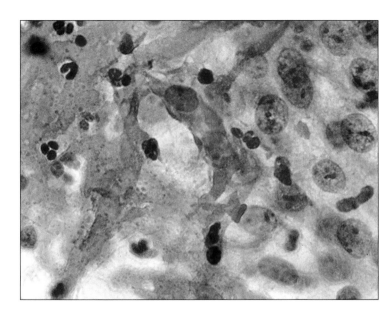

337 These cells represent a cervical scrape and endocervical brushing in a 23-year-old female. These cells are:

   a endometrial stromal cells
   b endocervical glandular cells
   c immature metaplastic cells
   d mature metaplastic cells

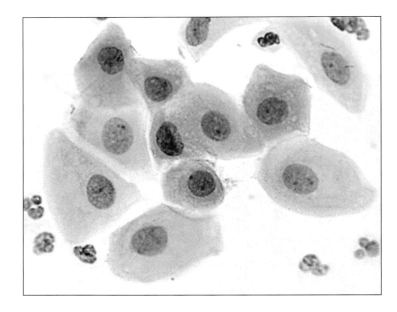

338 An 18-year-old female presents with primary amenorrhea and webbing of the neck. These cells are from a vaginal smear. The hormonal analysis is compatible with a clinical diagnosis of:

   a feminizing testicular syndrome/androgen insensitivity syndrome
   b Stein-Leventhal syndrome
   c Turner syndrome
   d polycystic ovaries

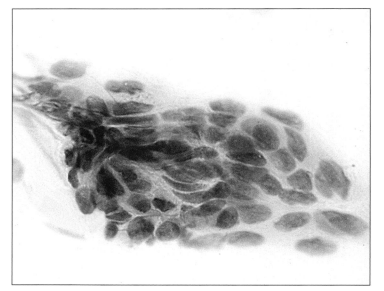

339 Which of the following criteria would help to classify these cells as metastatic rather than primary?

   a presence of columnar configuration
   b absence of a diathesis
   c cytoplasmic texture
   d nuclear characteristics

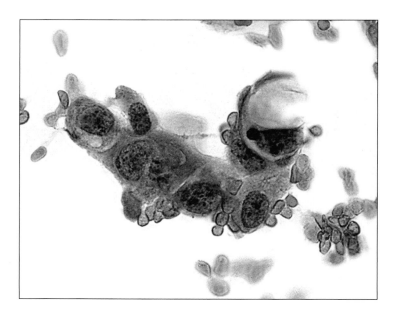

ISBN 978-089189-6357　©ASCP 2015

340 What clinical condition may be associated with this vaginal smear taken from a 30-year-old female (taken 8 weeks after her last menstrual period)?
- **a** follicular cytosis
- **b** ovarian eunuchoidism
- **c** Turner syndrome
- **d** Chiari-Frommel syndrome

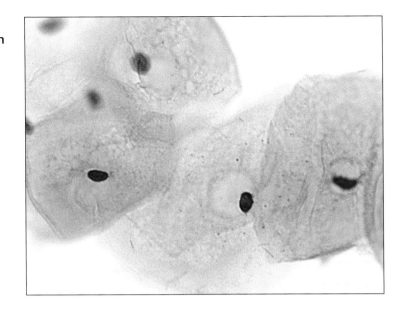

341 The most important criterion for distinguishing these cells from mild dysplasia is the:
- **a** N:C ratio
- **b** hyperchromasia
- **c** nucleoli
- **d** nuclear membrane

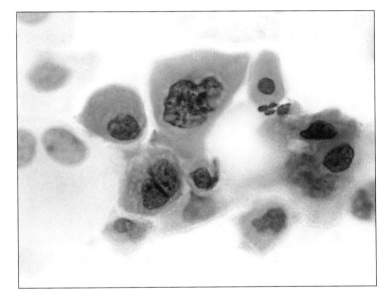

342 These cells are from a cervical scrape and an endocervical brushing from a 41-year-old female who presented for an annual Pap smear. These cells suggest a diagnosis of:
- **a** mild nonkeratinizing dysplasia, LSIL
- **b** moderate nonkeratinizing dysplasia, HSIL
- **c** severe nonkeratinizing dysplasia, HSIL
- **d** carcinoma in situ, intermediate cell type, HSIL

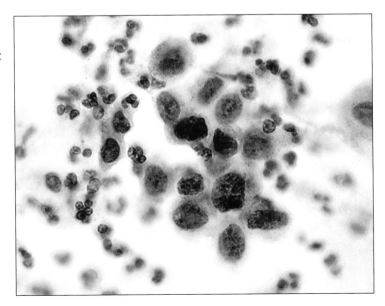

343 These cells are identified in a cellular sample obtained by an ectocervical scrape and endocervical aspiration from a 44-year-old female. The diagnosis is:

a normal immature squamous metaplasia
b low grade squamous intraepithelial lesion
c high grade squamous intraepithelial lesion
d birth control pill changes

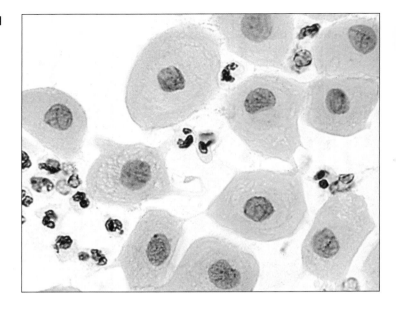

344 One criterion used to distinguish these cells from their precursor lesion includes the presence of:

a diathesis
b coarse, irregular chromatin
c nucleoli
d coarse, regular chromatin

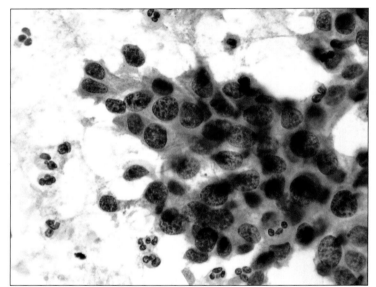

345 Which of the following papillomavirus types is etiologically related to these cells?

a HPV11
b HPV16
c HPV6
d HPV2

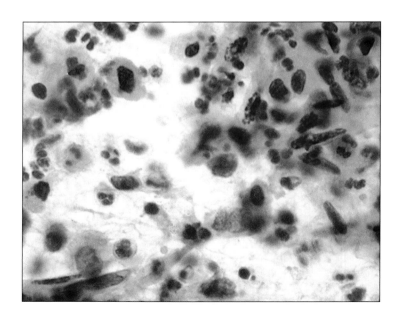

ISBN 978-089189-6357 ©ASCP 2015

346 These cells were taken from a 21-year-old female who presented with a fungating mass protruding from the anterior cervical lip. Cervical scrapings suggest a diagnosis of:

a squamous cell carcinoma, large cell variety
b HSIL, consistent with carcinoma in situ
c HSIL, consistent with moderate dysplasia
d LSIL, consistent with HPV

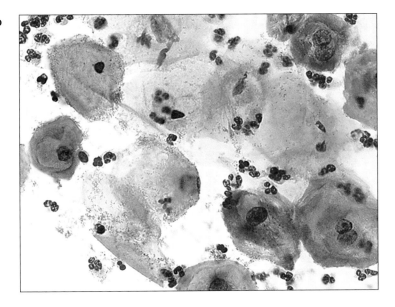

347 An 18-year-old female presents with primary amenorrhea. Which clinical condition may be associated with the cellular findings?

a congenital absence of the uterus
b Chiari-Frommel syndrome
c ovarian eunuchoidism
d gonadal dysgenesis

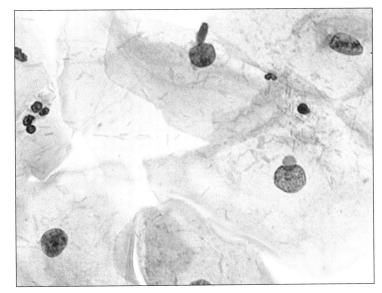

348 These cells represent a cervical/endocervical scraping taken from a 33-year-old female. The diagnosis is:

a negative for squamous intraepithelial lesion
b ASCUS, dyskeratocytes (pleomorphic parakeratosis) most likely associated with HPV infection
c LSIL, mild dysplasia, keratinizing type
d HSIL, severe dysplasia, keratinizing type

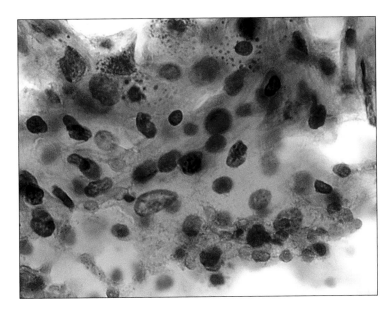

349 Which of the following is commonly associated with these cells?

   a Arias-Stella reaction
   b hyperkeratosis
   c reserve cell hyperplasia
   d follicular cervicitis

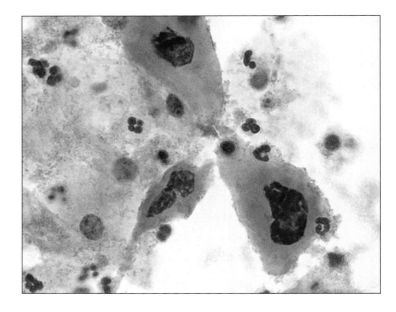

350 Based on these histologic tissue findings, the appropriate diagnosis is:

   a mild dysplasia, LSIL
   b severe dysplasia, HSIL
   c squamous metaplasia
   d reactive/reparative changes

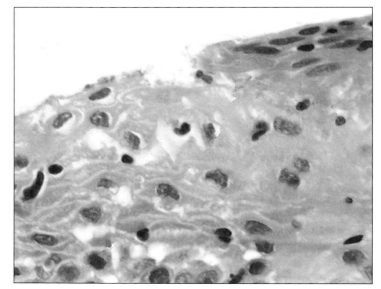

351 These cells are from an endocervical aspirate from a 32-year-old female with a recent history of conization for endocervical adenocarcinoma in situ. The cellular findings:

   a are representative of recurrent disease
   b would mandate a biopsy
   c are consistent with a reparative/regenerative process, endocervical origin
   d are consistent with invasive adenocarcinoma, endocervical type

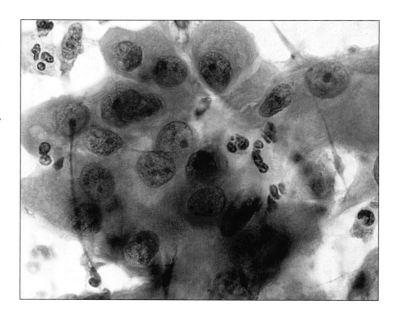

ISBN 978-089189-6357 ©ASCP 2015

352 These cells are from an asymptomatic patient presenting for a routine Pap smear. The diagnosis is:

   a squamous atypia/mature metaplastic ASCUS (mimicking mature native squames)
   b moderate metaplastic dysplasia (HSIL)
   c herpes genitalis
   d human papillomavirus infection

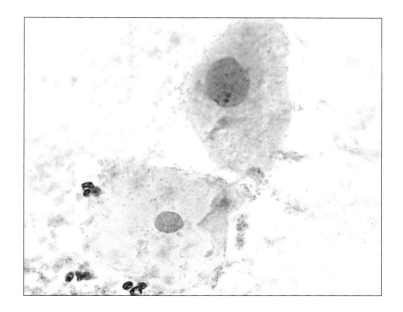

353 These cells represent a cervical/endocervical smear from a 43-year-old asymptomatic woman with no previous abnormal cytologic findings. The diagnosis is:

   a endocervical adenocarcinoma, well differentiated
   b AGUS, endocervical glandular dysplasia
   c tubal metaplasia
   d endocervical adenocarcinoma, poorly differentiated

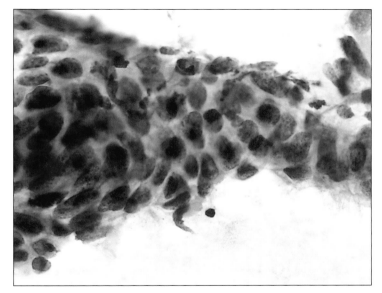

354 These cells represent a cervical/endocervical brushing from a 19-year-old female. The diagnosis is:

   a reactive/reparative changes
   b adenocarcinoma, endocervix
   c AGUS, endocervical glandular dysplasia
   d ASCUS

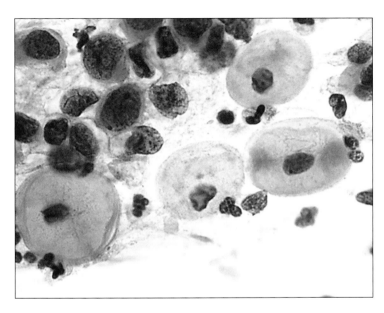

355 These cells are from a cervical/endocervical brushing from a 28-year-old female, LMP 12 days ago. The diagnosis is:

   a reactive/reparative endocervical cells
   b squamous carcinoma in situ
   c squamous cell carcinoma, nonkeratinizing
   d adenocarcinoma in situ, endocervix

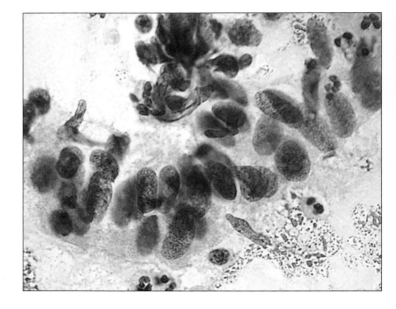

356 These cells are seen from a 57-year-old nulliparous woman with a history of obesity and postmenopausal bleeding. A vaginal/cervical/endocervical smear reveals:

   a atypical endometrial hyperplasia
   b low grade squamous intraepithelial lesion
   c mixed mesodermal tumor, homologous
   d papillary serous adenocarcinoma, endometrium

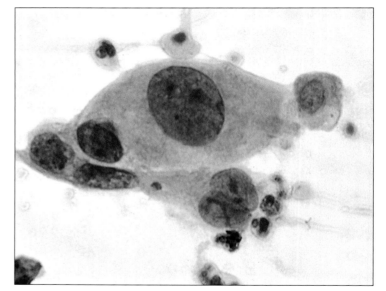

357 These cells were identified in a cellular sample obtained by an endometrial aspiration from a postmenopausal patient. The findings represent:

   a rhabdomyosarcoma
   b leiomyosarcoma
   c osteosarcoma
   d endometrial stromal sarcoma

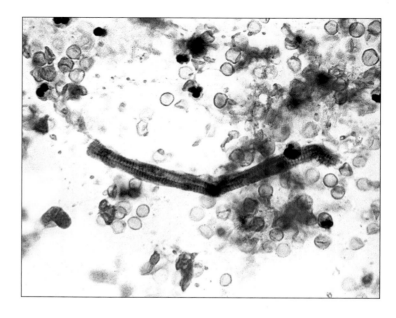

ISBN 978-089189-6357 ©ASCP 2015

358 These cellular findings represent a vaginal/cervical/ endocervical (VCE) sample taken from a 25-year-old asymptomatic woman presenting for a routine annual Pap smear. The findings are most consistent with:

  a reactive/reparative squamous cells
  b ASCUS: atypical squamous metaplasia/immature metaplastic variety
  c LSIL, mild dysplasia
  d normal squamous cells

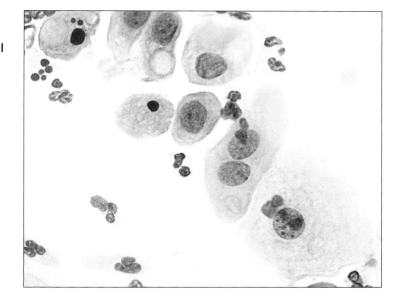

359 The presence of these structures in a Pap smear indicates:

  a a malignant ovarian process
  b a benign ovarian process
  c a malignant metastatic process
  d nonspecific findings

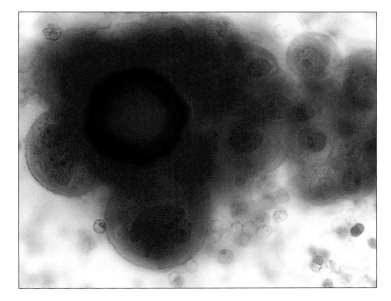

360 Culdocentesis and laparoscopic findings reveal the following structures in the presence of a malignant ovarian tumor. The most likely diagnosis is:

  a papillary serous cystadenocarcinoma
  b mucinous cystadenocarcinoma
  c endometrioid type adenocarcinoma
  d Brenner tumor

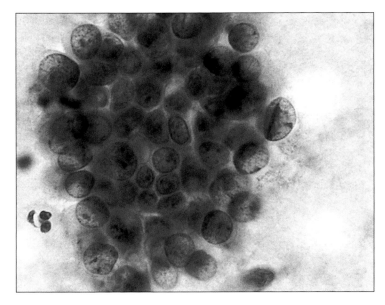

361 A 44-year-old female presents with a decrease in weight, abdominal distention, ascites, and malaise. A routine Pap smear reveals:

    a normal endometrial cells
    b tubal metaplasia
    c papillary serous cystadenocarcinoma, ovarian
    d nonkeratinizing squamous cell carcinoma

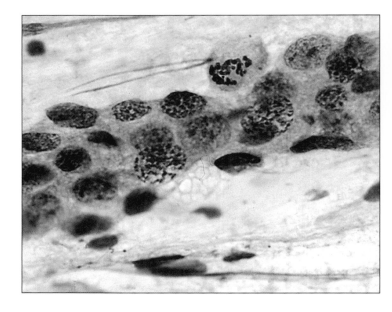

362 A 41-year-old patient suffering from oligomenorrhea presents for a Pap smear. Clinically, an ectocervical lesion is identified. A cervical scraping and endocervical brushing are performed. Based on the cellular findings, the diagnosis is:

    a nonkeratinizing squamous cell carcinoma
    b keratinizing squamous cell carcinoma
    c endocervical adenocarcinoma
    d LSIL, consistent with mild dysplasia

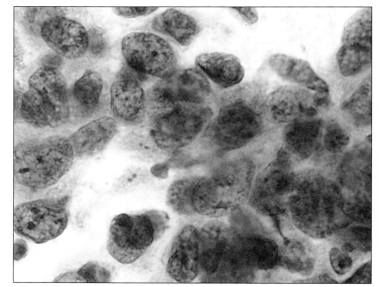

363 These cells are observed in a cervical/endocervical smear from a 58-year-old patient. The diagnosis is:

    a nonkeratinizing squamous cell carcinoma
    b ovarian adenocarcinoma
    c endocervical adenocarcinoma
    d mixed Müllerian tumor

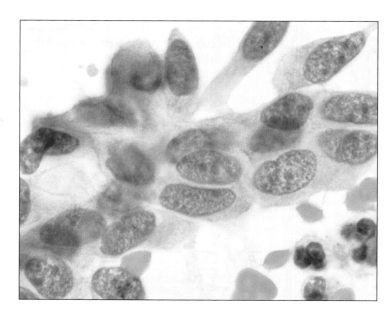

ISBN 978-089189-6357 ©ASCP 2015

364 These cells are from a vaginal smear from a 61-year-old postmenopausal woman with a history of ovarian disease. The findings are consistent with:

a adenocarcinoma, ovarian
b poorly differentiated endocervical carcinoma
c poorly differentiated squamous cell carcinoma
d endometrial polyp

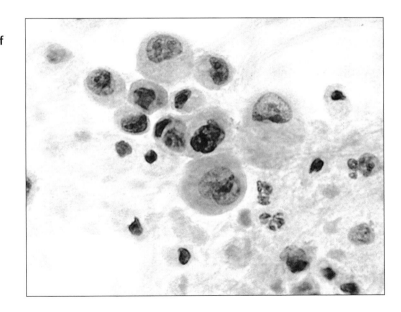

365 The cellular changes noted in this image are most likely related to:

a HPV11 or 6 infections
b herpesvirus infection
c HPV18 infection
d CMV infection

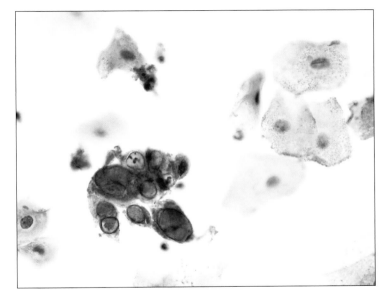

366 These cells are present in a cervical sample from a 39-year-old female on day 10 of her menstrual cycle. There is no history of previous abnormality. The best interpretation is:

a atypical endocervical cells
b metastatic adenocarcinoma
c normal endometrial cells
d atypical endometrial cells

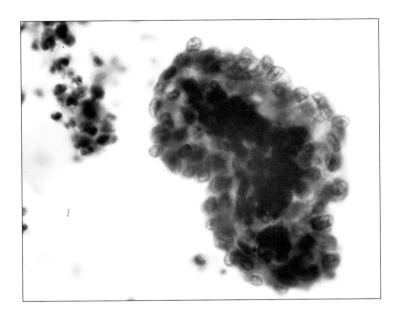

367 This smear is from a 69-year-old female with a history of vaginal bleeding. The cells are most consistent with origin from:

   a small cell carcinoma
   b endocervical adenocarcinoma
   c high grade squamous intraepithelial lesion
   d endometrial stroma

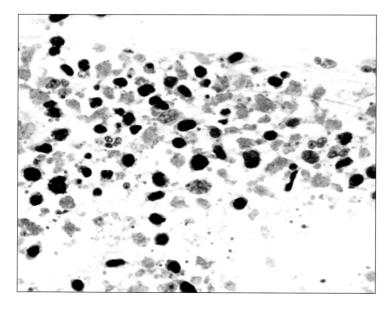

368 The cytologic features in this image from a cytologic sample from a 28-year-old female are most likely related to:

   a HPV infection
   b trichomoniasis
   c folate deficiency
   d *Candida* infection

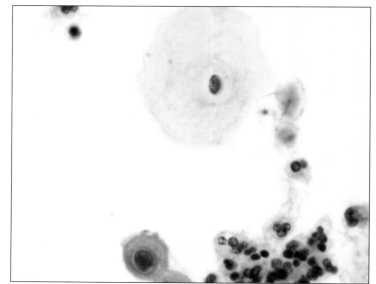

369 These cells are present in a cervical sample from a 65-year-old female with postmenopausal vaginal bleeding. The most likely origin is:

   a squamous cell carcinoma
   b endocervical repair reaction
   c endometrial adenocarcinoma
   d endocervical polyp

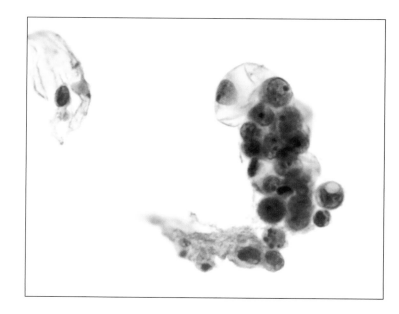

ISBN 978-089189-6357 ©ASCP 2015

370 The cells shown here are from a Pap smear from a 32-year-old female. The best diagnosis is:

   a nonkeratinizing squamous cell carcinoma
   b microinvasive squamous cell carcinoma
   c repair/regeneration
   d endocervical adenocarcinoma

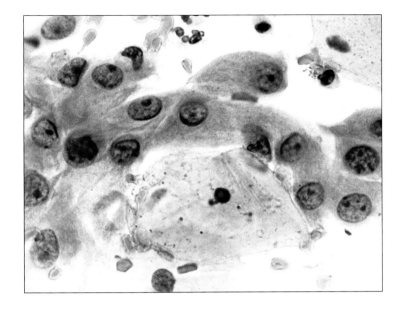

371 Consider the cells of interest in the Pap test from this 28-year-old female:

   a these cells are highly productive of HPV virions
   b these cells are being driven to proliferate by the interaction of HPVE2 and E4 with p53 and pRB in the host cell
   c these cells are being driven to proliferate by the interaction of HPVE6 and E7 with p53 and pRB in the host cell
   d the patient's risk of developing invasive cervical cancer in the next 5 years is over 50%

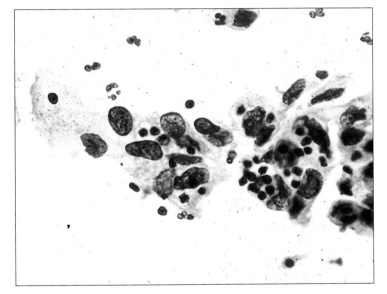

372 Which cytologic feature is represented in this endocervical brushing of a 36-year-old female with a last menstrual period 2 weeks ago?

   a ground glass nuclei with Cowdry type A inclusions
   b large nuclear inclusion surrounded by a halo
   c multinucleate, molded cells with chromatin margination
   d large nuclear inclusion surrounded by a halo

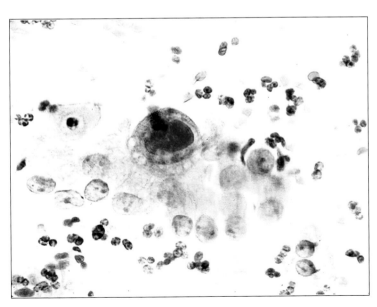

373 The best interpretation as to the origin of these cells in a cervical sample from a 40-year-old female is:

a endometrial adenocarcinoma
b high grade squamous intraepithelial lesion
c invasive squamous cell carcinoma
d endometrial stromal cells

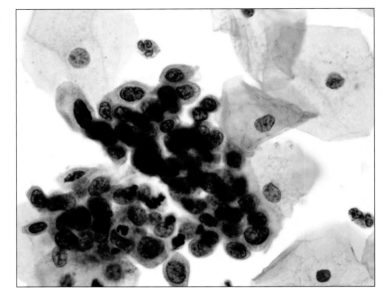

374 These cells are present in a cervical smear from a 52-year-old female. The patient has been radiated for cervical carcinoma. The best interpretation is:

a recurrent carcinoma
b radiation changes
c high grade squamous intraepithelial lesion
d low grade squamous intraepithelial lesion

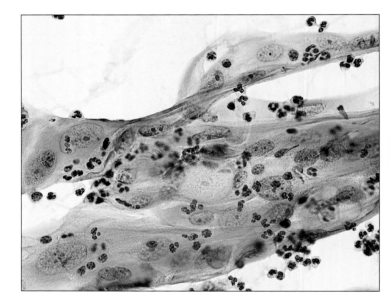

375 Consider a 35-year-old female with these diagnostic cells on her Pap test. What statement is true?

a she has more than a 95% chance of having a low risk HPV type
b her colposcopic biopsy is CIN1, so she can just be followed by repeat Paps
c she has a 50% chance of concurrent AIS
d she needs an ablative procedure regardless of the result of her colposcopy

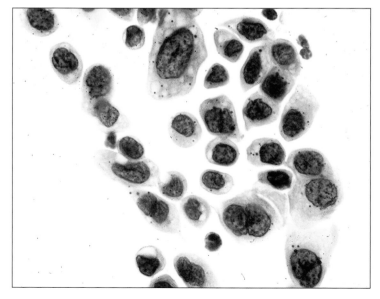

ISBN 978-089189-6357 ©ASCP 2015

376 These cells were present in a cervical smear from a 19-year-old female. These changes can be linked to which of the following?

a human papillomavirus type 6/11
b human papillomavirus type 16/18
c human papillomavirus type 31/33/35
d cytomegalovirus

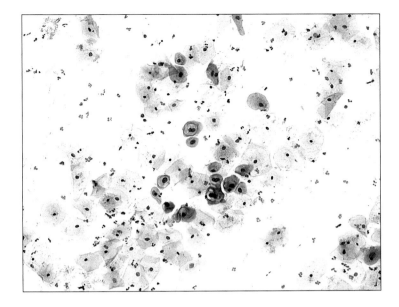

377 Which statement below is most correct concerning the diagnostic changes in this image?

a the nuclear enlargement is due to the nucleus being filled with HPV virions
b the cytoplasmic vacuolization is due to HPV oncogene expression
c the most common cause for this change is high risk HPV infection
d high risk HPV types only rarely induce this morphology

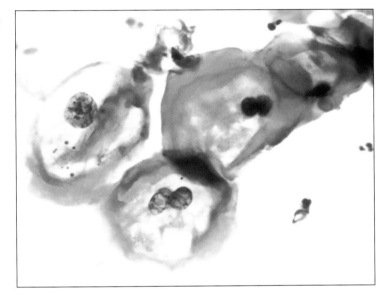

378 In this example of endocervical AIS, which criterion is most supportive of that interpretation?

a nuclear feathering
b syncytial aggregate
c 3D groups
d cohesive monolayered sheets

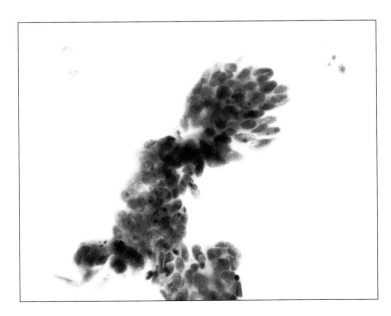

379 These cells were collected from the cervix/ endocervix of a 62-year-old female with complaints of postmenopausal bleeding. The most appropriate interpretation is:

a unsatisfactory for interpretation (lack of squamous component)
b atypical glandular cells
c high grade squamous intraepithelial lesion
d small cell undifferentiated carcinoma

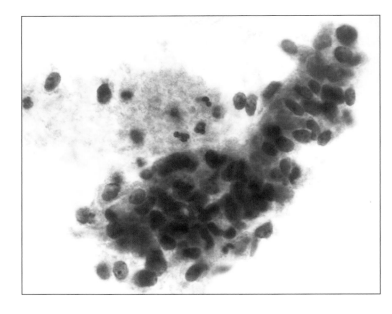

380 These cells were seen in this Pap from a 35-year-old female. Which of the following statements are most correct considering this entity?

a the Pap test is proven to decrease the risk of the cancer caused by this precancerous lesion
b this type of abnormality is seen in ~1% of Pap tests in an average laboratory
c patients with this lesion have a relatively high frequency of HPV type 18 compared to HPV type 16 infection
d the established precursor of this lesion is low grade glandular dysplasia

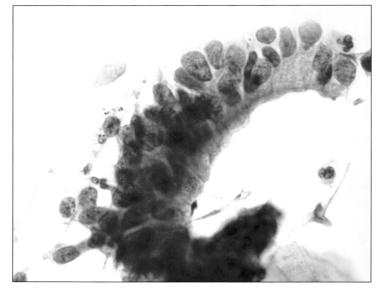

381 These cells were derived from a cervical/endocervical scraping/brushing from a 35-year-old female with a history of cervicitis and some spotting. The cytologic findings:

a are most consistent with herpes simplex infection
b should reflex to high risk HPV testing based on current ASCCP guidelines
c require pathologist review under CLIA '88 rules
d are most consistent with squamous cell carcinoma

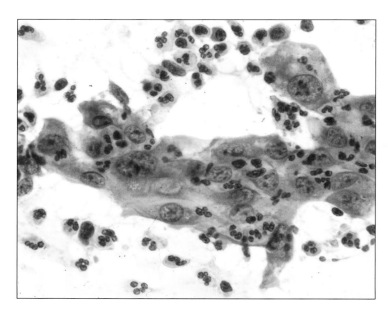

ISBN 978-089189-6357 ©ASCP 2015

382 A postpartum patient has a Pap test demonstrating this cytologic abnormality. Her history is significant for LSIL diagnosed 5 years ago, followed by 4 NILM Pap tests. Which of the following is true?

a what should be done next depends on the patient's age

b reflex HPV testing can be used to decide whether or not she needs colposcopy

c this patient is almost certainly positive for high risk HPV

d if colposcopy demonstrates only CIN1, she is most likely infected with low risk HPV

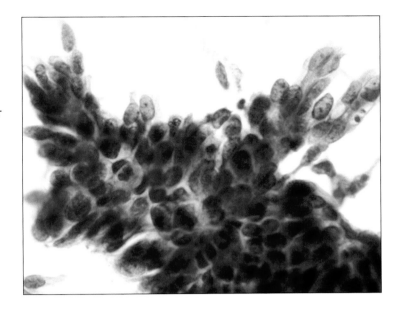

383 These cells were seen in the endocervical brushing of a 53-year-old female who is 6 months s/p radiation therapy for stage I squamous cell carcinoma of the cervix. The most appropriate cytologic interpretation is:

a atypical glandular cells

b postradiation squamous intraepithelial lesion, high grade

c endocervical adenocarcinoma in situ

d residual squamous cell carcinoma

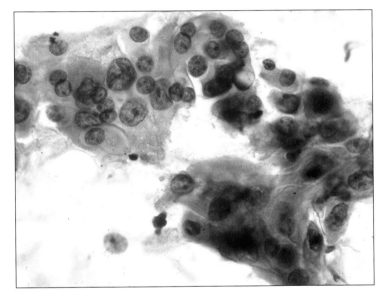

©ASCP 2015 ISBN 978-089189-6357

Female Reproductive Tract *Answer Key*

1 b secretory
The secretory or luteal phase lasts 14 days due to a programmed life/death span of 14 days for the corpus luteum/corpus albicans.
DeMay, A&S 2e. The menstrual cycle, p21-22

2 a luteinizing hormone
Luteinizing hormone (LH) and follicle stimulating hormone (FSH) are pituitary gonadotropins associated with the menstrual cycle. Estrogen and progesterone are produced within the ovary as a result of these pituitary gonadotropins.
DeMay, A&S 2e. Intermediate predominant maturation index, p13

3 a reserve cells
Reserve cells usually occur high in the endocervical canal. The presence of these cells occurs normally in response to squamous differentiation, but they may also serve as the stem cell for initiation of preneoplastic conditions. Histiocytic in appearance, they may be linked to endocervical mucosal cells, be associated with squamous metaplastic cells, or lie singularly.
DeMay, A&S 2e. Reserve cell hyperplasia, p24-25

4 c 14
The surge of luteinizing hormone (LH) occurs at ovulation.
DeMay, A&S 2e. Superficial predominant maturation index, p13-14

5 d no pathologic information
Mitotic figures are normal findings in benign, reactive/reparative, premalignant, or malignant processes. Their presence merely infers metabolic activity, protein synthesis, and cell viability. Abnormal mitotic figures, though, may be occasionally found in association with premalignant or malignant processes.
DeMay, A&S 2e. Benign cellular changes, p23

6 a hyperkeratosis
Hyperkeratosis is a condition of overall greater epithelial thickness (hyperdifferentiation). A stratum corneum (anucleate squames) replaces the normally nonkeratinized superficial cells/layer. Leukoplakia, clinically defined as a white patch, is the gross pathologic counterpart of hyperkeratosis acanthosis. This condition denotes the hard cornified visible area located either on the ectocervix or vagina.
DeMay, A&S 2e. Keratosis, p26-27

7 c large cells with multiple, tightly clustered nuclei
The presence of syncytiotrophoblasts found in vaginal/cervical smears of pregnant patients may indicate a threatened abortion. In addition, increased superficial cell maturation is also considered an indication of abnormal pregnancy.
DeMay, A&S 2e. Trophoblasts, p51-52

8 c vaginal adenosis
Vaginal adenosis is defined as the presence of ectopic glandular epithelium or squamous metaplastic cells within the normally gland free or squamous lined vagina. Their presence is increased in those patients who were exposed to diethylstilbestrol (DES) in utero.
DeMay, A&S 2e. Hormone therapy related cytology, p47

9 b 14
Serum estrogen levels peak at ovulation (generally day 14).
DeMay, A&S 2e. Superficial predominant maturation index, p13-14

10 a Sertoli-Leydig cell tumors
Sertoli-Leydig cell tumors, masculinizing tumors of the ovarian stroma, produce increased serum androgen levels, which in turn create atrophic vaginal smear patterns.
DeMay, A&S 2e. Intermediate predominant maturation index, p13

11 a corpus luteum
The corpus luteum degenerates to become a corpus albicans, and this ischemic structure allows for reinitiation of menstruation.
DeMay, A&S 2e. The menstrual cycle, p21-22

12 b inverse
As the serum estrogen levels increase, the follicular cells have increased sensitivity to follicle stimulating hormone (FSH). The direct feedback to the pituitary gland decreases the levels of FSH in the bloodstream.
DeMay, A&S 2e. Superficial predominant maturation index, p13-14

13 c oral contraceptives
Synonyms include birth control pill changes, pseudoparakeratosis (pseudokeratosis) and microglandular hyperplasia. These cells represent degenerating forms of hyperplastic endocervical glandular mucosa. The finding has been associated with patients taking oral contraceptives, late luteal phase, and late pregnancy. They are benign cellular findings; however, the differentiation from true parakeratosis is imperative. Cells from microglandular hyperplasia generally have eosinophilic or basophilic cytoplasm, contain eccentric nuclei, or resemble reactive endocervical cells, whereas true parakeratosis represents a keratinizing process (orangeophilia) with centrally located pyknotic nuclei in polygonal "waxy" cytoplasm (possibly with accompanying HPV changes).
DeMay, A&S 2e. Microglandular endocervical hyperplasia, p47-48

14 a menses
The corpus albicans in the late secretory phase of the menstrual cycle represents an ischemic corpus luteum. Subsequently, when ischemia of the endometrium occurs, the menstrual cycle is reinitiated.
DeMay, A&S 2e. The menstrual cycle, p21-22

ISBN 978-089189-6357 ©ASCP 2015

15 b FSH

The development of the primitive primordial follicles of the ovary is related to the release of follicle stimulating hormone (FSH) from the pituitary gland.

DeMay, A&S 2e. Superficial predominant maturation index, p13-14

16 d 100/0/0

Turner syndrome patients are ahormonal due to ovarian agenesis. A predominant population of basal to parabasal cells would be characteristic of the disease. Choices a, b, and c are all associated with hyperestrinism. Deep parabasal cells in sheets may represent an atrophic smear taken from a post pubertal patient with hyperestrinism. Conditions such as Turner syndrome may explain these findings. Turner syndrome is a nondisjunction of the X chromosome. These patients are described as sex chromatin negative, or 45XO. Occasionally, mosaicism may be found. These patients have a low hairline, pigmented nevi, and increased carrying angle of their arms. Ovarian agenesis leaves streaks of connective tissue instead of viable ovaries. The vaginal smear pattern is atrophic.

DeMay, A&S 2e. Hormonal cytology, p10-13

17 a increased vascularization near the basal lamina in women with intermediate cell atrophy

The increased vascularization may increase the permeability of the circulating endogenous androgens, which affects the overlying mucosa, creating an intermediate cell level of atrophy.

DeMay, A&S 2e. Intermediate predominant maturation index, p13

18 b 75/25/0

Parabasal or mixed intermediate cell patterns may be found in vaginal smears taken from postmenopausal patients. In addition, intermediate cell predominance may be observed in these patients (in the absence of hormonal therapy) due to endogenous androgens from the ovarian stroma or the adrenal cortex.

DeMay, A&S 2e. Parabasal predominant maturation index (atrophy), p12-13

19 c *Trichomonas vaginalis* infection

Patients with vaginal infections should not have hormone analyses performed due to the false sensitivity of this test. Inflammatory agents such as *Candida* species or *Trichomonas vaginalis* often present with a false increased cellular maturation.

DeMay, A&S 2e. Trichomonas vaginalis, p40-41

20 a increased estrogenic effect

An increased maturation index may be seen in patients with advanced liver cirrhosis due to the inability of the diseased liver to degrade estrogen, thus throwing it back into the bloodstream where estrogen sensitive tissues respond by maturing or differentiating.

DeMay, A&S 2e. Superficial predominant maturation index, p13-14

21 d cannot be determined based on the above clinical information

It is impossible to determine the vaginal smear pattern of a patient with secondary amenorrhea unless clinical history is provided.

DeMay, A&S 2e. Hormonal cytology, p10-12

22 a may overlie and/or be associated with a possible lesion

Hyperkeratosis is a condition of overall greater epithelial thickness (hyperdifferentiation). A stratum corneum (anucleate squames) replaces the normally nonkeratinized superficial cells/layer. Hyperkeratosis and parakeratosis may overlie a serious abnormality such as infection by human papillomavirus (HPV), dysplasia, or even invasive carcinoma. The diagnosis is important and should be correlated with the surrounding cytologic findings.

DeMay, A&S 2e. Keratosis, p26

23 d 75/25/0

In addition to hypothyroidism, other conditions that create parabasal predominant maturation indices include androgenic therapy, intrauterine fetal demise, hypopituitarism (starvation), and cervicovaginal ulceration.

DeMay, A&S 2e. Parabasal predominant maturation index (atrophy), p12-13

24 a increases cellular maturation

Increased maturation may result due to administration of this antiestrogen due to its ability to bind to estrogen receptors of hormonally receptive cells, such as squamous mucosal cells.

DeMay, A&S 2e. Superficial predominant maturation index, p13-14

25 c immature metaplastic cells

Immature metaplasia is usually parabasal in size with basophilic cytoplasm, well defined borders, and vesicular nuclei. Often a pavement configuration, remnants of cobblestone patterns, or the "cookie cutter" look is seen. These cells may possess spinelike or "spider cell" cytoplasmic processes when forcibly removed, or have ectoplasm/endoplasm rims when exfoliated. Squamous metaplasia, a common protective reaction found in mature cycling females, is a result of transformation of one adult type of epithelial tissue to another adult epithelial tissue via reserve cell hyperplasia. Squamous metaplasia is often associated with trauma, inflammation, or other endocrine disturbances. Squamocolumnar junctions, abrupt junctions occurring in young children, do not have associated transitional or transformational metaplastic zones.

DeMay, A&S 2e. Squamous metaplasia, p23-26

26 a *Torulopsis glabrata* lacks hyphae

Torulopsis or *Candida glabrata* presents as yeast forms (stones) without the pseudohyphae (sticks). Sticks and stones are both seen with *Candida albicans;* however, culture analysis is preferred if speciation is necessary.

DeMay, A&S 2e. Candida species, p39-40

27 **c** parakeratosis

Parakeratosis, an abortive attempt at keratinization, may overlie a serious abnormality such as infection by human papillomavirus (HPV), dysplasia, or even invasive carcinoma. The diagnosis is important and should be correlated with the surrounding cytologic findings. The finding of parakeratosis should be discriminated from related changes occurring in dyskeratocytes/atypical parakeratosis (atypical squamous cells suggestive of an HPV infection). Dyskeratosis or atypical parakeratosis is considered an ASCUS under the Bethesda System terminology, and is not specific for the determination of an HPV infection. Only the presence of koilocytes is a sensitive diagnostic indicator of HPV.

DeMay, A&S 2e. Keratosis, p26-27

28 **b** decreased maturation to the intermediate cell level

The overriding effects of progesterone on an estrogen primed epithelium should allow for decreased maturation to the intermediate cell level.

DeMay, A&S 2e. Hormonal cytology, p13-14

29 **a** pituitary hypogonadism

Pituitary hypogonadism is usually related to trauma or damage to the gland. The degree of pituitary damage is related to its ability to release FSH. Deficient FSH levels lead to an inadequate estrogen balance; therefore, these patients will have a vaginal smear pattern that is parabasal to intermediate cell maturation.

DeMay, A&S 2e. Hormonal cytology, p10-13

30 **c** coarse, irregular chromatin in carcinoma

Sheets of cells with well defined cytoplasmic borders, preserved nuclear polarity, predictable nuclear features, fine regular chromatin patterns, micro- to macronucleoli, and characteristic cytoplasmic streaming are diagnostic of reparative processes. This process is often associated with trauma, cervicitis, and inflammatory etiology. Although anisocytosis and anisonucleosis are common morphologic features seen with atypical reparative processes, predictability is maintained between cell groupings. In squamous carcinomas, lack of predictability and single scattered cells with coarse irregular chromatin and hyperchromasia are predominant. In addition, the background of reparative/regenerative conditions is clean and free of necrosis. Malignancy associated cellular backgrounds are generally composed of diathesis consisting of old and fresh blood, degenerated surrounding tissue, necrotic tumor cells, and assorted white blood cells.

DeMay, A&S 2e. Repair/regeneration, p30-31

31 **c** follicular cervicitis

Chronic follicular cervicitis is a diffuse or localized lymphocytic infiltration as identified in cervical/vaginal smears. Small (mature) and large (immunoblastic) lymphocytes, plasma cells, and tingible body macrophages (intracytoplasmic inclusions) are necessary for the establishment of this diagnosis. The diagnosis of follicular cervicitis must be discriminated from other benign conditions including microglandular hyperplasia, degenerating neutrophils, and small cell histiocytes.

DeMay, A&S 2e. Follicular cervicitis, p31-32

32 **a** superficial predominance, intermediate cells without folding or clustering

Stein-Leventhal syndrome is associated with a thickening of the tunica albuginea of the ovary, resulting in inability to expel the ovum. Patients with this condition are often overweight and have secondary amenorrhea. Vaginal smear patterns in these patients show generally intermediate to superficial cell maturation.

DeMay, A&S 2e. Intermediate & superficial predominant maturation index, p13-14

33 **d** pemphigus vulgaris

A bullous disease of the skin, pemphigus vulgaris is a condition that destroys the tonofilaments of the squamous mucosa, thus producing a sloughing of the skin. Reactive/reparative cells with bullet shaped nucleoli are generally found, as are fine, even chromatin patterns. Clinical history is essential to rule out a possible adenocarcinoma. Tzanck tests are negative.

DeMay, A&S 2e. Miscellaneous nonneoplastic conditions, p52-53

34 **a** folic acid

Folic acid deficiency (FAD) is a common water soluble vitamin deficiency state among pregnant women. FAD is related to deficient ingestion, absorption and the increased demands of folic acid required during pregnancy. Folic acid deficiency produces cytomegaly (an increase in the cell volume without cytokinesis) and karyomegaly, changes similar to those seen in radiation cellular injury. Multinucleation and nuclei with fine regular chromatin are observed. Cytoplasmic vacuolization may mimic a "swiss cheese" effect, indicating the cells' degenerative qualities.

DeMay, A&S 2e. Diet, p136-137

35 **d** reparative/regenerative process

Sheets of cells with well defined cytoplasmic borders, preserved nuclear polarity, predictable nuclear features, fine regular chromatin patterns, micro- to macronucleoli, and characteristic cytoplasmic streaming are diagnostic of repair. This process is often associated with trauma, cervicitis, and inflammatory etiology. The background of reparative/regenerative conditions is clean and free of necrosis. Malignancy associated cellular backgrounds are generally composed of diathesis consisting of old and fresh blood, degenerated surrounding tissue, necrotic tumor cells, and assorted white blood cells.

DeMay, A&S 2e. Repair/regeneration, p30-31

ISBN 978-089189-6357 ©ASCP 2015

36   **b**   macrocytic changes, polychromasia

The cytologic changes associated with radiation include cytomegaly (macrocytic changes) and karyomegaly. The maintenance of normal N:C ratios and the evidence of cytoplasmic vacuolization (related to degeneration) are characteristic of these cells. The nuclei associated with radiation cell changes are often degenerative or preserved and multinucleated, while the cytoplasmic staining is polychromatic and amphophilic.

DeMay, A&S 2e. Radiation cytology, p42-44

37   **a**   serous

2/3 of serous surface mesothelial tumors of the ovary may be bilateral. Cytologic identification reveals papillary fragments and possible psammoma bodies.

DeMay, A&S 2e. Serous adenocarcinoma, p98-99

38   **d**   nonglycogenated areas that do not stain with iodine

The Schiller test uses iodine to help identify abnormal lesions within the female reproductive tract by outlining nonglycogenated areas.

DeMay, A&S 2e. Intermediate cells, p8-10

39   **a**   *Lactobacillus acidophilus*

Bacillus vaginalis, or *Lactobacillus acidophilus,* is considered normal vaginal flora that flourishes under progesterone stimulated conditions (intermediate cell maturation). Lactic acid is produced and an acidic pH is maintained under normal conditions (pH 3.8-4.5). Döderlein bacilli predominate in the secretory phases of the menstrual cycle.

DeMay, A&S 2e. Normal flora & cytolysis, p32

40   **c**   expression of HPV16, 18 viral DNA

High risk viral types (HPV16, 18) integrate their viral genes into the host cellular DNA, creating malignant transformation.

DeMay, A&S 2e. HPV in cervical carcinogenesis, p131-134

41   **b**   mature cystic teratoma

A benign (mature) cystic teratoma, or dermoid cyst, is an ovarian tumor found generally in young females that is composed of germ cell tissues such as epithelial sebaceous glands, hair, sweat glands, or intestinal epithelium.

DeMay, A&S 2e. Mature teratoma, p310

42   A. all cases of atypical squamous cells of undetermined significance (ASCUS) are considered part of the 5 year retrospective review process

CLIA '88 mandates a retrospective review of the patient's previous smears be performed if the current cytologic findings are a high grade intraepithelial lesion or worse. The intent of the requirement is to rule out the possibility of missed abnormal cells in cases previously diagnosed as negative for squamous intraepithelial lesion; however, if abnormal cells are detected in a previous case falsely diagnosed as "benign," documentation is required so that appropriate quality assurance measures may be employed to help avert a future false negative occurrence. Because of the equivocal nature and poor interobserver reproducibility with the diagnosis of ASCUS, these diagnoses are not considered part of the 5 year retrospective review process.

DeMay, A&S 2e. CLIA '88, p1583-1588

43   **c**   endometrial hyperplasia

An increase in estrogen, unopposed estrogen stimulation, or pathological entities such as granulosa-theca cell tumors may be predisposing conditions for endometrial hyperplasia. Other risk factors for premalignant corpus disease include obesity, hypertension, nulliparity, and diabetes mellitus. Patients with these clinical histories are at a higher risk for developing invasive endometrial adenocarcinoma.

DeMay, A&S 2e. Histology of endometrial hyperplasia and carcinoma, p102-103

44   **a**   presence of granular cytoplasm and columnar cellular shape

The number of cells found in well differentiated endocervical adenocarcinoma (ECA) is typically greater than that found in endometrial adenocarcinomas (EMAs). Cell sizes associated with ECA are larger, contain more abundant cytoplasm, retain columnar configuration, and have finely granular, irregularly distributed chromatin with micronucleoli. EMAs are diffusely vacuolated and often contain engulfed polymorphonuclear cells, the opposite of the granular cytoplasm generally found in lesions arising from the endocervical glands. Endometrial adenocarcinoma cytologically presents with fewer numbers of cells on the slide (as opposed to endocervical adenocarcinomas), cell clusters with scalloping borders and 3D tissue fragments, high N:C ratios, and frothy, delicate, lacy, vacuolated cytoplasm. One of the key differential features between this lesion and endocervical adenocarcinoma is the cytoplasmic texture. Finally, the presence of a watery diathesis with associated lipophages may be helpful in discriminating endometrial adenocarcinomas from other epithelial malignancies.

DeMay, A&S 2e. Endocervical vs endometrial adenocarcinoma, p105-106

45 b   endometrial carcinoma + osteosarcoma

A heterologous mixed Müllerian tumor is diagnosed by the identification of well differentiated endometrial adenocarcinoma plus a nonindigenous sarcomatous element. These heterologous connective tissue malignancies may include osteosarcoma, chondrosarcoma, or rhabdomyosarcoma.

DeMay, A&S 2e. Mixed Müllerian tumors, p112-113

46 b   adjunctive methods that currently lack the specificity needed to determine the progression rate of any one lesion

To date, molecular determination of HPV is unable to provide predictable factors that can distinguish progression or regression of precancerous cervical lesions. Current studies focus on the interruption of antioncogenes such as p53 and the retinoblastoma gene.

DeMay, A&S 2e. Molecular model of cervical carcinogenesis, p132-134

47 b   mesoderm

The vagina, uterus, and ovaries are formed chiefly from embryological mesoderm.

DeMay, A&S 2e. Anatomy and embryology of the female genital tract, p4

48 b   nonkeratinizing dysplasia, severe (high grade squamous intraepithelial lesion)

Severe nonkeratinizing dysplasia cytologically presents as small immature metaplastic cells with hyperchromasia, high N:C ratios, and a thin rim of cytoplasm. The absence of coarse or irregular chromatin, nucleoli, and/or diathesis should help discriminate these cells from a carcinoma in situ or an invasive malignancy.

DeMay, A&S 2e. General features of dysplasia, p65-66

49 b   poorly differentiated type

Poorly differentiated endometrial adenocarcinomas (PDAs), in contrast with well differentiated lesions (most common), do not follow the typical natural history of hyperestrinism and endometrial hyperplasia. Instead, PDAs arise spontaneously in the atrophic epithelium of older, postmenopausal females and are preceded only by an endometrial adenocarcinoma in situ.

DeMay, A&S 2e. High grade endometrial adenocarcinoma, p104-105

50 b   pleomorphism

Pleomorphism is the single most important criterion in establishing a diagnosis of a keratinizing process.

DeMay, A&S 2e. Keratinizing squamous cell carcinoma, p74-75

51 d   Bowen disease

Bowen disease is a synonym for carcinoma in situ of the vulva. This disease should not be confused with Paget disease, a malignant glandular tumor of extra mammary origin, or Gartner disease, remnants of the Wolffian duct.

Raju RR, Goldblum JR, Hart WR. Pagetoid squamous cell carcinoma in situ (pagetoid Bowen's disease) of the external genitalia. Int J Gynecol Pathol 2003;22(2):127-35 [PMID 12649666]

52 a   reserve cell hyperplasia

Reserve cells usually occur high in the endocervical canal. These cells occur normally in response to squamous differentiation, but they may also serve as the stem cell for initiation of preneoplastic conditions. Histiocytic in appearance, they may be linked to endocervical mucosal cells, be associated with squamous metaplastic cells, or lie singularly.

DeMay, A&S 2e. Reserve cell hyperplasia, p24-25, 159

53 c   smudged nuclear features and cavelike perinuclear vacuoles

The histologic diagnosis of human papillomavirus infection of the cervix is based on the presence of superficial dyskeratosis or abnormal parakeratosis, middle layers of koilocytes (containing smudged nuclear chromatin and cytoplasmic margination), and deeper layers containing normal appearing parabasal and basal cells. Mitoses are frequently identified.

DeMay, A&S 2e. Cervical cytology and HPV-DNA, p57-59

54 a   Gartner cysts

Gartner cysts are remnants of the mesonephric system found within the lateral vaginal walls.

Molina Escudero R, Navas Martinez MC, Castillo OA. Vaginal Gartner cysts: clinical report of four cases and a bibliographic review. Arch Esp Urol 2014;67(2):181-4 [PMID 24691040]

55 c   pyknosis, karyorrhexis, karyolysis

Nuclear shrinking (pyknosis) is often followed by a rupture of the nuclear membrane (karyorrhexis) with subsequent dissolution of the nuclear material (karyolysis).

DeMay, A&S 2e. Inflammatory change and repair, p137-138

56 b   HPV6, HPV11

Human papillomavirus types 6 and 11 are considered low risk virotypes with episomal replication, an inability to transform cellular DNA in situ.

DeMay, A&S 2e. Human papillomavirus, p124-126

57 d   normochromasia, cytoplasmic streaming

Reparative/regenerative changes must be discriminated from low grade epithelial lesions or those of more significance. Sheets of cells with distinct cytoplasmic borders and/or cytoplasmic streaming may be helpful in establishing the benign nature of these cells. Additional criteria include preserved nuclear polarity, predictable nuclear features, fine regular chromatin patterns, and micro to macronucleoli. This process is often associated with trauma, cervicitis, and inflammatory etiology.

DeMay, A&S 2e. Repair/regeneration, p30-31

58 b   diabetes mellitus

Pregnancy, patients with diabetes mellitus, or those taking birth control pills have an increased susceptibility to *Candida* infections.

DeMay, A&S 2e. Fungi, p39-40

ISBN 978-089189-6357 ©ASCP 2015

59 b bicornuate uterus

A malfusion of the Müllerian ducts may result in a dual horned uterus (one with 2 cavities).

Fedele L, Bianchi S, Frontino G. Septums and synechiae: approaches to surgical correction. Clin Obstet Gynecol 2006;49(4):767-788 [PMID 17082672]

60 b *Trichomonas vaginalis* infection

Trichomonas vaginalis infection appears clinically as petechial hemorrhagic mucosa, often referred to as a strawberry cervix.

DeMay, A&S 2e. Protozoa, p40-41

61 a reactive trophoblasts

This bacterial related endometritis may occur postabortion or postpartum. Cytology reveals reactive trophoblasts, red and white blood cells, and multinucleated histiocytes.

DeMay, A&S 2e. Trophoblasts, p51-53

62 d hematoidin crystals

Hematoidin crystals are associated with the degradation of hemoglobin secondary to hemorrhage. In contrast to true hematoidin cockleburs, hematoidin crystals are less common and are cytologically identified as radiate, spherical, or rhomboid structures. In addition, these entities are generally smaller than true cockleburs and possess crystalline rays that are fine (instead of clublike).

DeMay, A&S 2e. Cockleburs, p52-53

63 a increased deposition of glycogen in the cytoplasm

Glycogen is gradually deposited within the cytoplasm of squamous cells during the proliferative phase of the menstrual cycle.

DeMay, A&S 2e. Hormonal cytology, p13-14

64 b glycogenated navicular cells

"Boat," or navicular, cells are glycogenated cells associated with an increase in progesterone. These cells are normally found during pregnancy or the secretory phase of the menstrual cycle.

DeMay, A&S 2e. Intermediate cells, p9-10

65 a dilation and curettage to rule out hyperplasia of the endometrium

The presence of endometrial cells out of cycle may be associated with abnormal proliferation of glandular tissue such as endometrial hyperplasia, atypical hyperplasia, or an invasive malignant lesion. Dilation and curettage is often necessary to rule out a disease process.

DeMay, A&S 2e. Abnormal shedding of endometrial cells, p20-21

66 c cockleburs

Hematoidin cockleburs may be seen in late pregnancy, patients taking birth control pills, or those using an IUD. The cytology reveals radiate arrays of golden refractile crystals with club shaped spokes surrounded by histiocytes. These structures do not possess the visible central filaments associated with actinomycotic sulfur granules.

DeMay, A&S 2e. Cockleburs, p52-53

67 b nulliparous

Several factors may contribute to the development of endometrial adenocarcinoma, including granulosa-theca cell tumors of the ovary, obesity, diabetes, unopposed estrogen stimulation, nulliparity, hypertension, and menopause.

DeMay, A&S 2e. Endometrial cervical adenocarcinoma, p98

68 a oncogene activation secondary to HPV

As indicated in the previous question, high risk viral types have been associated with the development of cervical cancer. In this sequence of events, the E1-E2 region (early genes) are disrupted, interfering with the ability of the virus to transcribe its late genes, thus creating a biologic dead end for the viral life cycle. However, without transcription of these late genes, the feedback mechanism that controls the transcription of the E6-E7 genes (the viral region that codes for proteins that regulate viral growth) is lost. E6-E7 genes may bind antioncogenes or tumor suppressor genes such as p53 or Rb (retinoblastoma), which serve as protective genes that prevent transcription of cancer-causing oncogenes.

DeMay, A&S 2e. t1.9 Cervical cytology and HPV-DNA, p57-59

69 a produced by the corpus luteum in early pregnancy

The emergence of human chorionic gonadotropin is important in maintaining the corpus luteum of pregnancy for 3 months until the placenta has developed.

DeMay, A&S 2e. Hormonal cytology (of pregnancy), p14

70 c paramesonephric

The paramesonephric ducts are responsible for the development of the female genital system. The mesonephric system develops the external male genitalia.

71 c syncytiotrophoblasts

The presence of large, poorly preserved, multinucleated cells, often with degenerated nuclei, may represent syncytiotrophoblasts of the placenta. These cells when identified in a pregnant woman may suggest a threatened abortion. The emergence of an estrogenic stimulation upon the vagina mucosa may be a concomitant finding.

DeMay, A&S 2e. Syncytiotrophoblasts, p52

72 d gastrointestinal epithelium

Radiosensitive tissues are considered those that will suffer severe damage when exposed to 2,500 roentgens or less. Cells of bone marrow origin, gastrointestinal epithelium, and germ cells are considered highly radiosensitive.

Qui W, Carson-Walter E, Liu H, et al. PUMA regulates intestinal progenitor cell radiosenstivity and gastrointestinal syndrome. Cell Stem Cell 2008;2:576-583 [PMID 18522850]

73 a   basophilic watery diathesis

A watery vaginal discharge associated with endometrial adenocarcinoma is represented by a finely granular, basophilic diathesis. Choice b represents a squamous cell carcinoma, choice c represents a poorly differentiated lesion, and choice d may represent a poorly differentiated papillary serous carcinoma.

DeMay, A&S 2e. Histology of endometrial hyperplasia and carcinoma, p103

74 c   granulosa-theca cell tumor

Granulosa-theca cell tumors are benign estrogen producing tumors that, unless removed, may predispose the patient to endometrial adenocarcinoma. Their presence has also been linked to precocious puberty. An increase in estrogen, unopposed estrogen stimulation, or pathological entities such as granulosa-theca cell tumors may be predisposing conditions for endometrial hyperplasia. Other risk factors for premalignant corpus disease include obesity, hypertension, nulliparity, and diabetes mellitus.

DeMay, A&S 2e. Endometrial adenocarcinoma, p100-105

75 a   ovarian

The diagnosis of papillary serous adenocarcinoma of the ovary in a Pap test is centered around the finding of 3D aggregates with hyperchromatic nuclei and finely granular, irregularly distributed chromatin with a cervical/endocervical/endometrial biopsy negative and colposcopy negative examination. The presence of papillary groups of malignant cells and psammoma bodies may help in identifying these lesions as ovarian origin, but are not specific findings. A history of ascites is helpful. Mucinous adenocarcinomas of the ovary present with signet ring morphology and may recapitulate signet ring endometrial adenocarcinomas. Clinical history is paramount in establishing an ovarian primary tumor. A tumor diathesis is usually absent in cases of metastatic carcinoma unless the lesion has seeded at the secondary site.

DeMay, A&S 2e. Metastatic adenocarcinoma, p85

76 a   colon for malignancy

The diagnosis of metastatic colon cancer in gynecological specimens is related to the presence of abundant abnormal palisading cells with basophilic granular cytoplasm and cigar shaped nuclei. Presence of finely granular, regularly distributed chromatin is important in the diagnosis of this disease. A diathesis may be visualized if the tumor has metastasized by direct extension or seeded within the vagina. The diagnosis of this lesion may be difficult to distinguish from endocervical adenocarcinoma; therefore, a history of normal pelvic examinations may be necessary.

DeMay, A&S 2e. Metastatic adenocarcinoma, p85

77 d   tubal metaplasia

Tubal metaplasia (TM) is a benign condition that may be confused with a true abnormal process such as adenocarcinoma in situ (AIS) of the endocervix, with the exception that TM presents with cilia and/or terminal bars/webs. Crowded sheets of glandular cells and anisokaryosis are common findings, mimicking the feathering effect seen in AIS.

DeMay, A&S 2e. Tubal metaplasia, p82-83

78 b   serous adenocarcinoma, ovarian

Psammoma bodies are 3D structures with concentric ringing containing calcified secretions of mucus. These structures are often found associated with papillary lesions of the ovary, including papillary serous adenocarcinoma. However, these are nonspecific findings and are not pathognomonic of malignancy.

DeMay, A&S 2e. Ovary, p300

79 c   ovary

The diagnosis of papillary serous adenocarcinoma of the ovary in a Pap test is centered around the finding of 3D aggregates with hyperchromatic nuclei and finely granular, irregularly distributed chromatin with a cervical/endocervical/endometrial biopsy negative and colposcopy negative examination. The presence of papillary groups of malignant cells and psammoma bodies may help in identifying these lesions as ovarian origin, but are not specific findings. A history of ascites is helpful.

DeMay, A&S 2e. Ovary, p300

80 c   round to oval

Vulvar intraepithelial neoplasia (VIN) has been associated with exposure to the human papillomavirus. These lesions may cytologically be identified using criteria similar to those necessary to diagnose nonkeratinizing cervical lesions. Round to oval cells with high N:C ratios, hyperchromasia, and finely granular, evenly distributed chromatin are suggestive of a high grade VIN.

Keebler CM, Somrak TM. The Manual of Cytotechnology. Nonneoplastic vulvar intraepithelial neoplasia, p150

81 c   columnar configuration and granular cytoplasm are observed in endocervical adenocarcinoma

The number of cells found in well differentiated endocervical adenocarcinoma (ECA) are typically greater than those found in endometrial adenocarcinomas (EMAs). Cell sizes associated with ECA are larger, contain more abundant cytoplasm, retain columnar configuration, and have finely granular, irregularly distributed chromatin with micronucleoli. EMAs are diffusely vacuolated and often contain engulfed polymorphonuclear cells, the opposite of the granular cytoplasm generally found in lesions arising from the endocervical glands. Finally, the presence of a watery diathesis with associated lipophages may be helpful in discriminating endometrial adenocarcinomas from other epithelial malignancies.

DeMay, A&S 2e. Endocervical vs endometrial adenocarcinoma, p105

ISBN 978-089189-6357 ©ASCP 2015

82 d *Haemophilus ducreyi*

Gram– bacilli found in the cytoplasm of leukocytes may suggest the diagnosis of *Haemophilus ducreyi*. Isolation of the bacillus in culture is imperative.

DeMay, A&S 2e. Bacterial vaginosis, p36-37

83 c leiomyosarcoma

Cytology reveals spindle cells with pleomorphic features, giant cells, isolated, fibrillar cytoplasm, and oval nuclei. The chromatin is finely granular, irregularly distributed, and may or may not contain nuclei. Leiomyosarcomas represent the most common sarcomatous lesion of the uterus. These lesions represent a malignant transformation of the indigenous smooth muscle elements.

DeMay, A&S 2e. Leiomyosarcoma, p110

84 a dyskeratosis

Dyskeratocytes are small cells with pleomorphic orangeophilic cytoplasm and smudged irregular nuclei. These cells may also be larger in size, making their differentiation from keratinizing dysplasia virtually impossible. Keratinizing or pleomorphic dysplasia (CIN mimicking keratosis) cytologically presents with well defined borders, dense refractile cytoplasm, and hyperchromatic, coarse, irregular chromatin or India ink pyknosis. These cells may often stain orangeophilic. However, the degree of pleomorphism is more important when establishing the severity of keratinizing dysplasia. Associated changes include hyperkeratosis, parakeratosis, and dyskeratosis. Dyskeratocytes, or pleomorphic parakeratosis, are classified as atypical squamous cells of undetermined significance under the Bethesda System. Their presence is suggestive but not pathognomonic for human papillomavirus (HPV) infection.

DeMay, A&S 2e. Dyskeratocytes, p69-70

85 a atypia of atrophy and maturity

The presence of bare nuclei seen in postmenopausal patients may be autolytic cells associated with atrophy or degenerated endocervical cell nuclei. Endocervical nuclei are oval in shape, possessing well preserved or degenerative chromatin. They may lie free or be trapped in streams of mucin. Atypia of atrophy represent low level parabasal to basal cells and often may mimic more significant disorders such as carcinoma in situ or endocervical dysplasia. These cells are basal to parabasal cells in syncytial-like arrangements or hyperchromatic crowded groups (HCGs) found among a granular precipitate containing degenerated epithelial cells and scattered red and white blood cells. The chromatin, if visible, is fine and evenly distributed. More commonly, the chromatin of these atypical cells is poorly preserved, smudged and indistinct. Clinical history should be evaluated before rendering a diagnosis.

DeMay, A&S 2e. Atypia of atrophy and maturity, p60-61

86 c endometrial biopsy to rule out cystic hyperplasia

An increase in estrogen, unopposed estrogen stimulation, or pathological entities such as granulosa-theca cell tumors may be predisposing conditions for endometrial hyperplasia. Other risk factors for premalignant corpus disease include obesity, hypertension, nulliparity, and diabetes mellitus. Patients with these clinical histories are at higher risk for developing invasive endometrial adenocarcinoma. The presence of normal endometrial cells at times other than days 1-14 of the menstrual cycle may be related to a hyperplastic endometrium. Cytologic features are those of normal endometrial cells. A tumor diathesis is absent. Endometrial cells identified outside of the proliferative phase of the menstrual cycle (days 14-28) are considered abnormal in the absence of clinical history. Normal appearing endometrial cells may be associated with hyperplasia, a predisposing condition for endometrial adenocarcinoma. An endometrial biopsy is often necessary to rule out a disease process.

DeMay, A&S 2e. Histology of endometrial hyperplasia and carcinoma, p102-103

87 c degenerated parabasal cells of atrophy

Sheets of lower level parabasal to basal cells with autolytic features, degenerating karyolytic cells ("blue blobs"), and the finding of pyknotic parabasal cells with eosinophilic cytoplasm (often referred as "mummified cells") are characteristic of deep atrophy as found in postmenopausal or postpartum patients. Care should be taken to discriminate these findings from more significant conditions such as parakeratosis or dyskeratosis, lesions associated with true keratinizing processes.

DeMay, A&S 2e. Atypia of atrophy and maturity, p60-61

88 d malignant lymphoma

Malignant lymphoma may mimic follicular cervicitis (FC); however, the findings of a polytypic cell population, which includes lymphocytes (mature, immunoblasts), plasma cells, and tingible body macrophages, are indicative of FC. In contrast, classic malignant lymphoma presents as a monomorphic population of immature lymphocytes. Furthermore, lymphoma presents with a gross cervical abnormality and generally an established history.

DeMay, A&S 2e. Lymphoma and leukemia, p114-115

89 b sheets of cells without single cells in repair

Sheets of cells with well defined cytoplasmic borders, preserved nuclear polarity, predictable nuclear features, fine regular chromatin patterns, micro- to macronucleoli, and characteristic cytoplasmic streaming are diagnostic of repair. This process is often associated with trauma, cervicitis, and inflammatory etiology.

DeMay, A&S 2e. Repair/regeneration, p30-31

90 d mucinous endometrial adenocarcinoma

These well differentiated endometrial adenocarcinomas resemble intestinal type adenocarcinomas. The cytology reveals mucin intracytoplasmically and contained within the background.

DeMay, A&S 2e. Variants of endometrial carcinoma, p106-107

91 c a squamous metaplastic component

These cells are round to oval in shape, possess acidophilic cytoplasm, and resemble oncocytes found in the salivary glands or thyroid. They are thought to be of squamous metaplastic origin and may cover the surface of normal or cancerous cells within the uterus. Their presence is necessary in establishing a diagnosis of adenoacanthoma. The clinical management of pure endometrial adenocarcinoma and adenoacanthoma is essentially the same.

DeMay, A&S 2e. Histology of endometrial hyperplasia and carcinoma, p102-103

92 c AGUS/endocervical dysplasia

Endocervical cells with slightly enlarged hyperchromatic nuclei with inconspicuous nucleoli, loss of polarity, and rosette formations are helpful in establishing a diagnosis of atypical glandular cells of undetermined significance (AGUS), in this case, referred to as endocervical columnar dysplasia (ECD). Its differential diagnosis is endocervical adenocarcinoma in situ (AIS); however, ECD has fine, regular chromatin whereas endocervical AIS contains coarse chromatin features. The identification of endocervical adenocarcinoma is grounded upon the findings of increased endocervical nuclear size, stratification of the cells, a feathering and splattering effect, frequent nucleoli, and the presence of finely granular, irregularly distributed chromatin. Columnar shaped morphology is maintained in these malignancies. Endocervical adenocarcinoma must be discriminated from atypical glandular cells of undetermined significance, endocervical origin. These "endocervical dysplasias" do not have classic malignant chromatin features of adenocarcinoma and do not present with true tissue fragments.

DeMay, A&S 2e. Differential of early endocervical glandular neoplasia, p90-91

93 b endocervical adenocarcinoma

The identification of endocervical adenocarcinoma is grounded upon the findings of increased endocervical nuclear size, stratification of the cells, a feathering and splattering effect, frequent nucleoli, and the presence of finely granular, irregularly distributed chromatin. Columnar shaped morphology is maintained in these malignancies. Endocervical adenocarcinoma must be discriminated from atypical glandular cells of undetermined significance, endocervical origin. "Endocervical dysplasias" do not have classic malignant chromatin features of adenocarcinoma and do not present with true tissue fragments. The presence of columnar morphology in the presence of obvious malignant criteria may help one to distinguish endocervical adenocarcinomas from those of endometrial origin. Other criteria that help discriminate the cells of endocervical adenocarcinoma (EA) from endometrial adenocarcinoma (EM) include the presence of rosettes vs cell balls and elongated, hyperchromatic, multinucleated cells with prominent multiple nucleoli vs rounded, finely granular chromatin and conspicuous nucleoli. EA possesses a granular cytoplasmic texture, whereas EM lesions have a lacy, frothy, vacuolated cytoplasmic texture. Lastly, EA tends to stain eosinophilic while EM is generally basophilic.

DeMay, A&S 2e. Endocervical carcinoma, p91-95

94 c large, distended vacuoles

Patients with an intrauterine device (IUD) may often present with proliferative or secretory endometrial cells that are reactive in nature. These cells are often single or in clusters, have large distended vacuoles, and contain finely granular, evenly distributed chromatin.

DeMay, A&S 2e. Intrauterine contraceptive device (IUD) changes, p49-50

95 d endometrial polyps

Endometrial polyps have not been established as precursor lesions within the morphogenesis or development of endometrial adenocarcinoma.

DeMay, A&S 2e. Histology of endometrial hyperplasia and carcinoma, p102-103

96 d mucinous cystadenocarcinoma/ovary

Mucinous adenocarcinomas of the ovary present with signet ring morphology and may recapitulate signet ring endometrial adenocarcinomas. Clinical history is paramount in establishing an ovarian primary tumor. A tumor diathesis is usually absent in cases of metastatic carcinoma unless the lesion has seeded at the secondary site.

DeMay, A&S 2e. Metastases, p115-116

97 a hyperkeratosis, plasma cells

Lichen sclerosus is a dermatologic hyperplastic disease that primarily affects postmenopausal females. The cytologic diagnosis requires the presence of hyperkeratosis, plasma cells, and mixed inflammatory cells. Parakeratotic cells may also be seen.

Ganovska A, Kovachev S, Nikolov A. Diagnosis and treatment of lichen sclerosus—review. Akush Ginekol (Sofiia) 2014;53(4):32-9 [PMID 25510069]

ISBN 978-089189-6357 ©ASCP 2015

98 a granular cell tumor (myoblastoma)

Granular cell tumors represent a small percentage of the primary vulval tumors. These lesions cytologically yield large cells containing intracytoplasmic eosinophilic granules and finely granular, eccentrically placed nuclei. The finding of a submucosal mass with overlying pigmented mucosa on the labia majora is essential in establishing the diagnosis of this neoplasm.

Domínguez-González M, Nogales-Pérez A, Vázquez Navarrete S.Granular cell tumor of the vulva. J Low Genit Tract Dis 2013;17(1):82-4 [PMID 22885645]

99 a an increase in sheets over gland formation

As adenocarcinoma of the endometrium becomes less differentiated, the ability to cytologically diagnose the presence of glandular formation is diminished. These cells are predominantly found in sheets, as single cells, or in syncytia. Obvious malignant morphology is present, such as an increase in size and number of nucleoli, coarse irregular chromatin, and anisonucleosis. It is important to correctly identify the nature and texture of the cytoplasm as adenocarcinoma rather than of squamous origin. Poorly differentiated glandular lesions lack the ability to form glandular groupings as seen in well differentiated tumors.

DeMay, A&S 2e. Histology of endometrial hyperplasia and carconoma, p102-105

100 c serous adenocarcinoma of the ovary

The diagnosis of papillary serous adenocarcinoma of the ovary in a Pap test is centered on the finding of 3D aggregates with hyperchromatic nuclei and finely granular, irregularly distributed chromatin with a cervical/endocervical/endometrial biopsy negative and colposcopy negative examination. The presence of papillary groups of malignant cells and psammoma bodies may help in identifying these lesions as ovarian origin, but are not specific findings. A history of ascites is helpful.

DeMay, A&S 2e. Metastases, p115-116

101 a increase

As adenocarcinoma of the endometrium becomes less differentiated, the ability to cytologically diagnose the presence of glandular formation is diminished. These cells are predominantly found in sheets, as single cells, or in syncytia. Obvious malignant morphology is present, such as an increase in size and number of nucleoli, coarse irregular chromatin, and anisonucleosis. It is important to correctly identify the nature and texture of the cytoplasm as adenocarcinoma rather than of squamous origin. Poorly differentiated glandular lesions lack the ability to form glandular groupings as seen in well differentiated tumors.

DeMay, A&S 2e. Histology of endometrial hyperplasia and carcinoma, p102-105

102 a folic acid deficiency

Folic acid deficiency (FAD) produces cytomegaly (an increase in the cell volume without cytokinesis) and karyomegaly, changes similar to those seen in radiation cellular injury. Multinucleation and nuclei with fine regular chromatin are observed. Cytoplasmic vacuolization may mimic a "swiss cheese" effect, indicating the cells' degenerative qualities. Folic acid deficiency (FAD) is a common water soluble vitamin deficiency state among pregnant women. FAD is related to deficient ingestion, absorption and the increased demands of folic acid required during pregnancy.

DeMay, A&S 2e. Diet, p116

103 a Donovan bodies, *Calymmatobacterium granulomatis*

Donovan bodies represent histiocytic inclusions or Gram– bacilli, also identified as *Calymmatobacterium granulomatis*. The morphologic identification of Donovan bodies is based on their "safety pin" appearance. Special staining with Romanowsky may be necessary to establish this diagnosis.

DeMay, A&S 2e. Granulomatous cervicitis, p32

104 b del Castillo syndrome

Patients with del Castillo syndrome may have previously taken birth control pills, and a milky discharge may be elaborated from the breast. The pituitary gland shuts down the production of follicle stimulating hormone and luteinizing hormone. Therefore, these patients are atrophic.

Keebler CM, Somrak TM. The Manual of Cytotechnology. Endocrinopathies, p74-78

105 a mosaic patterns

Mosaic patterns and punctuated mucosa are colposcopic findings associated with HPV.

DeMay, A&S 2e. Human papillomavirus, p124-126

106 b koilocytosis

Diagnosis of human papillomavirus infection is made based on the presence of koilocytes with or without associated dyskeratosis and/or immature metaplastic infected cells. The cytomorphologic diagnosis provides no information on whether the viral type is low risk (episomal) or high risk (transforming); therefore, risk prediction is not possible. Sophisticated molecular tests, including polymerase chain reaction and Southern blot analysis, may be employed to help decipher the biology of the disease. The Bethesda System classifies condyloma acuminata (human papillomavirus [HPV]) as a low grade squamous epithelial lesion. The pathognomonic cell for establishing an HPV infection is the koilocyte. This cell possesses large perinuclear halos (often referred to as cytoplasmic margination or large halo) or craterlike morphology. The nuclei may be well preserved with fine even chromatin or hyperchromatic and smudged, representing a degenerative quality.

DeMay, A&S 2e. Condyloma, p68-69

107 c an abrupt increase in squamous cell maturation

Patients who have an abrupt rise in maturation or hyperdifferentiation of the squamous mucosa after receiving radiation therapy for squamous carcinoma are at an increased risk for recurrence. Other key indicators include the presence of spindle cells and tissue necrosis.

DeMay, A&S 2e. Radiation cytology (persistent vs recurrent carcinoma), p45

108 a LEEP/LLETZ

In most instances, treatment for high grade lesions includes cryotherapy, laser ablation, endocervical curettage, large loop excision of the transformation zone (LLETZ), loop electrosurgical excision procedure (LEEP), or a cold knife conization.

DeMay, A&S 2e. f1.19, p152

109 a changes associated with *Trichomonas* infections

Perinuclear (inflammatory) halos may be found within squamous cells associated with *Trichomonas* or other inflammatory infections. These inflammatory halos are related to alcoholic fixation of an inflamed nucleus, whereas true koilocytic halos are large "cavelike" halos that are at least the width of an intermediate cell nucleus or larger.

DeMay, A&S 2e. Trichomonas vaginalis, p40

110 a parabasal cell predominance

Patients suffering from anorexia nervosa commonly have markedly atrophic vaginal smear patterns due to pituitary inhibition, which in turn, results in its inability to release FSH and LH.

DeMay, A&S 2e. Parabasal predominant maturation index (atrophy), p12-13

111 d high risk HPV types inducing exophytic lesions

Exophytic lesions are those that create condylomatous or papillary lesions. These histologic HPV types are more often associated with low risk viral types 6 and 11. High risk viral types have been associated with the development of cervical cancer. In this sequence of events, the E1-E2 region (early genes) are disrupted, interfering with the ability of the virus to transcribe its late genes, thus creating a biologic dead end for the viral life cycle. However, without transcription of these late genes, the feedback mechanism that controls the transcription of the E6-E7 genes (the viral region that codes for proteins that regulate viral growth) is lost. E6-E7 genes may bind antioncogenes or tumor suppressor genes such as p53 or Rb (retinoblastoma), which serve as protective genes that prevent transcription of cancer causing oncogenes.

DeMay, A&S 2e. Microbiology and molecular biology of HPV, p103-104

112 d 8 weeks postirradiation

Should malignant cells with radiation changes be found 8 weeks postirradiation therapy, it is considered persistent. However, should malignant cells without radiation effect be found 8 weeks postirradiation therapy, it is considered recurrent malignancy.

DeMay, A&S 2e. Radiation cytology, persistent vs recurrent carcinoma, p45

113 a endocervical reserve cell

The stem cell (if initiated) for nonkeratinizing, metaplastic squamous, and small cell lesions of the uterine cervix is the endocervical reserve cell. Mature metaplastic epithelium may give rise to nonkeratinizing dysplasia, immature squamous metaplasia may give rise to metaplastic dysplasia, and atypical reserve cells may give rise to small cell squamous carcinoma.

DeMay, A&S 2e. Reserve cell hyperplasia, p71

114 a macrocytes, kite, polka dot, and balloon cells

Markedly enlarged cells (macrocytes), the presence of nuclear smudging without cavelike cytoplasmic margination, and cells with long cytoplasmic tails (kite cells) are nonspecific cells associated with HPV infection. Other minor changes include cells with small globules of condensed cytoplasm (polka dot cells), tone cells, cracked cells, and squamous cells that resemble adipocytes possessing clear cytoplasm and peripheralized nuclei (balloon cells). These nonclassical, minor, or "soft" criteria may serve as antecedent cytomorphologic changes to a "classical" (koilocytic) HPV diagnosis.

DeMay, A&S 2e. Condyloma, p68-69

115 d intermediatelike cells in cobblestone pattern

Choice d suggests a mature metaplastic cell. Syncytial-like aggregates, hyperchromatic crowded "chaotic" groups with indistinct cell borders are associated with squamous carcinoma in situ.

DeMay, A&S 2e. General features of arcinoma in situ, p76-79

116 a large, round to oval stripped nuclei

These nuclei are often variable in size and contain "washed out" nuclear chromatin and prominent nucleoli. Their presence represents recurrence and may predate the findings of classic adenocarcinoma, which presents in clusters and glandular formations.

DeMay, A&S 2e. Radiation cytology (persistent vs recurrent carcinoma), p115

117 a flat

HPV viral types 16 and 18 are more commonly associated with planum (flat) cervical lesions and occur in mature metaplastic epithelium. The acuminatum variety (cauliflowerlike) is associated with keratinized lesions.

DeMay, A&S 2e. Condyloma, p68-69

118 b intermediate cell predominance

Long term, low dose estrogen replacement produces intermediate level maturation instead of the superficial level maturation associated with short term estrogen therapy.

DeMay, A&S 2e. Intermediate predominant maturation index, p13

ISBN 978-089189-6357 ©ASCP 2015

119 d pseudokeratosis

Synonyms include birth control pill changes, microglandular hyperplasia, and pseudoparakeratosis (pseudokeratosis). These cells represent degenerating forms of hyperplastic endocervical glandular mucosa. The finding has been associated with patients taking oral contraceptives, late luteal phase, and late pregnancy. They are benign cellular findings; however, the differentiation from true parakeratosis is imperative. Cells from microglandular hyperplasia generally have eosinophilic or basophilic cytoplasm, contain eccentric nuclei, or resemble reactive endocervical cells, whereas parakeratosis represents a true keratinizing process (orangeophilia) with centrally located pyknotic nuclei in polygonal "waxy" cytoplasm (possibly with accompanying HPV changes).

DeMay, A&S 2e. Microglandular endocervical hyperplasia, p17-18

120 a smaller than the original tumor cells

The small cell sizes associated with recurrent carcinoma are due in part to their anaplastic nature. These cells may also lack the pleomorphism commonly associated with the primary diagnosis of cervical carcinoma. In comparison, an indication of postirradiation dysplasia of the cervix (small cell type) may be the presence of small cells with high N:C ratios and hyperchromatic nuclei. The nuclear chromatin pattern is often too dense to interpret. small cell type postirradiation dysplasia is more likely to be found in older age groups. These cells mimic small cell carcinoma in situ; however, any grade of postirradiation dysplasia recurring before 3 years postirradiation therapy carries a poor prognosis.

DeMay, A&S 2e. Radiation cytology (persistent vs recurrent carcinoma), p45

121 b abnormal cells replacing the full thickness of the squamous mucosa; no differentiation at the surface

Carcinoma in situ of the cervix replaces the full epithelial thickness of the squamous mucosa with primitive cells, resulting in a total loss of cellular maturation throughout the epithelial strata.

DeMay, A&S 2e. Carcinoma in situ, p71-72

122 c dyskeratocytes

These pleomorphic cells with elongated nuclei, often described as dyskeratocytes or pleomorphic parakeratosis, are classified as atypical squamous cells of undetermined significance under the Bethesda System. Their presence is suggestive but not pathognomonic for human papillomavirus (HPV) infection.

DeMay, A&S 2e. Condyloma, p68-69

123 c increased nuclear to cytoplasmic area in high grade lesions

One of the most important criteria for distinguishing low grade squamous epithelial lesions from those of high grade variety is the N:C ratio. As the N:C ratio increases, so does the severity of dysplasia.

DeMay, A&S 2e. Introduction to diagnosis of squamous intraepithelial lesions, p64-65

124 d high grade squamous intraepithelial neoplasia, carcinoma in situ

Abnormal cells lacking nuclear polarity, containing hyperchromatic nuclei with fine to coarse and even chromatin and arranged in single cells or syncytia, are suggestive of an in situ lesion. The differential diagnosis between squamous and endocervical in situ lesions depends on many features, including the cell shape (columnar-endocervical) and/or accompanying dysplasia (squamous). Feathering or splattering cytoplasmic processes are often associated with endocervical lesions. One of the hallmarks of squamous carcinoma in situ is its coarse, regular chromatin distribution. Chromatin patterns found in dysplasia are typically finely granular and evenly distributed. Syncytial-like aggregates, hyperchromatic crowded "chaotic" groups with indistinct cell borders are associated with squamous carcinoma in situ. Distinguishing these aggregates from true papillary tissue fragments with community borders, well formed glandular structures, or HCGs with feathery edges may help in differentiating glandular lesions from those of squamous origin.

DeMay, A&S 2e. Carcinoma in situ, p76-79

125 b CIN3

Cervical intraepithelial neoplasia (CIN) is a diagnostic classification system that has 3 classifications: CIN1 (mild dysplasia or low grade intraepithelial lesion), CIN2 (moderate dysplasia or high grade intraepithelial lesion), and CIN3 (severe dysplasia, carcinoma in situ, or high grade intraepithelial lesion).

DeMay, A&S 2e. General features of carcinoma in situ, p66

126 a diathesis, increased cellular pleomorphism in carcinoma

A diathesis is defined as the tissue necrosis associated with an invasive malignancy. The debris includes hemolyzed red blood cells, degenerated epithelial cells, and inflammatory cells in a granular or "sandy" background.

DeMay, A&S 2e. Keratinizing squamous cell carcinoma, p74-75

127 a *Chlamydia trachomatis*

This obligate intracellular bacterium is the most common cause of nongonococcal cervicitis. Cytologic changes are nonspecific and may range from cytoplasmic inclusions with fine vacuolization that do not displace the nucleus or cytoplasm (nebular bodies) to dysplastic mimicking morphology. Because these findings are neither sensitive nor specific, cytology should not be the method of detection.

DeMay, A&S 2e. Chlamydia trachomatis, p39-40

128 a karyomegaly and macrocytosis

Benign radiation changes include vacuolization of the cytoplasm, macrocytosis, amphophilia, nucleomegaly, and well preserved N:C ratios. Nuclear pyknosis and karyorrhexis are degenerative changes associated with benign radiation changes.

DeMay, A&S 2e. Radiation cytology, p42-44

129 a irradiation

Benign radiation changes include vacuolization of the cytoplasm, macrocytosis, amphophilia, nucleomegaly, and well preserved N:C ratios. Nuclear pyknosis and karyorrhexis are degenerative changes associated with benign radiation changes.

DeMay, A&S 2e. Radiation cytology, p42-44

130 b squamous cell carcinoma, keratinizing type

These cells are demonstrating cellular pleomorphism, orangeophilia, and irregular, hyperchromatic, opaque nuclei. The background contains a granular diathesis. The presence of single cells with these characteristics is diagnostic of a squamous cell carcinoma. Keratinizing squamous carcinomas generally originate on the anterior cervical lip. The single or syncytial-like pleomorphic to bizarre tadpole or spindle cell formations are the trademarks of this lesion. The cells may stain orangeophilic or cyanophilic; however, eosinophilia is more often seen. Pyknotic hyperchromatic nuclei are more common due to its degenerative features; however, when better preserved, the chromatin is considered coarsely granular and irregularly distributed with nucleoli. A granular diathesis may or may not be present due to the exophytic nature of this lesion. Pearl formations, parakeratosis, and hyperkeratosis may accompany the malignant cells.

DeMay, A&S 2e. Keratinizing squamous cell carcinoma, p74-75

131 d atypical reserve cell hyperplasia

Immature metaplastic cells may give rise (if initiated) to metaplastic dysplasias, whereas mature metaplastic cells are linked to nonkeratinizing dysplasia. Atypical reserve cell hyperplasia is related to the development of small cell lesions, and small cell carcinomas in situ give rise to small cell carcinomas.

DeMay, A&S 2e. Reserve cell hyperplasia, p24-25

132 b reserve cells

Replication of the virus begins in the reserve cell or squamous basal cell.

DeMay, A&S 2e. Squamous metaplasia, p23-24

133 b nonkeratinizing squamous cell carcinoma

Single cells, syncytial fragments, and naked nuclei exhibiting hyperchromasia and coarse irregular chromatin with macronucleoli are diagnostic criteria of nonkeratinizing squamous cell carcinoma of the uterine cervix. A tumor diathesis is more commonly seen with nonkeratinizing carcinomas than in keratinizing malignancies.

DeMay, A&S 2e. Nonkeratinizing squamous cell carcinoma, p73-74

134 d early region 6, 7

These early genomic regions are found within cervical carcinomas and their metastases. High risk viral types have been associated with the development of cervical cancer. In this sequence of events, the E1-E2 region (early genes) are disrupted, interfering with the ability of the virus to transcribe its late genes, thus creating a biologic dead end for the viral life cycle. However, without transcription of these late genes, the feedback mechanism that controls the transcription of the E6-E7 genes (the viral region that codes for proteins that regulate viral growth) is lost. E6-E7 genes may bind antioncogenes or tumor suppressor genes such as p53 or Rb (retinoblastoma), which serve as protective genes that prevent transcription of cancer causing oncogenes.

DeMay, A&S 2e. HPV in cervical carcinogenesis, p131-132

135 b folic acid deficiency

Folic acid deficiency (FAD) produces cytomegaly (an increase in the cell volume without cytokinesis) and karyomegaly, changes similar to those seen in radiation cellular injury. Multinucleation and nuclei with fine regular chromatin are observed. Cytoplasmic vacuolization may mimic a "swiss cheese" effect, indicating the cells' degenerative qualities. Folic acid deficiency (FAD) is a common water soluble vitamin deficiency state among pregnant women. FAD is related to deficient ingestion, absorption, and the increased demands of folic acid required during pregnancy.

DeMay, A&S 2e. Diet, p136-137

136 c keratinizing processes, nonspecific

Pearl formations, parakeratosis, and hyperkeratosis often accompany keratinizing processes.

DeMay, A&S 2e. Parakeratosis, p27-28

ISBN 978-089189-6357 ©ASCP 2015

137 a   small cell neuroendocrine carcinoma, cervix
Small cell lesions arise from atypical reserve cells, foregoing the morphologic spectrum associated with dysplastic lesions arising from the mature and immature metaplastic zones. Small cell neuroendocrine carcinoma is a highly malignant neuroendocrine neoplasm that is ultrastructurally part of the amine precursor uptake and decarboxylation (APUD) tumors due to its cytoplasmic evidence of androgenic amines (membrane bound membrane granules). These cells contain hyperchromatic stippled chromatin, coarse clumping, nuclear molding, scanty cytoplasm, and micronucleoli. They have characteristic vertebral column formation, microbiopsy aggregates, cords, nests, or ribbons. In 1/3 of the cases, neuroendocrine differentiation may be demonstrated by immunocytochemical staining with chromogranin, neuron specific enolase, or synaptophysin. Neuroendocrine differentiation (argyrophilia) may also be demonstrated. Small cell carcinomas may be poorly differentiated squamous lesions or neuroendocrine tumors, both of which arise within the endocervical canal. Poorly differentiated squamous carcinomas are composed of small cells with high N:C ratios, uniform cellular sizes with well defined borders, coarse chromatin with nucleoli, but little to absent "crush" artifact. An abnormal host response or necrotic tumor diathesis often accompanies these squamous lesions. The oval nature of the nuclei in small cell squamous carcinoma reflects its high mitotic rate.
DeMay, A&S 2e. Small cell neuroendocrine carcinoma, p107-108

138 d   nucleic acid analysis
Hybrid Capture 2 (Digene Corp) is the only commercially approved in vitro HPV virotyping test for determining low or high risk infections. The test uses microplates for capturing RNA hybrids and has an analytical sensitivity of 1.0 pg/mL (5,000 HPV genomes per test). The test is approved direct to vial or can be tested off liquid based medium (ThinPrep Pap Test only as of March 2002).
DeMay, A&S 2e. DNA hybrid capture, p128

139 a   synaptophysin
Small cell neuroendocrine carcinoma is a highly malignant neuroendocrine neoplasm that is ultrastructurally part of the amine precursor uptake and decarboxylation (APUD) tumors due to its cytoplasmic evidence of androgenic amines (membrane bound membrane granules). These cells contain hyperchromatic stippled chromatin, coarse clumping, nuclear molding, scanty cytoplasm, and micronucleoli. They have characteristic vertebral column formation, microbiopsy aggregates, cords, nests, or ribbons. In 1/3 of the cases, neuroendocrine differentiation may be demonstrated by immunocytochemical staining with chromogranin, neuron specific enolase, or synaptophysin. Neuroendocrine differentiation (argyrophilia) may also be demonstrated.
DeMay, A&S 2e. Small cell neuroendocrine carcinoma, p107-108

140 c   immunohistochemistry
Immunocytochemistry may be helpful in differentiating metastatic lesions. Special staining with chromogranin (neuroendocrine lesions), S100 (melanoma), leukocyte common antigen (lymphoma), and α-fetoprotein (GI tract lesions) are some examples of its utility.
DeMay, A&S 2e. Metastasis, p115-117

141 a   greater
Immature metaplastic cells may give rise (if initiated) to metaplastic dysplasias, a variant that more commonly progresses to cancer (untreated) than nonkeratinizing dysplasia.
DeMay, A&S 2e. Metaplastic dysplasia, p67

142 a   1
Intestinal or mucinous endometrial adenocarcinoma usually presents as a grade I (well differentiated) lesion. The cells contain abundant mucin secretion as represented by the distended cytoplasmic vacuolization. The differential diagnosis is mucinous adenocarcinoma of the ovary, but the presence of a pale sticky diathesis will help establish this lesion as primary.
DeMay, A&S 2e. Histology of endometrial hyperplasia and carcinoma, p102-103

143 a   diathesis related changes with malignancies involving direct extension
Metastatic carcinomas usually lack a notable diathesis unless tumor seeding has occurred within the ectopic area.
DeMay, A&S 2e. Metastasis, p115-117

144 c   few "atypical" cells, associated benign epithelial elements
This degenerative artifactual change may show hyperchromatic crowded groups; however, these groups are generally sparse when compared with true neoplasia. Furthermore, cellular crowding is less pronounced as compared with neoplasia, and the chromatin is fine and regular. Mitotic figures are rare. Ciliated cells may be seen in conjunction with benign endometrial or endocervical elements.
DeMay, A&S 2e. Differential diagnosis of atypical glandular cells, p79-80

145 d   carcinoma in situ
Syncytial-like aggregates, hyperchromatic crowded "chaotic" groups with indistinct cell borders, are associated with squamous carcinoma in situ. Distinguishing these aggregates from true papillary tissue fragments with community borders, well formed glandular structures, or HCGs with feathery edges may help in differentiating glandular lesions from those of squamous origin.
DeMay, A&S 2e. General features of carcinoma in situ, p66

146 b 8th week of gestation

Vaginal adenosis is defined as the presence of ectopic glandular epithelium or squamous metaplastic cells within the normally gland free or squamous lined vagina. Their presence is increased in those patients who were exposed to diethylstilbestrol (DES) in utero.

DeMay, A&S 2e. Diethylstilbestrol, p47

147 a *Vorticella* species

In addition to *Vorticella*, other examples of uncommon protozoa include *Entamoeba histolytica* and *Balantidium coli*. Choices b, c, and d represent contaminants of vaginal smears.

Keebler CM, Somrak TM. The Manual of Cytotechnology. Microbiologic classification, p90

148 b myofibroblasts

Fibroblasts are common findings represented in cervical/vaginal specimens from patients who have received radiation for epithelial malignancies. Ulceration or epithelial fragility secondary to radiation is responsible for their presence. Differentiation from recurrent squamous carcinoma (SC) is based on the findings of single cells without opaque/nuclear hyperchromasia or coarse, irregular chromatin. In addition, the cytoplasm of fibroblasts is described as sparse, wispy, or vacuolated, whereas cells from SC typically possess abundant pleomorphic and/or orangeophilic dense cytoplasm.

DeMay, A&S 2e. Radiation cytology, p42-44

149 b rhabdomyosarcoma

Rhabdomyosarcoma is a heterologous sarcoma of the uterus that presents itself cytologically similar to leiomyosarcoma; however, this malignancy represents a striated muscle rather than a smooth muscle origin. The findings of "strap cells" are diagnostic of malignant blasts; however, strap cells represent only 1% of the total malignant population. It is important, though, to find these striations to help elucidate the origin of these cells. Multinucleated tumor giant cells are also observed with these malignancies. A heterologous mixed Müllerian tumor is diagnosed by the identification of well differentiated endometrial adenocarcinoma plus a nonindigenous sarcomatous element. Heterologous connective tissue malignancies may include osteosarcoma, chondrosarcoma, or rhabdomyosarcoma.

DeMay, A&S 2e. Rhabdomyosarcoma, p111

150 b poorly differentiated, delicate cytoplasm, prominent nucleoli

Clear cell adenocarcinomas of the endometrium are poorly differentiated tumors, which may have glycogenated cytoplasm. Classic malignant nuclear features are represented.

DeMay, A&S 2e. Histology of endometrial hyperplasia and carcinoma, p102-103

151 b small cell carcinoma

Small cell neuroendocrine carcinoma is a highly malignant neuroendocrine neoplasm that is ultrastructurally part of the amine precursor uptake and decarboxylation (APUD) tumors due to its cytoplasmic evidence of androgenic amines (membrane bound membrane granules). These cells contain hyperchromatic stippled chromatin, coarse clumping, nuclear molding, scanty cytoplasm, and micronucleoli. They have characteristic vertebral column formation, microbiopsy aggregates, cords, nests, or ribbons. In 1/3 of the cases, neuroendocrine differentiation may be demonstrated by immunocytochemical staining with chromogranin, neuron specific enolase, or synaptophysin. Neuroendocrine differentiation (argyrophilia) may also be demonstrated.

DeMay, A&S 2e. Small cell neuroendocrine carcinoma, p107-108

152 a CIS involves the underlying glandlike spaces

Glandular or microacinar differentiation within the syncytial-like aggregates may be seen if the squamous carcinoma in situ extends into the endocervical glands.

DeMay, A&S 2e. General features of carcinoma in situ, p66

153 a secretory adenocarcinoma

Secretory adenocarcinoma of the endometrium cytologically recapitulates well differentiated adenocarcinoma features, making these 2 conditions extremely difficult to differentiate using conventional cytopathology. With few exceptions, the cytologic manifestations do not reveal the secretory nature of these cells. Glycogen-positive cytoplasm is a feature of these tumors, but cytoplasmic vacuolization may not be a reliable distinguishing feature due to the shared morphology with mucinous adenocarcinomas of the endometrium. On the other hand, serous lesions often lack a tumor diathesis or the mucinous background associated with mucinous adenocarcinomas.

DeMay, A&S 2e. Endometrial adenocarcinoma, p103-104

154 c micronucleoli, diathesis

Microinvasive carcinomas of the cervix may be discriminated from carcinoma in situ by the presence of irregular chromatin distribution and micronucleoli. The cells are isolated, have syncytial-like arrangement, or are arranged in hyperchromatic crowded groups. The background contains a diathesis in up to 35% of the cases.

DeMay, A&S 2e. Cytology of squamous cell carcinoma, p72

155 a radiation

Granulomatous cervicitis may be related to tuberculosis, sutures, radiation, granuloma inguinale, lymphogranuloma venereum, schistosomiasis, syphilis, and possibly *Chlamydia*. The cytologic identification of this nonspecific condition is dependent upon the findings of foreign body giant cells (often with intracytoplasmic antigenic substance), epithelioid cells, and an inflammatory background.

DeMay, A&S 2e. Granulomatous cervicitis, p32

ISBN 978-089189-6357 ©ASCP 2015

156 b multinucleated giant histiocyte

Multinucleated histiocytes are often identified in vaginal smears taken from postmenopausal patients. Their presence is a normal finding in conjunction with epithelial atrophy.

DeMay, A&S 2e. Granulomatous cervicitis, p32

157 b vitamins A, B, and C deficiency

Other cofactors may include smoking, cervical trauma, cytomegalovirus, *Chlamydia*, smoking, steroids, pregnancy (immunodeficiency), decreased cellular immunity, or genetic susceptibility.

DeMay, A&S 2e. Possible cofactors in cervical carcinogenesis, p134-135

158 d squamous cell carcinoma, keratinizing type

Primary carcinoma of the vulva, a disease predominantly affecting elderly women, is cytologically diagnosed as keratinizing or pleomorphic squamous carcinoma. Cytoplasmic pleomorphism, India ink nuclei, decreased polarity, and coarse irregular chromatin are cytologic hallmarks of this disease.

DeMay, A&S 2e. Rare variants of squamous cell carcinoma, p75-77

159 c Bartholin gland adenocarcinoma

Bartholin gland adenocarcinomas are submucosal lesions that cytologically present as typical mucous glands possessing classic malignant criteria. Aspiration cytology may be necessary to diagnose this rare tumor.

DeMay, A&S 2e. Anatomy and embryology of the female genital tract, p4-5

160 a serous cystadenocarcinoma

The diagnosis of papillary serous adenocarcinoma of the ovary in a Pap test is centered on the finding of 3D aggregates with hyperchromatic nuclei and finely granular, irregularly distributed chromatin with a cervical/ endocervical/endometrial biopsy negative and colposcopy negative examination. The presence of papillary groups of malignant cells and psammoma bodies may help in identifying these lesions as ovarian origin, but are not specific findings. A history of ascites is helpful.

DeMay, A&S 2e. Metastases, p115-116

161 b endometrial stromal sarcoma

Endometrial stromal sarcoma is a homologous sarcoma found as small cells or groups with high N:C ratios and coarse hyperchromatic nuclei. The cytoplasmic morphology recapitulates that of benign endometrial superficial stromal cells.

DeMay, A&S 2e. Endometrial stromal sarcoma, p111

162 d Sertoli-Leydig cell tumor

The presence of psammoma bodies may be associated with most papillary lesions of the female genital tract. Endometrial adenocarcinomas, tubal malignancies, and reactive endometrium secondary to IUD implants may produce psammoma bodies in vaginal/cervical smears. The finding of these entities is not pathognomonic for malignancy.

DeMay, A&S 2e. Psammoma bodies, p122-123

163 b little pleomorphism

Adenocarcinoma in situ of the endocervix is identified cytologically with hyperchromasia, predictable nuclear sizes, loss of polarity, and irregular nuclear sizes and shapes, all in the presence of feathering effects. Large numbers of atypical cells will be found in comparison with normal endocervical cells. Abnormal cells lacking nuclear polarity, containing hyperchromatic nuclei with fine to coarse and even chromatin, and arranged in single cells or syncytia, are suggestive of an in situ lesion. The differential diagnosis between squamous and endocervical in situ lesions depends on many features, including the cell shape (columnar-endocervical) and/or accompanying dysplasia (squamous). Feathering or splattering cytoplasmic processes are often associated with endocervical lesions.

DeMay, A&S 2e. Cytology of adenocarcinoma in situ, p87-89

164 b not before 6-8 weeks postadministration

The acute phase of postirradiation consists of an admixture of necrotic tumor cells, white blood cells, and regenerative/ reparative changes amongst a diathesis laden background. Due to the smear's degenerative nature and the lingering malignant cells, effective analysis of these smears is best at least 6-8 weeks postirradiation. Should malignant cells with radiation changes be found 8 weeks postirradiation therapy, it is considered persistent. However, should malignant cells without radiation effect be found 8 weeks postirradiation therapy, it is considered recurrent malignancy.

DeMay, A&S 2e. Radiation cytology, p42

165 a atypical glandular cells (AGUS) often accompany squamous dysplasia

The presence of atypical (dysplastic) endocervical glandular cells found in concert with squamous dysplasia is not an unusual finding, primarily due to their shared HPV etiology.

DeMay, A&S 2e. Early endocervical glandular neoplasia, p77-80

166 c atypical glandular cells of undetermined significance, favor neoplastic

Adenocarcinoma in situ of the endocervix is identified cytologically with hyperchromasia, predictable nuclear sizes, loss of polarity, and irregular nuclear sizes and shapes, all in the presence of feathering effects. Large numbers of atypical cells will be found in comparison with normal endocervical cells. Abnormal cells lacking nuclear polarity, containing hyperchromatic nuclei with fine to coarse and even chromatin, and arranged in single cells or syncytia, are suggestive of an in situ lesion. The differential diagnosis between squamous and endocervical in situ lesions depends on many features, including the cell shape (columnar-endocervical) and/or accompanying dysplasia (squamous). Feathering or splattering cytoplasmic processes are often associated with endocervical lesions.

DeMay, A&S 2e. Atypical glandular cells, p77-80

167 c granular

One of the key differential features between endometrial adenocarcinoma and endocervical adenocarcinoma is the cytoplasmic texture. Endocervical adenocarcinoma tends to have granular cytoplasm.

DeMay, A&S 2e. Endocervical vs endometrial carcinoma, p105-106

168 d Arias-Stella reaction

Arias-Stella changes involve endometrial and endocervical cells and are seen in late pregnancy (high levels of HCG/ prolonged progesterone stimulation). The endocervical cells possess pale PAS+ cytoplasm and hyperchromatic nuclei with macronucleoli. Intranuclear cytoplasmic inclusions may also be seen. This "atypical reparative" morphology needs to be discriminated from clear cell adenocarcinoma; however, correlation of these changes with the clinical history will help define these changes as benign.

DeMay, A&S 2e. Arias-Stella reaction, p50-51

169 a cells with columnar morphology arranged into rosettes and crowded sheets with holes for endocervical adenocarcinoma compared with round, plump cells arranged into balls and molded groups for endometrial adenocarcinoma

The number of cells found in well differentiated endocervical adenocarcinoma (ECA) is typically greater than that found in endometrial adenocarcinomas (EMAs). Cells associated with ECA are larger, contain more abundant cytoplasm, retain columnar configuration, and have finely granular, irregularly distributed chromatin with micronucleoli. EMAs are diffusely vacuolated and often contain engulfed polymorphonuclear cells, the opposite of the granular cytoplasm generally found in lesions arising from the endocervical glands. Endometrial adenocarcinoma cytologically presents with fewer numbers of cells on the slide (as opposed to endocervical adenocarcinomas), cell clusters with scalloping borders and 3D tissue fragments, high N:C ratios, and frothy, delicate, lacy, vacuolated cytoplasm. One of the key differential features between this lesion and endocervical adenocarcinomas is the cytoplasmic texture. Endocervical adenocarcinoma, as indicated earlier, tends to have granular cytoplasm. Finally, the presence of a watery diathesis with associated lipophages may be helpful in discriminating endometrial adenocarcinomas from other epithelial malignancies.

DeMay, A&S 2e. Endocervical vs endometrial carcinoma, p105-106

170 a prolonged progesterone stimulation

Arias-Stella changes involve endometrial and endocervical cells and are seen in late pregnancy (high levels of HCG/ prolonged progesterone stimulation). The endocervical cells possess pale PAS+ cytoplasm and hyperchromatic nuclei with macronucleoli. Intranuclear cytoplasmic inclusions may also be seen. This "atypical reparative" morphology needs to be discriminated from clear cell adenocarcinoma; however, correlation of these changes with the clinical history will help define these changes as benign.

DeMay, A&S 2e. Arias-Stella reaction, p50-51

171 d malignant melanoma

Melanoma typically presents in single cells, in aggregates, or as spindle cells with bizarre malignant nuclear features, macronucleoli, intranuclear cytoplasmic inclusions, and possibly intracytoplasmic golden-brown pigment. Due to the fact that these diseases may be amelanotic, it may be helpful to confirm this disease process with S100, HMB45, melan A or MITF (microphthalmia associated transcription factor)–all which preferentially react with melanoma cells.

DeMay, A&S 2e. Melanoma, p50-51

172 a increase in single cells, loosely arranged cell groups, macronucleoli, and diathesis present in endocervical adenocarcinoma

Endocervical adenocarcinoma must be discriminated from adenocarcinoma in situ. Endocervical adenocarcinoma in situ does not have the classic malignant chromatin features of adenocarcinoma and does not present in true tissue fragments, but rather with feathering cytoplasmic effects.

DeMay, A&S 2e. Differential of early endocervical glandular neoplasia, p90-91

173 a chromatin is fine to moderately granular, and cells present with minimal anisocytosis and lack pseudostratification in endocervical glandular dysplasia

Endocervical cells with slightly enlarged hyperchromatic nuclei with inconspicuous nucleoli, loss of polarity, and rosette formations are helpful in establishing a diagnosis of atypical glandular cells of undetermined significance, in this case, referred to as endocervical columnar dysplasia (ECD). Its differential diagnosis is endocervical adenocarcinoma in situ (AIS); however, ECD has fine, regular chromatin, whereas endocervical AIS contains coarse chromatin features and cellular pseudostratification (trailing, splattering, feathering patterns).

DeMay, A&S 2e. Differential of early endocervical glandular neoplasia, p90-91

174 b vacuolated cytoplasm, finely granular chromatin with macronucleoli in endometrial adenocarcinoma

Due to the lack of differentiation found in large cell/poorly differentiated squamous carcinomas, it if often difficult to distinguish these lesions from poorly differentiated adenocarcinoma (PDA). PDA, though, may present with vacuolated cytoplasm and finely granular chromatin, whereas large cell squamous lesions contain densely granular cytoplasm and coarse, irregular chromatin patterns. Special stains are ineffective due to the fact that many PDAs are nonmucus secreting lesions.

DeMay, A&S 2e. Histology of endometrial hyperplasia and carcinoma, p102-103

ISBN 978-089189-6357 ©ASCP 2015

175 b 20

The development of vaginal adenocarcinoma arising in patients exposed to diethylstilbestrol (DES) in utero usually occurs in the third decade. The precursor lesion is vaginal adenosis. Clear cell adenocarcinoma presents as a typical mucinous adenocarcinoma containing enlarged nuclei and hypochromatic irregularly distributed chromatin. The presence of "hobnail cells," in which the nuclei are peripherally oriented toward the glandular lumen, may be helpful in identifying this malignancy.

DeMay, A&S 2e. Diethylstilbestrol, p47

176 c "hobnail" serous adenocarcinoma, endometrium

Serous or "hobnail" adenocarcinoma of the endometrium is a poorly differentiated endometrial lesion. Cells found in papillary clusters with associated psammoma bodies scattered among a necrotic background may be helpful in discriminating these lesions from serous adenocarcinoma of the ovary, due to the clean background associated with metastatic tumors.

DeMay, A&S 2e. Serous adenocarcinoma, p107

177 d primary endometrioid endocervical adenocarcinoma

Primary endometrioid endocervical adenocarcinoma (EEA) may mimic true endometrial adenocarcinoma (EA) with the exception that many of the cells of endometrioid endocervical adenocarcinoma have columnar morphology as well as endometrioid features. In addition, EEA presents with an increased number of malignant cells when compared with EA. Care should be taken to rule out the possibility of an endometrial adenocarcinoma that directly extends into the cervical os.

DeMay, A&S 2e. Endocervical carcinoma, p128

178 d bowenoid papulosis

Bowenoid papulosis is often referred to as carcinoma in situ of the vulva. Human papillomavirus exposure has been implicated as causative etiology in its histogeneses, usually affecting young females. Cytologic criteria for diagnosing bowenoid papulosis are similar to those of cervical carcinoma in situ.

DeMay, A&S 2e. General features of carcinoma in situ, p66

179 d more irregular

Nuclear detail is better preserved; therefore, irregular nuclear membranes may have more clarity when visualizing liquid based Pap tests. The degree of nuclear membrane irregularity increases with significance of cervical disease.

DeMay, A&S 2e. Cytology of LBC, p140-141

180 a more detail

The chromasia is clearer and the distribution of the chromatin pattern is better visualized with liquid based Pap tests.

DeMay, A&S 2e. Cytology of LBC, p140-141

181 b clinging to cells

Although reduced when compared with conventional smears, the key difference when analyzing tumor necrosis or diathesis in liquid based Pap tests is the appearance of ratty material clinging to the cells throughout the preparation.

DeMay, A&S 2e. Cytology of LBC, p140-141

182 a thicker cytoplasm

A denser and thicker cytoplasm is common in parabasal and metaplastic cells with conventional Pap tests.

DeMay, A&S 2e. Cytology of LBC, p140-141

183 d more hyperchromatic

Due to the small cell size as well the lack of air drying features, the nuclei of endocervical cells may appear at first impression darker; however, closer inspection of the cytoplasmic polarity (honeycombing, picket fence) and well delineated cell borders that push the cells apart (as if someone "erased" in between the cells, thus allowing the observer the perception that he/she can "cut them out" with scissors) verifies the benignity of these cells.

DeMay, A&S 2e. Cytology of LBC, p140-141

184 c endocervical and/or squamous metaplastic cells

Cells found in the endocervical canal are both squamous metaplastic and endocervical glandular type.

DeMay, A&S 2e. Cytology of LBC, p140-141

185 b smaller nuclear diameter

Liquid based preparations tend to "shrink" the overall cell and nuclear size when compared with the air drying typically seen with conventional Pap tests.

DeMay, A&S 2e. Liquid based pap tests, p140

186 c irregular nuclear borders

N:C ratios and the irregular nuclear borders are important features for confirming the presence of a significant cervical disease process.

DeMay, A&S 2e. Cytology of LBC, p140-141

187 d sampling error

Sampling error accounts for ½ to ¾ of all the false negative Pap test diagnoses reported in the literature.

DeMay, A&S 2e. Data analysis, p1578

188 a limited cellularity

Obscuring cellular elements are commonplace when analyzing conventional Pap tests; however, these factors are minimized in liquid based preparation systems, thus providing the morphologist with a decreased probability that the slide has limited cellularity.

DeMay, A&S 2e. Liquid based pap tests, p140

189 c   glandular pathology

Better morphologic visualization of the atypical features (nuclear stratification and cellular feathering) is seen when analyzing true glandular abnormalities in liquid based preparation systems. This correlates with fewer false positive diagnoses and a higher propensity for a biopsy proven lesion.

DeMay, A&S 2e. Liquid based pap tests, p140

190 b   lysed

In liquid based Paps, red blood cell casts are dispersed throughout the slide and don't preclude the visualization of other cells as compared with the likelihood that obscuring blood will cover important cells (as often seen in conventional Pap tests).

DeMay, A&S 2e. Cytology of LBC, p140-141

191 a   greater depth of focus

True tissue fragments with community borders, such as those seen with adenocarcinoma, will round up in liquid based preparations and have a greater depth of focus as compared with the flattening of the cells seen in conventional Pap tests.

DeMay, A&S 2e. Cytology of LBC, p140-141

192 b   lack orangeophilia and keratinization

Orangeophilia and keratinization are often exaggerated in degenerative specimens, such as those that allow for more degeneration to occur after the cells are removed from the patient (as conventional Paps). The diagnosis of squamous cell carcinoma in liquid based Pap specimens is more akin to that seen in freshly prepared specimens, such as effusions and fine needle aspirations. It is important to point out that the diagnosis of squamous cell carcinoma is best determined by the degree of pleomorphism, rather than simply the color of the cell.

DeMay, A&S 2e. Cytology of LBC, p140-141

193 c   identical

The incidence and identification of microorganisms in liquid based specimens is comparable to that seen with conventional Pap smears. Although the amount and number of microorganisms may be reduced in liquid based Pap tests, the likelihood for identification remains good owing to the decreased inflammatory background in these specimens.

DeMay, A&S 2e. Liquid based pap tests, p140

194 d   often seen concurrent with squamous atypia or intraepithelial lesions

Some studies have reported coexisting SIL in up to ~40% of Pap tests with endocervical glandular atypia.

DeMay, A&S 2e. Endocervical cells, p14-18

195 b   granular intracytoplasmic inclusions

The morphologic detection of *Chlamydia* is based upon the identification of particular intracytoplasmic inclusions in endocervical or metaplastic cells.

DeMay, A&S 2e.

196 d   are pregnant

Cockleburs are radiate crystalline arrays found in a small number of pregnant women. They have club shaped spokes that stain reddish to golden-brown, and are typically surrounded by histiocytes. Their presence is not associated with any adverse effect on maternal or fetal prognosis.

DeMay, A&S 2e. Cockleburs, p52-53

197 c   ovarian carcinoma

Ovarian carcinoma, followed by breast carcinoma, is the most common source for metastatic cancer to the uterine cervix.

DeMay, A&S 2e. Metastases, p115-116

198 c   cell arrangements and architecture

Architectural features such as strips of palisading cells with nuclear pseudostratification, rosette or gland formation, columnar cell shapes, and crowded sheets with "feathered" edges are the most useful criteria to distinguish HSIL from AIS.

DeMay, A&S 2e. Differential of early endocervical glandular neoplasia, p90-91

199 b   intranuclear and intracytoplasmic inclusions

Cytomegalovirus infection is characterized by large intranuclear (owl's eye) inclusion bodies and small intracytoplasmic inclusions. Multinucleated cells, if present, are few in number.

DeMay, A&S 2e. Viruses, p34-35

200 c   clue cells

Squamous cells covered with coccoid bacteria (clue cells) are characteristic for the presence of bacterial vaginosis. Lactobacilli and an inflammatory background are typically not seen.

DeMay, A&S 2e. Bacterial vaginosis, p36-37

201 d   97%

HSIL is an intraepithelial lesion that carries a significant risk for progression to cervical cancer. Approximately, 90%-97% of women with a diagnosis of HSIL test positive for high risk HPV.

DeMay, A&S 2e. Human papillomavirus, p124-125

202 a   tumor diathesis and prominent nucleoli

The differential diagnosis of squamous cell carcinoma includes primarily high grade squamous intraepithelial lesion. Prominent nucleoli and tumor diathesis are the principal cytologic features that help distinguish these 2 entities. Tumor diathesislike debris can be seen in women with atrophic vaginitis and severe cervicitis, so one should avoid making an overcall in these cases.

DeMay, A&S 2e. General features of carcinoma in situ, p66

203 c   type 18

Endocervical adenocarcinoma in situ, along with invasive endocervical adenocarcinoma, is closely associated with HPV type 18 and slightly less likely HPV type 16.

DeMay, A&S 2e. Cervical adenocarcinoma in situ, p86

ISBN 978-089189-6357 ©ASCP 2015

204 d high grade squamous intraepithelial lesion

Small pale cells of a HSIL can be difficult to locate and even more difficult to interpret, once they have been identified. It is clear that there exists a subset of HSIL that is very difficult to interpret correctly. Errors may be either screening or interpretive in type.

DeMay, A&S 2e. Metaplastic dysplasia, p67

205 a her risk of having biopsy proven CIN2/3 identified in the next 2 years approaches 25%

ALTS established the risk for CIN2/3 in women with LSIL, with a 2 year risk approaching 25%.

Stoler MH. ASC, TBS, and the power of ALTS. Am J Clin Pathol. Apr 2007; 127(4):489-491

206 a atypical atrophy

The diagnosis of atypical squamous cells of undetermined significance (ASCUS) includes an alteration in the normal squamous nuclear size, possibly 2-3× greater than that of a normal intermediate cell nucleus. The chromatin is finely granular, regularly distributed, and generally hypochromatic (normochromatic). A true ASCUS is a noninflammatory related change that may be related to subclinical or early manifestations of the human papillomavirus infection or dysplasia; however, ASCUS may also involve immature squamous epithelial cells as well as basal and parabasal cells found in atrophic conditions. Based on the cytologic diagnosis and the negative HPV test, the appropriate management for this patient should be a repeat Pap test in 12 months.

DeMay, A&S 2e. Atypical squamous cells of undetermined significance (ASCUS), p138

207 c adenocarcinoma, endometrial origin

Endometrial adenocarcinomas have diffusely vacuolated cytoplasm and often contain engulfed polymorphonuclear cells. Endometrial adenocarcinomas often present with fewer numbers of cells on the slide (as opposed to endocervical adenocarcinomas), cell clusters with scalloping borders and 3D tissue fragments, high N:C ratios, and frothy, delicate, lacy, vacuolated cytoplasm. Finally, the presence of a watery diathesis with associated lipophages may be helpful in discriminating endometrial adenocarcinomas from other epithelial malignancies.

DeMay, A&S 2e. Endometrial adenocarcinoma, p100-102

208 d LSIL; repeat Pap in 12 months

Adolescents (women <20) with a cytologic diagnosis of LSIL have a high rate of regression; however, immunologic clearance, followed by regression, may take several years. Because of the regressive feature of LSIL in adolescents, follow-up with annual cytologic testing is only recommended. Upon annual follow-up, only those adolescents with a cytologic diagnosis of HSIL or greater should be referred to colposcopy.

DeMay, A&S 2e. f1.19 Management of adolescent women with either ASCUS or LSIL, p150

209 b squamous cell carcinoma, nonkeratinizing type

Syncytial fragments, and cannibalism, nuclei exhibiting hyperchromasia and coarse irregular chromatin with macronucleoli are diagnostic criteria of nonkeratinizing squamous cell carcinoma of the uterine cervix. A tumor diathesis, presenting as "cotton candy" like frothy material found in the background is commonly seen with liquid based preparations as compared with the granular diathesis typical represented in conventional Pap preparations.

DeMay, A&S 2e. Nonkeratinizing squamous cell carcinoma, p73-74

210 b small cell squamous carcinoma

p16 is a cyclin-dependent kinase-4 inhibitor that is expressed in HPV associated lesions, including invasive squamous carcinomas. Endometrial cells/lesions are negative for p16. Small cell carcinomas may be poorly differentiated squamous lesions or neuroendocrine tumors, both of which arise within the endocervical canal. Poorly differentiated squamous carcinomas, such as this case from a postmenopausal patient, are composed of small cells with high N:C ratios, uniform cellular sizes with well defined borders, coarse chromatin with nucleoli, but little to absent "crush" artifact. An abnormal host response or necrotic tumor diathesis often accompanies these squamous lesions. Conversely, and as depicted in this photomicrograph, neuroendocrine small cell tumors reveal fine chromatin, inconspicuous nucleoli, and distinguished vertebral-like arrangements and nuclear molding, recapitulating their lung counterparts. These cells contain hyperchromatic stippled chromatin, coarse clumping, nuclear molding, scanty cytoplasm, and micronucleoli. They have characteristic vertebral column formation, microbiopsy aggregates, cords, nests, or ribbons. In 1/3 of the cases, neuroendocrine differentiation may be demonstrated by immunocytochemical staining with chromogranin, neuron specific enolase, or synaptophysin. Neuroendocrine differentiation (argyrophilia) may also be demonstrated.

DeMay, A&S 2e. Small cell squamous carcinoma, p72-73

211 d adenocarcinoma in situ, endocervical type

The diagnosis of endocervical adenocarcinoma in situ (AIS) may often be difficult to differentiate from squamous carcinoma in situ (CIS) with the exception that AIS often possesses feathering or pseudostratified syncytial-like fragments, stratified strips, or rosettes. The maintenance of columnar morphology may also be a key feature in establishing the diagnosis of an atypical endocervical process.

DeMay, A&S 2e. Cytology of endocervical adenocarcinoma, p93-94

212 c NILM; inflammatory cells

These cells represent normal polymorphonuclear neutrophils found in a "cannonball" formation. This phenomenon is often seen as a result of the processing associated with liquid based ThinPrep specimens. Although the majority of inflammation is eliminated with from liquid based Pap tests, a notable quantity is still represented in patients with severe inflammation. The aggregation of inflammatory cells is found in a mucous wisp and allows the reviewer to comment on acute inflammation.

DeMay, A&S 2e. Cannonballs, p297

213 d vaginal delivery should be avoided

A caesarian section recommended due to the diagnosis of herpesvirus. The presence of "ground glass" chromatin, chromatinic margination, multinucleation, and nuclear molding, with or without intranuclear eosinophilic Cowdry type A inclusions, suggests a diagnosis of herpesvirus. Grossly, these lesions appear as erythematous papules or ulcerations. They must be distinguished from other multinucleated cells found within a liquid based Pap test.

DeMay, A&S 2e. Herpes simplex virus, p34-35

214 c metastatic endometrial stromal sarcoma

Endometrial stromal sarcoma is a homologous sarcoma found as small cells or groups with high N:C ratios and coarse hyperchromatic oval nuclei, spindle shaped cells with frothy wispy cytoplasm. Since a secondary lesion has developed, direct scrapings will likely produce a diathesis similar to the original primary lesion.

DeMay, A&S 2e. Endometrial stromal sarcoma, p111

215 a metastatic colon cancer

The diagnosis of metastatic colon cancer in gynecological specimens is related to the presence of abundant abnormal palisading cells with basophilic granular cytoplasm and cigar shaped nuclei. Presence of finely granular, regularly distributed chromatin is important in the diagnosis of this disease. A diathesis may be visualized if the tumor has metastasized by direct extension or seeded within the vagina. The diagnosis of this lesion may be difficult to distinguish from endocervical adenocarcinoma; therefore, a history of normal pelvic examinations may be necessary.

DeMay, A&S 2e. Metastases, p115-116

216 b use of an intrauterine device (IUD)

Actinomyces is associated with the use of an intrauterine device (IUD).

DeMay, A&S 2e. Actinomyces, p37

217 a a spore form predominates in this species

Torulopsis glabrata has uninterrupted outer walls as well as budding encapsulated yeast, whereas *Candida* species possess pseudohyphae.

DeMay, A&S 2e. Fungi, p39-40

218 a elementary bodies

This obligate intracellular bacterium (*Chlamydia trachomatis*) is the most common cause of nongonococcal cervicitis. Cytologic changes are nonspecific and may range from cytoplasmic inclusions with fine vacuolization that do not displace the nucleus or cytoplasm (nebular bodies) to dysplastic mimicking morphology. Because these findings are neither sensitive nor specific, cytology should not be the method of detection.

DeMay, A&S 2e. Chlamydia trachomatis, p39-40

219 d diathesis changes associated with an invasive primary malignancy

A diathesis is defined as the tissue necrosis associated with an invasive malignancy. The debris includes hemolyzed red blood cells, degenerated epithelial cells, and inflammatory cells scattered in a granular or "sandy" background. Care must be taken not to confuse this process with normal necrobiosis or coccoid bacteria, which often accompany *Trichomonas vaginalis*.

DeMay, A&S 2e. Cytology of squamous cell carcinoma, p72

220 a increased risk of fetal infection, possibly resulting in death in utero

Cells with large, basophilic inclusions suggestive of an "owl's eye" are diagnostic of infection with cytomegalovirus. Occasionally, eosinophilic intracytoplasmic inclusions are found. The diagnosis is imperative in pregnant females due to the increased risk of abortion or development of severe physical and mental malformations in the fetus.

DeMay, A&S 2e. Viruses, p34-35

221 d *Trichomonas vaginalis*

Leptothrix vaginalis are long hairlike structures that tend to aggregate in the presence of *Trichomonas vaginalis*.

DeMay, A&S 2e. Protozoa, p40; Other organisms, p41

222 d adenosis

The presence of glandular or squamous metaplastic epithelium in the vagina (normally lined by native squamous epithelium) is diagnostic of vaginal adenosis. This condition has been linked to in utero exposure to diethylstilbestrol (DES).

DeMay, A&S 2e. Diethylstilbestrol, p47

223 a these cells are indicative of infection by human papillomavirus

Parakeratosis is considered ASCUS under the Bethesda terminology and not specific for the determination of an HPV infection. Only the presence of koilocytes is a specific diagnostic indicator of HPV.

DeMay, A&S 2e. Keratosis, p26-27

ISBN 978-089189-6357 ©ASCP 2015

224 b cytomegalovirus

Cells with large, basophilic inclusions suggestive of an "owl's eye" are diagnostic of an infection with cytomegalovirus. Occasionally, eosinophilic intracytoplasmic inclusions are found. The correct diagnosis is imperative in pregnant females due to the increased risk of abortion or development of severe physical and mental malformation in the fetus.

DeMay, A&S 2e. Cytomegalovirus, p35

225 b use of birth control pills

Candida species is a common yeast found in pregnancy, late luteal phase, birth control pill users, patients with diabetes mellitus, immunosuppression, or those taking broad spectrum antibiotics. The characteristic pseudohyphae structures ("sticks") and/or the presence of small spores ("stones") are necessary to establish the diagnosis.

DeMay, A&S 2e. Fungi, p39-40

226 a hyperkeratosis

Leukoplakia, clinically defined as a white patch, is the gross pathologic counterpart of hyperkeratosis acanthosis. This condition denotes the hard, cornified visible area located either on the ectocervix or vagina.

DeMay, A&S 2e. Keratosis, p26-27

227 c Geotrichum candidum

Geotrichum candidum appears as a large fungal structure that often branches at 90° angles. Diagnosis is confirmed by the evaluation of true hyphae (not pseudohyphae as in *Candida albicans*) and/or arthrospores.

DeMay, A&S 2e. Fungi, p39-40

228 b postmenopausal patient with adrenal hyperplasia

An intermediate cell/level vaginal epithelial maturation will predominate in patients taking exogenous androgens. Choice a will create superficial cell/level maturation while choices c&d are associated with deep parabasal level dematuration.

DeMay, A&S 2e. Hormonal cytology, p14

229 d suggestive of pollen

Pollen is often found in cervical smears due to aerial contamination from plant sources within the laboratory or physician's office. These structures present as transparent oval structures with a refractile glassy capsule and a thick cell wall with spikes.

DeMay, A&S 2e. Other organisms, p41

230 a may mask an underlying pathologic condition

Parakeratosis, an abortive attempt at keratinization, may overlie a serious abnormality such as infection by human papillomavirus (HPV), dysplasia, or even invasive carcinoma. The diagnosis is important and should be correlated with the surrounding cytologic findings. The finding of parakeratosis should be discriminated from related changes occurring in dyskeratocytes, atypical squamous cells suggestive of an HPV infection.

DeMay, A&S 2e. Keratosis, p26-27

231 a benign protective reaction

Hyperkeratosis is a condition of overall greater epithelial thickness (hyperdifferentiation). A stratum corneum (anucleate squames) replaces the normally nonkeratinized superficial cell layer.

DeMay, A&S 2e. Keratosis, p26-27

232 c vaginal acidity

Döderlein bacillus, or *Lactobacillus acidophilus*, is considered normal flora of the vagina. Its production of lactic acid serves as an endogenous inhibitor of microbial growth by maintaining a low pH. The organism is commonly seen in the latter half of the menstrual cycle (days 15-28), at which time glycogenated cells predominate. These organisms produce lactic acid by destroying the intermediate cells, thus creating cytolysis.

DeMay, A&S 2e. Normal flora and cytolysis, p32-34

233 b use of intrauterine devices

Actinomyces species is a filamentous bacillus that branches at acute angles and clumps together to form structures known as "sulfur granules." These entities may be found in patients who have intrauterine devices (IUDs).

DeMay, A&S 2e. Actinomyces, p37-38

234 a atrophy

Sheets of lower level parabasal to basal cells with autolytic features and degenerating karyolytic cells or "blue blobs," and the finding of pyknotic parabasal cells with eosinophilic cytoplasm, often referred to as "mummified cells," are characteristic of deep atrophy, which is often found in postmenopausal or postpartum patients. Care should be taken to discriminate these findings from more significant conditions such as parakeratosis or dyskeratosis, lesions that are associated with true keratinizing processes.

DeMay, A&S 2e. Hormonal cytology, p12-13

235 c lubricant jelly

Lubricant jelly often appears in the background of cervical smears as a blue to purple haze or tint. Differential diagnosis would include "sticky" mucus from the endocervical canal; however, mucin usually stains eosinophilic. Clinicians should apply warm water instead of lubricant to the speculum before performing a Pap test.

DeMay, A&S 2e. Arthropods and contaminants, p1478

236 c late secretory

The predominance of intermediate cells and cytolysis suggests an increased progesterone stimulation, which in turn produces epithelial dedifferentiation of the vaginal mucosa. The presence of Döderlein bacillus will often accompany these cytologic findings.

DeMay, A&S 2e. Hormonal cytology, p12-13

237 d herpesvirus

The presence of "ground glass" chromatin, chromatinic margination, multinucleation, and nuclear molding, with or without intranuclear eosinophilic Cowdry type A inclusions, suggests a diagnosis of herpesvirus. Grossly, these lesions appear as erythematous papules or ulcerations. They must be distinguished from other multinucleated cells found within smears.

DeMay, A&S 2e. Herpes simplex virus, p34-35

238 b it is impossible to predict the progression rate of the lesion

Diagnosis of human papillomavirus infection is based on the presence of koilocytes with or without associated dyskeratosis and/or immature metaplastic infected cells. The cytomorphologic diagnosis provides no information on whether the viral type is low risk (episomal) or high risk (transforming); therefore, risk prediction is not possible. Sophisticated molecular tests, including polymerase chain reaction and Southern blot analysis, may be employed to help decipher the biology of the disease.

DeMay, A&S 2e. Condyloma, p68

239 a diabetes mellitus

Patients with diabetes mellitus are at an increased risk for endogenous and exogenous vaginal infections. Fungal infections, such as the *Candida* infection shown here, are common.

DeMay, A&S 2e. Candida species, p39

240 d too long between application of mounting medium and coverslipping

Improper coverslipping may lead to "corn flaking" or brown artifact, which is most likely caused by the drying of the mounting medium before the coverslip has been placed. Gill indicates an increased occurrence with the required small fume hoods (personal communication). Conversely, water in the xylene will cause a milky haze to appear on the slide, not a brown artifact.

DeMay, A&S 2e. Hyperkeratosis, p27

241 a perimenarche

3 cell patterns (ie, superficial, intermediate, and parabasal) found simultaneously in vaginal smears are often associated with perimenarchal early squamous maturation. Parabasal cells are generally not observed in mature cycling females (as in choices b & c) and the presence of a large population of superficial cells (estrogenic stimulation, choice d) is a contraindication in postmenopausal females unless the patient is under the administration of short term exogenous estrogen therapy, or if found with other pathologic disorders such as endometrial adenocarcinomas or granulosa-theca cell tumors of the ovary.

DeMay, A&S 2e. Hormonal cytology, p10-12

242 a 0/50/50

In this example, there is a 50% admixture of superficial (pyknotic) cells and intermediate (vesicular) cells.

DeMay, A&S 2e. Hormonal cytology, p10-12

243 b menopausal patient on high dose, short term estrogen therapy

Short term estrogen therapy in many atrophic patients will create a hyperdifferentiation of the squamous mucosa of the vagina, the result being a richly estrogen primed epithelium. A predominant population of superficial cells will be observed when hormonal smears are performed on these patients. Choices a, c, and d are associated with intermediate cell/level maturation.

DeMay, A&S 2e. Hormonal cytology, p10-12

244 b vaginal adenosis

Squamous metaplasia should not be observed in mucosa of the vagina. These findings suggest possible DES exposure in utero. The presence of glandular or squamous metaplastic epithelium in the vagina (normally lined by native squamous epithelium) is diagnostic of vaginal adenosis.

DeMay, A&S 2e. Diethylstilbestrol, p47

245 a 18-year-old female with primary amenorrhea

The cellular pattern, consistent with deep parabasal cells in sheets, may represent an atrophic smear taken from a postpubertal patient with hyperestrinism. Conditions such as Turner syndrome may explain these findings.

DeMay, A&S 2e. Hormonal cytology, p12-13

246 c alkalinity

When the pH of the vagina rises, organisms such as *Candida* species tend to proliferate. Changes in the hormonal status, administration of birth control pills, pregnancy, and antibiotic therapy are other situations in which these organisms tend to flourish. The characteristic pseudohyphae structures and/or the presence of small spores are necessary to establish the diagnosis.

DeMay, A&S 2e. Fungi, p39-40

247 b molluscum contagiosum

This disease, related to the poxvirus and sexually transmitted in cases of vaginal infections, presents clinically as papillomatous skin lesions. Cytologic identification of parabasal cells with large eosinophilic intracytoplasmic inclusions and degenerated (often karyolytic) nuclei are important for the diagnosis of molluscum contagiosum.

DeMay, A&S 2e. Other viral infections, p35

248 b good prognostic information

The cytologic picture is consistent with that of pregnancy or progesterone stimulated epithelium. The administration of estrogen has no effect upon a progesterone primed epithelium; therefore, no cytohormonal deviation will be found in a normal pregnancy. Should a hormonal imbalance exist, the estrogen test would promote cellular maturation.

DeMay, A&S 2e. Hormonal cytology, p10-14

ISBN 978-089189-6357 ©ASCP 2015

249 c treat and repeat due to presence of microbiologic agent

The presence of *Trichomonas vaginalis* precludes the possibility of rendering a hormonal evaluation due to the pseudoeosinophila (a false estrogenic maturation) that is associated with its presence.

DeMay, A&S 2e. Specific infections, p111

250 d late proliferative phase of the menstrual cycle

Choice d indicates a hyperestrogenic pattern which should predominate in a normal mature cycling female prior to ovulation. Estrogen primed epithelium should consist of a superficial cell/level maturation, whereas the hormonal pattern depicted in this photomicrograph is consistent with a progesterone stimulated mucosa, such as the maturation levels found in choices a, b, and c.

DeMay, A&S 2e. Hormonal cytology, p10-14

251 a pleomorphism/caudate shape/opaque, irregular chromatin distribution

The cytologic attributes described represent squamous cell carcinoma. Choice b represents an adenocarcinoma, choice c is diagnostic of immature metaplastic cells, and choice d represents a diagnosis of reparative/reactive changes.

DeMay, A&S 2e. Keratinizing squamous cell carcinoma, p74-75

252 c adenocarcinoma in situ/carcinoma in situ

Abnormal cells lacking nuclear polarity, containing hyperchromatic nuclei with fine to coarse and even chromatin, and arranged in single cells or syncytia are suggestive of an in situ lesion. The differential diagnosis between squamous and endocervical in situ lesions depends on many features, including the cell shape (columnar-endocervical) and/or accompanying dysplasia (squamous). Feathering or splattering cytoplasmic processes are often associated with endocervical lesions.

DeMay, A&S 2e. Differential diagnosis of carcinoma in situ, p90-91

253 d squamous cell carcinoma, keratinizing type

These cells are demonstrating cellular pleomorphism, orangeophilia, and irregular, hyperchromatic, opaque nuclei. The background contains a granular diathesis. The presence of single cells with these characteristics is diagnostic of a squamous cell carcinoma.

DeMay, A&S 2e. Keratinizing squamous cell carcinoma, p74-75

254 c endometrial adenocarcinoma

Stein-Leventhal disease (SLD) is associated with hyperestrinism. Endometrial adenocarcinoma (EA), a disease more commonly found in peri- and postmenopausal women, has been linked to excessive or unopposed estrogen levels. Patients with SLD are at a greater risk for carcinogenic development. The cells of EA are found in clusters, have nuclei similar to that of an intermediate squamous cell, and possess irregular chromatin, macronucleoli, and anisokaryosis. Often, a watery diathesis is present.

DeMay, A&S 2e. Endometrial adenocarcinoma, p103-105

255 d chronic lymphocytic cervicitis

Chronic lymphocytic cervicitis is associated with findings of small and large lymphocytes (immunoblasts), plasma cells, and tingible body macrophages. The cellular findings are always single cells without cohesiveness. In contrast, small cell neuroendocrine carcinoma maintains nuclear molding, vertebral column formation, and coarse chromatin patterns.

DeMay, A&S 2e. Follicular cervicitis, p31-32

256 d unsatisfactory for evaluation because of drying artifact

Air drying or inadequate fixation often creates cellular ballooning, karyorrhexis, karyolysis, and cytolytic features, thus preventing evaluation of the cellular sample.

DeMay, A&S 2e. Specimen adequacy, p145

257 b pouch of Douglas

The pouch of Douglas contains cells indigenous to body cavities such as mesenchymal elements.

DeMay, A&S 2e. Culdocentesis, p331

258 a radiation changes

Radiation changes include cytomegaly with proportionate karyomegaly, normal N:C ratios, and hypochromatic nuclei. Recurrent squamous carcinoma possesses true hyperchromasia and intact coarse irregular chromatin, often in the presence of accompanying diathesis.

DeMay, A&S 2e. Radiation cytology, p42-44

259 c endocervical area

Endocervical cells possess well defined borders with honeycombing, picket fence, or single columnar cell forms. The nuclei are vesicular and often contain micronucleoli. These cells must be distinguished from endometrial cells, which present in 3D clusters or as single cells with frothy cytoplasm.

DeMay, A&S 2e. Squamous metaplasia, p23-24

260 c endometrium

Normal endometrial glandular cells often occur in 3D ("double contour") cell balls, but often occur singly. The cells present with round to oval (often degenerated) nuclei and scanty ill defined basophilic cytoplasm.

DeMay, A&S 2e. Endometrial cells, p18-20

261 c mucinous cystadenocarcinoma, ovarian primary

The finding of large cells with distended, vacuolated cytoplasm, anisonucleosis, irregular nuclear membranes, irregular chromatin, hyperchromasia, macronucleoli, and signet ring morphology from a female with a peritoneal effusion suggests mucinous adenocarcinoma of the ovary. Special staining for mucin is necessary to confirm the diagnosis. Differential diagnoses include metastatic gastrointestinal tract malignancies (especially poorly differentiated adenocarcinoma of the stomach) and primary mucinous adenocarcinoma of the endometrium.

DeMay, A&S 2e. Metastases, p115-117

262 a erosion

The presence of endocervical components on the ectocervical region suggests a rolling out of these cells during processes such as erosion. This may occur as a normal process during menarche or as a result of pathogenic infection.

DeMay, A&S 2e. Endocervical cells, p14-17

263 b adenocarcinoma, fallopian tube

These cells possess typical features of an adenocarcinoma: 3D clusters, anisokaryosis, irregular chromatin, and nucleoli. The clinical feature of a profuse watery discharge and the negative clinical indicators suggest fallopian tube adenocarcinoma.

DeMay, A&S 2e. Odds and ends, p121

264 c LSIL; ablation without histologic confirmation is considered unacceptable

All low grade lesions (HPV changes, mild dysplasia/CIN1) should be histologically confirmed to rule out a more invasive process.

DeMay, A&S 2e. Algorithms for Pap test management from the ASCCP, p151

265 c endometrial adenocarcinoma, grade I

The depicted cells are diagnostic of well differentiated endometrial adenocarcinoma, grade I. These cells demonstrate cellular clusters with nuclear overlapping, anisonucleosis, irregular chromatin, and macronucleoli. A granular basophilic (watery) diathesis as well as the presence of old and fresh blood is often associated with these tumors.

DeMay, A&S 2e. Endometrial adenocarcinoma, p103-105

266 c navicular cells

Often referred as "boat shaped," these glycogenated cells are indicative of a progesterone stimulated epithelium. They must be differentiated from koilocytes infected by HPV, which have true cytoplasmic margination (cavelike), raisinoid nuclei, smudged degenerative chromatin, or well preserved nuclei with binucleation.

DeMay, A&S 2e. Cytology of pregnancy, p50

267 d endometrial adenocarcinoma

The presence of endometrial cells in a postmenopausal female raises suspicion of a possible endometrial neoplasm. These cells demonstrate cellular clusters with overlapping nuclei, anisonucleosis, irregular chromatin, and macronucleoli. A granular basophilic (watery) diathesis as well as the presence of old and fresh blood is often associated with these tumors.

DeMay, A&S 2e. Endometrial adenocarcinoma, p103-105

268 d immature metaplastic

Immature metaplasia is usually parabasal in size with basophilic cytoplasm, well defined borders, and vesicular nuclei. Often a pavement configuration, remnants of cobblestone patterns (not unlike those of Charleston's streets) or the "cookie cutter" look is seen. These cells may possess spinelike or "spider cell" cytoplasmic processes when forcibly removed, or have ectoplasm/endoplasm rims when exfoliated.

DeMay, A&S 2e. Squamous metaplasia, p23-24

269 c possible exposure to diethylstilbestrol (DES) in utero

Vaginal adenosis is defined as the presence of ectopic glandular epithelium or squamous metaplastic cells within the normally gland free or squamous lined vagina. The presence of these cells is increased in those patients who were exposed to diethylstilbestrol (DES) in utero.

DeMay, A&S 2e. Diethylstilbestrol, p47

270 a endometrial stromal cells, in cycle

The photomicrograph represents normal stromal cells from the endometrial cavity. These cells, both deep (stratum spongiosa) and superficial (stratum compacta), are normally present in the first half of the menstrual cycle. Deep stromal cells possess spindle shaped cytoplasm with oval nuclei whereas superficial stromal cells generally contain reniform, kidney bean or boomerang shaped nuclear features and frothy cytoplasm.

DeMay, A&S 2e. Endometrial stromal cells, p20

271 a within normal limits, negative for squamous intraepithelial lesion

Normal cellular elements from squamous and endocervical origin are necessary for a cell sample to be considered negative for squamous intraepithelial lesion.

DeMay, A&S 2e. General categorization, p145

272 b endometrial hyperplasia

The presence of normal endometrial cells at times other than days 1-14 of the menstrual cycle may be related to a hyperplastic endometrium. Cytologic features are those of normal endometrial cells. Atypical (complex) endometrial hyperplasia may be difficult to distinguish from a frankly invasive malignant process. Tissue confirmation is strongly suggested, especially in those women approaching menopause.

DeMay, A&S 2e. Histology of endometrial hyperplasia and carcinoma, p102-103

273 c mixed Müllerian tumor, homologous type

The identification of endometrial carcinoma with concomitant leiomyosarcoma or endometrial stromal sarcoma is necessary to establish the diagnosis of a homologous mixed Müllerian tumor.

DeMay, A&S 2e. Mixed Müllerian tumor, p112

ISBN 978-089189-6357 ©ASCP 2015

274 a   production of lactic acid

Döderlein bacillus, or *Lactobacillus acidophilus,* is considered normal flora of the vagina. Its production of lactic acid serves as an endogenous inhibitor of microbial growth by maintaining a low pH. The organism is commonly seen in the latter half of the menstrual cycle (days 15-28), at which time glycogenated cells predominate. These organisms produce lactic acid by utilizing the glycogen in intermediate cells, thus creating cytolysis.

DeMay, A&S 2e. Normal flora and cytolysis, p33

275 b   endometrial adenocarcinoma, grade I

Well differentiated endometrial adenocarcinomas (type I) often appear in patients with a history of hyperestrinism and endometrial hyperplasia. These lesions have enlarged nuclei, irregularly aggregated chromatin, and slight nucleolar enlargement. Neutrophils may be present within the cytoplasm of these neoplastic cells. A watery diathesis, presenting as a finely granular, basophilic diathesis, often accompanies the malignant cellular components.

DeMay, A&S 2e. Endometrial adenocarcinoma, p103-104

276 c   karyorrhectic

Chromatinic nuclear membranes and broken or interrupted nuclear membranes are associated with karyorrhexis. Other types of nuclear degeneration include karyopyknosis (condensed) and karyolysis (dissolution).

DeMay, A&S 2e. Inflammation and inflammatory change, p28-30

277 d   *Actinomyces* species

Actinomyces species is a filamentous bacillus that branches at acute angles and clumps together to form structures known as "sulfur granules." These entities are often associated with patients who have intrauterine devices (IUDs).

DeMay, A&S 2e. Other organisms and specific infections, p37-38

278 a   adenomyosis

The presence of ectopic normal endometrial glands embedded within the smooth muscular layer of the uterus is diagnostic of adenomyosis. Cytologic features are those of normal endometrial cells. Endometriosis may be intramural, submucosal, or subserosal.

DeMay, A&S 2e. Endometriosis, p81

279 b   deliver via cesarean

The cytologic findings are consistent with a herpetic infection. In this example, the fetus is at an increased risk of infection due to exposure to the mother's infected birth canal. Neonatal infection can be life threatening.

DeMay, A&S 2e. Other organisms and specific infections, p34

280 c   unopposed estrogen stimulation

Endometrial adenocarcinoma has been linked to increased exposure or unopposed estrogen. Estrogen most likely acts as a promoter in the development of this disease.

DeMay, A&S 2e. Endometrial adenocarcinoma, p103-105

281 d   leiomyosarcoma

These cells suggest a sarcomatous neoplasm, most consistent with a leiomyosarcoma. Cytology reveals spindle cells with pleomorphic features, giant cells, and isolated cells with fibrillar cytoplasm and oval nucleoli. The chromatin is finely granular and irregularly distributed, and may or may not contain nucleoli. Leiomyosarcomas represent the most common sarcomatous lesion of the uterus. These lesions represent a malignant transformation of the indigenous smooth muscle elements.

DeMay, A&S 2e. General features of sarcomas, p110

282 a   frothy, yellow-green discharge/strawberry cervix

Trichomonas vaginalis parasites are transmitted through sexual contact. Cytologically they appear as small gray to blue, faint staining, pear shaped structures with eccentric nuclei. Flagella are rare unless preparation is with cellular suspension process. These organisms are often accompanied by coccoid bacteria and *Leptothrix.*

DeMay, A&S 2e. Trichomonas vaginalis, p40-41

283 d   Turner syndrome

Turner syndrome patients are ahormonal due to ovarian agenesis. A predominant population of basal to parabasal cells would characterize the vaginal smear pattern. Choices a, b, and c are all associated with hyperestrinism.

DeMay, A&S 2e. Hormonal cytology, p13

284 b   nucleoli, diathesis, irregular chromatin distribution

These cells represent nonkeratinizing squamous cell carcinoma, a neoplasm that must be differentiated from that of its precursor, carcinoma in situ (CIS). CIS usually possesses regular chromatin, lacks nucleoli and has a clean "diathesis free" background.

DeMay, A&S 2e. Nonkeratinizing squamous cell carcinoma, p73-74

285 b   internal cervical os

These cells are diagnostic of a high grade squamous intraepithelial lesion of metaplastic origin. Metaplastic dysplasia arises from immature metaplastic areas within the endocervical canal, in contrast to nonkeratinizing dysplasias, which arise from mature areas of metaplasia, distal to the ectocervix.

DeMay, A&S 2e. Metaplastic dysplasia, p67-68

286 d   squamous atypia/mature metaplastic ASCUS (mimicking mature native squames)

The diagnosis of atypical squamous cells of undetermined significance (ASCUS) should be rendered when the cells lack the specific features necessary to diagnosis dysplasia, including hyperchromasia and increased N:C ratios. Cells diagnostic of ASCUS or squamous atypia (mature metaplastic derivative) typically have slightly increased nuclear sizes (2-3× that of a normal intermediate cell nucleus) and hypochromasia. In the absence of true inflammatory sequelae this diagnosis may be necessary. The diagnosis of ASCUS is considered a slight risk for the subsequent development of HPV or dysplasia.

DeMay, A&S 2e. Atypical squamous cells, p55-56

287 b low

Keratinizing and nonkeratinizing squamous carcinomas have a low mitotic rate in comparison with that of small cell squamous carcinomas.

DeMay, A&S 2e. Keratinizing squamous cell carcinoma, p74-75; Nonkeratinizing squamous cell carcinoma, p55-56

288 d reparative/regenerative changes secondary to therapy

Reparative changes secondary to cauterization must be discriminated from true dysplastic or invasive squamous processes. As described earlier, reparative/regenerative cells often contain macronucleoli, respectable polarity, and/or cytoplasmic streaming. The predictability of these cells is important in establishing their benignity. A necrotic background may be found secondary to cauterization, especially if smears are performed shortly after therapy.

DeMay, A&S 2e. Repair/regeneration, p30-31

289 b radiation induced cell changes

The cytologic changes associated with radiation include cytomegaly (macrocytic changes) and karyomegaly. The maintenance of normal N:C ratios and the evidence of cytoplasmic vacuolization (related to degeneration) are characteristic of these cells. The nuclei associated with radiation cell changes are often degenerative or preserved and multinucleated, while the cytoplasmic staining is polychromatic and amphophilic.

DeMay, A&S 2e. Radiation cytology, p42-44

290 c normal endometrial cells, possibly associated with endometrial hyperplasia

Endometrial cells identified outside of the proliferative phase of the menstrual cycle (days 14-28) are considered abnormal in the absence of appropriate clinical history. Normal endometrial cells may be associated with hyperplasia, a predisposing condition for endometrial adenocarcinoma.

DeMay, A&S 2e. Histology of endometrial hyperplasia and carcinoma, p102-103

291 d 100%

Carcinoma in situ of the cervix replaces the full epithelial thickness of the squamous mucosa with primitive cells, resulting in a total loss of cellular maturation throughout the epithelial strata.

DeMay, A&S 2e. Introduction to diagnosis of squamous intraepithelial lesions, p64-65

292 a atypia of atrophy

Atypical cells associated with atrophy are basal to parabasal cells in single syncytial-like arrangements or hyperchromatic crowded groups (HCGs) found amongst a granular precipitate containing degenerated epithelial cells and scattered red and white blood cells. The chromatin, if visible, is fine and evenly distributed. More commonly, the chromatin of these atypical cells is poorly preserved, smudged, and indistinct. In comparison with dysplasia or cancer, the chromatin of truly dysplastic lesions is described as distinct and "crisp," whereas malignant lesions generally possess coarsely granular, irregularly distributed chromatin.

DeMay, A&S 2e. Atypia of atrophy and maturity, p60-61

293 a normal endometrial cells

The finding of normal endometrial cells within the proliferative phase of the menstrual cycle is common. Parenchymal epithelial cells may present in 3D clusters or as single cells with normally high N:C ratios, nuclear hypochromasia, finely granular, evenly distributed chromatin, and micronuclei. Stromal cells are often seen between days 6 and 10. Deep stromal cells are fibroblastic, whereas superficial stromal cells resemble histiocytes (with reniform nuclei).

DeMay, A&S 2e. Endometrial cells, p18-20

294 a HSIL, moderate nonkeratinizing dysplasia

Nonkeratinizing dysplasias are the most common morphologic variant of dysplasia and less apt to progress to more invasive processes. The nuclei of these cells are large compared with immature metaplastic dysplasia, the texture of the cytoplasm is translucent, and the N:C ratios increase correspondingly with the degree of severity.

DeMay, A&S 2e. General features of dysplasia, p65-66

295 c immature metaplastic transformational zone

These cells are diagnostic of a high grade squamous intraepithelial lesion of metaplastic origin. Metaplastic dysplasia arises from immature metaplastic areas within the endocervical canal, in contrast to nonkeratinizing dysplasias, which arise from mature areas of metaplasia, distal to the ectocervix.

DeMay, A&S 2e. Metaplastic dysplasia, p67

296 c irregular chromatin

These cells are diagnostic of nonkeratinizing squamous cell carcinoma. Important features that are helpful in establishing the diagnosis of this lesion are the presence of irregularly distributed chromatin, nucleoli, and a diathesis—3 key features absent in squamous carcinoma in situ.

DeMay, A&S 2e. Nonkeratinizing squamous cell carcinoma, p73-74

ISBN 978-089189-6357 ©ASCP 2015

297 a squamous cell carcinoma, keratinizing type

Keratinizing squamous carcinomas generally originate on the anterior cervical lip. The single or syncytial-like pleomorphic to bizarre tadpole or spindle cell formations are the trademarks of this lesion. The cells may stain orangeophilic or cyanophilic; however, eosinophilia is more often seen. A granular diathesis may or may not be present due to the exophytic nature of this lesion. Pearl formations, parakeratosis, and hyperkeratosis may accompany the malignant cells.

DeMay, A&S 2e. Squamous cell carcinoma, p71-72; Keratinizing squamous cell carcinoma, p74-75

298 a pleomorphism

The more undifferentiated or anaplastic the squamous lesion becomes, the more likely the cells will begin to recapitulate each other and become more "clone" like. In keratinizing malignancies, pleomorphism will decrease with an increasing tumor grade.

DeMay, A&S 2e. Keratinizing squamous cell carcinoma, p74-75

299 b a hyperdifferentiation that places the patient at a higher risk for postirradiation dysplasia

Patients who have an abrupt rise in maturation or hyperdifferentiation of the squamous mucosa after receiving radiation therapy for squamous carcinoma are at an increased risk for recurrence. Other key indicators include the presence of spindle cells and tissue necrosis.

DeMay, A&S 2e. Postadiation dysplasia, p45-46

300 a strips of pseudostratified or "feathering" epithelium in glandular lesions

The diagnosis of endocervical adenocarcinoma in situ (AIS) may often be difficult to differentiate from squamous carcinoma in situ (CIS) with the exception that AIS often possesses feathering or pseudostratified syncytial-like fragments, stratified strips, or rosettes. The maintenance of columnar morphology may also be a key feature in establishing the diagnosis of an atypical endocervical process.

DeMay, A&S 2e. Cytology of adenocarcinoma in situ, p87-89

301 a coarse chromatin

Cells with coarse even chromatin patterns arranged within syncytial-like aggregates amongst a "clean" background are diagnostic of squamous carcinoma in situ. These cells must be discriminated from their precursor lesion–severe dysplasia–a process that possesses finely granular, evenly distributed chromatin.

DeMay, A&S 2e. General features of carcinoma in situ, p66

302 b it is less common

Immature metaplastic dysplasia is less frequent than nonkeratinizing squamous dysplasias, which arise from mature metaplastic epithelium.

DeMay, A&S 2e. Metaplastic dysplasia, p67-68

303 d rosettes, acinar morphology, feathering cytoplasmic borders

The diagnosis of endocervical adenocarcinoma in situ (AIS) may often be difficult to differentiate from squamous carcinoma in situ (CIS) with the exception that AIS often possesses feathering or pseudostratified syncytial-like fragments, stratified strips, or rosettes. The maintenance of columnar morphology may also be a key feature in establishing the diagnosis of an atypical endocervical process.

DeMay, A&S 2e. Cytology of adenocarcinoma in situ, p87-89

304 b small cell carcinoma in situ

The presence of small cell carcinoma in situ may be difficult to distinguish from frankly invasive small cell carcinoma in endocervical smears. The absence of a necrotic diathesis as well as the presence of coarse regular chromatin may help confirm small cell carcinoma in situ. Small cell lesions arise from atypical reserve cells, foregoing the morphologic spectrum associated with dysplastic lesions arising from the mature and immature metaplastic zones.

DeMay, A&S 2e. General features of carcinoma in situ, p66

305 d atrophic vaginitis

Sheets of lower level parabasal to basal cells with autolytic features and degenerating karyolytic cells ("blue blobs"), and the finding of pyknotic parabasal cells with eosinophilic cytoplasm, often referred to as "mummified cells," are characteristic of deep atrophy, as may be found in postmenopausal or postpartum patients. Care should be taken to discriminate these findings from more significant conditions such as parakeratosis or dyskeratosis, lesions associated with true keratinizing processes.

DeMay, A&S 2e. Atypia of atrophy and maturity, p60-61

306 d ectocervical, mature metaplastic

These cells represent a moderate nonkeratinizing dysplasia, a high grade squamous intraepithelial lesion. Their origin is distal to the ectocervical canal within areas of mature metaplastic epithelium. The clinical course for nonkeratinizing dysplasia is generally less severe.

DeMay, A&S 2e. Metaplastic dysplasia, p67-68

307 b pleomorphic, caudate, spindled

This tissue section reveals a keratinizing squamous carcinoma of the cervix. Histopathologic findings include pleomorphism, orangeophilia, pearl formation, and stromal invasion.

DeMay, A&S 2e. Squamous cell carcinoma, p72-73; Keratinizing squamous cell carcinoma, p74-75

308 b verrucous

Pleomorphic or keratinizing squamous carcinoma generally occurs as an exophytic (verrucous) lesion. The lesion may be papillary, cauliflower form, or everted.

DeMay, A&S 2e. Squamous cell carcinoma, p72-73; Keratinizing squamous cell carcinoma, p74-75

309 b no

Although the presence of koilocytes is a specific cytologic criterion for the detection of HPV, the specific histologic pattern cannot be predicted with cytology. HPV may manifest itself histologically as papillomatous, flat, or inverted. In addition, cytologic identification of HPV is neither sensitive nor specific in determining whether the patient is infected with a "low" or "high" risk viral type, nor can it help in predicting the possibility of progression to dysplasia or cancer.

DeMay, A&S 2e. Condyloma, p68-69

310 c nonkeratinizing squamous carcinoma, moderately differentiated

Moderately differentiated squamous carcinomas of the cervix present with classic malignant morphology. Numerous populations of single cells and/or syncytial aggregates with large nuclear sizes, coarse irregular chromatin patterns, and macronucleoli scattered amongst a granular diathesis validate the diagnosis. Stripped nuclei are often found in association with the above criteria.

DeMay, A&S 2e. Nonkeratinizing squamous cell carcinoma, p73-74

311 a follicular cervicitis

The diagnosis of follicular cervicitis must be discriminated from other benign conditions including microglandular hyperplasia, degenerating neutrophils, and small cell histiocytes. When establishing a diagnosis of follicular cervicitis, the presence of small mature lymphocytes and large immunoblasts in an admixture of plasma cells and tingible body macrophages identifies this process.

DeMay, A&S 2e. Follicular cervicitis, p31-32

312 d squamous cell carcinoma, nonkeratinizing type

Single cells, syncytial fragments, and naked nuclei exhibiting hyperchromasia and coarse irregular chromatin with macronucleoli are diagnostic criteria of nonkeratinizing squamous cell carcinoma of the uterine cervix. A tumor diathesis is more commonly seen in nonkeratinizing carcinomas than in keratinizing malignancies.

DeMay, A&S 2e. Nonkeratinizing squamous cell carcinoma, p73-74

313 d postirradiation dysplasia

An indication of postirradiation dysplasia of the cervix may be the presence of dysplastic cells with high N:C ratios and hyperchromatic nuclei. The nuclear chromatin pattern is often too dense to interpret. Small cell type postirradiation dysplasia is more likely to be found in older age groups. These cells mimic small cell carcinoma in situ; however, any grade of postirradiation dysplasia recurring within 3 years carries a poor prognosis.

DeMay, A&S 2e. Postradiation dysplasia, p45-46

314 d small cell neuroendocrine carcinoma

Small cell carcinomas may be poorly differentiated squamous lesions or neuroendocrine tumors, both of which arise within the endocervical canal. Poorly differentiated squamous carcinomas are composed of small cells with high N:C ratios, uniform cellular sizes with well defined borders, coarse chromatin with nucleoli, but little to absent "crush" artifact. An abnormal host response or necrotic tumor diathesis often accompanies these squamous lesions. Conversely, and as depicted in this photomicrograph, neuroendocrine small cell tumors reveal fine chromatin, inconspicuous nucleoli, and distinguished vertebral-like arrangements and nuclear molding, recapitulating their lung counterparts. These cells contain hyperchromatic stippled chromatin, coarse clumping, nuclear molding, scanty cytoplasm, and micronucleoli. They have characteristic vertebral column formation, microbiopsy aggregates, cords, nests, or ribbons. In 1/3 of the cases, neuroendocrine differentiation may be demonstrated by immunocytochemical staining with chromogranin, neuron specific enolase, or synaptophysin. Neuroendocrine differentiation (argyrophilia) may also be demonstrated.

DeMay, A&S 2e. Small cell neuroendocrine carcinoma, p107-108

315 a benign radiation cellular changes

The cells depicted in this photomicrograph are consistent with the benign cellular changes associated with radiation cell injury. The cytologic changes associated with radiation include cytomegaly (macrocytic changes) and karyomegaly. The maintenance of normal N:C ratios and the evidence of cytoplasmic vacuolization (related to degeneration) are characteristic of these cells. The nuclei associated with radiation cell changes are often degenerative or preserved and multinucleated, while the cytoplasmic staining is polychromatic and amphophilic. Recurrent squamous carcinoma possesses true hyperchromasia and intact coarse irregular chromatin, often in the presence of accompanying diathesis.

DeMay, A&S 2e. Radiation cytology, p42-44

316 b negative for squamous intraepithelial lesion with radiation induced cellular changes

Benign radiation changes include vacuolization of the cytoplasm, macrocytosis, amphophilia, nucleomegaly, and well preserved N:C ratios. Nuclear pyknosis and karyorrhexis are degenerative changes associated with benign radiation changes. The cytoplasmic staining is polychromatic and amphophilic.

DeMay, A&S 2e. Radiation cytology, p42-44

317 a postirradiation dysplasia

The cytology of postirradiation dysplasia mirrors that found in ordinary dysplasia. The large cell type is generally seen in younger women, whereas a small cell type may be more common in older women.

DeMay, A&S 2e. Radiation cytology, p42-44

ISBN 978-089189-6357 ©ASCP 2015

318 b syncytial-like

Syncytial-like aggregates, or hyperchromatic crowded "chaotic" groups (HCGs), with indistinct cell borders are associated with squamous carcinoma in situ. Distinguishing these aggregates from true papillary tissue fragments with community borders, well formed glandular structures, or HCGs with feathery edges may help in differentiating glandular lesions from those of squamous origin.
DeMay, A&S 2e. Carcinoma in situ, p70-71

319 d in the transformation zone

Squamous metaplasia, a common protective reaction found in mature cycling females, is a result of transformation of one adult type of epithelial tissue to another adult epithelial tissue via reserve cell hyperplasia. The finding of parabasal to intermediate cells in pavement or "cobblestone" configuration, either in pools or as single cells, is diagnostic. Squamous metaplasia is often associated with trauma, inflammation, or other endocrine disturbances. Squamocolumnar junctions, abrupt junctions occurring in young children, do not have associated transitional or transformational metaplastic zones.
DeMay, A&S 2e. Squamous metaplasia, p23-24

320 c chronic follicular cervicitis

Chronic follicular cervicitis is a diffuse or localized lymphocytic infiltration as identified in cervical/vaginal smears. Small (mature) and large (immunoblastic) lymphocytes, plasma cells, and tingible body macrophages (intracytoplasmic inclusions) are necessary to establish this diagnosis.
DeMay, A&S 2e. Follicular cervicitis, p31-32

321 c severe cervicitis

These cells are representative of a severe inflammatory exudate associated with acute inflammations. A hypercellular population of polymorphonuclear neutrophils is seen.
DeMay, A&S 2e. Background features of inflammation, p30

322 b possible fetal death in utero

A pure population of superficial cells suggests an estrogenic effect that is contraindicative for a normal pregnancy.
DeMay, A&S 2e. Cytology of pregnancy, p50

323 b clean—no tumor diathesis

The background in this benign condition is clean and free of necrosis. Malignancy associated cellular backgrounds are generally composed of diathesis consisting of old and fresh blood, degenerated surrounding tissue, necrotic tumor cells, and assorted white blood cells.
DeMay, A&S 2e. Intermediate predominant maturation index, p13

324 a microglandular hyperplasia

Synonyms include birth control pill changes and pseudoparakeratosis (pseudokeratosis). These cells represent degenerated forms of hyperplastic endocervical glandular mucosa. The findings are often associated with patients taking oral contraceptives, late luteal phase, and late pregnancy. They are benign cellular findings; however, the differentiation from true parakeratosis is imperative. Cells from microglandular hyperplasia generally have eosinophilic or basophilic cytoplasm, contain eccentrically located nuclei, or resemble reactive endocervical cells. Parakeratosis represents a true keratinizing process (orangeophilia) with centrally located pyknotic nuclei in polygonal "waxy" cytoplasm (possibly with accompanying HPV changes).
DeMay, A&S 2e. Microglandular endocervical hyperplasia, p47-48

325 c serum levels

A serum analysis is considered the gold standard for determining hormonal levels.
DeMay, A&S 2e. Hormonal cytology, p10-12

326 a Cushing syndrome

Cushing syndrome is a physiologic condition related to an overproduction of cortisol by the adrenal gland. This effect may be secondary to hyperplasia, pheochromocytoma, or adrenal cortical adenoma. Afflicted women present with buffalo obesity, a moon shaped face, and hirsutism. The vaginal smear pattern is generally intermediate maturation but may be atrophic.
Keebler CM, Somrak TM. The Manual of Cytotechnology. Endocrinopathies, p74-78

327 a reparative/regenerative process

Squamous reparative/regenerative changes must be discriminated from low grade squamous epithelial lesions or those of more significance. Sheets of cells with distinct cytoplasmic borders and/or cytoplasmic streaming may be helpful in establishing the benign nature of these cells. Normal N:C ratios, normochromasia, and nucleoli are also helpful diagnostic features.
DeMay, A&S 2e. Repair/regeneration, p30-31

328 c pemphigus vulgaris

A bullous disease of the skin, pemphigus vulgaris is a condition that destroys the squamous tonofilaments, producing a sloughing of the skin. Reactive/reparative cells with bullet shaped nucleoli are generally found amongst fine, even chromatin patterns. Clinical history is essential to rule out a possible abnormality. Tzanck tests are negative.
DeMay, A&S 2e. Pemphigus vulgaris, p53

329 a   correlates with history

Stein-Leventhal syndrome is associated with a thickening of the tunica albuginea of the ovary, resulting in the inability to expel the ovum. Patients with this condition are often overweight and have secondary amenorrhea. Vaginal smear patterns in these patients show intermediate to superficial cell maturation.

Keebler CM, Somrak TM. The Manual of Cytotechnology. Endocrinopathies, p74-78

330 c   HSIL, keratinizing variety

Keratinizing or pleomorphic dysplasia (CIN mimicking keratosis) cytologically presents with well defined borders, dense refractile cytoplasm, and hyperchromatic, fine to coarse, regular chromatin or India ink pyknosis. These cells may often stain orangeophilic. The degree of pleomorphism is most important when establishing the severity of keratinizing dysplasia. Associated changes include hyperkeratosis, parakeratosis, and dyskeratosis.

DeMay, A&S 2e. Keratinizing dysplasia, p68

331 c   LSIL, HPV

The identification of koilocytes are compulsory findings for establishing the diagnosis of HPV. The 2001 Bethesda System classifies condyloma acuminata (human papillomavirus [HPV]) as a low grade squamous epithelial lesion.

DeMay, A&S 2e. Condyloma, p68-70

332 a   del Castillo syndrome

Patients with del Castillo syndrome present with a milky discharge in the absence of recent delivery. These patients may have previously taken birth control pills and a milky breast discharge may be elaborated. The pituitary gland shuts down the production of follicle stimulating hormone and luteinizing hormone. Therefore, the hormonal pattern of these patients is atrophic.

Keebler CM, Somrak TM. The Manual of Cytotechnology. Endocrinopathies, p74-78

333 b   the hormonal analysis is not compatible with history

Patients with feminizing testicular syndrome are responsive to the endogenous effects of estrogens; therefore, a hormonal analysis would show a maturation pattern consisting of mixed intermediate and superficial cells. Instead, this photomicrograph reveals a deep atrophic condition, suggesting male pseudohermaphroditism.

Keebler CM, Somrak TM. The Manual of Cytotechnology. Endocrinopathies, p74-78

334 b   high grade intraepithelial lesion, metaplastic dysplasia

Immature metaplastic cells may give rise (if initiated) to metaplastic dysplasias, whereas mature metaplastic cells are linked to nonkeratinizing dysplasia. Atypical reserve cell hyperplasia is related to the development of small cell lesions (choice c), and small cell carcinoma in situ gives rise to small cell carcinoma (choice d).

DeMay, A&S 2e. Metaplastic dysplasia, p67

335 d   granulosa-theca cell tumor

Feminizing tumors, such as granulosa-theca cell tumors, overproduce estrogen, hence typically increased maturation on the vaginal smear. These tumors may be related to precocious puberty as well as endometrial adenocarcinoma.

Keebler CM, Somrak TM. The Manual of Cytotechnology. Endocrinopathies. p74-78

336 b   reparative/regenerative process

These cells are representative of squamous reparative/ regenerative changes. Sheets of cells with well defined cytoplasmic borders, preserved nuclear polarity, predictable nuclear features, fine regular chromatin patterns, micro- to macronucleoli, and characteristic cytoplasmic streaming are diagnostic of repair. This process is often associated with trauma, cervicitis, and inflammatory etiology. The background of reparative/regenerative conditions is clean and free of necrosis.

DeMay, A&S 2e. Repair/regeneration, p30-31

337 d   mature metaplastic cells

Nonkeratinizing dysplasias (CIN mimicking mature squamous metaplasia) arise from mature metaplastic areas of the transformational zone.

DeMay, A&S 2e. Squamous metaplasia, p23-24

338 c   Turner syndrome

Turner syndrome is a nondisjunction of the X chromosome. These patients are described as sex chromatin negative, or 45XO. Occasionally, mosaicism may be found. These patients have a low hairline, pigmented nevi, and increased carrying angle of their arms. Ovarian agenesis leaves streaks of connective tissue instead of viable ovaries. The vaginal smear pattern is atrophic.

Keebler CM, Somrak TM. The Manual of Cytotechnology. Endocrinopathies, p74-78

339 b   absence of a diathesis

Metastatic carcinomas usually lack a notable diathesis unless tumor seeding has occurred within the ectopic area.

DeMay, A&S 2e. Metastases, p115-116

340 a   follicular cytosis

Follicular cytosis is associated with ovarian follicle persistence, thus forming cystic structures. The increase in endogenous estrogen produces a vaginal smear pattern with a predominant superficial cell pattern.

Keebler CM, Somrak TM. The Manual of Cytotechnology. Endocrinopathies, p74-78

341 a   N:C ratio

One of the most important criteria for distinguishing low grade squamous epithelial lesions from those of high grade variety is the N:C ratio. As the N:C ratio increases, so does the severity of dysplasia. The cells depicted in this photomicrograph represent a moderate dysplastic process.

DeMay, A&S 2e. Morphology of dysplasia and carcinoma in situ, p65-66

ISBN 978-089189-6357 ©ASCP 2015

342 c severe nonkeratinizing dysplasia, HSIL

Severe nonkeratinizing dysplasia cytologically presents as small immature metaplastic cells with hyperchromasia, high N:C ratios, and a thin rim of cytoplasm. The absence of coarse and irregular chromatin, nucleoli and/or diathesis should help discriminate these cells from a carcinoma in situ or an invasive malignancy.

DeMay, A&S 2e. Morphology of dysplasia and carcinoma in situ, p65-68

343 a normal immature squamous metaplasia

Immature metaplastic cells or "spider cells" are found proximal to the endocervical glandular mucosa. Their nuclei often appear darker due to the increased nucleoprotein and dark cytoplasmic nature. A 1:1 staining N:C ratio may aid the cytologist in defining these cells as normal.

DeMay, A&S 2e. Squamous metaplasia, p23-24

344 d coarse, regular chromatin

One of the hallmarks of carcinoma in situ is its coarse, regular chromatin distribution. Chromatin patterns found in dysplasia are typically finely granular and evenly distributed.

DeMay, A&S 2e. Morphology of dysplasia and carcinoma in situ, p65-68

345 b HPV16

Using molecular biological techniques, the presence of HPV16, 18, 31, 33, 35, and 39, and other viral sequences has been shown to transform keratinocyte cancer cell lines in vitro and to be integral in the etiology of squamous carcinoma of the uterine cervix.

DeMay, A&S 2e. Methods of detection of HPV, p126-128

346 d LSIL, consistent with HPV

The Bethesda System classifies condyloma acuminata (human papillomavirus [HPV]) as a low grade squamous epithelial lesion. The pathognomonic cell for establishing an HPV infection is the koilocyte. This cell possesses large perinuclear halos (often referred to as cytoplasmic margination or large halo) or craterlike morphology. The nuclei may be well preserved with fine even chromatin or hyperchromatic and smudged, representing a degenerative quality.

DeMay, A&S 2e. Koilocytes, p69

347 a congenital absence of the uterus

Patients with congenital absence of the uterus usually present with normal secretory patterns (normal ovaries). Although these patients lack menstrual cycles, the vaginal mucosa is hormonally receptive.

Keebler CM, Somrak TM. The Manual of Cytotechnology. Endocrinopathies, p74-78

348 b ASCUS, dyskeratocytes (pleomorphic parakeratosis) most likely associated with HPV infection

These pleomorphic cells with elongated nuclei, often described as dyskeratocytes or pleomorphic parakeratosis, are classified as atypical squamous cells of undetermined significance under the Bethesda System. Their presence is suggestive but not pathognomonic for human papillomavirus (HPV) infection.

DeMay, A&S 2e. Atypical parakeratosis, p59

349 b hyperkeratosis

Hyperkeratosis and parakeratosis are protective reactions often associated with keratinizing lesions such as this example of keratinizing dysplasia.

DeMay, A&S 2e. Keratinizing dysplasia, p68

350 a mild dysplasia, LSIL

The histologic findings in dysplasia show some degree of cellular abnormality throughout the entire epithelial thickness. In this example of mild dysplasia, the more primitive basal cells replace up to 25% of the lower epithelial surface, and more differentiated abnormal cells are seen in the upper 75% of the epithelial thickness. Nuclear sizes are variable, hyperchromasia is evident, and an increased mitotic activity may be observed.

DeMay, A&S 2e. Introduction to diagnosis of squamous intraepithelial lesions, p64-65

351 c are consistent with a reparative/regenerative process, endocervical origin

Reactive/reparative endocervical cells may at times be difficult to distinguish from endocervical atypia. These cells have normochromic enlarged nuclei and possess well defined borders and maintenance of polarity.

DeMay, A&S 2e. Repair/regeneration, p30-31

352 a squamous atypia/mature metaplastic ASCUS (mimicking mature native squames)

The diagnosis of atypical squamous cells of undetermined significance (ASCUS) is an alteration in the normal squamous nuclear size, possibly 2-3× greater than that of a normal intermediate cell nucleus. The chromatin is finely granular, regularly distributed, and generally hypochromatic (normochromic). A true ASCUS is a noninflammatory related change that may be related to subclinical or early manifestations of the human papillomavirus infection or dysplasia. Illustrated is an example of squamous atypia occurring in mature metaplastic squamous cells. ASCUS may also involve immature squamous epithelial cells as well as basal and parabasal cells found in atrophic conditions.

DeMay, A&S 2e. Atypical squamous cells, p55-59

353 c tubal metaplasia

Tubal metaplasia (TM) is a benign condition that may be confused with a true abnormal process, such as adenocarcinoma in situ (AIS) of the endocervix, with the exception that TM presents with cilia and/or terminal bars/webs. Crowded sheets of glandular cells and anisokaryosis are common findings, mimicking the feathering effects seen in AIS.

DeMay, A&S 2e. Tubal metaplasia, p82-83

354 c   AGUS, endocervical glandular dysplasia

Endocervical cells with slightly enlarged hyperchromatic nuclei with inconspicuous nucleoli, loss of polarity, and rosette formations are helpful in establishing a diagnosis of atypical glandular cells of undetermined significance (AGUS), in this case, referred to as endocervical columnar dysplasia (ECD). Its differential diagnosis is endocervical adenocarcinoma in situ (AIS); however, ECD has fine, regular chromatin, whereas endocervical AIS contains coarse chromatin features.

DeMay, A&S 2e. Differential of early endocervical glandular neoplasia, p90-91

355 d   adenocarcinoma in situ, endocervix

The diagnosis of endocervical adenocarcinoma in situ (AIS) may often be difficult to differentiate from squamous carcinoma in situ (CIS) with the exception that AIS often possesses feathering or pseudostratified syncytial-like fragments, stratified strips, or rosettes. The maintenance of columnar morphology may also be a key feature in establishing the diagnosis of an atypical endocervical process.

DeMay, A&S 2e. Differential of early endocervical glandular neoplasia, p90-91

356 c   mixed mesodermal tumor, homologous

The diagnosis of mixed mesodermal/Müllerian tumor is determined by the cytologic identification of endometrial adenocarcinoma (usually well differentiated) with a concomitant homologous or heterologous sarcomatous element. The findings represented by this photomicrograph indicate the sarcomatous element composed of isolated spindle cells with classic malignant criteria, suggesting leiomyosarcoma. Also identified are epithelial cells with enlarged nuclei, macronucleoli, and irregular chromatin.

DeMay, A&S 2e. Mixed Müllerian tumors, p112-113

357 a   rhabdomyosarcoma

Rhabdomyosarcoma is a heterologous sarcoma of the uterus that presents itself cytologically similar to leiomyosarcoma; however, this malignancy originates from striated muscle rather than smooth muscle. The findings of "strap cells" are diagnostic of malignant blasts; however, strap cells represent only 1% of the total malignant population. Multinucleated tumor giant cells also may be observed with these malignancies.

DeMay, A&S 2e. Rhabdomyosarcoma, p111

358 b   ASCUS: atypical squamous metaplasia/immature metaplastic variety

The diagnosis of atypical squamous cells of undetermined significance (ASCUS) includes an alteration in the normal squamous nuclear size, possibly 2-3× greater than that of a normal intermediate cell nucleus. The chromatin is finely granular, regularly distributed, and generally hypochromatic (normochromic). A true ASCUS is a noninflammatory related change that may be related to subclinical or early manifestations of the human papillomavirus infection or dysplasia. ASCUS may also involve immature squamous epithelial cells as well as basal and parabasal cells found in atrophic conditions.

DeMay, A&S 2e. Atypical squamous cells, p55-59

359 d   nonspecific findings

Psammoma bodies are 3D structures with concentric ringing containing calcified secretions of mucus. These structures are often found associated with papillary lesions of the ovary, including papillary serous adenocarcinoma. However, these are nonspecific findings and are not pathognomonic of malignancy.

DeMay, A&S 2e. Psammoma bodies, p122-123

360 a   papillary serous cystadenocarcinoma

The diagnosis of papillary serous adenocarcinoma of the ovary in a Pap test is centered on the finding of 3D aggregates with hyperchromatic nuclei and finely granular, irregularly distributed chromatin. Cervical/endocervical/endometrial biopsies and colposcopy findings are negative. The presence of papillary groups of malignant cells and psammoma bodies may help in identifying these lesions as ovarian, but are not specific findings. A history of ascites is helpful.

DeMay, A&S 2e. Psammoma bodies, p122-123

361 c   papillary serous cystadenocarcinoma, ovarian

The diagnosis of papillary serous adenocarcinoma of the ovary in a Pap test is centered around the finding of 3D aggregates with hyperchromatic nuclei and finely granular, irregularly distributed chromatin. Cervical/endocervical/endometrial biopsies and colposcopy findings are negative. The presence of papillary groups of malignant cells and psammoma bodies may help in identifying these lesions as ovarian, but are not specific findings. A history of ascites is helpful.

DeMay, A&S 2e. Metastases, p115-116

362 c   endocervical adenocarcinoma

The cellular morphology suggests an endocervical adenocarcinoma. Cells with palisading features, overlapping nuclei, irregular chromatin, and columnar morphology demonstrate invasive endocervical morphology.

DeMay, A&S 2e. Cytology of endocervical adenocarcinoma, p93-96

ISBN 978-089189-6357   ©ASCP 2015

363 c   endocervical adenocarcinoma

The presence of columnar morphology in the presence of obvious malignant criteria may help one to distinguish endocervical adenocarcinomas from those of endometrial origin. Other criteria that help discriminate the cells of endocervical adenocarcinoma (EA) from endometrial adenocarcinoma (EM) include the presence of rosettes vs cell balls and elongated, hyperchromatic, multinucleated cells with prominent multiple nucleoli vs rounded, finely granular chromatin and conspicuous nucleoli. EA possesses a granular cytoplasmic texture whereas EM lesions have lacy, frothy, vacuolated cytoplasm. Last, EA tends to stain eosinophilic while EM shows generally basophilic cytoplasm.

DeMay, A&S 2e. Cytology of endocervical adenocarcinoma, p93-96

364 a   adenocarcinoma, ovarian

Mucinous adenocarcinomas of the ovary present with signet ring morphology and may recapitulate signet ring endometrial adenocarcinomas. Clinical history is paramount in establishing an ovarian primary tumor. A tumor diathesis is usually absent in cases of metastatic carcinoma unless the lesion has seeded at the secondary site. A vaginal smear, rather than a directed cervical smear and endocervical brushing, also helps rule out the other processes.

DeMay, A&S 2e. Female genital tract, p300-301

365 b   herpesvirus infection

This image depicts some classic features of herpesvirus cytopathic effect, particularly the "ground glass" appearance of the nuclei and the intranuclear inclusions. Another common feature (not as well depicted in this image) is multinucleation with nuclear molding.

DeMay, A&S 2e. Herpes simplex virus, p34-35

366 c   normal endometrial cells

Exfoliated endometrial cells occur in ball-like clusters. During the first half of the menstrual cycle, double contoured clusters of endometrial cells ("exodus" pattern) may be seen.

DeMay, A&S 2e. Endometrial cells, p18-20

367 a   small cell carcinoma

Small cell undifferentiated carcinoma (neuroendocrine carcinoma, grade III) comprises a small minority of cervical carcinoma. Small cell undifferentiated carcinoma is composed of small, relatively uniform cells with nuclear molding, with "crush artifact" being a frequent finding. The nuclei are hyperchromatic. Background tumor diathesis is common. The differential includes poorly differentiated squamous carcinoma with small cells, poorly differentiated adenocarcinoma, low grade endometrial stromal sarcoma and lymphoma.

DeMay, A&S 2e. Small cell neuroendocrine carcinoma, p107-108

368 b   trichomoniasis

Trichomonas vaginalis are anaerobic, parasitic flagellated protozoa that present as pear shaped, oval or round cyanophilic organisms with a single, eccentrically located slitlike nucleus and eosinophilic cytoplasmic granules.

DeMay, A&S 2e. Trichomonas vaginalis, p40-41

369 c   endometrial adenocarcinoma

The cytologic findings in endometrial adenocarcinoma are largely dependant upon the grade of the tumor. Nuclei in higher grade tumors are larger and display moderate hyperchromasia with irregular chromatin distribution and prominent nuclei.

DeMay, A&S 2e. Endometrial adenocarcinoma, p100-102

370 c   Repair/regeneration

Repair is characterized by flat cohesive sheets of well ordered cells; single reparative cells are usually absent and, when present, are found in the vicinity of the sheets. The nuclei tend to line up in orderly rows ("nuclear streaming"). Although prominent nucleoli, or macronucleoli, typically are present, the chromatin is fine and pale. An inflammatory reaction often is present in the background, and it is common to see neutrophils in the cytoplasm of the reparative cells. The major differential is with carcinoma, which is characterized by poorly cohesive, disorderly cells with a conspicuous component of atypical single cells. The malignant chromatin is abnormal, often hyperchromatic and irregularly distributed.

DeMay, A&S 2e. Repair/regeneration, p30-31

371 c   these cells are being driven to proliferate by the interaction of HPVE6 and E7 with p53 and pRB in the host cell

High risk HPV E6 binds to and degrades p53. E7 binds to and degrade pRB causing uncontrolled cell proliferation that manifests itself as HSIL as in this image.

DeMay, A&S 2e. Pap test management guidelines, p137-139

372 d   large nuclear inclusion surrounded by a halo

Cytomegalovirus (CMV) is a DNA virus that is a member of the herpesvirus family. Classic cytologic features of CMV include cellular enlargement, nuclear enlargement, large nuclear inclusion surrounded by a halo ("owl's eye"), and small satellite nuclear or cytoplasmic inclusions.

DeMay, A&S 2e. Cytomegalovirus, p35

373 b   high grade squamous intraepithelial lesion

Abnormal cells lacking nuclear polarity, containing hyperchromatic nuclei with fine to coarse uniformly distributed chromatin, arranged as single cells or in syncytia, are suggestive of an in situ lesion. Syncytial-like aggregates, hyperchromatic crowded "chaotic" groups with indistinct cell borders are associated with squamous carcinoma in situ. Distinguishing these aggregates from true papillary tissue fragments with community borders, well formed glandular structures, or "HCGs" with feathery edges may help in differentiating glandular lesions from those of squamous origin.

DeMay, A&S 2e. Carcinoma in situ, p70-71

374 b radiation changes

Cells with enlarged nuclei, increased cell size, abundant vacuolated polychromatic cytoplasm and mild nuclear hyperchromasia are reactive cellular changes associated with radiation. Bizarre cell shapes may occur. Prominent single or multiple nucleoli may be seen if coexisting repair is present.

DeMay, A&S 2e. Radiation cytology, p42-44

375 d she needs an ablative procedure regardless of the result of her colposcopy

The cells demonstrate severe dysplasia/CIN3/HSIL. This lesion needs ablation to prevent the patient from developing invasive cancer.

DeMay, A&S 2e. Pap test management guidelines, p137-139

376 a human papillomavirus type 6/11

Koilocytes are diagnostic of HPV infection and condyloma, which is considered an LSIL in the Bethesda System.

DeMay, A&S 2e. Koilocytes, p69-70

377 c the cytoplasmic vacuolization is due to HPV oncogene expression

High risk HPVs account for >80% of cervical infections and most LSILs are due to this group.

DeMay, A&S 2e. Human papillomavirus, p124-126

378 a nuclear feathering

Cytologic features of endocervical adenocarcinoma in situ include columnar cells arranged in strips and/or rosettes, nuclear feathering around the edges and hyperchromatic nuclei with apoptotic bodies

DeMay, A&S 2e. Cytology of adenocarcinoma in situ, p87-89

379 b atypical glandular cells

A cluster of glandular cells showing crowding and overlapping, slight nuclear enlargement, mild hyperchromasia, and vacuolated cytoplasm in a symptomatic postmenopausal patient is strongly suggestive of endometrial disease.

DeMay, A&S 2e. Endometrial glandular cells, p18-19

380 c patients with this lesion have a relatively high frequency of HPV type 18 compared to HPV type 16 infection

AIS is enriched in HPV18 compared to HPV16.

DeMay, A&S 2e. Cervical adenocarcinoma in situ, p86

381 c require pathologist review under CLIA '88 rules

CLIA'88 requires that all Pap tests with reactive/reparative changes must be reviewed by a pathologist.

DeMay, A&S 2e. CLIA '88, p1583-1588

382 c this patient is almost certainly positive for high risk HPV

The image demonstrates adenocarcinoma in situ (AIS). All patients with a cytologic diagnosis of AIS require colposcopy. This patient is almost certainly positive for high risk HPV.

DeMay, A&S 2e. Cervical adenocarcinoma in situ, p86

383 a atypical glandular cells

Irradiated endocervical cells may show marked cell and nuclear enlargement, variation in cell and nuclear size, prominent nucleoli, and clumped chromatin, especially in smears taken with 3-6 months post therapy.

DeMay, A&S 2e. Radiation cytology, p43-44

ISBN 978-089189-6357 ©ASCP 2015

Reporting, Screening & Management Guidelines

Chapter 2

2014 Bethesda System for Reporting Cervical Cytology

2012 ACS, ASCCP & ASCP Screening Guidelines for the Prevention & Early Detection of Cervical Cancer

2012 ASCCP Updated Consensus Guidelines for the Management of Abnormal Cervical Cancer Screening Tests & Cancer Precursors

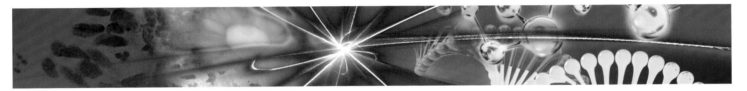

All questions in this section make use of the publications noted above; see individual question references for detail.

1   Which of the following are considered pertinent for issuing a final report of "satisfactory for evaluation?"
a   at least 2 microscopic fields of squamous cells found in liquid based preparation
b   presence or absence of endocervical/transformation zone component
c   specimen not processed
d   inflammation obscures all but 2% of squamous cells in a conventional slide

2   Which of the following is considered acceptable terminology when rendering a diagnosis of benign or negative?
a   class 1
b   benign cellular changes
c   WNL (within normal limits)
d   NILM (negative for intraepithelial lesion or malignancy)

3   Which of the following statements is acceptable Bethesda System terminology classification of GYN cytology slides?
a   satisfactory, but limited by lack of endocervical cell component
b   benign cellular changes (as a separate category)
c   "other" category to include endometrial cells in women at least 40 years of age
d   atypical squamous cells of undetermined significance (ASCUS), favor reactive

4   Which of the following statements is acceptable terminology for classification of GYN cytology slides?
a   ASCUS, favor neoplastic
b   endocervical adenocarcinoma in situ
c   atypical glandular cells of undetermined significance (AGUS), favor reactive
d   AGUS, favor dysplasia

5   Which of the following is an acceptable report category for classification of GYN cytology slides?
a   hormonal evaluation
b   ancillary testing
c   organisms and other nonneoplastic findings mandatory under "negative for intraepithelial lesion or malignancy"
d   conventional cytologic review

6   The presence of endometrial cells on cervical cytology in women who are at least 45 years of age is more often associated with endometrial hyperplasia or even adenocarcinoma as opposed to benign endometrium.
a   true
b   false

7   The Pap test is reliable for the detection of endometrial lesions and can be used to evaluate suspected endometrial abnormalities.
a   true
b   false

8   If automated computer systems are used to scan slides, the type of system used and the result should be reported.
a   true
b   false

©ASCP 2015   ISBN 978-089189-6357

9 How many cells must be confirmed on a liquid based Pap slide to establish a satisfactory specimen for diagnosis?
   a 1,000
   b 2,500
   c 5,000
   d 10,000

10 How many transformational zone cells must be confirmed on a liquid based Pap slide to establish an adequate specimen?
   a 5
   b 10
   c 20
   d 0

11 Which is considered unsatisfactory for evaluation under the specimen adequacy clause of the Bethesda System?
   a 50% of the cellular material is obscured by inflammation
   b air drying that obscures evaluation of at least 75% of the epithelial cells
   c air drying that obscures evaluation of at least 30% of the epithelial cells
   d 25% of the cells are obscured by blood

12 Which professional organization sets the guidelines for the management of women with abnormal cervical cancer screening tests?
   a ASCCP
   b ACOG
   c ASC
   d ASCP

13 Which of the following management recommendations is appropriate for women with an initial diagnosis of atypical squamous cells of undetermined significance (ASCUS):
   a high risk HPV test−; repeat cytology at 6 & 12 months
   b high risk HPV test−; repeat cytology in 12 months
   c triage to colposcopy, regardless of HPV test status
   d high risk HPV test+; perform conization

14 Which of the following is the appropriate management algorithm for patients with ASCUS?
   a high risk HPV test+; requires repeat in HPV test in 6 months
   b high risk HPV test+; requires colposcopy
   c ASCUS requires immediate colposcopy regardless of HPV risk status
   d 3 consecutive cytologic diagnoses of ASCUS diagnoses at 6, 12 and 18 months are recommended before colposcopy

15 A patient with ASCUS and a positive HPV test was referred to colposcopy. The colposcopy was negative; therefore, the appropriate follow-up would be:
   a repeat cytology at 6 & 12 months or HPV test in 12 months
   b immediate conization
   c immediate repeat high risk HPV test
   d repeat high risk HPV in 6 months

16 A patient with an initial diagnosis of ASCUS was eventually referred to colposcopy due to a cotest HPV result that was high risk positive. Colposcopy showed CIN1. The management paradigm should be:
   a repeat HPV test
   b repeat cytology at 6 & 12 months or HPV test in 12 months
   c perform diagnostic excision procedure
   d return the patient to routine cytologic testing in 12 months

17 What is the appropriate management for women with a cytologic diagnosis of LSIL?
   a immediate colposcopy
   b perform diagnostic excision procedure
   c confirm with HPV test; if HPV test is positive, perform LEEP
   d repeat Pap in 6 months

18 What is the management for women with LSIL who are confirmed as negative by colposcopy and for whom the endocervical curettings (ECCs) were negative?
   a cotesting at 12 months
   b repeat colposcopic examination
   c repeat immediately with an HPV test; if HPV test is positive, perform a LEEP
   d routine screening in 12 months

19 What is the management for women who have LSIL and are confirmed by colposcopy as CIN1 (with a negative ECC)?
   a perform an HPV test; if HPV test is positive, perform a LEEP
   b repeat colposcopic examination
   c cotesting at 12 months
   d routine screening in 12 months

20 What is the management for women who have LSIL and are confirmed by colposcopy as CIN2 or 3?
   a hysterectomy
   b repeat colposcopy in 6 months to determine regression of disease
   c repeat immediately with an HPV test; if HPV test is positive, perform a LEEP
   d with adequate colposcopy, either excision or ablation of T zone

21 What is the recommended management for women <20 with a cytologic diagnosis of ASCUS?
   a repeat Pap in 6 months
   b repeat Pap in 12 months (acceptable) or HPV testing (preferred)
   c immediate colposcopy
   d high risk HPV test recommended, if positive, immediate colposcopy

22 What is the recommended management for women <20 with a cytologic diagnosis of LSIL?
   a repeat Pap in 6 months
   b repeat Pap in 12 months
   c immediate colposcopy
   d high risk HPV test recommended; if positive, immediate colposcopy

ISBN 978-089189-6357 ©ASCP 2015

23 Which of the following statements is correct regarding an 18-year-old female with LSIL and a positive HPV test?
    a   repeat Pap in 6 months; if LSIL, perform immediate colposcopy
    b   immediate colposcopy
    c   2 consecutive positive HPV tests are required in adolescents with LSIL at 6 month intervals before colposcopy is warranted
    d   inadvertent HPV test should be ignored regardless of positivity; colposcopy is not warranted; repeat Pap in 12 months

24 What is the recommended management for women <20 with a cytologic diagnosis of HSIL?
    a   repeat Pap test in 6 months
    b   colposcopy
    c   immediate loop electrosurgical excision (LEEP)
    d   high risk HPV test recommended, then follow as clinically indicated

25 What of the following is a recommended management for women age 21-24 with a cytologic diagnosis of atypical squamous cells: cannot rule out high grade SIL (ASC-H) who has received a negative colposcopy?
    a   immediate HPV test
    b   repeat colposcopy
    c   cotesting at 12 and 24 months
    d   conization

26 What is the recommended management for women over 30 who are cytology negative, but HPV positive?
    a   immediate HPV test
    b   repeat cotesting in 12 months
    c   repeat colposcopy
    d   conization

27 What is the preferred method for a 30-year-old pregnant patient with a cytologic diagnosis of LSIL?
    a   colposcopy
    b   perform HPV testing postpartum
    c   repeat Pap at 6 weeks postpartum
    d   immediate loop electrosurgical excision (LEEP)

28 What is the preferred management for a 16-year-old female with a cytologic diagnosis of HSIL followed by a negative colposcopic evaluation?
    a   D&C
    b   repeat colposcopy in 3 months
    c   repeat colposcopy and cytology in 3 and 6 months
    d   repeat colposcopy and cytology in 6 month intervals for up to 2 years

29 What is the management paradigm for a 17-year-old patient with HSIL, followed by a negative colposcopy at 6 & 12 months, but with an HSIL cytologic diagnosis that persists for a year?
    a   conization
    b   HPV testing to confirm HSIL
    c   repeat colposcopy in 3 months
    d   biopsy

30 What is the appropriate management for a 34-year-old patient with an initial cytologic diagnosis of atypical glandular cells (AGC) of undetermined significance, endocervical cells NOS?
    a   follow-up Pap every 6 months to determine if progression to adenocarcinoma in situ occurs
    b   colposcopy with ECC, HPV testing
    c   immediate loop electrosurgical excision (LEEP)
    d   HPV testing in 12 months

31 What is the appropriate management for a 48-year-old patient with a cytologic diagnosis of atypical glandular cells (AGC), endometrial cells favor neoplastic?
    a   follow-up Pap every 6 months to determine if progression to adenocarcinoma in situ occurs
    b   endometrial and endocervical sampling
    c   immediate loop electrosurgical excision (LEEP)
    d   hysterectomy

32 What is the appropriate management for a 37-year-old patient with an initial cytologic diagnosis of atypical glandular cells (AGC), glandular cells, NOS ?
    a   follow-up Pap every 6 months to determine if progression to adenocarcinoma in situ occurs
    b   immediate loop electrosurgical excision (LEEP)
    c   colposcopy with ECC, HPV testing, and endometrial sampling
    d   hysterectomy

33 What is the appropriate management for a 29-year-old patient with an initial cytologic diagnosis of adenocarcinoma in situ (AIS)?
    a   HPV testing followed by colposcopy
    b   hysterectomy
    c   repeat Pap in 6 months; if AIS persists by cytology, perform a conization
    d   diagnostic excisional procedure

34 What is the appropriate management for a 37-year-old patient who received cotesting with HPV as a primary screening tool where the cytology is negative but the HPV test is positive?
    a   immediate colposcopy
    b   repeat HPV test immediately
    c   repeat HPV and Pap test every 6 months
    d   repeat HPV and Pap test at 12 months

35 After appropriate follow-up of a 37-year-old patient with negative cytology and a positive HPV test, a repeat HPV test proved negative but the cytology was ASCUS. What is the appropriate management for the patient at this point?
    a   repeat cytology at 12 months
    b   colposcopy
    c   repeat HPV test immediately
    d   immediate loop electrosurgical excision (LEEP)

36 The intent of the 2012 Updated American Society for Colposcopy and Cervical Pathology (ASCCP) Consensus Guidelines for the Management of Abnormal Cervical Cancer Screening Tests and Cancer Precursors (2012 ASCCP Consensus Management Guidelines) is to:
    a present a patient management strategy that will eliminate cervical cancer risk in older women
    b prescribe patient management algorithms that should always be followed
    c promote best clinical practices focused on efficiently identifying women at highest risk
    d discourage the use of HPV testing in women over 30 years old

37 What is the role for HPV testing in the initial evaluation of patients with atypical glandular cells (AGC)?
    a HPV testing alone is "recommended" for triage
    b HPV testing may be useful in conjunction with colposcopy and endocervical and/or endometrial sampling
    c HPV testing has no role in the initial evaluation of patients with AGC
    d HPV testing should be performed for both low and high risk serotypes

38 According to the 2012 ASCCP Consensus Management Guidelines, what is the recommended management for young women (age <21) diagnosed with either ASCUS or LSIL?
    a HPV testing for ASCUS triage
    b repeat cytology at 12 months
    c repeat cytology at 6 months
    d colposcopy, HPV testing and repeat cytology at 6 & 12 months are all acceptable options

39 2 patients with LSIL are referred to colposcopy. Patient A has biopsy proven CIN1, while patient B has a normal colposcopy with biopsies demonstrating only cervicitis. If both patients are followed for 24 months, what do you expect to find?
    a patient A has a 12% risk of being diagnosed with CIN2/3, while the risk for patient B is 5%
    b patients A and B both have a 5% risk of being diagnosed with CIN2/3
    c neither patient will develop a CIN2/3; only CIN1 has been identified and will likely regress
    d patients A and B both have a 12% risk of being diagnosed with CIN2/3

40 If the cytologic interpretation is ASCUS, then:
    a reflex testing for both low risk and high risk HPV DNA is useful for triage to colposcopy
    b reflex high risk HPV testing is more useful than a repeat Pap test for triage to colposcopy
    c at least 90% should test positive for high risk HPV DNA
    d triage HPV testing should be performed irrespective of patient's age

41 Which of the following is true about a cytologic interpretation of ASC-H?
    a reflex HPV testing efficiently determines which patients require colposcopy
    b ASC-H should account for ~20% of a laboratory's ASC interpretations
    c ~25% of ASC-H cases are positive for high risk HPV serotypes
    d the positive predictive value of ASC-H for CIN2/3 approaches 50%

42 A 25-year-old female with ASCUS positive for high risk HPV has a colposcopy demonstrating CIN1. The recommended follow-up is:
    a treatment of this lesion by either laser or cryoablation
    b follow-up with repeat Pap and HPV testing at 6 months
    c dependent on a "satisfactory" colposcopy
    d repeat cotesting at 12 months

43 A 30-year-old female who has had 3 prior NILM Paps tests in the last 5 years has a current Pap test interpreted as ASC-H. Her high risk HPV DNA test is negative. Which of the following statements is true?
    a this patient does not need colposcopy
    b this patient should have colposcopy
    c if colposcopy, biopsy and ECC are all normal, the ASC-H diagnosis was an overcall
    d HPV testing is the recommended triage for ASC-H in women 30 and older

44 According to the 2012 Updated ASCCP Consensus Guidelines, follow-up for a 35-year-old patient with a negative Pap test and a positive high risk HPV test should be
    a repeat cytology at 6 months
    b colposcopy
    c repeat cytology and HPV testing at 12 months
    d repeat cytology at 3 years

45 According to the 2012 Updated ASCCP Consensus Guidelines, how should women with atypical squamous cells, cannot exclude high grade SIL (ASC-H) be managed?
    a next step in patient management depends on patient's age
    b all patients should have colposcopy
    c HPV test results should be used to determine if colposcopy is indicated
    d if colposcopy and biopsies show no CIN2/3, conization should be performed

46 Per 2012 Updated ASCCP Consensus Guidelines, high risk HPV DNA testing is recommended for:
    a precolopscopic triage of ASCUS for women 21 and older, laboratory QC and primary screening of women <30
    b precolopscopic triage of ASC-H, laboratory QC and primary screening of women >30
    c precolopscopic triage of AGUS, laboratory QC and primary screening of women >30
    d precolopscopic triage of ASCUS for women 21 and older, laboratory QC and primary screening of women >30

ISBN 978-089189-6357   ©ASCP 2015

47 The 2012 Updated ASCCP Consensus Guidelines state that testing for high risk HPV is "acceptable" as triage for postmenopausal women with cytologic diagnosis of LSIL. In this context "acceptable" means
   a HPV triage is the best option available
   b HPV triage is one of multiple available options, none of which is considered "best"
   c HPV triage is the only acceptable option
   d HPV testing is indicated for all postmenopausal women diagnosed with LSIL

48 Based on Bethesda System criteria, for liquid based Pap tests, which of the following must be identified to document transformation zone sampling?
   a 1 endocervical and/or metaplastic squamous cell
   b 10 endocervical cells
   c 20 endocervical and/or metaplastic squamous cells
   d 10 endocervical and/or metaplastic squamous cells

49 Based on Bethesda System criteria how many squamous cells are required for a liquid based Pap test to be considered satisfactory for evaluation for epithelial abnormality?
   a 5,000
   b 7,500
   c 2,500
   d 10,000

50 Under 2012 Updated ASCCP Consensus Guidelines, the correct follow-up for an adolescent woman with a cytologic interpretation of atypical squamous cells of undetermined significance (ASCUS) is:
   a repeat cytologic exam in 12 months
   b colposcopic examination
   c testing for high risk HPV
   d repeat cytologic exam in 3 months

51 In the Bethesda System for reporting cervical/vaginal cytologic diagnoses, a specimen is unsatisfactory for evaluation if which of the following is present?
   a a conventional specimen with 12,000-15,000 squamous epithelial cells
   b a liquid based specimen with 10,000 squamous epithelial cells
   c obscuring inflammation that precludes interpretation of 75% or more of the epithelial cells
   d presence of abnormal cells (atypical squamous cells of undetermined significance [ASCUS] or atypical glandular cells [AGC])

52 According to 2012 Updated ASCCP Consensus Guidelines, the preferred treatment for biopsy confirmed endocervical adenocarcinoma in situ is:
   a cryotherapy
   b laser therapy
   c topical 5FU
   d hysterectomy

53 The June 2009 Practice Improvement in Cervical Screening and Management (PICSM) Symposium on Management of Cervical Abnormalities in Adolescents and Young Women made a recommendation for cervical cancer screening prior to age 21. Which of the following statements is true?
   a women under 21 years of age should not be screened regardless of the age of sexual initiation or other risk factors
   b screening should commence after sexual initiation, even if the patient is <21 years of age
   c HPV vaccination in adolescence increases the age of initial screening from age 21-30
   d HPV primary screening is recommended for women younger than 21 in lieu of a Pap test

54 According to 2012 collaborative Screening Guidelines for the Prevention and Early Detection of Cervical Cancer, which statement is false regarding circumstances for which women can be exited from Pap test screening?
   a age older than 65 years; and evidence of prior negative screening (adequate negative prior screening is defined as 3 consecutive negative cytology results or 2 consecutive negative cotests within the 10 years before ceasing screening, with the most recent test occurring within the past 5 years); and no history of CIN2+ within the last 20 years
   b women at any age following a hysterectomy with removal of the cervix who have no history of CIN2+ should not be screened for vaginal cancer using any modality; evidence of adequate negative prior screening is not required
   c once screening is discontinued, it should not resume for any reason
   d report of a new sexual partner warrants a return to active screening

55 According to 2012 collaborative Screening Guidelines for the Prevention and Early Detection of Cervical Cancer, screening recommendations following vaccination for HPV:
   a increase the initial age of initial screening from age 21 to age 30
   b lengthen the window between negative Pap tests from 3 years to 5 years
   c lengthen the window between negative Pap tests from 5 years to 10 years
   d should not change on the basis of HPV vaccination status

56 According to the 2012 Updated ASCCP Consensus Guidelines, how should this patient be managed?
   a colposcopy is recommended
   b HPV testing should be done
   c depends on patient's age
   d HPV testing is never indicated

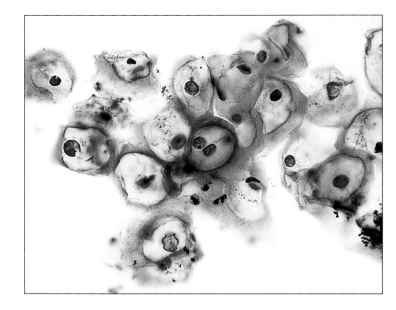

57 According to the 2012 Updated ASCCP Consensus Guidelines, follow-up for a 35-year-old patient with this Pap test and a positive high risk HPV test should be
   a repeat cytology at 6 months
   b colposcopy
   c repeat cotesting at 12 months
   d repeat cytology at 3 years

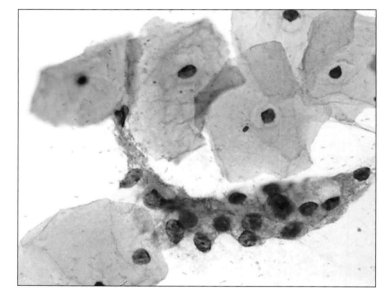

58 According to the 2012 Updated ASCCP Consensus Guidelines, what is the best management option for this patient?
   a colposcopic examination
   b immediate LEEP
   c depends on patient age
   d colposcopic examination with endocervical assessment

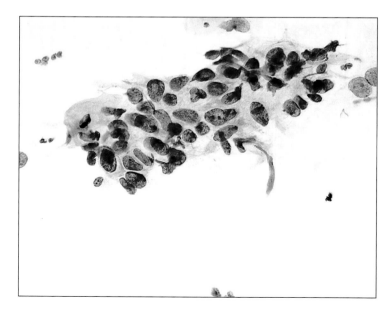

ISBN 978-089189-6357 ©ASCP 2015

59 These cells were seen in the liquid based Pap test taken during a normal examination of an 18-year-old female with an LMP date of 2 weeks ago. The appropriate management for these findings according to 2012 Updated ASCCP Consensus Guidelines, is:

a immediate colposcopy and cervical biopsy
b repeat cytology in 12 months
c excision or ablation of the T zone
d endocervical and endometrial tissue sampling

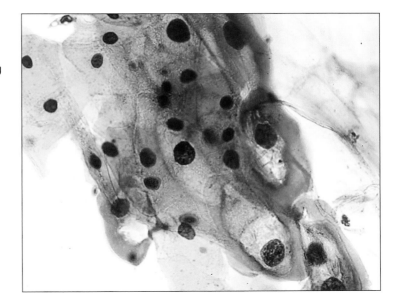

Guidelines for Cervical Cancer *Answer Key*

1 **b** presence or absence of endocervical/transformational zone component

The Bethesda System includes specific statements about specimen adequacy. Studies have not proven that a lack of transformation zone components (in a specimen that would otherwise be diagnosed as negative) places the patient at a subsequent higher risk for a high grade squamous intraepithelial lesion (HSIL).

Nayar R, Wilbur D, eds. The Bethesda System for Reporting Cervical Cytology 2015 [in press]

2 **d** NILM (negative for intraepithelial lesion or malignancy)

Pap slides that have no epithelial abnormalities are listed under the category NILM (negative for intraepithelial lesion or malignancy). If present, organisms may be included as a comment in the NILM category. The presence of atrophy, radiation, and inflammation may also be optionally included.

Nayar R, Wilbur D, eds. The Bethesda System for Reporting Cervical Cytology 2015 [in press]

3 **c** "other" category to include endometrial cells in women at least 40 years of age

The Bethesda System of classification has an "other" category for reporting normal or abnormal endometrial cells in females over the age of 40. This is paramount because the presence of endometrial cells (even normal by morphology) seen from women 45 years or older may be associated with endometrial hyperplasia or even adenocarcinoma as opposed to a benign endometrium.

Nayar R, Wilbur D, eds. The Bethesda System for Reporting Cervical Cytology 2015 [in press]

4 **b** endocervical adenocarcinoma in situ

Criteria of adenocarcinoma in situ have been well established, and it is now included as a descriptive diagnosis as well as the diagnosis of "AGC, favor neoplasia," indicating those cells that have clear morphologic features (overlapping cells, hyperchromasia) but lack full spectrum of diagnostic criteria for AIS (stratification of the cells, or a feathering and splattering effect with abnormal nuclear features).

Nayar R, Wilbur D, eds. The Bethesda System for Reporting Cervical Cytology 2015 [in press]

5 **b** ancillary testing

Should HPV DNA cotesting be performed (concurrent with the Pap slide from a liquid based specimen) this should be reported in parallel with the cytology results. In addition, if the laboratory utilizes an automated (computer-assisted) screening system, the specific type of system used and the result should be provided on the final report.

Nayar R, Wilbur D, eds. The Bethesda System for Reporting Cervical Cytology 2015 [in press]

6 **a** true

The Bethesda System of classification has an "other" category for reporting normal or abnormal endometrial cells in females over the age of 40. This is paramount because the presence of endometrial cells (even normal by morphology) seen from women 45 years or older may be associated with endometrial hyperplasia or even adenocarcinoma as opposed to a benign endometrium.

Nayar R, Wilbur D, eds. The Bethesda System for Reporting Cervical Cytology 2015 [in press]

7 **b** false

The Pap test is primarily considered a screening test for squamous epithelial lesions and cancer but should not be used for the detection of endometrial adenocarcinoma. A NILM Pap does not imply absence of an endometrial lesion due to the fact that the endometrium is not sampled by the clinician during the Pap test and the fact that many endometrial lesions do not shed.

Nayar R, Wilbur D, eds. The Bethesda System for Reporting Cervical Cytology 2015 [in press]

8 **a** true

If the laboratory utilizes an automated (computer assisted) screening system, the specific type of system used and the result should be provided on the final report.

Nayar R, Wilbur D, eds. The Bethesda System for Reporting Cervical Cytology 2015 [in press]

9 **c** 5,000

A minimum of 5,000 cells are required to render a liquid based Pap specimen adequate for evaluation, whereas 8,000-12,000 cells are considered optimal for analyzing conventional Pap tests.

DeMay, A&S 2e. Specimen adequacy, p145

ISBN 978-089189-6357 ©ASCP 2015

10 b 10

The presence or absence of a transformational zone component should be reported in the specimen adequacy section of the cytology report, as should presence of a minimum of 10 well preserved transformation zone cells (endocervical and/or squamous metaplastic cells) as individuals and/or groups. Mucus or parabasal cells do not count in this computation.

DeMay, A&S 2e. Specimen adequacy, p145

11 b air drying that obscures evaluation of at least 75% of the epithelial cells

If air drying, or any other factor, obscures 75% or more of the epithelial cells on the surface of the slide, the case is rendered unsatisfactory.

DeMay, A&S 2e. Specimen adequacy, p145

12 a ASCCP

In 2005, the American Society for Colposcopy and Cervical Pathology (ASCCP), along with its partner societies (as well as federal and international organizations) developed the new guidelines at an NIH conference in September 2006. "Consensus Guidelines for the Management of Women with Abnormal Cervical Cancer Screening Tests" as first published in 2006, with a subsequent update in 2012, "2012 Updated Consensus Guidelines for the Management of Abnormal Cervical Cancer Screening Tests and Cancer Precursors."

Massad LS, Einstein MH, Huh WK, et al. 2012 Updated consensus guidelines for the management of abnormal cervical cancer screening tests and cancer precursors. J Low Genit Tract Dis 2013;17(3):367 [PMID 23519301]

13 b high risk HPV test–; repeat cytology in 12 months

HPV cotesting with cytology eliminates the need for women to return to the office for an additional DNA test. Moreover, women with HPV– Paps diagnosed as ASCUS are allowed to be re-evaluated by the clinician in 12 months as opposed to undergoing unnecessary colposcopy (which would otherwise affect 40%-60% of women).

Saslow D, Solomon D, Lawson HW, et al. American Cancer Society, American Society for Colposcopy and Cervical Pathology, and American Society for Clinical Pathology screening guidelines for the prevention and early detection of cervical cancer. Am J Clin Pathol 2012;137:516-542 [PMID 22431528]

14 b high risk HPV test+; requires colposcopy

HPV cotesting with cytology eliminates the need for women to return to the office for an additional DNA test. Moreover, women with HPV+ Paps diagnosed as ASCUS are forwarded to the clinician for immediate colposcopy.

Saslow D, Solomon D, Lawson HW, et al. American Cancer Society, American Society for Colposcopy and Cervical Pathology, and American Society for Clinical Pathology screening guidelines for the prevention and early detection of cervical cancer. Am J Clin Pathol 2012;137:516-542 [PMID 22431528]

15 a repeat cytology at 6 & 12 months or HPV test in 12 months

HPV testing performed 12 months after the initial colposcopy or 2 repeat cytology examinations performed at 6 month intervals are both equally effective means for following a patient with an HPV+ ASCUS Pap for which colposcopy reveals no lesion.

Massad LS, Einstein MH, Huh WK, et al. 2012 Updated consensus guidelines for the management of abnormal cervical cancer screening tests and cancer precursors. J Low Genit Tract Dis 2013;17(3):367 [PMID 23519301]

16 b repeat cytology at 6 & 12 months or HPV test in 12 months

HPV testing performed 12 months after the initial colposcopy or 2 repeat cytology examinations performed at 6 month intervals are both equally effective means for following a patient with an HPV+ ASCUS Pap for which colposcopy reveals LSIL, due to the fact that LSIL is likely to regress and may involve nononcogenic HPV virotypes.

Massad LS, Einstein MH, Huh WK, et al. 2012 Updated consensus guidelines for the management of abnormal cervical cancer screening tests and cancer precursors. J Low Genit Tract Dis 2013;17(3):367 [PMID 23519301]

17 a immediate colposcopy

Among women with LSIL, the prevalence of CIN2,3 identified at colposcopy is 12%-16%–the same as women with ASCUS and HPV positivity; ergo, managing both groups of women in similar fashion is recommended (except in postmenopausal women).

Massad LS, Einstein MH, Huh WK, et al. 2012 Updated consensus guidelines for the management of abnormal cervical cancer screening tests and cancer precursors. J Low Genit Tract Dis 2013;17(3):367 [PMID 23519301]

18 a cotesting at 12 months

Cotesting at 12 months is recommended for following a patient with a LSIL Pap for which colposcopy was negative.

Massad LS, Einstein MH, Huh WK, et al. 2012 Updated consensus guidelines for the management of abnormal cervical cancer screening tests and cancer precursors. J Low Genit Tract Dis 2013;17(3):367 [PMID 23519301]

19 c cotesting at 12 months

Cotesting at 12 months is recommended for following a patient with an LSIL Pap for which colposcopy was CIN1.

Massad LS, Einstein MH, Huh WK, et al. 2012 Updated consensus guidelines for the management of abnormal cervical cancer screening tests and cancer precursors. J Low Genit Tract Dis 2013;17(3):367 [PMID 23519301]

20 **d** with adequate colposcopy, either excision or ablation of T zone

With adequate colposcopy, either excision or ablation of T zone should be immediately implemented for women with colposcopically confirmed CIN2 or 3 (except when pregnant).

Massad LS, Einstein MH, Huh WK, et al. 2012 Updated consensus guidelines for the management of abnormal cervical cancer screening tests and cancer precursors. J Low Genit Tract Dis 2013;17(3):367 [PMID 23519301]

21 **b** repeat Pap in 12 months (acceptable) or HPV testing (preferred)

Follow-up with annual cytologic testing is recommended (acceptable) or HPV testing (preferred). Upon follow-up, only those adolescents with a cytologic diagnosis of HSIL or greater should be referred to colposcopy.

Massad LS, Einstein MH, Huh WK, et al. 2012 Updated consensus guidelines for the management of abnormal cervical cancer screening tests and cancer precursors. J Low Genit Tract Dis 2013;17(3):367 [PMID 23519301]

22 **b** repeat Pap in 12 months

Adolescents (women <20) with a cytologic diagnosis of LSIL have a high rate of regression; however, immunologic clearance, followed by regression, may take several years. Because of the regressive feature of LSIL in adolescents, follow-up with annual cytologic testing is only recommended. Upon annual follow-up, only those adolescents with a cytologic diagnosis of HSIL or greater should be referred to colposcopy.

Massad LS, Einstein MH, Huh WK, et al. 2012 Updated consensus guidelines for the management of abnormal cervical cancer screening tests and cancer precursors. J Low Genit Tract Dis 2013;17(3):367 [PMID 23519301]

23 **d** inadvertent HPV test should be ignored regardless of positivity; colposcopy is not warranted; repeat Pap in 12 months

HPV DNA testing and colposcopy is not warranted for adolescents with ASCUS or LSIL. Inadvertent HPV testing should be ignored and not considered when managing the patient.

Saslow D, Solomon D, Lawson HW, et al. American Cancer Society, American Society for Colposcopy and Cervical Pathology, and American Society for Clinical Pathology screening guidelines for the prevention and early detection of cervical cancer. Am J Clin Pathol 2012;137:516-542 [PMID 22431528]

24 **b** colposcopy

Colposcopy is warranted if the patient has a cytologic diagnosis of HSIL. If confirmed by colposcopy as CIN2 or 3, a loop electrosurgical excision (LEEP) with endocervical curettage should be immediately implemented (except when pregnant).

Massad LS, Einstein MH, Huh WK, et al. 2012 Updated consensus guidelines for the management of abnormal cervical cancer screening tests and cancer precursors. J Low Genit Tract Dis 2013;17(3):367 [PMID 23519301]

25 **c** cotesting at 12 & 24 months

Cotesting performed at 12 and 24 months is recommended for following a patient with an ASC-H Pap for which colposcopy was negative.

Massad LS, Einstein MH, Huh WK, et al. 2012 Updated consensus guidelines for the management of abnormal cervical cancer screening tests and cancer precursors. J Low Genit Tract Dis 2013;17(3):367 [PMID 23519301]

26 **b** repeat cotesting in 12 months

Repeat cotesting performed 12 months after the initial colposcopy is recommended for women over 30 who are cytology–, but HPV+

Massad LS, Einstein MH, Huh WK, et al. 2012 Updated consensus guidelines for the management of abnormal cervical cancer screening tests and cancer precursors. J Low Genit Tract Dis 2013;17(3):367 [PMID 23519301]

27 **a** colposcopy

For pregnant (nonadolescent) patients with a cytologic diagnosis of LSIL, colposcopy is recommended, but an endocervical curettage (ECC) is not recommended. If the patient or the clinician chooses, postponing the follow-up colposcopy until 6 weeks postpartum is considered an acceptable management paradigm for patients with this diagnosis.

Massad LS, Einstein MH, Huh WK, et al. 2012 Updated consensus guidelines for the management of abnormal cervical cancer screening tests and cancer precursors. J Low Genit Tract Dis 2013;17(3):367 [PMID 23519301]

28 **d** repeat colposcopy and cytology in 6 month intervals for up to 2 years

Should a patient have a negative colposcopy and endocervical curetting after a cytologic diagnosis of HSIL, the recommended management is for clinical observation with colposcopy and repeat cytology at 6 month intervals for up to 2 years .

Massad LS, Einstein MH, Huh WK, et al. 2012 Updated consensus guidelines for the management of abnormal cervical cancer screening tests and cancer precursors. J Low Genit Tract Dis 2013;17(3):367 [PMID 23519301]

29 **d** biopsy

A biopsy should be performed on adolescent patients with persistent HSIL after repeated negative colposcopies. If the biopsy is subsequently positive, the management should follow ASCCP guidelines as related to the severity of disease.

Massad LS, Einstein MH, Huh WK, et al. 2012 Updated consensus guidelines for the management of abnormal cervical cancer screening tests and cancer precursors. J Low Genit Tract Dis 2013;17(3):367 [PMID 23519301]

ISBN 978-089189-6357 ©ASCP 2015

30 b   colposcopy with ECC, HPV testing

HPV testing and/or a repeat Pap test have poor sensitivity in the initial triage for AGC; therefore, multiple clinical modalities are recommended, including colposcopy, endocervical curetting, HPV testing, and endometrial evaluation (if the patient is over the age of 35).

Massad LS, Einstein MH, Huh WK, et al. 2012 Updated consensus guidelines for the management of abnormal cervical cancer screening tests and cancer precursors. J Low Genit Tract Dis 2013;17(3):367 [PMID 23519301]

31 b   endometrial and endocervical sampling

Both of these clinical modalities are recommended for patients with cytologic diagnoses of AGC specifying endometrial morphology. Colposcopy may be concomitantly performed or deferred until determination of its relevance is established after the histologic results have been analyzed from the endometrial and endocervical sampling.

Massad LS, Einstein MH, Huh WK, et al. 2012 Updated consensus guidelines for the management of abnormal cervical cancer screening tests and cancer precursors. J Low Genit Tract Dis 2013;17(3):367 [PMID 23519301]

32 c   colposcopy with ECC, HPV testing, endometrial sampling

HPV testing and/or a repeat Pap test have poor sensitivity in the initial triage for AGC; therefore, multiple clinical modalities are recommended, including colposcopy, endocervical curetting, HPV testing, and in this case of a 37-year-old female, endometrial evaluation (included in the workup for patients over the age of 35).

Massad LS, Einstein MH, Huh WK, et al. 2012 Updated consensus guidelines for the management of abnormal cervical cancer screening tests and cancer precursors. J Low Genit Tract Dis 2013;17(3):367 [PMID 23519301]

33 d   diagnostic excisional procedure

Confirmation that there is no invasive disease is followed by an immediate excisional procedure for these adenocarcinomas in situ glandular lesions, based on cytology alone.

Massad LS, Einstein MH, Huh WK, et al. 2012 Updated consensus guidelines for the management of abnormal cervical cancer screening tests and cancer precursors. J Low Genit Tract Dis 2013;17(3):367 [PMID 23519301]

34 d   repeat HPV and Pap test at 12 months

Conservative follow-up with repeat cytology and HPV testing at 12 months is the best management paradigm due to the fact that these may be subclinical lesions that are not clinically detectable. Should repeat test results be persistently HPV+ and cytology negative, colposcopy is warranted.

Saslow D, Solomon D, Lawson HW, et al. American Cancer Society, American Society for Colposcopy and Cervical Pathology, and American Society for Clinical Pathology screening guidelines for the prevention and early detection of cervical cancer. Am J Clin Pathol 2012;137:516-542 [PMID 22431528]

35 a   repeat cytology at 12 months

Considering the HPV test is now negative, the patient should be managed per ASCCP protocol. In that case, management recommendations would be to repeat cytology in 12 months with or without an HPV test.

Saslow D, Solomon D, Lawson HW, et al. American Cancer Society, American Society for Colposcopy and Cervical Pathology, and American Society for Clinical Pathology screening guidelines for the prevention and early detection of cervical cancer. Am J Clin Pathol 2012;137:516-542 [PMID 22431528]

36 c   promote best clinical practices focused on efficiently identifying women at highest risk

No management strategy will ever eliminate all cancer risk, and management algorithms should never be used as a substitute for clinical judgment. The 2012 Updated ASCCP Consensus Guidelines seek to minimize overall cancer risk, while at the same time minimizing cost, complications and anxiety for women at low risk.

Massad LS, Einstein MH, Huh WK, et al. 2012 Updated consensus guidelines for the management of abnormal cervical cancer screening tests and cancer precursors. J Low Genit Tract Dis 2013;17(3):367 [PMID 23519301]

37 b   HPV testing may be useful in conjunction with colposcopy and endocervical and/or endometrial sampling

For all subcategories of AGC (excluding atypical endometrial cells), the initial evaluation should include colposcopy (with endocervical sampling) and HPV testing, and endometrial sampling (if >35 years of age or at risk for endometrial neoplasia).

Massad LS, Einstein MH, Huh WK, et al. 2012 Updated consensus guidelines for the management of abnormal cervical cancer screening tests and cancer precursors. J Low Genit Tract Dis 2013;17(3):367 [PMID 23519301]

38 **b** repeat cytology at 12 months

ASCUS and LSIL in young women generally reflect transient HPV infections, which can and should be managed conservatively. Since 90 % of these infections clear spontaneously within 12-24 months, recommended follow-up is repeat cytology at 12 months. HPV testing is "unacceptable" for women age 21.

Saslow D, Solomon D, Lawson HW, et al. American Cancer Society, American Society for Colposcopy and Cervical Pathology, and American Society for Clinical Pathology screening guidelines for the prevention and early detection of cervical cancer. Am J Clin Pathol 2012;137:516-542 [PMID 22431528]

39 **d** patients A and B both have a 12% risk of being diagnosed with CIN2/3

From the ALTS trial we know that an initial colposcopy is only 65% sensitive for the detection of an underlying CIN2/3, and both patients have a similar risk (12%-14%) of being diagnosed with CIN2/3 over the next 24 months. The recommended follow-up for both patients is repeat cytology at 6 & 12 months or HPV testing alone at 12 months; a repeat Pap showing more than ASCUS or a positive HPV test both trigger repeat colposcopy.

Massad LS, Einstein MH, Huh WK, et al. 2012 Updated consensus guidelines for the management of abnormal cervical cancer screening tests and cancer precursors. J Low Genit Tract Dis 2013;17(3):367 [PMID 23519301]

40 **b** reflex high risk HPV testing is more useful than a repeat Pap test for triage to colposcopy

A single high risk HPV test is more effective than 2 repeat Pap tests in identifying an underlying CIN2/3. Per 2012 Updated ASCCP Consensus Guidelines, HPV testing is not indicated for women younger than age 21.

Massad LS, Einstein MH, Huh WK, et al. 2012 Updated consensus guidelines for the management of abnormal cervical cancer screening tests and cancer precursors. J Low Genit Tract Dis 2013;17(3):367 [PMID 23519301]

41 **d** the positive predictive value of ASC-H for CIN2/3 approaches 50%

ASC-H identifies a patient population at high risk for underlying CIN2/3, with a positive predictive value approaching 50%. Colposcopy is mandatory and not based on HPV triage. Initial colposcopy, biopsies and endocervical sampling may be falsely negative though, and these patients should be followed with repeat Pap tests at 6 & 12 months or HPV testing at 12 months.

Massad LS, Einstein MH, Huh WK, et al. 2012 Updated consensus guidelines for the management of abnormal cervical cancer screening tests and cancer precursors. J Low Genit Tract Dis 2013;17(3):367 [PMID 23519301]

42 **d** repeat cotesting at 12 months

For women with a colposcopy diagnosis of CIN1, preceded by ASCUS, ASC-H or LSIL cytology, the recommended management is repeat cotesting at 12 months

Massad LS, Einstein MH, Huh WK, et al. 2012 Updated consensus guidelines for the management of abnormal cervical cancer screening tests and cancer precursors. J Low Genit Tract Dis 2013;17(3):367 [PMID 23519301]

43 **b** this patient should have colposcopy

Since ASC-H identifies a patient population at high risk for CIN2/3, colposcopy is mandatory and not based on HPV triage. Initial colposcopy, biopsies and endocervical sampling may be falsely negative though, and these patients should be followed with repeat Pap tests at 6 & 12 months or HPV testing at 12 months.

Stoler MH. Testing for human papillomavirus: data driven implications for cervical neoplasia management. Clin Lab Med 2003;23(3):569-583 [PMID 14560529]

44 **b** colposcopy

According to 2012 Updated ASCCP Consensus Guidelines, patients with NILM cytology and a positive high risk HPV test should return for repeat cytology and HPV testing at 12 months

Massad LS, Einstein MH, Huh WK, et al. 2012 Updated consensus guidelines for the management of abnormal cervical cancer screening tests and cancer precursors. J Low Genit Tract Dis 2013;17(3):367 [PMID 23519301]

45 **b** all patients should have colposcopy

Initial management for all patients, regardless of age, should be colposcopy.

Massad LS, Einstein MH, Huh WK, et al. 2012 Updated consensus guidelines for the management of abnormal cervical cancer screening tests and cancer precursors. J Low Genit Tract Dis 2013;17(3):367 [PMID 23519301]

46 **d** precolopscopic triage of ASCUS for women 21 and older, laboratory QC and primary screening of women >30

HPV testing is the most effective tool for the triage of ASCUS, and in combination with the Pap it improves the sensitivity and negative predictive value of screening of women over 30.

Stoler MH. ASC, TBS, and the power of ALTS. Am J Clin Pathol 2007;127(4):489-491 [PMID 17369124]

ISBN 978-089189-6357 ©ASCP 2015

47 b HPV triage is one of multiple available options, none of which is considered "best"

The terms "recommended," "preferred," "acceptable" and "unacceptable," are used to describe each of the clinical interventions described in the Guidelines, and these terms are clearly defined.

Massad LS, Einstein MH, Huh WK, et al. 2012 Updated consensus guidelines for the management of abnormal cervical cancer screening tests and cancer precursors. J Low Genit Tract Dis 2013;17(3):367 [PMID 23519301]

48 d 10 endocervical and/or metaplastic squamous cells

A minimum of 10 endocervical and/or metaplastic squamous cells is required.

Nayar R, Wilbur D, eds. The Bethesda System for Reporting Cervical Cytology 2015 [in press]

49 a 5,000

A minimum of 5,000 unobscured squamous cells are required to consider a liquid based Pap test satisfactory for evaluation for an epithelial cell abnormality. However, under certain clinical circumstances, lower cell counts due to cell clustering, atrophy or autolysis may still be considered adequate.

Nayar R, Wilbur D, eds. The Bethesda System for Reporting Cervical Cytology 2015 [in press]

50 a repeat cytologic exam in 12 months

The vast majority of adolescents with a cytologic finding of ASCUS or LSIL will have the lesion regress regardless of their HPV status. Follow-up with cytologic testing at the 12 month interval is recommended. Only adolescents with HSIL or greater on repeat cytology should be referred for colposcopy. HPV testing is not recommended for adolescents with ASCUS or LSIL per 2012 Updated ASCCP Consensus Guidelines.

Saslow D, Solomon D, Lawson HW, et al. American Cancer Society, American Society for Colposcopy and Cervical Pathology, and American Society for Clinical Pathology screening guidelines for the prevention and early detection of cervical cancer. Am J Clin Pathol 2012;137:516-542 [PMID 22431528]

51 c obscuring inflammation that precludes interpretation of 75% or more of the epithelial cells

The current recommendations, based on preliminary scientific evidence, are a minimum cellularity of 5,000 cells for a liquid based preparation and 8,000-12,000 minimum cellularity for conventional smears. These minimum cell ranges should estimated and compared to reference images. Studies show that reference images are quickly learned and have better interobserver reproducibility than the previous Bethesda criterion of 10% slide coverage. Specimens with >75% of squamous cells obscured should be termed unsatisfactory, assuming that no abnormal cells are identified. Any specimen with abnormal cells (ASCUS or AGC) is by definition satisfactory for evaluation.

Nayar R, Wilbur D, eds. The Bethesda System for Reporting Cervical Cytology 2015 [in press]

52 d hysterectomy

Hysterectomy is considered appropriate for diagnosis and treatment of endocervical adenocarcinoma in situ.

Massad LS, Einstein MH, Huh WK, et al. 2012 Updated consensus guidelines for the management of abnormal cervical cancer screening tests and cancer precursors. J Low Genit Tract Dis 2013;17(3):367 [PMID 23519301]

53 a women under 21 years of age should not be screened regardless of the age of sexual initiation or other risk factors

Cervical cancer is rare in young women and may not be prevented by cytology screening. In addition, there is a potential for relative net harm due to intervention for abnormal Pap test results in women under age 21, in which preinvasive lesions have a high probability of spontaneous regression. Therefore, women aged younger than 21 years should not be screened by any modality regardless of the age of sexual initiation or other risk factors.

Saslow D, Solomon D, Lawson HW, et al. American Cancer Society, American Society for Colposcopy and Cervical Pathology, and American Society for Clinical Pathology screening guidelines for the prevention and early detection of cervical cancer. Am J Clin Pathol 2012;137:516-542 [PMID 22431528]

54 d report of a new sexual partner warrants a return to active screening

Once screening is discontinued, it should not resume for any reason, even if a woman reports having a new sexual partner.

Saslow D, Solomon D, Lawson HW, et al. American Cancer Society, American Society for Colposcopy and Cervical Pathology, and American Society for Clinical Pathology screening guidelines for the prevention and early detection of cervical cancer. Am J Clin Pathol 2012;137:516-542 [PMID 22431528]

55 d should not change on the basis of HPV vaccination status

Guideline participants judged that it is premature to modify screening in the United States based on HPV vaccination history, and doing so would require epidemiologic studies on an optimally vaccinated subset of women.

Saslow D, Solomon D, Lawson HW, et al. American Cancer Society, American Society for Colposcopy and Cervical Pathology, and American Society for Clinical Pathology screening guidelines for the prevention and early detection of cervical cancer. Am J Clin Pathol 2012;137:516-542 [PMID 22431528]

56 c depends on patient's age

For women under the age of 21, the recommended follow-up for LSIL is repeat cytology at 12 months. For other patients, colposcopy is generally indicated, although HPV testing may be a useful triage tool in postmenopausal women.

Saslow D, Solomon D, Lawson HW, et al. American Cancer Society, American Society for Colposcopy and Cervical Pathology, and American Society for Clinical Pathology screening guidelines for the prevention and early detection of cervical cancer. Am J Clin Pathol 2012;137:516-542 [PMID 22431528]

57 c   repeat cotesting at 12 months

According to 2012 Updated ASCCP Consensus Guidelines, patients with NILM cytology and a positive high risk HPV test should return for repeat cytology and HPV testing at 12 months.

Massad LS, Einstein MH, Huh WK, et al. 2012 Updated consensus guidelines for the management of abnormal cervical cancer screening tests and cancer precursors. J Low Genit Tract Dis 2013;17(3):367 [PMID 23519301]

58 c   depends on patient age

Colposcopic examination with endocervical assessment and immediate LEEP conization are both acceptable management options; however, immediate LEEP conization is unacceptable in young women under age 21.

Massad LS, Einstein MH, Huh WK, et al. 2012 Updated consensus guidelines for the management of abnormal cervical cancer screening tests and cancer precursors. J Low Genit Tract Dis 2013;17(3):367 [PMID 23519301]

59 b   repeat cytology in 12 months

2012 Updated ASCCP Consensus Guidelines recommend repeat cytology at 12 months for adolescents with a cytologic interpretation of LSIL.

Massad LS, Einstein MH, Huh WK, et al. 2012 Updated consensus guidelines for the management of abnormal cervical cancer screening tests and cancer precursors. J Low Genit Tract Dis 2013;17(3):367 [PMID 23519301]

ISBN 978-089189-6357 ©ASCP 2015

Chapter 3
Body Fluids

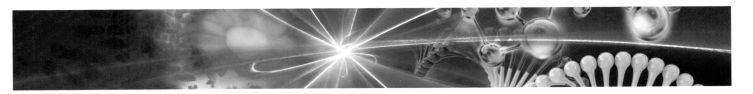

1   In gouty arthritis, which type of crystal may be visualized under polarized microscopy?
a   calcium phosphate
b   monosodium urate
c   triple phosphate
d   calcium carbonate

2   A synovial disease often found in elderly women that manifests cytologically as multiple fragments of chondrocytes, osteoclasts, lymphocytes, and reactive synovial lining cells is:
a   rheumatoid arthritis
b   septic arthritis
c   osteoarthritis
d   osteocalcinosis

3   The most common metastatic tumor diagnosed by cerebrospinal fluid cytology is:
a   lung
b   liver
c   stomach
d   colon

4   Which of the following tumors has the greatest predisposition for brain metastasis?
a   choriocarcinoma
b   clear cell carcinoma
c   cholangiocarcinoma
d   adenoid cystic carcinoma

5   Polymorphonuclear neutrophils, trapezoidal histiocytes, cholesterol crystals, cells with intracytoplasmic inclusions, and a dense eosinophilic granular background in synovial fluid are diagnostic of:
a   osteoarthritis
b   rheumatoid arthritis
c   Reiter syndrome
d   gout

6   The presence of siderophages (hemosiderin laden macrophages) in CSF could be related to:
a   post oil myelogram
b   subdural hematoma
c   tuberculosis
d   bacterial meningitis

7   A tumor often involving the long bones and found in children in their second decade cytologically presents in synovial fluid as small, mononuclear cells scattered among blood vessels and fibrous stroma. The diagnosis is:
a   villonodular synovitis
b   giant cell tumor
c   Ewing sarcoma
d   gout

8   A synonym for pseudogout is:
a   osteochondritis
b   acidosis
c   sodium biuratosis
d   chondrocalcinosis

9   A plasma cell infiltrate seen in a CSF specimen may be related to:
a   acute bacterial meningitis
b   epileptic seizure
c   hemorrhage
d   multiple sclerosis

10 The cytologic/histologic pattern of cells from an intraventricular mass in the choroid plexus reveals which architecture pattern?
a   papillary
b   acinar
c   sheets
d   signet ring

11 A pea sized lesion composed of anaplastic cells located posterior to the third ventricle over the brain stem is diagnostic of:
a   medulloblastoma
b   retinoblastoma
c   meningioma
d   pineoblastoma

12 In cerebrospinal fluid, round to cuboidal neuronal elements with vacuolated and pigmented cytoplasm exhibiting small, eccentric, vesicular nuclei are identified as:
a   ependymal cells
b   nucleus pulposus cells
c   chondrocytes
d   leptomeningeal cells

©ASCP 2015   ISBN 978-089189-6357

13 A CSF specimen shows numerous blood cells, neutrophils, lymphocytes, and a few single cells exhibiting giant cell features and multinucleation. These cells are diagnostic of:
  a peripheral blood contamination
  b chronic lymphocytic leukemia
  c metastatic sarcoma
  d metastatic giant cell carcinoma

14 A 41-year-old female presents with a meningeal tumor contained within the cerebral hemispheres. Cytology shows cells in a whorl-like formation and cigar shaped cells with delicate chromatin, micronucleoli, and intranuclear inclusions. The diagnosis is:
  a meningioma
  b schwannoma
  c pituitary adenoma
  d Rathke pouch cyst

15 What infectious agent in cerebrospinal fluid stains positively with mucicarmine?
  a *Blastomyces dermatitidis*
  b *Cryptococcus neoformans*
  c *Candida albicans*
  d cytomegalovirus

16 Which tumor is neural crest in origin?
  a oligodendroglioma
  b astrocytoma
  c meningioma
  d medulloblastoma

17 A circumscribed tumor found in adolescents, which may arise in the fourth ventricle of the posterior fossa, comprises elongated cells and rosettes with round, eccentric nuclei and micronucleoli. These cells are diagnostic of:
  a medulloblastoma
  b neuroblastoma
  c astrocytoma
  d ependymoma

18 A cerebellar neoplasm identified in a 5-year-old male sheds cells into the CSF. Lumbar puncture reveals small spindle cells with fibrillar, fine, and lacy cytoplasm. The nuclei have a bland appearance. These cells are representative of:
  a ependymoma
  b medulloblastoma
  c astrocytoma
  d glioblastoma multiforme

19 A patient receiving intrathecal therapy for acute lymphocytic leukemia has a lumbar puncture 2 weeks after treatment. Cytology reveals a heterogeneous population of lymphocytes, many of which have nucleoli. The diagnosis is:
  a reactive pleocytosis
  b recurrent leukemia
  c atypical changes suggestive of recurrent leukemia
  d peripheral blood contamination

20 Lipid laden histiocytes found in a CSF specimen may be related to:
  a post oil myelogram
  b melanoma
  c neurosyphilis
  d viral meningitis

21 A disease of young adults that may involve the knee is cytologically diagnosed as a highly cellular anaplastic tumor. Histologically, slitlike spaces are found within the tissue. The cellular findings suggest:
  a Ewing sarcoma
  b villonodular synovitis
  c giant cell tumor of tendon sheath
  d synovial sarcoma

22 A primary tumor of the cerebellum, usually found in children, that sheds small cells with hyperchromatic nuclei forming pseudorosettes is characteristic of:
  a medulloblastoma
  b oligodendroglioma
  c glioblastoma multiforme
  d pituitary adenoma

23 A benign tumor of neural sheath arising predominantly in adults is termed:
  a meningioma
  b schwannoma
  c pituitary adenoma
  d craniopharyngioma

24 A periorbital mass infiltrating the optic tract and shedding cells into CSF is:
  a medulloblastoma
  b retinoblastoma
  c neuroblastoma
  d pinealoma

25 A 3-year-old female presents with evaluated catecholamines in the urine and abdominal enlargement. CSF cytology reveals anaplastic cells forming rosettes. Electron microscopy reveals secretory granules. The diagnosis is:
  a nephroblastoma
  b medulloblastoma
  c neuroblastoma
  d schwannoma

26 A 68-year-old male presents with diplopia. CSF analysis reveals a population of pleomorphic cells with large, eccentrically located, hyperchromatic nuclei with irregular chromatin and dense, hard, refractile cytoplasm. A previous pleural fluid was malignant. The most likely diagnosis/primary site of this malignancy is:
  a metastatic carcinoma, lung
  b metastatic carcinoma, pancreas
  c metastatic carcinoma, colon
  d metastatic carcinoma, prostate

ISBN 978-089189-6357 ©ASCP 2015

27 An elderly woman with a previously diagnosed extra-CNS malignancy currently presents with hemiparesis and disorientation. A lumbar puncture is performed. The CSF reveals cells in 3D groupings and loose clusters with fine chromatin, macronucleoli, and granular cytoplasm. Which of the following most likely represents the primary site?

a muscle
b skin
c breast
d liver

28 A joint related disease that is related to chlamydial infection is referred to as:

a rheumatoid arthritis
b Reiter syndrome
c gout
d chondrocalcinosis

29 Which of the following may present as neutrophilia in a cerebrospinal fluid specimen?

a viral encephalitis
b acute bacterial meningitis
c neurosyphilis
d metastatic carcinoma

30 A small group of cohesive cells with macronucleoli is seen in synovial fluid from an elderly male. Elevated acid phosphatase is noted. The diagnosis/origin is:

a squamous carcinoma/lung (parathormone+)
b adenocarcinoma/kidney (lipid+)
c adenocarcinoma/prostate (PSA+)
d osteogenic sarcoma/bone (vimentin−)

31 A 32-year-old male presents with frequent headaches and a recent onset of seizures. Nuclear magnetic resonance reveals a 3 cm mass located in the left cerebral hemisphere. A ventricular tap reveals a pleomorphic sample with stellate bipolar cells exhibiting hyperchromatic nuclei, anisocytosis, and multinucleated giant cells scattered in a granular background. Many single cells as well as aggregates are seen. Based on the cytologic findings, the diagnosis is:

a astrocytoma
b glioblastoma multiforme
c oligodendroglioma
d ependymoma

32 What special stain might prove useful in distinguishing oligodendrogliomas from other primary brain tumors?

a PAS
b oil red O
c mucicarmine
d Giemsa

33 A benign congenital nest intracranial cystic tumor shedding keratin pearls and anucleate squames into the CSF is diagnostic of:

a meningioma
b craniopharyngioma
c pinealoma
d ependymoma

34 A 22-year-old HIV+ patient with meningoencephalitis and myocarditis submits for a lumbar puncture because of a spiking fever. Cytology reveals mononuclear pleocytosis. Giemsa staining reveals many crescent shaped cystic structures within the cytoplasm of histiocytes. The diagnosis is:

a *Cryptosporidium*
b *Toxoplasma gondii*
c *Entamoeba histolytica*
d Kaposi sarcoma

35 A 44-year-old male with a previously diagnosed extra-CNS malignancy presents for CSF analysis. Cytology reveals large cells containing large, eccentrically located hyperchromatic nuclei and double mirror image nuclei with macronucleoli. Intranuclear cytoplasmic invaginations are present in many of the cells. Which of the following is the most likely diagnosis?

a adenocarcinoma, bronchogenic
b adenocarcinoma, stomach
c malignant melanoma
d histiocytic lymphoma

36 A patient with pleurisy secondary to pneumonia presents with a 500 mL pleural effusion. A large population of cells are present in the cytology analysis of a filter preparation. Cells have frothy cytoplasm and eccentrically located vesicular/reniform nuclei. These cells are:

a macrophages
b mesothelial cells
c associated with Hodgkin disease
d atypical mesothelial cells

37 The most commonly identified fungus found in cerebrospinal fluid specimens is:

a *Blastomyces dermatitidis*
b *Cryptococcus neoformans*
c *Histoplasma capsulatum*
d *Candida albicans*

38 The presence of mitotic figures in effusion cytology:

a is of little significance
b most likely represents malignancy
c suggests an infectious process
d should recommend a biopsy

39 In differentiating metastatic adenocarcinoma from malignant mesothelioma in a pleural fluid, which special stains would confirm metastatic adenocarcinoma?

a D-PAS+
b D-PAS−
c hyaluronic acid+
d alcian blue-hyaluronidase−

40 Which of these cytologic findings favors a metastatic effusion over a benign condition?

a "knobby" cytoplasmic borders
b community borders
c prominent nucleoli
d monolayer sheets

©ASCP 2015 ISBN 978-089189-6357

41 A 69-year-old male with a 2 pack per day history of cigarette smoking presents with a pleural effusion. A thoracentesis reveals cells in vertebral column formation with molding and coarse irregular chromatin. Which of the following is the most likely diagnosis?
a squamous carcinoma, nonkeratinizing
b sclerosing hemangioma
c small cell carcinoma
d bronchioloalveolar adenocarcinoma

42 Cells presenting with increased nuclear sizes, micronucleoli, round and uniform nuclear contours, and "knobby" cytoplasmic borders in an ascitic fluid specimen are diagnostic of:
a lymphocytic lymphoma
b reactive mesothelial cells
c small cell carcinoma
d Hodgkin disease

43 A young child with a history of embryonal rhabdomyosarcoma presents with a peritoneal effusion. Which stain may confirm a metastatic neoplasm?
a PAS
b melanin
c lipid
d amyloid

44 A 44-year-old female presents with a butterfly rash on her face and a pleural effusion. Cytology reveals severe acute inflammation. Many cells contain eosinophilic intracytoplasmic inclusions. The diagnosis is:
a rheumatoid pleuritis
b systemic lupus erythematosus
c tuberculous effusion
d eosinophilic pleural effusion

45 The organism most commonly associated with elephantiasis of the genitalia or extremities is:
a Echinococcus granulosus
b Paragonimus westermani
c Mycobacterium tuberculosis
d Nocardia asteroides

46 When discriminating adenocarcinoma from mesothelioma, which of the following is true?
a mesothelioma is positive for vimentin
b adenocarcinoma is positive for vimentin
c mesothelioma is positive for LeuM1 and secretory component
d adenocarcinoma is positive for β human chorionic gonadotropin

47 A pleural effusion from a 51-year-old female reveals a foreign population of multiple 3D round, cohesive tissue fragments resembling "cannonballs," blastulas, or proliferation spheres with community borders. Multiple Barr bodies are identified. The likely diagnosis/origin of these cells is:
a poorly differentiated adenocarcinoma/lung
b adenocarcinoma/breast
c adenocarcinoma/colon
d adenocarcinoma/ovary

48 Effusions that are composed predominantly of eosinophils are:
a most often related to Wegener granulomatosis
b specific for tuberculosis
c idiopathic
d diagnostic of sarcoidosis

49 Which of the following organisms is highly antigenic, often resulting in anaphylaxis when aspirated?
a Mycobacterium tuberculosis
b Wuchereria bancrofti
c Echinococcus granulosus
d Nocardia asteroides

50 Cells staining positive for D-PAS and mucicarmine in an effusion could be diagnostic of:
a mesothelioma
b adenocarcinoma
c lymphoma
d squamous carcinoma

51 A 65-year-old shipyard worker with a history of asbestos exposure and persistent pleural effusions currently presents with shortness of breath. Sputum and bronchoscopic analyses show no evidence of malignancy. Pleural fluid cytology reveals abundant single cells with nuclear enlargement, multiple macronucleoli, hyperchromasia, and coarse irregular chromatin. The cytoplasm has a dense nature with an ectoplasm/endoplasm 2-toned staining. Which special stain would have a negative reaction with these cells?
a alcian blue
b alcian blue-hyaluronidase
c PAS
d cytokeratin

52 In the evaluation of malignant processes involving the serous cavities, what factor is essential before rendering a diagnosis?
a identification of a blood cell component
b patient history
c special stains for mucin
d cytochemical staining

53 A malignant teratoid renal tumor found in children is:
a Grawitz tumor
b Wilms tumor
c neuroblastoma
d embryonal rhabdomyosarcoma

54 One of the most helpful criteria in determining malignancy in effusion cytology is:
a a single cell population of abnormal cells
b a discrete population of foreign cells and normal cells
c identification of nucleoli
d presence of mitotic figures

ISBN 978-089189-6357 ©ASCP 2015

55 A pleural fluid reveals many large elongated "snake" cells exhibiting basophilia, well defined cell borders, finely granular regularly distributed chromatin, and round to oval well preserved nuclei. Another population of multinucleated cells with cytoplasmic inclusions were found. The background exhibits an eosinophilic granular debris. The cytologic findings suggest:

a metastatic squamous cell carcinoma
b synovial sarcoma
c systemic lupus erythematosus
d rheumatoid pleuritis

56 A malignant population of cohesive cells staining mucicarmine negative may represent:

a a poorly differentiated adenocarcinoma, not otherwise specified
b ductal carcinoma of the breast
c well differentiated adenocarcinoma of the lung
d colonic adenocarcinoma

57 A 41-year-old female presents with abdominal ascites. Cytologic analysis of the effusion reveals large clusters of transparent, elongated cells with distended vacuoles and community borders staining positive with mucicarmine. The origin of these cells is most likely:

a liver
b colon
c ovary
d kidney

58 A 62-year-old female with a history of radiation exposure to the head and neck presents with a 300 mL pleural effusion. Cytologic analysis reveals clusters of malignant cells and many eosinophilic, calcifying structures with concentric rings. What may be the site of origin?

a thyroid
b trachea
c salivary glands
d esophagus

59 A peritoneal effusion from a 72-year-old male is represented by a heterogeneous population of cells possessing central granular and clear peripheral cytoplasm and large, hyperchromatic nuclei with macronucleoli. Clinical symptoms include hypercalcemia, hypertension, and polycythemia. Prostatic acid phosphatase and mucicarmine stains were negative. Special staining with oil red O was strongly positive. The most likely diagnosis/origin is:

a adenocarcinoma/colon
b renal cell carcinoma/kidney
c hepatocellular carcinoma/liver
d melanoma/skin

60 An abdominal centesis from a 56-year-old male yields an abundant population of cohesive cells in papillary clusters with tall, columnar morphology, irregular chromatin, and nucleoli. The most likely diagnosis/ origin of these cells is:

a adenocarcinoma/pancreas
b cholangiocarcinoma/bile duct
c mesothelioma/parietal peritoneal
d adenocarcinoma/colon

61 A chylous effusion may be associated with:

a scleroderma
b rheumatoid arthritis
c cirrhosis
d systemic lupus erythematosus

62 Septic arthritis in a synovial fluid is related to:

a a generalized body infection
b an autoimmune disease
c *Chlamydia*
d trauma

63 What type of cell found in an ascitic fluid might suggest extramedullary hematopoiesis associated with myeloid metaplasia?

a plasma cell
b megakaryocyte
c immunoblasts
d reticulocyte

64 Which of the following diagnoses has an associated hyaluronic acid background and does not stain positive with alcian blue hyaluronidase?

a adenocarcinoma, pancreas
b carcinoid tumor, lung
c hepatocellular carcinoma
d mesothelioma, carcinomatous

65 A 44-year-old male with a known primary malignancy presents with a 400 mL pleural effusion. The cells are predominantly single in nature with large, eccentrically located nuclei and intranuclear cytoplasmic invaginations. Many cells have multiple nuclei as well as macronucleoli. Which of the following is most likely represented?

a melanoma
b poorly differentiated adenocarcinoma
c squamous cell carcinoma
d pancreatic adenocarcinoma

66 A 4-year-old female presents with an abdominal mass and a peritoneal effusion. Analysis of the serous fluid reveals small, immature cells with high N:C ratios. The cells are found in small aggregates with a central lumen, resembling rosettes. Special stains for chromogranin are positive. The most likely diagnosis/ origin is:

a Wilms tumor/kidney
b Ewing sarcoma/bone
c embryonal rhabdomyosarcoma/vagina
d neuroblastoma/adrenals

67 Which of the following is associated with septic arthritis in a synovial fluid?
a decrease in fibrin
b sarcoid
c rheumatoid factor
d tuberculosis

68 Normal mesothelial cells are:
a positive for neutral mucin
b positive for DPAS
c negative for neutral mucin
d always positive with LeuM5

69 Single cells with "windows" and dense endoplasm/ pale ectoplasm features seen in serous fluids are characteristic of:
a macrophages
b mesothelial cells
c lymphocytes
d oat cell carcinoma

70 The diagnosis of traumatic arthritis in a synovial fluid specimen is associated with the cytologic identification of:
a immunoblasts
b lymphocytic effusion
c hemosiderin laden macrophages
d chlamydial inclusions

ISBN 978-089189-6357 ©ASCP 2015

71 These cells, identified in a pleural effusion from a 53-year-old male with a history of a gastrointestinal disorder, represent:

a metastatic squamous cell carcinoma
b pleuroesophageal fistula
c skin contaminant
d collagen balls

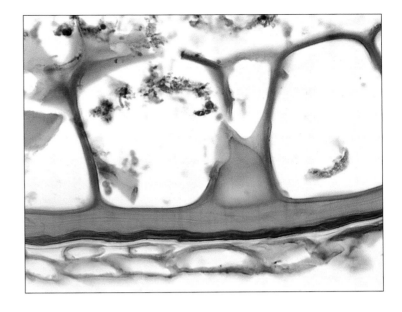

72 A 44-year-old male, after intrathecal therapy for chronic myelogenous leukemia, presents for follow-up analysis via the ventricular shunt. These cells are diagnostic of:

a reactive lymphocytosis
b recurrent CML
c viral meningitis
d acute bacterial meningitis

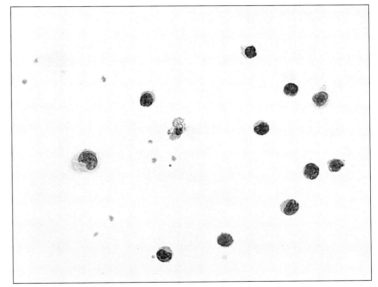

73 The cellular process as demonstrated in this lumbar puncture specimen (stained with mucicarmine) represents:

a starch
b *Cryptococcus neoformans*
c *Taenia solium*
d coxsackievirus infection

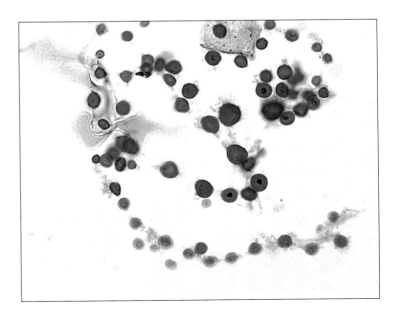

74 These cells are from a 63-year-old alcoholic male with
    a left sided pleural effusion. Clinical findings include a
    low hematocrit value and high amylase levels. 800 mL
    of a dark brown fluid was obtained for evaluation.
    Cytology reveals:
    a normal/reactive mesothelial cells
    b normal/reactive hepatocytes
    c mesothelioma
    d pancreatic adenocarcinoma

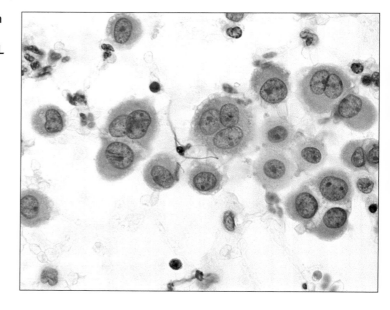

75 These cells are from the CSF specimen of a 5-year-old
    child previously diagnosed with acute lymphoblastic
    leukemia and now presenting with a spiking fever and
    malaise. What special stain would aid in establishing
    the possibility of recurrence?
    a tumor marker: terminal deoxytransferase
    b S100
    c α-fetoprotein
    d chromogranin

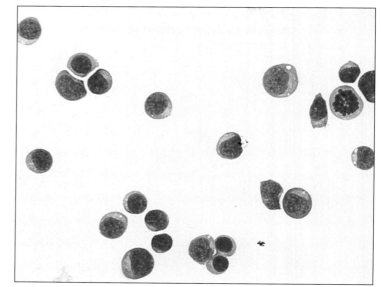

76 A 44-year-old male with recent fainting spells presents
    with a large cerebral mass. No history of cancer is
    noted. A ventricular aspiration is performed. Based on
    the cytologic findings, the diagnosis is:
    a astrocytoma, grade I
    b glioblastoma multiforme
    c ependymoma
    d oligodendroglioma

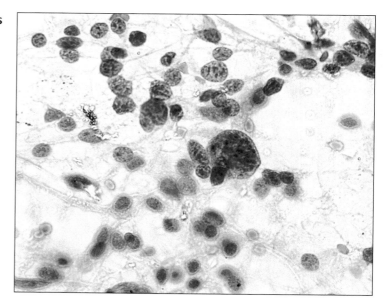

ISBN 978-089189-6357 ©ASCP 2015

77 A 44-year-old female with joint inflammation, multiple tophi deposits, and a history of an inborn uric acid metabolism disorder undergoes synovial fluid analysis. These structures were found with polarized light. Cytology reveals:

a chondrocalcinosis/monosodium urate monohydrate
b gout/monosodium urate monohydrate
c chondrocalcinosis/bisodium urate monohydrate
d gout/bisodium urate bihydrate

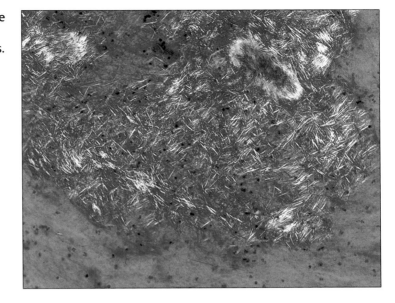

78 A lumbar puncture was performed on a 44-year-old AIDS patient. The cytologic pattern represents:

a bacterial meningitis
b viral meningitis
c lymphocytic lymphoma
d neuroblastoma

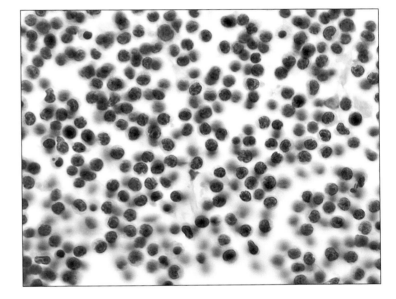

79 A ventricular tap from a 10-year-old child with a history of acute lymphocytic leukemia status post intrathecal therapy (via ventricular peritoneal shunt catheter) yields a 1 mL specimen for analysis. The findings are consistent with:

a recurrent leukemia
b acute inflammation, secondary to bacterial meningitis
c neural elements
d chronic inflammation, secondary to viral meningitis

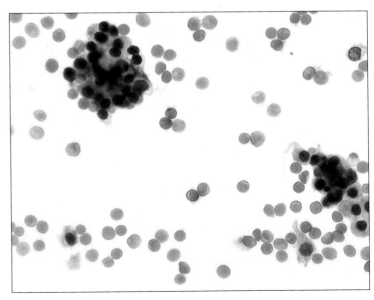

80 A lumbar puncture is performed on a 44-year-old male with a history of severe headaches. Cytology reveals:

    a normal cellular findings
    b hypocellular sample, suggest repeat
    c viral meningitis
    d leptomeningeal cells

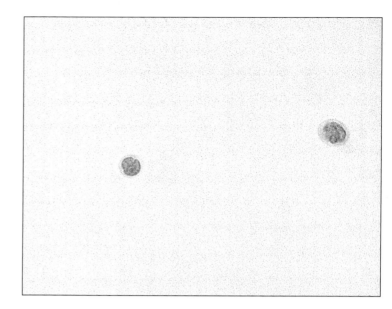

81 An 8-year-old female presents with a 2 cm midline cerebellar lesion. These cells are found on ventricular tap. They are diagnostic of:

    a neuroblastoma
    b lymphoma
    c astrocytoma
    d medulloblastoma

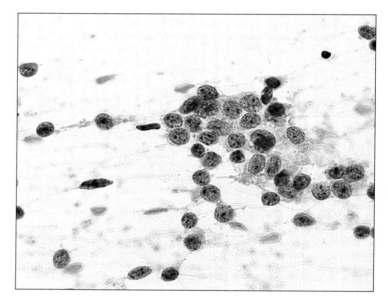

82 These cells were identified in a pleural effusion from a 55-year-old female with a bilateral 300 mL pulmonary effusion and a history of congestive heart failure. The diagnosis is:

    a mesothelioma
    b metastatic adenocarcinoma, breast
    c metastatic large cell carcinoma, lung
    d reactive mesothelial cells

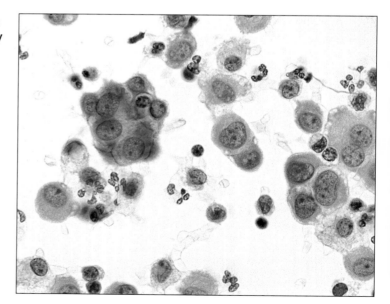

ISBN 978-089189-6357 ©ASCP 2015

83 A 40-year-old female with no history of malignancy presents with a midline tumor of the left cerebral hemisphere. These cells are detected in a lumbar puncture specimen. They are consistent with a diagnosis of:

a meningioma
b squamous cell carcinoma
c pinealoma
d pituitary adenoma

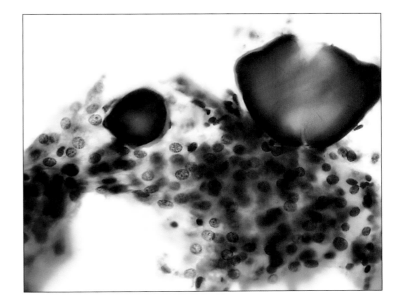

84 A 56-year-old female with a history of lung carcinoma presents with diplopia and vomiting. Lumbar puncture specimen reveals these cells. Suspicion of metastasis can be confirmed by positive immunocytochemical staining with:

a high molecular weight keratin
b chromogranin
c α-fetoprotein
d common leukocyte antigen

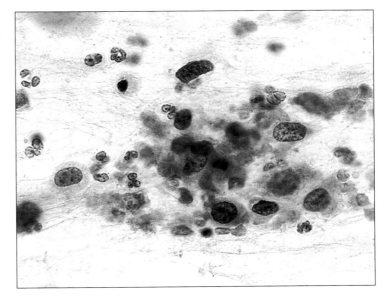

85 The depicted cells represent a pelvic washing specimen from a 48-year-old female who had undergone surgery for a 3 × 5 cm ovarian mass. The depicted cells represent:

a liver parenchyma
b mucinous cystadenocarcinoma of ovary
c normal mesothelial cells
d squamous cells, contaminant from the skin

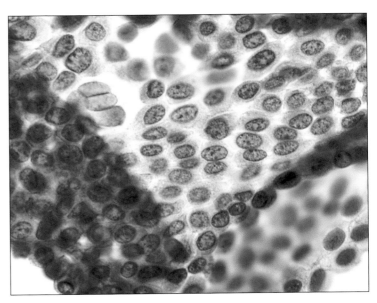

©ASCP 2015 ISBN 978-089189-6357

86 A 67-year-old male with a history of cancer presents with meningeal carcinomatosis. Based on the cellular morphology, the most likely primary site is:

a colon
b lung
c pancreas
d bladder

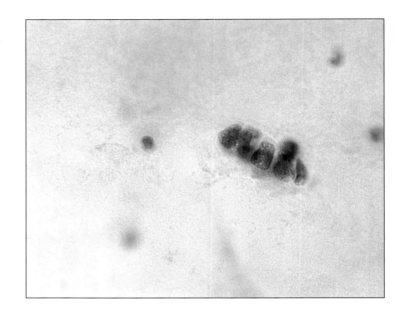

87 These cells, when detected in a pleural effusion, are:

a idiopathic
b suggestive of a parasitic effusion
c suggestive of a hypersensitivity reaction
d suggestive of asthma

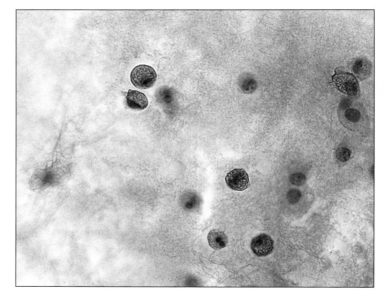

88 A 55-year-old male with a history of tuberculosis presents with dizziness and diplopia. Cytology reveals:

a viral meningitis
b acute bacterial meningitis
c intracranial hemorrhage
d lymphoma

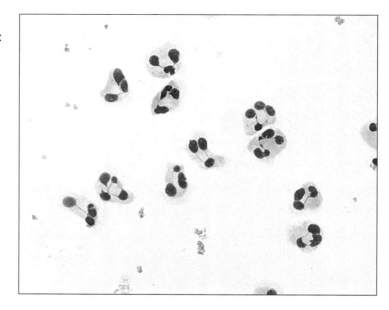

ISBN 978-089189-6357 ©ASCP 2015

89   A 66-year-old male presents with unilateral chest pain and shortness of breath. 300 mL of bloody pleural fluid underwent cytologic analysis. These cells represent a Papanicolaou stained smear. The findings are consistent with:

    a large cell carcinoma
    b mesothelioma
    c reactive mesothelial cells
    d poorly differentiated adenocarcinoma

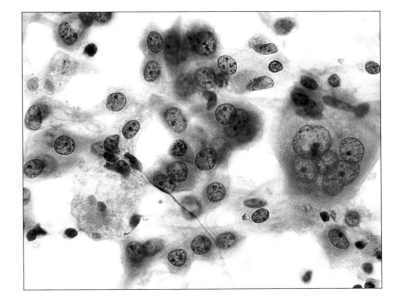

90   This cellular sample is from a 67-year-old male with a pulmonary disorder and a bilateral pleural effusion. Which of the following is supported by the cellular findings?

    a adenosquamous carcinoma
    b adenocarcinoma, bronchogenic type
    c large cell undifferentiated carcinoma
    d carcinosarcoma

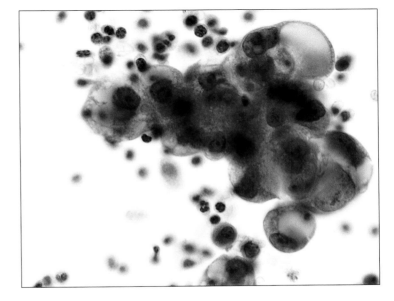

91   The presence of these cells from synovial fluid with D-PAS+ granules is often diagnostic of a(n):

    a LE cell
    b macrophage
    c metastatic carcinoma, breast
    d Mott cell

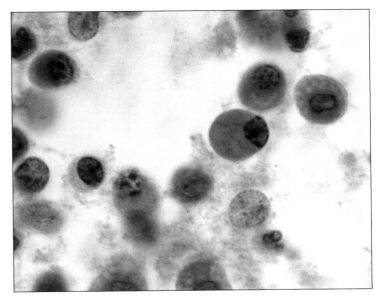

92   What would be the best stain to confirm a diagnosis of this pleural effusion from a 44-year-old male?
  a chromogranin
  b S100
  c common leukocyte antigen
  d α-fetoprotein

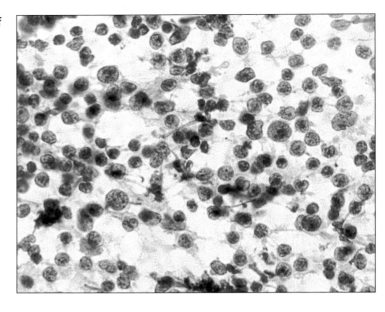

93   A 36-year-old female with swollen joints, subcutaneous nodules, and pain has 3 mL of synovial fluid submitted for evaluation. The cells suggest:
  a systemic lupus erythematosus
  b Reiter syndrome
  c gouty arthritis
  d rheumatoid arthritis

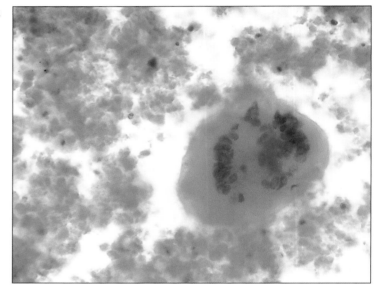

94   These cells were found in a 62-year-old female with an increasing abdominal girth. Ultrasonography revealed a 3×4 cm mass near the common bile duct. Paracentesis yielded 500 mL of proteinaceous fluid. The cytologic pattern represents:
  a pancreatobiliary carcinoma
  b epithelioid histiocytes
  c mesothelioma
  d reactive mesothelial cells

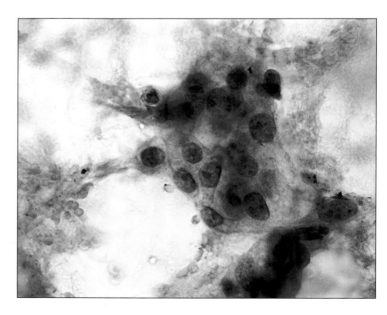

ISBN 978-089189-6357 ©ASCP 2015

95 These cells were observed in a pericardial effusion from a 44-year-old female suffering from an autoimmune disease. A serum specimen was positive for antinuclear antibodies. These findings are diagnostic of:

a acute inflammation with "tart cells"
b a Mallory body
c systemic lupus erythematosus
d rheumatoid arthritis

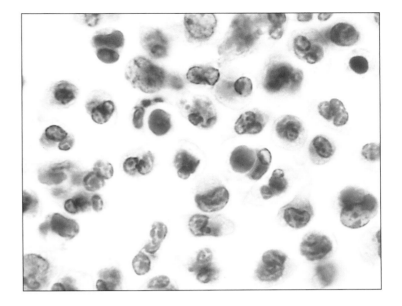

96 These cytologic findings represent a pleural effusion from a 57-year-old male suffering from a collagen disease. The cellular pattern represents:

a systemic lupus erythematosus
b rheumatoid pleuritis
c scleroderma
d tuberculosis

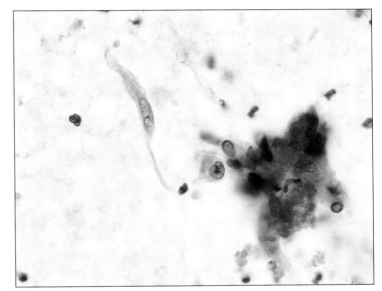

97 These cells were found in a pericardial effusion from a 60-year-old male. The cytologic pattern shows:

a small cell carcinoma
b large cleaved lymphoma
c lobular carcinoma, breast
d reactive lymphoid process

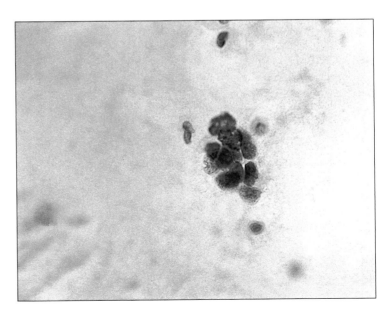

98   These cells, found in an ascitic fluid specimen from a
     50-year-old female, are often associated with:
     a   rheumatoid peritonitis
     b   mucicarmine–
     c   an ovarian mass
     d   an increase in ACTH

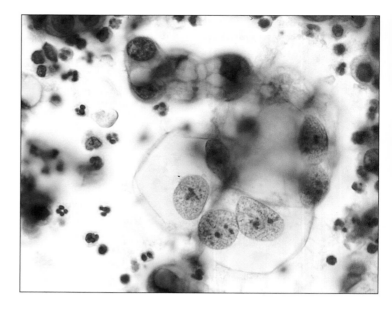

99   Represented is cerebrospinal fluid (CSF; lumbar
     puncture) from a 42-year-old male with AIDS. The
     patient presents to the clinician with weakness,
     malaise, a spiking fever, and cervical adenopathy. The
     diagnosis is:
     a   metastatic small cell carcinoma (pulmonary origin)
     b   small noncleaved lymphoma
     c   reactive lymphocytes secondary to viral meningitis
     d   bacterial meningitis

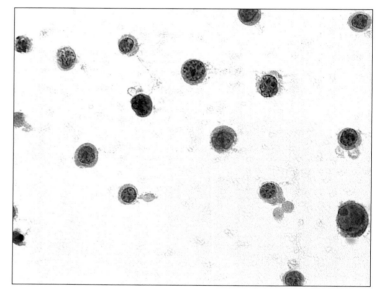

100 These cells were present in a peritoneal effusion from
     a 2-year-old female with a retroperitoneal tumor
     and increased levels of urine catecholamine and
     vanillylmandelic acid. The cytologic pattern represents:
     a   angiomyolipoma
     b   retroperitoneal sarcoma
     c   neuroblastoma
     d   Wilms tumor

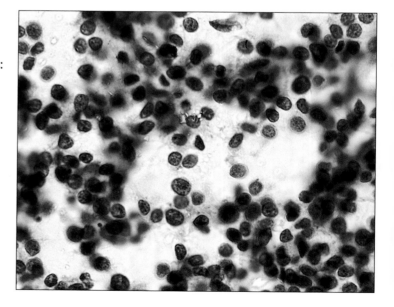

ISBN 978-089189-6357 ©ASCP 2015

101 What stain would help identify these cells obtained from a peritoneal effusion in a 50-year-old male?
  a chromogranin
  b α-fetoprotein
  c neuron specific enolase
  d S100

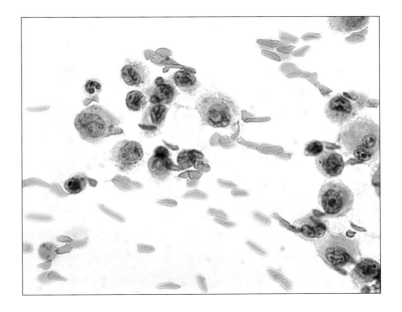

102 These cells were identified in a synovial fluid specimen from a 42-year-old athlete with joint pain. The findings are consistent with:
  a reactive synovial lining cells
  b histiocytes
  c cartilaginous material
  d synovial sarcoma

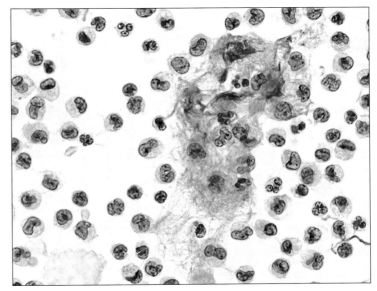

103 A peritoneal effusion from a 40-year-old female with an abdominal mass reveals these cells. They are diagnostic of:
  a adenocarcinoma, pancreatic
  b mucinous cystadenocarcinoma, ovarian
  c adenocarcinoma, endometrial
  d serous cystadenocarcinoma, ovarian

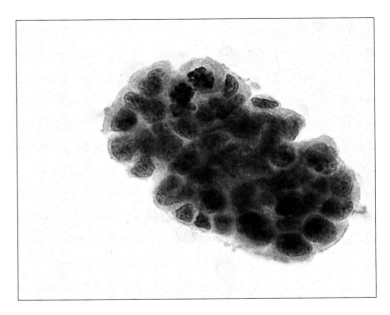

104 A 72-year-old male presents with a peritoneal effusion and a history of a genitourinary tract primary neoplasm. These cells:

a are reactive mesothelial in origin

b could be verified as renal cell carcinoma by using a Giemsa stain

c could be verified as prostatic adenocarcinoma by using a prostate specific antigen (PSA) immunohistochemical stain

d represent a chronic infectious process

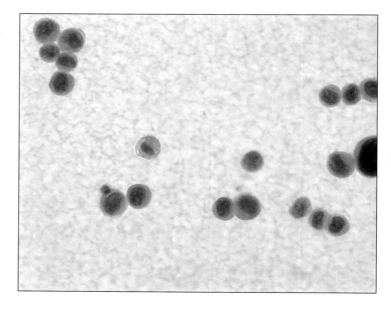

105 These cells were found in an ascitic effusion specimen from a 3-year-old male with a flank mass. Immunocytochemical staining for chromogranin is negative. The cellular findings are representative of:

a neuroblastoma

b Ewing sarcoma

c pheochromocytoma

d Wilms tumor

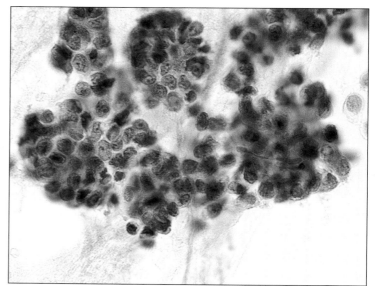

106 These cells were taken from a 52-year-old female presenting with a 300 mL pleural effusion. The cellular findings represent:

a mesothelial hyperplasia

b changes secondary to pulmonary infarct

c collagen balls

d metastatic breast carcinoma

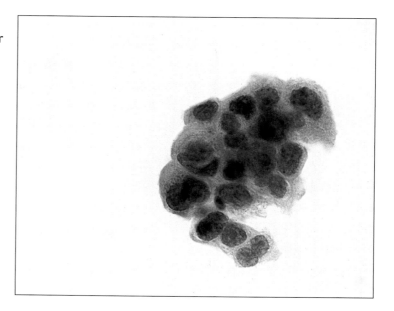

ISBN 978-089189-6357 ©ASCP 2015

107 A 38-year-old female underwent exploratory laparotomy for a right adnexal mass. Peritoneal washings were performed and processed as a liquid based cytology specimen. The best diagnosis is:

   a endometriosis
   b ovarian carcinoma
   c normal mesothelial cells
   d benign cystic teratoma of ovary

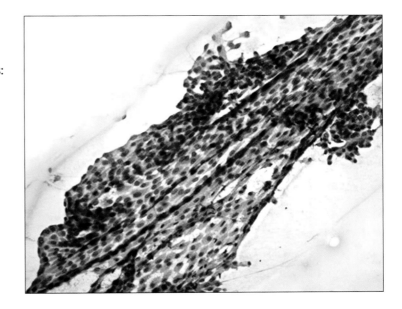

108 A pelvic wash was procured on a 35-year-old female who underwent a right oophorectomy for an ovarian mass. What is the diagnosis?

   a negative for malignancy
   b papillary carcinoma
   c adenoid cystic carcinoma
   d mucinous carcinoma

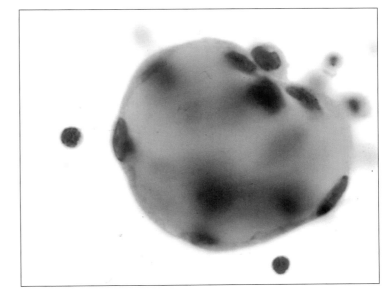

109 Pleural effusion from a 57-year-old female. The most probable diagnosis is:

   a collagen balls
   b marked mesothelial cell hyperplasia
   c metastatic melanoma
   d metastatic breast carcinoma

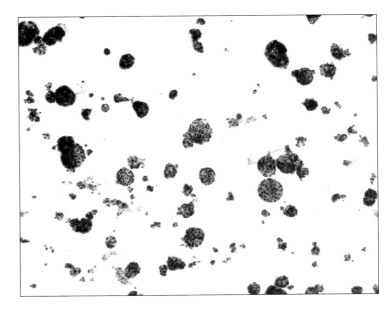

110 This pleural fluid is from a 63-year-old female with a history of joint pains and shortness of breath. What is the most likely diagnosis?

  a squamous cell carcinoma
  b tuberculosis
  c systemic lupus erythematosus
  d rheumatoid arthritis

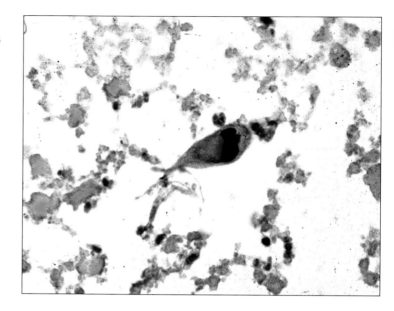

111 This cell block obtained from a pelvic wash on a 65-year-old female who underwent total abdominal hysterectomy with bilateral oophorectomy for an ovarian cystic neoplasm. How would you interpret this specimen?

  a papillary serous neoplasm of low malignant potential
  b benign mesothelial cells
  c papillary serous adenocarcinoma
  d mucinous adenocarcinoma

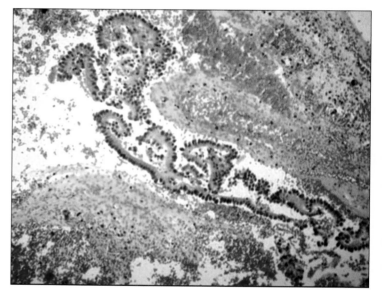

112 This pleural effusion is from a 27-year-old female. What is the most probable cause of her effusion?

  a plasma cell dyscrasia/multiple myeloma
  b lymphoma
  c signet ring carcinoma
  d systemic lupus erythematosus

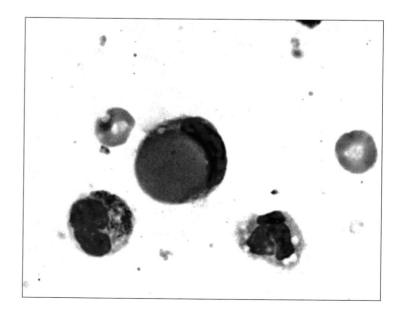

ISBN 978-089189-6357 ©ASCP 2015

113 This CSF from a 5-year-old male with a history of hydrocephalus shows:
 a medulloblastoma
 b pilocytic astrocytoma
 c brain tissue
 d germinoma

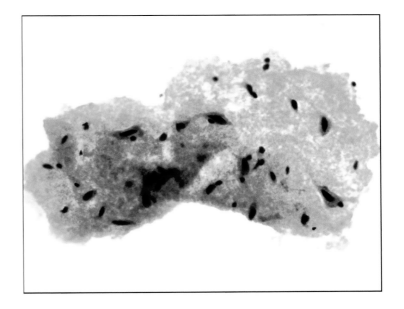

114 This cerebrospinal fluid is from a 43-year-old male with history of HIV. What is the correct interpretation?
 a lymphoma
 b pollen
 c corpora amylacea
 d *Cryptococcus* species

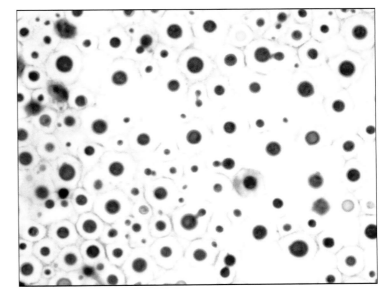

115 A 5-year-old male was referred to a neurologist who identified a midline cerebellar mass on CT scan. As part of the clinical workup, cerebrospinal fluid was obtained by lumbar puncture. What is the most likely diagnosis?
 a viral meningitis
 b ependymoma
 c astrocytoma
 d medulloblastoma

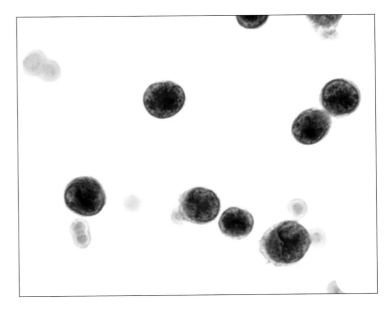

116 A 41-year-old male was seen by a neurologist for extremity numbness. CSF was submitted to hematology and cytology. What is your interpretation?
   a metastatic adenocarcinoma
   b benign chronic inflammation
   c malignant lymphoma
   d metastatic small cell carcinoma

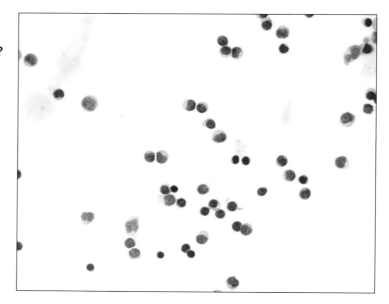

117 This CSF fluid was most likely obtained from:
   a an 83-year-old female with a history of melanoma
   b a 21-year-old male with a V-P shunt
   c a 5-year-old male with Burkitt lymphoma
   d a 57-year-old female with a history of breast carcinoma

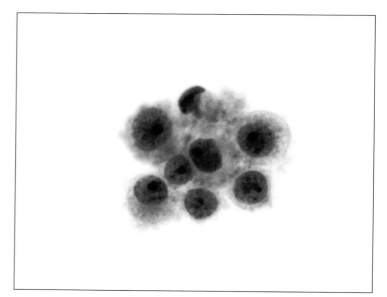

118 With these findings in a CSF specimen, what should you convey to a clinician?
   a obtain specimen for culture
   b obtain specimen for flow cytometry
   c reassure that this is reactive process
   d do nothing

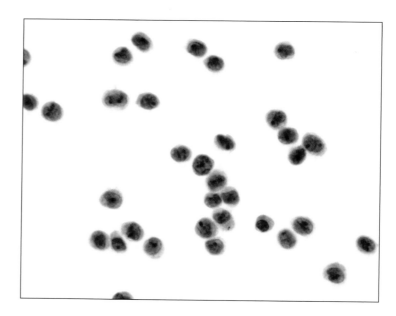

ISBN 978-089189-6357 ©ASCP 2015

119 This 73-year-old female presented with pleural fluid. What should be the next procedure to explain these findings?
  a CT scan of the brain
  b EUS of the pancreas
  c pelvic ultrasound
  d mammogram

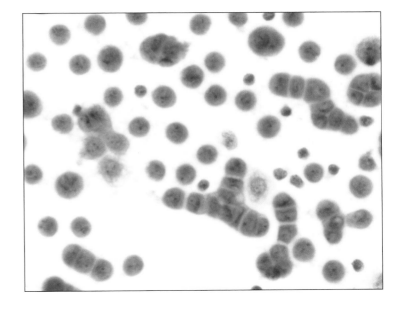

120 This ascitic fluid was obtained from a 67-year-old female. What is your diagnosis?
  a endosalpingiosis
  b endometriosis
  c papillary adenocarcinoma
  d collagen ball

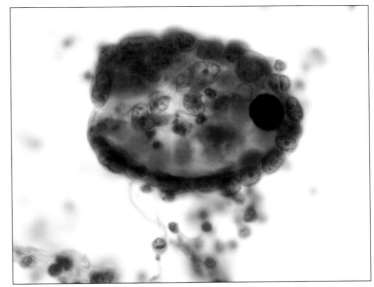

121 A 70-year-old female with a history of a lung tumor developed cauda equina syndrome. The image is representative of a cytospin of cerebrospinal fluid. The best diagnosis is:
  a myxopapillary ependymoma
  b meningioma
  c glioblastoma multiforme
  d metastatic adenocarcinoma

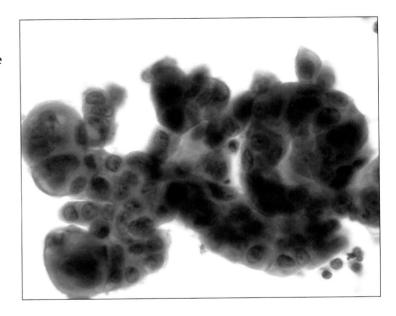

©ASCP 2015 ISBN 978-089189-6357

122 A 50-year-old female, a heavy smoker, presented with dyspnea and a large right pleural effusion. Thoracentesis was performed. The image shows a representative field, high magnification, Pap stain. The best diagnosis is:

a reactive mesothelial cells
b mesothelioma
c lobular carcinoma
d small cell carcinoma

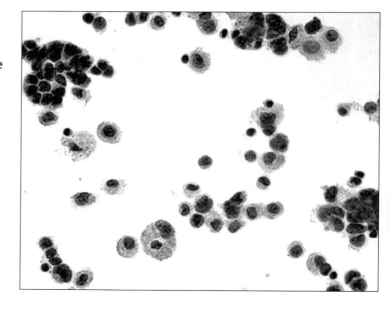

123 The following represents a pelvic washing from a 45-year-old female, post surgery for a Sertoli-Leydig cell tumor of the ovary. The diagnosis is consistent with:

a Sertoli-Leydig cell tumor
b malignant mesothelioma
c endometriosis
d benign collagen balls

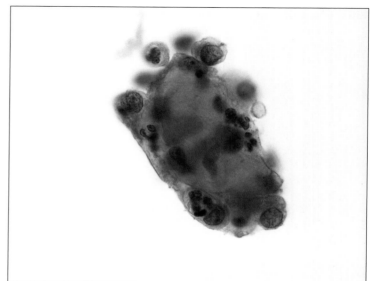

124 The patient represented in the previous question also had the following cellular components represented in the ThinPrep processed specimen of the pelvic washing. Based on the previous, the diagnosis is:

a reactive mesothelial cells
b Sertoli-Leydig cell tumor
c endometriosis
d malignant mesothelioma

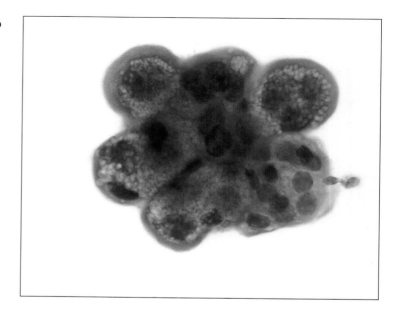

ISBN 978-089189-6357 ©ASCP 2015

Body Fluids *Answer Key*

1 b   monosodium urate

Monosodium urate crystals (strongly negative birefringence with pointed ends) polarize and help confirm the presence of gouty arthritis. The differential diagnosis includes pseudogout/chondrocalcinosis, which is marked by calcium phosphate crystals that are not enhanced by polarized light.

DeMay, A&S 2e. Gout, p342

2 c   osteoarthritis

A degenerative joint disease, osteoarthritis usually occurs in the weight bearing joints due to repeated trauma to the articular cartilage.

DeMay, A&S 2e. Degenerative arthritis (osteoarthritis), p341

3 a   lung

The most common metastatic carcinoma to the brain is lung cancer. Of these lesions, adenocarcinoma is the most frequently diagnosed tumor, followed by small cell and squamous carcinomas, respectively. In addition to lung cancer, other common metastatic lesions include carcinoma of the breast, malignant melanoma, and adenocarcinoma of the stomach.

DeMay, A&S 2e. Metastatic malignancy, p248

4 a   choriocarcinoma

Choriocarcinomas are placental lesions that metastasize to the brain. Cytologic findings consist of mononuclear and multinucleated cells with high N:C ratios, granular chromatin, anisonucleosis, and prominent nucleoli. Clinical history is important as well as positive staining with β-human chorionic gonadotropin.

DeMay, A&S 2e. Metastatic malignancy, p248

5 b   rheumatoid arthritis

This collagen disease may be identified by the presence of multinucleated histiocytes and epithelioid histiocytes ("snake cells") among a granular, "sandy" or "fluffy" eosinophilic necrotic background. Large numbers of ragocytes, which represent mono- or multilobulated neutrophils with dark blue cytoplasmic inclusions (immunoglobulin) are specific for this disease. These findings are consistent with a necrotizing granuloma. Clinical symptoms include joint pain and/or synovitis and a positive serum test for rheumatoid factor. Rheumatoid arthritis usually affects women; nevertheless, effusion related disease is seen more often in men.

DeMay, A&S 2e. Rheumatoid arthritis, p341

6 b   subdural hematoma

Intracranial hemorrhaging will often result in cytologic presence of hemosiderin laden macrophages or siderophages, which are macrophages with a refractile, gold intracytoplasmic pigment. The differential diagnosis of siderophages may include metastatic melanoma, which can be excluded based on their negative reaction with S100, HMB45, melan A or positivity with an iron stain.

DeMay, A&S 2e. Siderophages, p213

7 c   Ewing sarcoma

Ewing sarcoma cytologically presents as small, round cells with granular cytoplasm found in clusters or rosette formations. The nuclei contain coarsely granular, irregularly distributed chromatin with nucleoli. Tumor diathesis is a reliable cytomorphologic feature of these lesions. Differentiation of synovial sarcoma, osteogenic sarcoma, and other neuroendocrine lesions is permitted by the positive staining of intracytoplasmic glycogen, as demonstrated with periodic acid-Schiff. Ewing sarcoma lesions are found in serous or synovial effusions.

DeMay, A&S 2e. Ewing/PNET, p111

8 d   chondrocalcinosis

Pseudogout/chondrocalcinosis is marked by calcium phosphate crystals that are not enhanced by polarized light.

DeMay, A&S 2e. Pseudogout/chrondrocalcinosis, p342

9 d   multiple sclerosis

The mere presence of plasma cells in CSF specimens represents a pathologic process. Some of the disease processes include neurosyphilis, multiple sclerosis, viral infections, sarcoidosis, or sclerosing panencephalitis. Answers a, b, and c are conditions associated with neutrophilic infiltrates.

DeMay, A&S 2e. Plasma cells, p498

10 a   papillary

Cells derived from choroid plexus papillomas appear in papillary cohesive clusters with irregular nuclear membranes. The cytoplasm is generous and basophilic. These cells are often difficult to distinguish from normal choroid plexus cells, ependymomas, and pineocytomas; therefore, the clinical history of an intraventricular mass is imperative.

DeMay, A&S 2e. Choroid plexus tumors, p511-512

11 d   pineoblastoma

Pineoblastomas present cytologically with "small blue cell" tumor morphology. The cells may be either pleomorphic or monomorphic, with scanty, ill defined cytoplasm and hyperchromasia. The differential diagnosis includes pineocytoma, its benign counterpart (which lacks malignant criteria), and medulloblastoma (differentiated by location).

DeMay, A&S 2e. Pineal gland tumors, p514

12 d   leptomeningeal cells

These cells resemble mesothelial cells or monocytes and are derived from the pia-arachnoid layers of the brain covering.

DeMay, A&S 2e. Pia-arachnoid (leptomeningeal) cells, p499-500

13 a   peripheral blood contamination

Peripheral blood contamination in a CSF specimen renders it unsatisfactory. The presence of megakaryocytes may at first seem alarming based on their giant cell size, multinucleation, and coarse appearing chromatin patterns. However, these sparse cells found in conjunction with other peripheral blood cells should suggest their blood derived origin.

DeMay, A&S 2e. Giant cells, p501

14   a   meningioma

Cells with fibroblastic appearance found in whorls and sheets with benign nuclear features represent meningioma. These meningeal tumors are generally found in adolescents. These benign lesions need to be discriminated from their malignant counterpart, meningiosarcoma, a tumor that presents with classic sarcomatous features.

DeMay, A&S 2e. Meningiomas, p248

15   b   *Cryptococcus neoformans*

The presence of single, yeastlike structures (5-15 µm) with mucinous capsules is diagnostic of *Cryptococcus neoformans*. These organisms reproduce by teardrop budding. Special staining with mucicarmine will help elucidate the distinctive capsule. Differentiation includes starch crystals, which possess a Maltese cross birefringence.

DeMay, A&S 2e. Cryptococcus, p505

16   d   medulloblastoma

The finding of small, anaplastic cells ("small blue cell tumors") in the CSF of children may indicate the presence of medulloblastoma, neuroblastoma, or retinoblastoma. Special attention should focus on possible clinical history. Medulloblastomas are neural crest tumors that arise from the cerebellum and are found in children or adolescents. Neuroblastomas (rare in the brain) typically arise within the cerebral hemisphere. Retinoblastomas involve the orbit and optic tract.

DeMay, A&S 2e. Medulloblastoma, p512-513

17   d   ependymoma

Ependymoma, a benign common spinal cord lesion that generally occurs in children and adolescents, presents readily in CSF specimens due to its ventricular origin. Cytologically, the cells demonstrate columnar morphology and possess finely granular, evenly distributed chromatin patterns with occasional nucleoli. Small clusters or rosettes may be seen; furthermore, the presence of blepharoplasts (basal bodies), which are positive with phosphotungstic acid hematoxylin, is a confirmatory finding. Differential diagnosis must exclude neural crest tumors, the cells of which stain positive for chromogranin.

DeMay, A&S 2e. Ependymoma, p511

18   c   astrocytoma

Astrocytomas are the most common primary brain neoplasm found in children. Uniform cells with oval nuclei and hypochromasia mimic their normal benign counterparts. Because the cytology may be difficult to distinguish from normal astrocytes, the history of a radiographically identified cerebellar lesion is extremely important.

DeMay, A&S 2e. Astrocytoma, p509-510

19   a   reactive pleocytosis

Severe inflammation/reactive lymphocytosis is often difficult to distinguish from recurrent leukemia, with the exception that reactive changes consist of a polytypic population of small mature lymphocytes and immunoblasts (often containing prominent nucleoli), as well as plasma cells. The absence of malignant blasts with irregular, notched, or cleaved nuclear membranes and hyperchromatic, coarse, irregular chromatin with prominent nucleoli is important when differentiating reactive processes secondary to intrathecal therapy or infection from recurrent leukemic involvement. A negative reaction with tumor marker terminal deoxytransferase is useful in ruling out recurrent leukemia.

DeMay, A&S 2e. Inflammatory cells, p214-215

20   a   post oil myelogram

When lipophages are observed, a differential diagnosis may include metastatic adenocarcinoma. Confirmation with oil red O and clinical history of a recent oil myelogram or pneumoencephalogram are key in corroborating the benign nature of these cells.

DeMay, A&S 2e. Lipophages, p213

21   d   synovial sarcoma

Malignant synovioma or synovial sarcoma is an extremely aggressive neoplasm that presents as a very cellular monotonous population of anaplastic cells. Differential staining will differentiate it from metastatic neuroendocrine tumors (latter stains positive for chromogranin). Although these lesions represent indigenous neoplasms, they rarely arise in the joints.

DeMay, A&S 2e. Tumors, p343

22   a   medulloblastoma

The finding of small, anaplastic cells ("small blue cell tumors") in the CSF of children may indicate the presence of medulloblastoma, neuroblastoma, or retinoblastoma. Special attention should focus on possible clinical history. Medulloblastomas are neural crest tumors that arise from the cerebellum and are found in children or adolescents. Neuroblastomas (rare in the brain) typically arise within the cerebral hemisphere. Retinoblastomas involve the orbit and optic tract.

DeMay, A&S 2e. Medulloblastoma, p512-513

23   b   schwannoma

Schwannomas cytologically present as hypocellular, monotonous clusters of spindle-appearing cells. The presence of Verocay bodies, clusters of cells with peripherally palisading nuclei, central fibrillar cores, and "flamelike" cytoplasm, is an essential component in diagnosing a primary schwannoma.

DeMay, A&S 2e. Nerve sheath tumors (schwannoma & neurofibroma), p585-587

ISBN 978-089189-6357 ©ASCP 2015

24 **b** retinoblastoma

The finding of small, anaplastic cells ("small blue cell tumors") in the CSF of children may indicate the presence of medulloblastoma, neuroblastoma, or retinoblastoma. Special attention should focus on possible clinical history. Medulloblastomas are neural crest tumors that arise from the cerebellum and are found in children or adolescents. Neuroblastomas (rare in the brain) typically arise within the cerebral hemisphere. Retinoblastomas involve the orbit and optic tract.

DeMay, A&S 2e. Retinoblastoma, p513

25 **c** neuroblastoma

Should small, anaplastic cells be identified in serous effusions from children, the diagnostic focus should be differentiating between neuroblastoma of adrenal origin and Wilms tumor (nephroblastoma). The former is a neuroendocrine lesion that will immunologically stain positive for chromogranin. Wilms tumors are negative for chromogranin.

DeMay, A&S 2e. Neuroblastoma, p513

26 **a** metastatic carcinoma, lung

Cytology reveals pleomorphic cells with hyperchromatic, eccentrically located nuclei, irregular nuclear membranes, macronucleoli, and dense, hard cytoplasm. Positive staining with high molecular weight keratin would indicate a squamous cell carcinoma (the most common lung neoplasm).

DeMay, A&S 2e. Metastatic malignancy, p248

27 **c** breast

Metastatic carcinoma of the breast is the most common malignancy of the CNS. The most common morphologic variant, ductal adenocarcinoma, may be cytologically identified as "cannonballs," 3D proliferation spheres, or morula formations. However, metastatic adenocarcinoma of the breast in the CSF can also present as single cells with cohesive features with plasmacytoid morphology. In this case, the presence of these true tissue fragments with community cell borders is strongly suggestive of breast metastasis.

DeMay, A&S 2e. Metastatic malignancy, p248

28 **b** Reiter syndrome

Reiter syndrome is associated with polyarthritis and is diagnosed cytologically by the finding of intracytoplasmic eosinophilic inclusions within synovial cells. Mononucleate leukocytes and fibrinous protein are found within the background. A clinical history of conjunctivitis or nongonococcal urethritis is important in correlating the disease process.

DeMay, A&S 2e. Reiter syndrome, p341-342

29 **b** acute bacterial meningitis

A hypercellular population of neutrophilic leukocytes are commonly associated with acute bacterial infections. Culture analysis should be performed to specify the etiology of the infection. Differential diagnosis includes a tuberculous effusion. Clinical history is imperative in discriminating these 2 diagnoses.

DeMay, A&S 2e. Bacterial meningitis, p503

30 **c** adenocarcinoma/prostate (PSA+)

Prostatic adenocarcinomas present in serous effusions as small cells in microacinar clusters containing hyperchromatic nuclei and macronucleoli. A history of prostate cancer is helpful in conjunction with immunohistochemical staining with prostatic specific antigen or acid phosphatase.

DeMay, A&S 2e. Prostatic adenocarcinoma, p476

31 **b** glioblastoma multiforme

Glioblastomas (grade IV astrocytomas) represent the most common primary brain neoplasm (often contained within the frontal lobes) detected in adults. The cytomorphologic criteria associated with this lesion are the finding of pleomorphic, bizarre, frankly malignant cells with opaque or lacy cytoplasm and wispy cytoplasmic appendages, either singularly or in cell balls. These cells are easily recognized as malignant; however, the differential diagnosis may include a pleomorphic carcinoma or sarcoma. Immunocytochemical staining with glial fibrillary acidic protein will confirm CNS origin.

DeMay, A&S 2e. Glioblastoma multiforme, p510

32 **a** PAS

Oligodendrogliomas appear benign by cytomorphologic criteria, possessing round, uniform shapes, and are found in sheets or syncytial aggregates with predictable patterns and finely granular, evenly distributed chromatin. Special staining with PAS is positive for intracytoplasmic glycogen and may be a key differential feature in discriminating these lesions from other adult glial tumors.

DeMay, A&S 2e. Oligodendroglioma, p510

33 **b** craniopharyngioma

These supracellular cystic tumors, which arise within the Rathke pouch, are cytologically diagnosed only after rupture of the cyst into the meninges. Cells lining the cyst are composed of columnar cells, anucleate squames, and/or keratin pearls. Occasionally, degenerative components and cholesterol crystals may be seen.

DeMay, A&S 2e. Craniopharyngioma, p514

34 **b** *Toxoplasma gondii*

Toxoplasma gondii is an intracellular parasite acquired by exposure to uncooked meats or blood transfusions. 20%-70% of Americans have antibody titers but are asymptomatic, unless there is a reactivation of a dormant disease secondary to failed cell mediated immunity. Cerebrospinal fluid infections may be seen in patients with AIDS. The cysts are readily demonstrated by staining with PAS, Giemsa, Romanowsky (Diff-Quik), or immunocytochemistry.

DeMay, A&S 2e. Toxoplasma, p505

35 c malignant melanoma

Melanoma typically presents in single cells, in aggregates, or as spindle cells with bizarre malignant nuclear features, macronucleoli, intranuclear cytoplasmic inclusions, and possibly intracytoplasmic golden-brown pigment. Due to the fact that these diseases may be amelanotic, it may be helpful to confirm this disease process with S100, HMB45, melan A or MITF (microphthalmia associated transcription factor)–all which preferentially react with melanoma cells.

DeMay, A&S 2e. Metastatic malignancy (melanoma), p248

36 a macrophages

Macrophages are commonly identified elements in serous effusions. These cells are roughly the same size as mesothelial cells but possess frothy, indistinct cytoplasm with eccentric, bean shaped, reniform, boomerang, or round nuclei. The chromatin is fine and regular in Papanicolaou stained specimens while resembling "raked sand" in air dried material. These phagocytes may have intracytoplasmic inclusions often containing the phagosome, such as hemosiderin laden macrophages or siderophages. Histiocytes stain positive for neutral red and Janus green (supravital stains), whereas mesothelial cells are negative.

DeMay, A&S 2e. Histiocytes, p77-278

37 b *Cryptococcus neoformans*

The presence of single, yeastlike structures (5-15 μm in diameter) with mucinous capsules is diagnostic of *Cryptococcus neoformans*. These organisms reproduce by teardrop budding. Special staining with mucicarmine will help elucidate the distinctive capsule. Differentiation includes starch crystals, which possess a Maltese cross birefringence.

DeMay, A&S 2e. Cryptococcus, p505

38 a is of little significance

Mitotic figures are common findings in effusion cytology. Their presence is related to hyperplastic and/or reactive as well as malignant conditions. Mesothelial cells have the ability to proliferate within the fluid matrix.

DeMay, A&S 2e. The cells, p274-275

39 a D-PAS+

Identifying the cells as mesothelial cell lineage is the first step in establishing the diagnosis of carcinomatous mesothelioma. Cytology reveals many cells possessing homogeneous cytoplasm with "skirts" or "blebs," multinucleation, single cells and clusters, and coarse, irregular chromatin with multiple macronucleoli. Irregular papillae and knobby 3D clusters with cytoplasmic vacuolation are found among a metachromatic precipitous background (demonstrated with Diff-Quik staining). The differential diagnosis is metastatic adenocarcinoma; however, special staining with alcian blue-hyaluronidase and D-PAS is negative for carcinomatous mesothelioma, but positive for adenocarcinoma. Immunocytochemical staining with CEA and B72.3 is also negative for mesothelioma but positive for adenocarcinoma.

DeMay, A&S 2e. Special studies in diagnosis of mesothelioma, p321-322

40 b community borders

Benign reactive mesothelial cells may present with pseudoacinar or papillae structures; however, the cytoplasmic borders are described as "knobby" or flowerlike. In contrast, the most common metastatic malignancies to the serous cavities are adenocarcinomas, which present as 3D true acinar, papillary, or morula groupings with smooth community borders.

DeMay, A&S 2e. Reactive mesothelial cells, p274

41 c small cell carcinoma

Metastatic small cell carcinoma presents with hyperchromatic, stippled chromatin, coarse clumping, nuclear molding, scanty cytoplasm, and micronucleoli. The cells are arranged characteristically in vertebral column formation ("stack of dishes"), microbiopsy aggregates, and as cords, nests, or ribbons.

DeMay, A&S 2e. Small cell carcinoma, p241

42 b reactive mesothelial cells

Reactive mesothelial cells (reactive hyperplasia) show papillae and pseudoacini with knobby borders instead of true community borders, and single cells with "windows" between adjacent cells–a result of centrifugation and maintenance of the cytoplasmic brush border. The finding of a brush border infers benignity and is often described as indistinct or fuzzy in appearance. The nuclei of these cells are round and centrally located with well defined, regular nuclear membranes and finely granular, regularly distributed chromatin with nucleoli. The cytoplasmic morphology is homogeneous and dense with peripheral fading, often demonstrating an endo-ectoplasmic demarcation. The density of the cytoplasm may give a false "atypical" impression of hyperchromatic nuclei; however, when the nuclear intensity is compared with that of the cytoplasm, there is little divergence. The presence of psammoma bodies may also be seen in reactive conditions such as mesothelial hyperplasia and endosalpingiosis. Psammoma bodies are more commonly seen in benign effusions than in malignant effusions (eg, ovarian cancer).

DeMay, A&S 2e. Reactive mesothelial cells, p274

43 a PAS

Embryonal rhabdomyosarcoma is considered an uncommon vaginal lesion affecting young girls generally <5 years of age. The cytologic identification of small single cells, clusters, and cells with elongated tadpolelike morphology with broad bands ("strap cells") is helpful in identifying this lesion. Special staining for PAS and myoglobulin may help confirm these lesions.

DeMay, A&S 2e. Rhabdomyosarcoma, p111

ISBN 978-089189-6357 ©ASCP 2015

44   b   systemic lupus erythematosus

Systemic lupus erythematosus may be cytologically confirmed by finding characteristic LE cells, a neutrophil containing a large hematoxylin inclusion consisting of antinuclear antibody coated, degenerative nuclear material. This disease, generally affecting women in childbearing years, presents with idiopathic pleural effusions. It must be confirmed with antinuclear antibodies and clinical manifestations such as a butterfly facial rash and joint pain. In the absence of a previously established clinical and serological diagnosis, the diagnosis may be difficult and suggestive only. The differential diagnosis includes the more commonly found tart cell; however, this cell does not have discernible chromatin within the hematoxylin body.

DeMay, A&S 2e. Systemic lupus erythematosus, p287

45   b   *Paragonimus westermani*

This unusual parasite has been described in effusion cytology as yellowish ova with a flat, thick operculum at one end and a rounded, thickened shell on the opposite end. It should be differentiated from *Echinococcus granulosus,* a cestode which often presents with hydatid sand consisting of associated scoleces and hooks.

DeMay, A&S 2e. Microorganisms, p281

46   a   mesothelioma is positive for vimentin

Vimentin is an intermediate filament that immunocytochemically will stain positive in mesenchymal cells (mesothelial) but negative in epithelial cells.

DeMay, A&S 2e. Vimentin, p323

47   b   adenocarcinoma/breast

Metastatic carcinoma of the breast is the most common malignancy involving the pleural cavity in women. The most common morphologic variant, ductal adenocarcinoma, may be cytologically identified as "cannonballs," 3D proliferation spheres, or morula formations. The presence of these true tissue fragments with community cell borders is strongly suggestive of breast metastasis in light of the clinical history.

DeMay, A&S 2e. Breast, p296-297

48   c   idiopathic

The presence of a vast majority of eosinophils in serous fluids may be idiopathic in the absence of a specific clinical history such as trauma, hypersensitivity, pneumothorax, or pulmonary infarct. Idiopathic eosinophilia is self limiting and tends to spontaneously resolve.

DeMay, A&S 2e. Eosinophils, p279

49   c   *Echinococcus granulosus*

Echinococcus granulosus is a cestode that often presents with hydatid sand consisting of associated scoleces and hooks. Aspiration of *Echinococcus granulosus* is a contraindication due to the possibility of creating anaphylactic shock.

DeMay, A&S 2e. Microorganisms, p281

50   b   adenocarcinoma

Mesothelial cells do not contain neutral mucin but rather mesenchymal mucin or hyaluronic acid; therefore, neutral mucin positivity as identified by special staining with mucicarmine or alcian blue would indicate an adenocarcinoma. Mesothelial cells may be peripherally positive with PAS, but after digestion with diastase the cells are negative, whereas adenocarcinomas will remain positive.

DeMay, A&S 2e. Special studies in diagnosis of mesothelioma, p321-322

51   b   alcian blue-hyaluronidase

Mesotheliomas stain negative with alcian blue-hyaluronidase, whereas adenocarcinomas are positive. Both mesotheliomas and adenocarcinomas may be positive for alcian blue (without hyaluronidase), PAS (mesotheliomas peripherally positive), and immunostaining with cytokeratin. Therefore, the latter stains will be of little value in differentiating the 2 tumor types.

DeMay, A&S 2e. Special studies in diagnosis of mesothelioma, p321-322

52   b   patient history

It is imperative to have appropriate clinical history to correctly identify the origin of a metastatic neoplasm. Correlation with the original primary tissue is also of great utility in establishing metastasis. In the absence of clinical history, special stains and immunocytochemical marking may be useful, but oftentimes are not reliable.

DeMay, A&S 2e. Malignant effusions, p289

53   b   Wilms tumor

Wilms tumors cytologically present as small cells with anaplastic features and infrequent spindle cells, often mimicking neuroblastoma of the adrenal gland. The clinical history is important, as well as the use of adjunctive immunocytochemistry.

DeMay, A&S 2e. Wilms tumor), p311

54   b   a discrete population of foreign cells and normal cells

A foreign population of cells with foreign features may suggest a metastatic malignant process when found in association with a benign population of mesothelial cells and histiocytes.

DeMay, A&S 2e. General patterns of adenocarcinoma, p294-296

55   d   rheumatoid pleuritis

This collagen disease may be identified by the presence of multinucleated histiocytes and epithelioid histiocytes ("snake cells") in a granular, "sandy" or "fluffy" eosinophilic necrotic background. These findings are consistent with a necrotizing granuloma. Occasional cholesterol crystals and multinucleated or trapezoidal histiocytes are seen in rheumatoid pleuritis. Large numbers of ragocytes, which represent mono- or multilobulated neutrophils with dark blue cytoplasmic inclusions (immunoglobulin), are specific for this disease. Serum confirmation of rheumatoid factor is necessary to establish this disease process.

DeMay, A&S 2e. Rheumatoid effusion, p286-287

56 **a** **poorly differentiated adenocarcinoma, not otherwise specified**

Poorly differentiated adenocarcinomas (PDA) may not actively produce mucin. Therefore, the possibility of PDA cannot be ruled out when the cells are negative for mucicarmine staining. Immunocytochemical staining with CEA and B72.3 is positive for adenocarcinoma.

DeMay, A&S 2e. Special studies in diagnosis of mesothelioma, p321-322

57 **c** **ovary**

These cells represent metastatic mucinous cystadenocarcinoma of the ovary. The presence of irregular, transparent clusters with large distended, degenerated cytoplasmic vacuoles, "signet ring" morphology, and classic malignant nuclear features often suggests this metastatic neoplasm. Although ovarian tumors often produce peritoneal effusions, pleural effusions may be seen without ascites. Staining with alcian blue-hyaluronidase will be positive for most mucinous adenocarcinomas.

DeMay, A&S 2e. Ovary, p300

58 **a** **thyroid**

Psammoma bodies are common findings associated with papillary carcinomas of the thyroid; however, the presence of psammoma bodies per se is neither sensitive nor specific in the differentiation of benign and malignant disease.

DeMay, A&S 2e. Psammoma bodies, p280

59 **b** **renal cell carcinoma/kidney**

Renal cell carcinomas contain intracytoplasmic lipids that stain positive with oil red O or Sudan black. Colonic adenocarcinoma, hepatocellular carcinoma, and melanoma will all be negative for lipid.

DeMay, A&S 2e. Renal cell carcinoma, p475

60 **d** **adenocarcinoma/colon**

Tall columnar cells in clusters with granular cytoplasm and hyperchromatic nuclei containing finely granular, irregularly distributed chromatin with macronucleoli are suggestive of metastatic colonic adenocarcinoma. Special emphasis should be placed on the columnar or cigar shaped cellular morphology when differentiating these lesions from other possible metastatic sites.

DeMay, A&S 2e. Colon/rectum, p298

61 **a** **scleroderma**

Chylous effusions, those containing emulsified neutral lipids, are milky in nature and often associated with diseases such as scleroderma, tuberculosis, or cancer (most commonly lymphoreticular malignancies).

DeMay, A&S 2e. Chylous effusion, p282

62 **a** **a generalized body infection**

The diagnosis of septic arthritis in synovial fluid specimens is grounded upon the finding of an admixture of neutrophils, fibrin, and sheets of synovial cells. The etiology is usually related to bacteria (often mycobacteria or pyogenic), a virus, or fungus; however, the exact etiology of the disorder must be ascertained.

DeMay, A&S 2e. Septic arthritis, p341

63 **b** **megakaryocyte**

The presence of numerous megakaryocytes might raise suspicion of a possible myeloid metaplasia, a condition considered a precursor for myelocytic leukemia. Care must be taken not to overestimate the importance of these findings, especially if peripheral blood contamination is present.

DeMay, A&S 2e. Megakaryocytes, p281

64 **d** **mesothelioma, carcinomatous**

Identifying the cells as mesothelial cell lineage is the first step in establishing the diagnosis of carcinomatous mesothelioma. Cytology reveals many cells possessing homogeneous cytoplasm with "skirts" or "blebs," multinucleation, single cells and clusters, and coarse, irregular chromatin with multiple macronucleoli. Irregular papillae and knobby 3D clusters with cytoplasmic vacuolation are found among a metachromatic precipitous background (demonstrated with Diff-Quik staining). The differential diagnosis is metastatic adenocarcinoma; however, special staining with alcian blue-hyaluronidase and D-PAS is negative for carcinomatous mesothelioma, but positive for adenocarcinoma. Immunocytochemical staining with CEA and B72.3 is also negative for mesothelioma, but positive for adenocarcinoma.

DeMay, A&S 2e. Morphology of mesothelioma, p316-318

65 **a** **melanoma**

Melanoma typically presents in single cells, aggregates, or as spindle cells with bizarre malignant nuclear features, macronucleoli, intranuclear cytoplasmic inclusions, and possibly intracytoplasmic golden-brown pigment. Due to the fact that these diseases may be amelanotic, it may be helpful to confirm this disease process with S100, HMB45, melan A or MITF (microphthalmia associated transcription factor)—all which preferentially react with melanoma cells.

DeMay, A&S 2e. Melanoma, p309

66 **d** **neuroblastoma/adrenals**

Should the presence of small anaplastic cells be identified in serous effusions from children, the diagnostic focus should be discriminating between neuroblastoma of adrenal origin and Wilms tumor (nephroblastoma) of kidney origin. The former is a neuroendocrine lesion that will immunologically stain positive for chromogranin. Wilms tumors are negative for chromogranin.

DeMay, A&S 2e. Malignant effusions in children, p311

67 **d** **tuberculosis**

The diagnosis of septic arthritis in synovial fluid specimens is grounded upon the finding of an admixture of neutrophils, fibrin, and sheets of synovial cells. The etiology is usually related to bacteria (often mycobacteria or pyogenic), a virus, or fungus; however, the exact etiology of the disorder must be ascertained.

DeMay, A&S 2e. Septic arthritis, p341

ISBN 978-089189-6357 ©ASCP 2015

68 c negative for neutral mucin

Mesothelial cells do not contain neutral mucin but rather mesenchymal mucin or hyaluronic acid; therefore, neutral mucin positivity as identified by special staining with mucicarmine or alcian blue would indicate an adenocarcinoma. Mesothelial cells may be peripherally positive with PAS, but after digestion with diastase, the cells are negative, whereas adenocarcinomas will remain positive.

DeMay, A&S 2e. Mesothelial cells, p274-277

69 b mesothelial cells

Mesothelial cells show papillae and pseudoacini with knobby borders instead of true community borders, and single cells with "windows" between adjacent cells—a result of centrifugation and maintenance of the cytoplasmic brush border. The finding of a brush border infers benignity and is often described as indistinct or fuzzy in appearance. The nuclei of these cells are round and centrally located with well defined, regular nuclear membranes and finely granular, regularly distributed chromatin with nucleoli. The cytoplasmic morphology is homogeneous and dense with peripheral fading, often demonstrating an endo-ectoplasmic demarcation. The density of the cytoplasm may give a false "atypical" impression of hyperchromatic nuclei; however, when the nuclear intensity is compared with that of the cytoplasm, there is little divergence. The presence of psammoma bodies may also be seen in reactive conditions such as mesothelial hyperplasia and endosalpingiosis. Psammoma bodies are more commonly seen in benign effusions than in malignant effusions (eg, ovarian cancer).

DeMay, A&S 2e. Mesothelial cells, p334

70 c hemosiderin laden macrophages

Hemosiderin macrophages (siderophages), neutrophils, cartilaginous elements, sheets of synovial lining cells, and multinucleated histiocytes, in a plethora of proteinaceous debris, are descriptive of traumatic arthritis.

DeMay, A&S 2e. Traumatic arthritis, p342

71 b pleuroesophageal fistula

The depicted cells represent vegetable material from a pleuroesophageal fistula. A fistula may be suspected should the cytology contain benign glandular cells (perirectal), squamous cells (periesophageal), bacteria, or detritus. Cells with double cell walls, squared off cytoplasm containing smudgy nuclei and intracytoplasmic granules are diagnostic of vegetable contaminant.

DeMay, A&S 2e. Nonreactive mesothelial cells, p334

72 a reactive lymphocytosis

Severe inflammation/reactive lymphocytosis is often difficult to distinguish from recurrent leukemia, with the exception that reactive changes consist of a polytypic population of small mature lymphocytes and immunoblasts (often containing prominent nucleoli) as well as plasma cells. The absence of malignant blasts with irregular, notched, or cleaved nuclear membranes and hyperchromatic, coarse, irregular chromatin with prominent nucleoli is important when differentiating reactive processes secondary to intrathecal therapy or infection from recurrent leukemic involvement. A negative reaction with tumor marker terminal deoxytransferase is useful in ruling out recurrent leukemia.

DeMay, A&S 2e. Lymphocytes, p278

73 b *Cryptococcus neoformans*

The presence of single, yeastlike structures (5-15 μm) with mucinous capsules is diagnostic of *Cryptococcus neoformans*. These organisms reproduce by teardrop budding. Special staining with mucicarmine will help elucidate the distinctive capsule. Differentiation includes starch crystals, which have a Maltese cross birefringence.

DeMay, A&S 2e. Cryptococcus, p505

74 a normal/reactive mesothelial cells

Pancreatitis may often be associated with a hemorrhagic effusion. In such cases, a bloody or dark "chocolate" effusion, representative of old blood, may be withdrawn along with a population of normal mesothelial cells and inflammatory cells. The depicted mesothelial cells possess distinct cell windows between adjacent cells that are representative of the microvillus borders. An endo-ectoplasmic demarcation is seen and the cytoplasm is homogeneous. The nuclei are variable, round to oval, and possess well defined smooth nuclear membranes. The chromatin is finely granular, evenly distributed, with variable nucleoli. An occasional multinucleated or "atypical" mesothelial cell with aberrant nuclear features may be seen. However, in benign processes, a 1 cell population is seen instead of the typical 2 cell population associated with metastatic carcinomatosis (normal mesothelial cells and a second population of "foreign" cells).

DeMay, A&S 2e. t3.3 Gross examination of effusion fluid, p272

75 a tumor marker: terminal deoxytransferase

The cellular findings are consistent with recurrent acute lymphoblastic leukemia (ALL). Recurrent leukemia may often be difficult to separate from benign/reactive processes. Terminal deoxytransferase is a DNA polymerase leukemic marker that is absent in normal or reactive lymphocytes; therefore, a positive reaction may help confirm the emergence of recurrent ALL.

DeMay, A&S 2e. Acute lymphoblastic leukemia, p517-518

76 b glioblastoma multiforme

Glioblastomas (grade IV astrocytomas) represent the most common primary brain neoplasm (often contained within the frontal lobes) detected in adults. The cytomorphologic criterion associated with this lesion is the finding of pleomorphic, bizarre, frankly malignant cells with opaque or lacy cytoplasm and wispy cytoplasmic appendages, either singularly or in cell balls. These cells are easily recognized as malignant; however, the differential diagnosis may include a pleomorphic carcinoma or sarcoma. Immunocytochemical staining with glial fibrillary acidic protein will confirm CNS origin.

DeMay, A&S 2e. Glioblastoma multiforme, p510

77 b gout/monosodium urate monohydrate

Monosodium urate crystals (strongly negative birefringence with pointed ends) polarize and help confirm the presence of gouty arthritis. The differential diagnosis includes pseudogout/chondrocalcinosis, a condition that features calcium phosphate crystals that are not enhanced by polarized light.

DeMay, A&S 2e. Gout, p342

78 b viral meningitis

A hypercellular population of polytypic reactive lymphocytes in this patient suggests a possible viral meningitis. Care should be taken to discriminate these cells from those of a primary leukemia/lymphoma, which are usually monomorphic. It may be difficult if not impossible to discriminate these cells as benign if a lymphopoietic malignancy had been diagnosed in the past.

DeMay, A&S 2e. Viral meningitis, p504

79 c neural elements

Choroid/ependymal cells may be seen following intrathecal therapy. The cells present as single cells and in microacinar or papillary clusters. They have moderate lacy cytoplasm (often containing a yellow pigment) and uniform nuclear sizes with fine, even chromatin. Although cilia are generally absent, club shaped microvilli may be present.

DeMay, A&S 2e. Choroid plexus cells, p499

80 a normal cellular findings

Normal cerebrospinal fluid taken from lumbar taps reveals a hypocellular population of small round mature lymphocytes or monocytes (0-5 cells/μL, or 20-70 if cytocentrifuged). Rarely, leptomeningeal, ependymal, or neuronal elements are identified in lumbar taps, but appear more frequently in ventricular taps.

DeMay, A&S 2e. Normal cells, p495-498

81 d medulloblastoma

The finding of small anaplastic cells ("small blue cell tumors") in the CSF of children may indicate the presence of medulloblastoma, neuroblastoma, or retinoblastoma. Special attention should focus on possible clinical history. Medulloblastomas are neural crest tumors that arise from the cerebellum and are found in children or adolescents. Neuroblastomas (rare in the brain) typically arise within the cerebral hemisphere. Retinoblastomas involve the orbit and optic tract.

DeMay, A&S 2e. Medulloblastoma, p512-513

82 d reactive mesothelial cells

Reactive mesothelial cells (reactive hyperplasia) occur as papillae and pseudoacini with knobby borders (instead of true community borders) and as single cells with "windows" between adjacent cells–a result of centrifugation and maintenance of the cytoplasmic brush border. The finding of a brush border infers benignity and is often described as indistinct or fuzzy in appearance. The nuclei of these cells are round and centrally located with well defined, regular nuclear membranes and finely granular, regularly distributed chromatin with nucleoli. The cytoplasmic morphology is homogeneous and dense with peripheral fading, often demonstrating an endo-ectoplasmic demarcation. The density of the cytoplasm may give a false "atypical" impression of hyperchromatic nuclei; however, when the nuclear intensity is compared to that of the cytoplasm, there is little divergence. The presence of psammoma bodies may also be seen in reactive conditions such as mesothelial hyperplasia and endosalpingiosis. Psammoma bodies are more commonly seen in benign effusions than in malignant effusions (eg, ovarian cancer).

DeMay, A&S 2e. Reactive mesothelial cells, p334

83 a meningioma

Small cells found in whorls and sheets with benign nuclear features (often accompanied by psammoma bodies) indicate meningioma. These meningeal tumors are generally found in adolescents. These benign lesions need to be discriminated from their malignant counterpart, meningiosarcoma, a tumor that presents with classic sarcomatous features.

DeMay, A&S 2e. Meningioma, p521

84 a high molecular weight keratin

Cytology reveals pleomorphic cells with hyperchromatic, eccentrically located nuclei, irregular nuclear membranes, macronucleoli, and dense, hard cytoplasm. Positive staining with high molecular weight keratin would indicate a squamous cell carcinoma (the most common lung neoplasm).

DeMay, A&S 2e. Metastatic malignancy, p521-522

85 c normal mesothelial cells

The depicted cells are representative of normal or nonreactive mesothelial cells from body cavity washings. The cells are usually seen in flat sheets with polygonal cytoplasm and polygonal borders (stripped away by the saline jet). The nuclei are usually single and often paracentrally located with fine, regular chromatin. "Daisy cells," benign cells with lobulated nuclei that may be seen in women at midcycle, may also be found in body cavity washings. In addition to the normal mesothelial cells, body cavity washings may have associated white and red blood cells, starch granules (from gloves), and debris. In contrast to body cavity washings, serous effusions often contain mesothelial cells with reactive features.

DeMay, A&S 2e. Nonreactive mesothelial cells, p334

86 b lung

These cells are consistent with small cell carcinoma of the lung. Cytology reveals the typical presentation of anaplastic cells with nuclear molding and vertebral column formation arranged in cords, nests, or ribbons. The nuclei exhibit coarse, irregular chromatin and hyperchromasia. Extreme importance should be given to correlative studies with the original tissue section, or a previous history. Differential diagnoses include undifferentiated gliomas, large cell lymphomas, lobular carcinoma of the breast in women, and Merkel cell tumor of the skin.

DeMay, A&S 2e. Lung, p297-298

87 a idiopathic

The presence of a very large number of eosinophils in serous fluids may be idiopathic in the absence of a specific clinical history such as trauma, hypersensitivity, pneumothorax, or pulmonary infarct. Idiopathic eosinophilia is self limiting and tends to spontaneously resolve.

DeMay, A&S 2e. Eosinophils, p279

88 b acute bacterial meningitis

A hypercellular population of neutrophilic leukocytes is commonly associated with acute bacterial infections. Culture analysis should be performed to specify the etiology of the infection.

DeMay, A&S 2e. Bacterial meningitis, p503

ISBN 978-089189-6357 ©ASCP 2015

89 b mesothelioma

Identifying the cells as mesothelial cell lineage is the first step in establishing the diagnosis of carcinomatous mesothelioma. Cytology reveals many cells possessing homogeneous cytoplasm with "skirts" or "blebs," multinucleation, single cells and clusters, and coarse, irregular chromatin with multiple macronucleoli. Irregular papillae and knobby 3D clusters with cytoplasmic vacuolation are found among a metachromatic precipitous background (demonstrated with Diff-Quik staining). The differential diagnosis is metastatic adenocarcinoma; however, special staining with alcian blue-hyaluronidase and D-PAS is negative for carcinomatous mesothelioma, but positive for adenocarcinoma. Immunocytochemical staining with CEA and B72.3 are also negative for mesothelioma but positive for adenocarcinoma.
DeMay, A&S 2e. Cytologic diagnosis, p317

90 b adenocarcinoma, bronchogenic type

Metastatic bronchogenic adenocarcinoma cytologically presents in clusters and as single cells with vacuolated cytoplasm positive for mucin, hyperchromatic nuclei with irregular nuclear membranes, fine to coarse chromatin with irregular distribution, and macronucleoli. Clinical history and tissue comparison with the original primary site is important in confirming this metastatic process.
DeMay, A&S 2e. Bronchogenic adenocarcinoma, p238

91 d Mott cell

Mott cells are of plasma cell lineage with PAS+ intracytoplasmic granules (Russell bodies).
DeMay, A&S 2e. Mott cells, p339

92 c common leukocyte antigen

Immunocytochemical confirmation with common leukocyte antigen separates a lymphopoietic malignancy (lymphoma) from a metastatic carcinoma such as small cell carcinoma or other neuroendocrine metastases.
DeMay, A&S 2e. Lymphoma/leukemia, p515-516

93 d rheumatoid arthritis

A predominance of neutrophilic inflammatory cells among a fibrinous, granular or "sandy" necrotic background (which stain from blue to pink to orange) with occasional cholesterol crystals and multinucleated or trapezoidal histiocytes is suggestive of rheumatoid arthritis. Serum confirmation of rheumatoid factor is necessary to establish this disease process.
DeMay, A&S 2e. Rheumatoid arthritis, p341

94 a pancreaticobiliary carcinoma

Cells in vertebral column formations or 3D clusters containing pleomorphic cytoplasm, classic malignant nuclear features, prominent nucleoli, and evidence of mucus secretion or papillary formation are helpful features in establishing the diagnosis of metastatic pancreatic and biliary adenocarcinoma. The morphologic differentiation between pancreatic and biliary duct carcinoma is difficult; however, pancreatic lesions are generally less differentiated. The diagnosis, though, must be correlated with a previously established malignancy or related clinical history as indicated by this question.
DeMay, A&S 2e. Pancreatobiliary tract, p299

95 c systemic lupus erythematosus

Systemic lupus erythematosus may be cytologically confirmed by finding the characteristic LE cell, a neutrophil containing a large hematoxylin inclusion consisting of antinuclear antibody coated, degenerated nuclear material. This disease, generally affecting women in childbearing years, presents with idiopathic pleural effusions, and must be clinically diagnosed with antinuclear antibodies and clinical manifestations such as a butterfly facial rash and joint pain. In the absence of a previously established clinical and serological diagnosis, the diagnosis may be difficult.
DeMay, A&S 2e. Systemic lupus erythematosus, p287

96 b rheumatoid pleuritis

This collagen disease may be identified by the presence of multinucleated histiocytes and epithelioid histiocytes ("snake cells") amongst a granular, "sandy" or "fluffy" eosinophilic necrotic background. Large numbers of ragocytes, which represent mono- or multilobulated neutrophils with dark blue cytoplasmic inclusions (immunoglobulin), are specific for this disease. These findings are consistent with a necrotizing granuloma. Clinical symptoms include joint pain and/or synovitis and a positive serum test for rheumatoid factor. Rheumatoid pleuritis usually affects women; nevertheless, effusion related disease is seen more often in men.
DeMay, A&S 2e. Rheumatoid effusion, p286-287

97 a small cell carcinoma

Metastatic small cell carcinoma presents with hyperchromatic, stippled chromatin, coarse clumping, nuclear molding, scanty cytoplasm, and micronucleoli. The cells are arranged characteristically in vertebral column formation ("stack of dishes"), microbiopsy aggregates, and in cords, nests, or ribbons.
DeMay, A&S 2e. Small cell carcinoma, p241-242

98 c mucicarmine–

These cells represent metastatic mucinous cystadenocarcinoma of the ovary. The presence of irregular transparent clusters with large distended, degenerated cytoplasmic vacuoles, "signet ring" morphology and classic malignant nuclear features, in combination with the clinical history, suggests this metastatic neoplasm. Although ovarian tumors suggest peritoneal effusions, pleural effusions may often be seen without ascites. Staining with alcian blue-hyaluronidase will be positive for most mucinous adenocarcinomas.

DeMay, A&S 2e. Ovary, p300

99 b small noncleaved lymphoma

Small noncleaved lymphomas may be secondary to AIDS or, more commonly, seen in children (Burkitt and non-Burkitt lymphoma). The cytology reveals a small to medium size population of immature lymphocytes with a monomorphic cellular pattern. The cells have round nuclei, moderately clumped chromatin, macronucleoli, and abundant cytoplasm.

DeMay, A&S 2e. Lymphoproliferative disease, p247

100 c neuroblastoma

The clinical findings suggest the adrenal neoplasm neuroblastoma. Small cells appear in clusters with rosette formations and anaplastic nuclear features. Immunocytochemical positivity for chromogranin and D-PAS negativity would help confirm the malignancy.

DeMay, A&S 2e. Neuroblastoma, p311

101 d S100

Amelanotic melanoma typically presents in single cells, in aggregates, or as spindle cells with bizarre malignant nuclear features, macronucleoli, intranuclear cytoplasmic inclusions. Due to the fact that these cells do not contain the melanin typically associated with metastatic melanoma, it becomes essential to attempt to confirm this disease process with immunocytochemistry markers such as S100, HMB45, melan A or MITF (microphthalmia associated transcription factor)–all which preferentially react with melanoma cells.

DeMay, A&S 2e. Melanoma, p389

102 a reactive synovial lining cells

Synovial cells resemble mesothelial cells, possessing round to oval, often eccentrically placed nuclei containing finely granular, regularly distributed chromatin and abundant basophilic cytoplasm. They are seen in sheets or in single cells, which resemble macrophages.

DeMay, A&S 2e. Synovial cells, p339

103 d serous cystadenocarcinoma, ovarian

The diagnosis of serous cystadenocarcinoma of the ovary cytologically presents as 3D aggregates with hyperchromatic nuclei and finely granular, irregularly distributed chromatin. The presence of psammoma bodies may help in identifying these lesions as ovarian primary. These cells recapitulate fallopian tube cells and may be difficult to distinguish from reactive or malignant mesothelial cells.

DeMay, A&S 2e. Ovary, p300

104 c could be verified as prostatic adenocarcinoma by using a prostate specific antigen (PSA) immunohistochemical stain

Prostatic carcinomas metastatic to the serous cavities are generally poorly differentiated lesions, presenting in small, microacinar groups and as single cells with hyperchromatic, irregular nuclei, and prominent nucleoli. Clinical history and special staining with prostatic specific antigen is important in confirming this disease process.

DeMay, A&S 2e. Prostatic adenocarcinoma, p476

105 d Wilms tumor

When small anaplastic cells are identified in serous effusions from children, the diagnostic focus should be discriminating between neuroblastoma of adrenal origin and Wilms tumor of kidney origin (nephroblastoma). The former is a neuroendocrine lesion that will immunologically stain positive for chromogranin. Wilms tumors are negative for chromogranin. Wilms tumors represent small blue cell tumors that present cytologically as anaplastic cells in clusters and balls. A spindle cell component may be identified (not seen in this photograph).

DeMay, A&S 2e. Wilms tumor, p311

106 d metastatic breast carcinoma

Metastatic carcinoma of the breast is the most common malignancy involving the pleural cavity in women. The most common morphologic variant, ductal adenocarcinoma, may be cytologically identified as "cannonballs," 3D proliferation spheres, or morula formations. The presence of these true tissue fragments with community cell borders is strongly suggestive of breast metastasis in light of provided clinical history.

DeMay, A&S 2e. Metastatic malignancy, p272

107 c normal mesothelial cells

The image shows flat, cohesive sheets of bland mesothelial cells. The flat sheets seen are typically associated with mechanical dislodgement, as compared to the spontaneous shedding of single mesothelial cells seen in effusions.

DeMay, A&S 2e. Cells, p275

108 a negative for malignancy

The image shows benign structure so called collagen ball. Core of collagen usually surrounded by benign mesothelial cells. More common in peritoneal washings than in effusions, due to their origin from microscopic adenofibromatous change on the ovarian surface.

DeMay, A&S 2e. Collagen balls, p280

ISBN 978-089189-6357 ©ASCP 2015

109 d metastatic breast carcinoma
This low magnification image shows 3 dimensional (cannonball) clusters characteristic for metastatic breast carcinoma.
DeMay, A&S 2e. Cannonballs, p297

110 d rheumatoid arthritis
This image shows all characteristic features of rheumatoid arthritis, such as a necroinflammatory background and a giant multinucleated epithelioid cell. These features are pathognomonic for this entity.
DeMay, A&S 2e. Rheumatoid arthritis, p341

111 b benign mesothelial cells
Vigorous washing can obtain large sheets of mesothelial cells that on cell block preparation can assume a pseudopapillary configuration.
DeMay, A&S 2e. Groups, p274

112 d systemic lupus erythematosus
The image shows a classic LE cell, which is a leukocyte with cytoplasm containing homogeneous material.
DeMay, A&S 2e. Systemic lupus erythematosus, p287

113 c brain tissue
Fragments of brain tissue may be seen in patients who have intracranial shunts. In this image you can appreciate fragments of brain matter with neurons and their dendritic processes.
DeMay, A&S 2e. Anatomy & physiology, p491

114 d *Cryptococcus* species
This image shows numerous yeast forms varying in size with thick mucoid capsules and single narrow necked budding.
DeMay, A&S 2e. Cryptococcus, p505

115 d medulloblastoma
Primary CNS neoplasms are the most common type of solid tumors in children; consequently neoplastic cells are more frequently identified in the CSF of children than adults. Lesions that are likely to shed cells into CSF include primary neuroectodermal tumors, or PNETs (including medulloblastoma, ependymomas, germ cell tumors, high grade gliomas and choroid plexus tumors). From a cytomorphologic perspective, the PNETs and many of the small round cell tumors are impossible to distinguish cytologically without clinical history and additional testing (eg, immunocytochemistry, electron microscopy, cytogenetics). Noting the dense, granular quality of the cytoplasm is useful in distinguishing these cells from lymphocytes or malignant lymphoma.
DeMay, A&S 2e. Medulloblastoma, p505

116 b benign chronic inflammation
A mixed lymphoid population of small to medium sized lymphocytes, as well as plasma cells, are seen. Mature lymphocytes are small and have dense chromatin with no discernible cytoplasm. Reactive lymphocytes have larger nuclei, more cytoplasm, prominent nucleoli, and may have a cleaved nuclear envelope. Plasma cells have a larger eccentrically placed nucleus with a more characteristic open chromatin pattern. A mixed lymphoid population in CSF suggests a benign inflammatory reaction and may further suggest viral meningitis or multiple sclerosis.
DeMay, A&S 2e. Medulloblastoma, p505

117 d a 57-year-old female with a history of breast carcinoma
The image shows a loose cluster of epithelial plasmacytoid cells with prominent nucleoli most consistent with breast carcinoma..
DeMay, A&S 2e. Breast, p296-297.

118 b obtain specimen for flow cytometry
This is a very cellular specimen showing numerous single, highly atypical lymphoid cells. Further classification of this lymphoproliferative disorder should be done by flow cytometry.
DeMay, A&S 2e. Lymphoreticular malignancies, p303-305

119 d mammogram
This image shows cells with characteristic features of a lobular breast carcinoma–single, fairly bland cells files (single files), plasmacytoid cells with occasional prominent nucleoli.
DeMay, A&S 2e. Breast cancer, p346

120 c papillary adenocarcinoma
The image shows a 3D cluster of malignant pleomorphic epithelial cells with very irregular nuclear membranes, cleared chromatin and prominent nucleoli. Note the psammoma body. Psammoma bodies may also be seen in a variety of benign lesions, including endosalpingiosis.
DeMay, A&S 2e. Psammoma bodies, p280

121 d metastatic adenocarcinoma
This CSF is very cellular and shows numerous multidimensional clusters of pleomorphic cells with intracytoplasmic mucin for adenocarcinoma.
DeMay, A&S 2e. Metastatic malignancy, p248

122 d small cell carcinoma
The image shows small, tight clusters arranged in single files of small cells with high N:C ratios, nuclear molding and "salt & pepper" chromatin. No prominent nucleoli are present.
DeMay, A&S 2e. Lung, p297-298

123 d benign collagen balls
Bland mesothelial cell nuclei arranged around a hyaline globule of collagen are described as "collagen balls." The use of peritoneal washings can help determine subclinical peritoneal dissemination by nonserous ovarian tumors.
DeMay, A&S 2e. Collagen balls, p280

124 a reactive mesothelial cells

Reactive hyperplasia shows papillae and pseudoacini with knobby borders instead of true community borders, and single cells with "windows" between adjacent cells—a result of ThinPrep processing—and maintenance of the cytoplasmic brush border. The finding of a brush border infers benignity and is often described as indistinct or fuzzy in appearance. The nuclei of these cells are round and centrally located with well defined, regular nuclear membranes and finely granular, regularly distributed chromatin with nucleoli. The cytoplasmic morphology is homogeneous and dense with peripheral fading, often demonstrating an endo-ectoplasmic demarcation. The density of the cytoplasm may give a false "atypical" impression of hyperchromatic nuclei; however, when the nuclear intensity is compared with that of the cytoplasm, there is little divergence.

DeMay, A&S 2e. Reactive mesothelial cells, p274-276

ISBN 978-089189-6357 ©ASCP 2015

Chapter 4

Gastrointestinal Tract

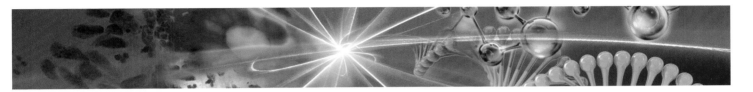

1   What places a patient at an increased risk for the development of colonic carcinoma?
  a   ulcerative colitis
  b   *Giardia lamblia*
  c   intestinal metaplasia
  d   chronic follicular colitis

2   Leiomyosarcoma is often differentiated histologically from its benign counterpart by:
  a   counting >10 mitotic figures per high power field
  b   enlarged nuclear features as determined cytologically
  c   presence of single cells
  d   fusiform appearance

3   A 44-year-old female presents with a polypoid mass in the rectum. Cytology reveals cells in sheets, elongated "trumpet" shaped cells with granular cytoplasm and basally located nuclei, and hypochromatic nuclei without nucleoli. The diagnosis is:
  a   villous adenoma
  b   adenocarcinoma
  c   ulcerative colitis
  d   reparative/regenerative changes

4   Which special stain would prove useful in the diagnosis of intestinal metaplasia as seen in gastric brushings?
  a   PAS
  b   oil red O
  c   GMS
  d   Congo red

5   A colonic brushing consists of abundant cells in cohesive, orderly sheets with hypochromatic nuclei and macronucleoli. Single cells are not identified. The diagnosis is:
  a   adenocarcinoma, well differentiated
  b   reparative/regenerative changes
  c   leiomyoma
  d   villous adenoma

6   A radioimmunoassay for carcinoembryonic antigen may be a false positive predictor of colonic adenocarcinoma if the patient has:
  a   cervical carcinoma
  b   mesothelioma
  c   cystitis
  d   alcoholic cirrhosis

7   Clusters of columnar cells with multiple distinct vacuoles, varying nuclear locations, hypochromatic nuclei, mild anisocytosis, naked nuclei, and the absence of single cells as found in duodenal specimens are diagnostic of:
  a   leiomyosarcoma
  b   adenocarcinoma, well differentiated
  c   hemangioma
  d   reactive/reparative changes

8   A 44-year-old female presents with chronic diarrhea, cyanotic flushing of the skin, and 5 hydroxyindoleacetic acid urinary changes. CAT scan reveals a 2 cm nodule located in the ileum. Brush cytology shows a population of monomorphic plasmacytoid appearing cells in loose aggregates. The diagnosis is:
  a   adenocarcinoma, well differentiated
  b   metastatic ovarian adenocarcinoma
  c   carcinoid tumor
  d   adenoma, Brunner gland

9   In comparison with other gastrointestinal neoplasms, cancer of the small bowel is:
  a   common
  b   rare
  c   most often sarcomatous
  d   most often lymphopoietic

10   A mixed population of lymphoid elements including small and large lymphocytes, tingible body macrophages, and plasma cells is diagnostic of:
  a   large cell lymphoma
  b   multiple myeloma
  c   Hodgkin disease
  d   chronic follicular gastritis

Cytopathology Review Guide 4e

11 Bipolar spindle cells in aggregates and overlapping single cells associated with ulcerative gastric specimens are:
a reparative/regenerative changes
b smooth muscle in origin
c adenocarcinoma, poorly differentiated
d carcinoid

12 Which of the following is associated with gastric and peptic ulcer disease?
a *Entamoeba histolytica*
b *Helicobacter pylori*
c *Mycobacterium* species
d Human papillomavirus

13 The most common primary neoplasm of the small intestine cytologically resembles:
a colorectal adenocarcinoma
b gastric type adenocarcinoma
c signet ring adenocarcinoma
d leiomyosarcoma

14 Clusters of cells with cyanophilic granular cytoplasm, enlarged hyperchromatic nuclei, macronucleoli, and tall columnar single cells with irregular chromatin and eccentrically located nuclei identified in colonic brushings represent:
a carcinoid tumor
b villous adenoma
c reparative/regenerative changes
d adenocarcinoma

15 What special stain is helpful in the diagnosis of carcinoid tumors of the intestinal tract?
a mucicarmine
b Fontana
c PAS
d alcian blue

16 A 42-year-old male presents with abdominal distention, nausea, and hemiparesis. A 2×3 cm periampullar lesion is identified in the small intestine. An intestinal brushing reveals many clusters of hyperchromatic cells with nuclear compression, irregular chromatin, macronucleoli, and cells with large distended vacuoles. A large population of single cells with abnormal features is present. The diagnosis is most consistent with:
a adenocarcinoma
b reactive/reparative cellular changes
c carcinoid
d adenoma

17 A patient with a dull right sided pain is evaluated for anemia. An ulcerative lesion is identified on endoscopic examination. Cytology reveals many single cells and epithelial aggregates with a high N:C ratio, granular and vacuolated cytoplasm, hyperchromasia, macronucleoli, and many cells with signet ring morphology. The diagnosis is:
a adenocarcinoma, well differentiated
b adenocarcinoma, poorly differentiated
c reparative/regenerative changes
d primary lymphoma

18 Which of the following is associated with steatorrhea and malnutrition?
a *Allescheria boydii*
b *Schistosoma haematobium*
c *Toxoplasma gondii*
d *Giardia lamblia*

19 A gastric brushing reveals normal cells with goblet cell features and windows between adjacent cells. The diagnosis is:
a respiratory contaminants
b normal gastric mucosa
c intestinal metaplasia
d chronic atrophic gastritis

20 An esophageal scraping reveals squamous cells with abundant cytoplasm, normal N:C ratios, degenerative nuclear features, and chromatic membranes. These cells are representative of:
a reparative/regenerative changes
b nonkeratinizing squamous cell carcinoma
c pernicious anemia
d granulomatous reaction

21 An esophageal brushing specimen from the distal third reveals squamous cells as well as nongoblet glandular cells. The presence of the glandular cells suggests:
a Barrett esophagitis
b normal representative findings
c reparative/regenerative cellular changes
d respiratory contaminants

22 The most common esophageal malignancy is:
a squamous carcinoma, nonkeratinizing
b adenocarcinoma, poorly differentiated
c adenocarcinoma, signet ring
d squamous carcinoma, keratinizing

23 Sheets of cells with abundant cytoplasm exhibiting hypochromasia, enlarged nuclei, well defined cellular borders, and cytoplasmic streaming and containing fine, regular chromatin patterns in esophageal specimens are diagnostic of:
a adenocarcinoma, well differentiated
b squamous carcinoma
c reparative/regenerative changes
d chronic atrophic gastritis

ISBN 978-089189-6357 ©ASCP 2015

24 What is considered an important feature in the cytologic diagnosis of gastric adenocarcinoma?
   a single cells
   b macronucleoli
   c bare nuclei
   d fibropurulent exudate

25 Poorly differentiated gastric adenocarcinoma of the stomach reveals which cytologic criteria?
   a 3D clusters of malignant cells
   b sheets of anaplastic cells
   c signet ring cells, single malignant cells
   d polygonal cells with hyperchromatic opaque nuclei

26 A 55-year-old male with a history of tobacco smoking and EtOH abuse presents with dysphagia. Esophageal brushing cytology reveals many clusters of cells with granular cytoplasm, fine, irregular chromatin patterns, nuclear compression, and macronucleoli in every cell. The diagnosis is:
   a squamous carcinoma
   b adenocarcinoma
   c reparative/regenerative changes
   d granulomatous reaction

27 Eosinophilic staining cells with intracytoplasmic granules and centrally located nuclei found in gastric specimens represent:
   a surface neck cells
   b chief cells
   c parietal cells
   d respiratory contaminants

28 The signet ring form of gastric adenocarcinoma is considered:
   a well differentiated
   b moderately well differentiated
   c moderately differentiated
   d poorly differentiated

29 Gastric adenomatous polyps:
   a have premalignant predisposition
   b have no premalignant predisposition
   c are inflammatory in nature
   d are hamartomatous

30 A 44-year-old female with a history of achlorhydria submits for evaluation. Gastric washings reveal numerous columnar appearing cells with karyolytic bland nuclear features, cytomegaly, karyomegaly, and nuclear folds. The diagnosis is:
   a pernicious anemia
   b intestinal metaplasia
   c reparative/regenerative changes
   d adenocarcinoma, well differentiated

31 The presence of small single cells without cohesive features, with scanty cytoplasm and lobulated nuclear features containing macronucleoli is diagnostic of:
   a metastatic small cell carcinoma
   b primary lymphoma
   c inflammatory changes
   d leiomyoma

32 Which is etiologically related to esophageal carcinoma?
   a tuberculosis
   b Plummer-Vinson syndrome
   c ulcerative esophagitis
   d herpetic esophagitis diverticula

33 The histologic representation most commonly associated with esophageal carcinoma is:
   a fungating
   b ulcerative
   c flat
   d inverted

34 A 55-year-old patient presents with GI bleeding and anemia. Gastric cytology reveals cells in well defined clusters, altered polarity, anisonucleosis, slight nuclear compression, hyperchromasia, and frequent macronucleoli. Few single cells are present. The diagnosis is:
   a reactive/reparative cellular changes
   b a malignant glandular tumor arising from intestinal metaplasia
   c a malignant glandular tumor that does not arise from intestinal metaplasia
   d leiomyosarcoma

35 The most common lymphoma involving the stomach is:
   a small cell cleaved
   b small cell noncleaved
   c large cell type
   d Burkitt lymphoma

36 Cells with well defined borders exhibiting good polarity, enlarged nuclei, and macronucleoli in an esophageal specimen are suggestive of:
   a pernicious anemia
   b squamous carcinoma, nonkeratinizing
   c herpetic esophagitis
   d reparative/regenerative cellular changes

37 Cells in sheets, single cells, and hyperchromatic syncytia with irregular chromatin, nucleoli, cellular cannibalism, and cytoplasmic ringing in esophageal brushings are representative of:
   a adenocarcinoma, poorly differentiated
   b squamous carcinoma, nonkeratinizing
   c squamous carcinoma, keratinizing
   d adenocarcinoma, well differentiated

38 These cells from a gastric brushing were most likely collected from a patient with a history of:
a intestinal metaplasia
b chronic follicular gastritis
c pernicious anemia
d hyperplastic polyps

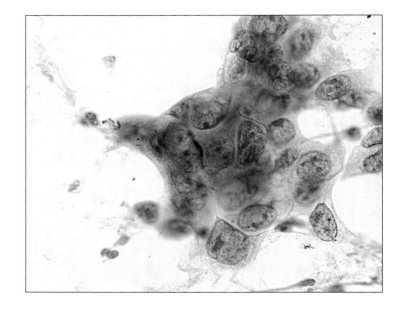

39 These cells were identified in a gastric washing specimen. They are diagnostic of:
a adenocarcinoma, well differentiated
b adenocarcinoma, poorly differentiated signet ring
c reactive/reparative process
d Crohn disease

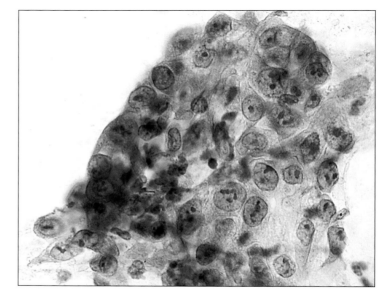

40 A 60-year-old male presents with unexplained nausea and vomiting. A barium swallow identified a 3 cm lesion in the ileum of the small intestine. Brushings revealed these cells, which represent
a adenomatosis
b hemangioma
c adenocarcinoma
d reactive/reparative process

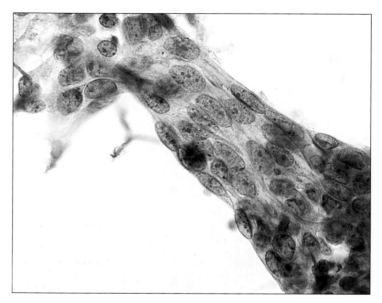

ISBN 978-089189-6357 ©ASCP 2015

41 A 67-year-old male with dysphagia, iron deficiency anemia, and positive guaiac testing results presents for a gastric brushing. Which of the following may give rise to the depicted cells?

   a intestinal metaplasia
   b native gastric epithelium
   c Peutz-Jeghers syndrome
   d aspirin gastritis

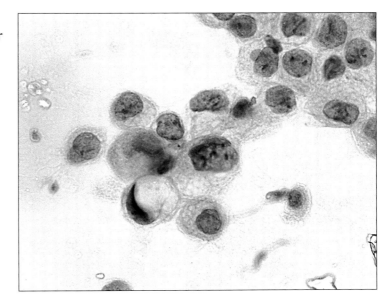

42 These cells were taken from a 45-year-old male with multiple ulcerative lesions of the rectum. A colonic brushing specimen reveals these cells. They are diagnostic of:

   a reactive/reparative changes
   b adenocarcinoma, well differentiated
   c carcinoid tumor
   d villous adenoma

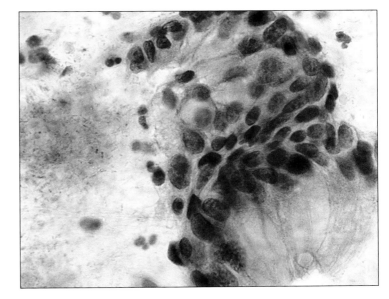

43 A 66-year-old female with a history of ulcerative colitis presents with a polypoid mass in the rectum. Colonic brushing specimen reveals:

   a adenocarcinoma, well differentiated
   b villous adenoma
   c hamartomatous polyp
   d reactive/reparative changes

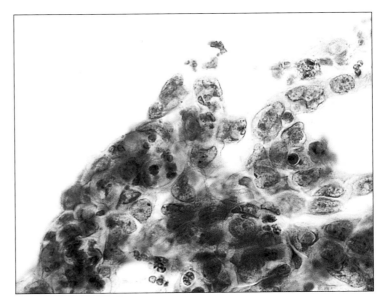

44 These cells were found in a gastric brushing specimen taken from a 55-year-old male with a history of celiac disease. They are diagnostic of:
a poorly differentiated adenocarcinoma
b pseudolymphoma
c small cell cleaved lymphoma
d large cell lymphoma

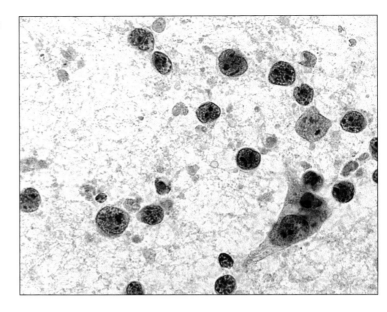

45 This structure was found in a duodenal brushing specimen from a 44-year-old female who had recently traveled abroad. The clinical finding/diagnosis is:
a vomiting/*Helicobacter pylori* infection
b nonspecific clinical findings/*Entamoeba histolytica* infection
c steatorrhea/*Giardia lamblia* infection
d bloody stool/*Strongyloides stercoralis* infection

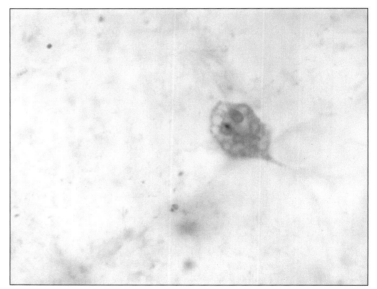

46 A 56-year-old male with a history of colonic adenocarcinoma presents with a 300 mL peritoneal effusion. Which of the following might aid in confirmation of a metastatic colonic adenocarcinoma?
a S100+
b vimentin+
c serotonin+
d carcinoembryonic antigen+

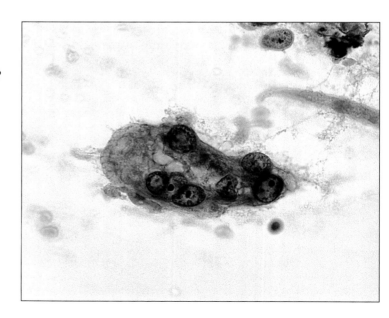

ISBN 978-089189-6357 ©ASCP 2015

47 The finding of these cells in an esophageal brushing specimen from the middle third of the esophagus is diagnostic of:
a villous adenoma
b reactive/reparative changes
c Barrett esophagus
d adenocarcinoma, well differentiated

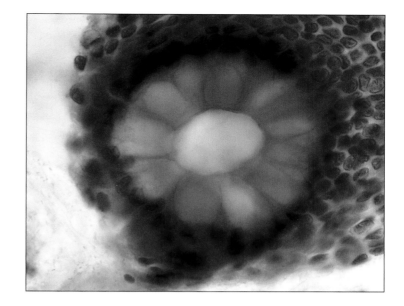

48 A 43-year-old female with unexplained gastritis undergoes gastric lavage. These cells represent:
a large cell lymphoma
b pseudolymphoma
c small cell lymphoma
d signet ring adenocarcinoma

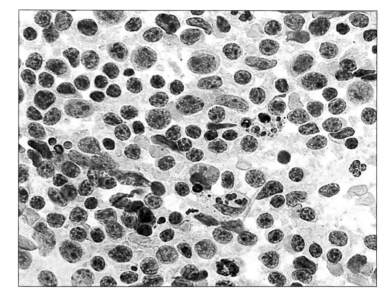

49 A 55-year-old Japanese farmer presents with vomiting of long duration. Results of a gastric lavage are diagnostic of:
a adenocarcinoma, well differentiated intestinal type
b adenocarcinoma, signet ring type
c intestinal metaplasia
d reactive/reparative process

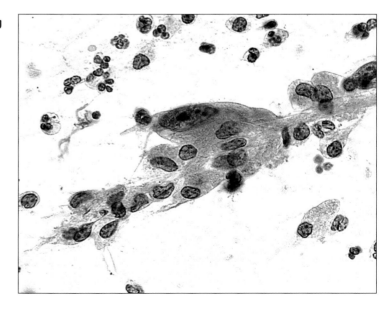

50　A 55-year-old male with a dull pain located on the right side of his abdomen presents for evaluation. The physician notes anorexia and anemia. Guaiac is positive for occult blood. Colonic brushings reveal these cells. The diagnosis is most consistent with:

a villous adenoma
b large cell lymphoma
c adenocarcinoma, poorly differentiated
d melanoma

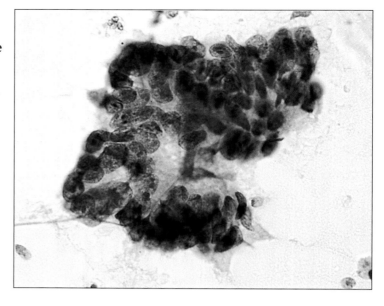

51　A 34-year-old AIDS patient presents with rectal adhesions. These cells, identified upon rectal swabbing, are diagnostic of:

a cytomegalovirus
b herpesvirus
c reactive/reparative changes
d adenocarcinoma

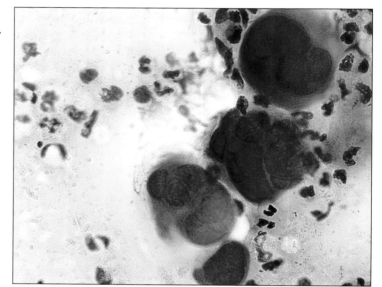

52　A 44-year-old male complaining of rectal bleeding presents with a 2 cm lesion of the sigmoid region of the colon. These cells, identified in a colonic brushing, are diagnostic of:

a adenocarcinoma, well differentiated
b normal colonic mucosa
c ulcerative colitis
d villous adenoma

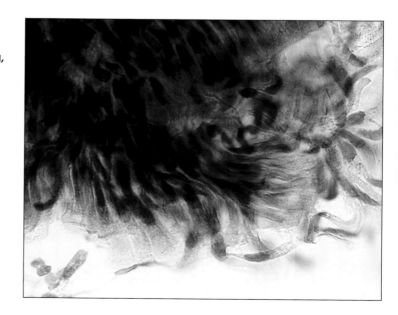

ISBN 978-089189-6357　©ASCP 2015

53 This photomicrograph is from a cell block of an alimentary tract neoplasm. A clinical symptom of this patient would be:

a longstanding dysphagia
b aspirin gastritis
c steatorrhea
d bloody stool

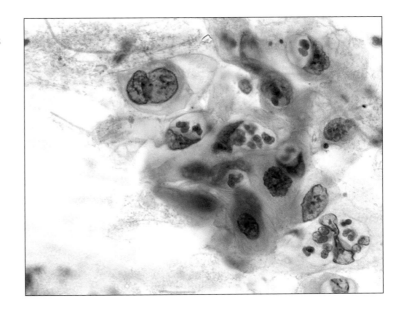

54 A 50-year-old female underwent an esophageal brushing. Which clinical condition best explains these cellular findings?

a chronic esophageal reflux
b herpetic esophagitis
c granulomatous esophagitis
d syphilitic esophagitis

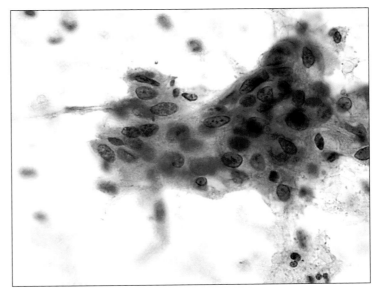

55 This is a histologic section of gastric mucosa stained with periodic acid-Schiff. The findings are consistent with:

a adenocarcinoma, well differentiated
b adenocarcinoma, poorly differentiated
c intestinal metaplasia
d normal mucus neck cells

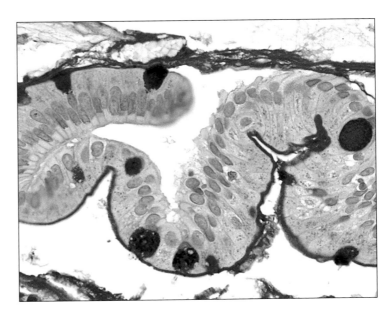

©ASCP 2015 ISBN 978-089189-6357

56   Represented is a gastric wash specimen taken from a
55-year-old male. The cellular finding is:
   a primary adenocarcinoma
   b reparative/regenerative changes
   c respiratory tract contaminants
   d pernicious anemia

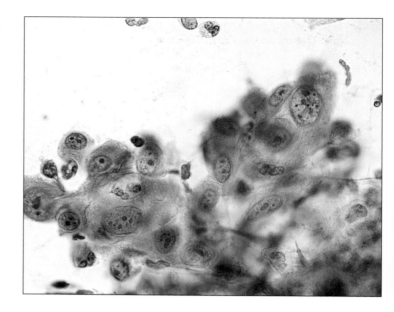

57   These elements identified in an esophageal brushing
from a 50-year-old male with dysphagia suggest:
   a leiomyosarcoma
   b food contamination
   c leiomyoma
   d metastatic sarcoma, not otherwise specified

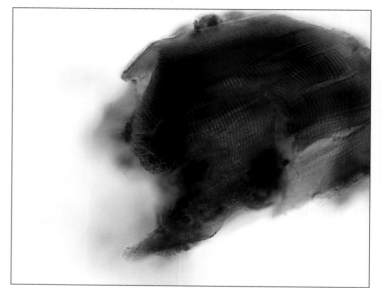

58   A 60-year-old male with a 20 year history of excessive
alcohol intake as well as smoking presents with a 2 cm
mucosal lesion. An esophageal brushing reveals:
   a squamous cell carcinoma, nonkeratinizing
   b atypical laryngeal cells, "Pap" cells
   c moderate keratinizing squamous dysplasia
   d squamous cell carcinoma, keratinizing

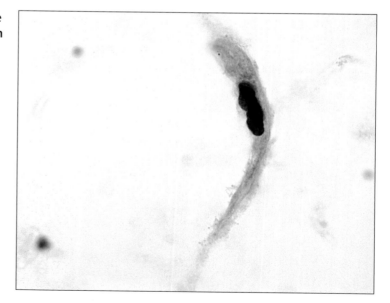

ISBN 978-089189-6357 ©ASCP 2015

59 A 62-year-old female previously diagnosed with reflux esophagitis presents with dysphagia. Esophageal brushings reveal these cells, which are compatible with:

a reactive/reparative changes
b squamous cell carcinoma
c atypical squamous cells
d squamous dysplasia

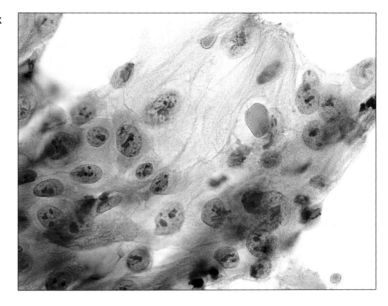

60 These cells represent a gastric brushing from a 65-year-old male with a history of chronic atrophic gastritis secondary to pernicious anemia. The cellular pattern represents:

a parietal cells
b intestinal metaplasia
c Crohn disease
d a gastric ulcer

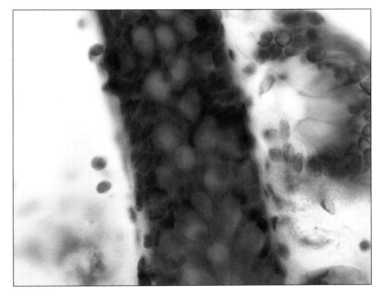

61 A 55-year-old male with Crohn disease presents for an esophageal brushing. The cytologic pattern depicted is:

a squamous cell carcinoma, nonkeratinizing
b granulomatous esophagitis
c pemphigus vulgaris
d Barrett metaplasia

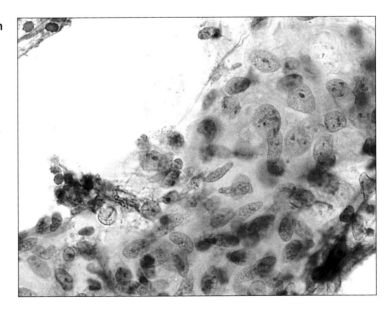

62 These cells were identified in a gastric washing specimen from a patient with hematemesis. The findings are consistent with:

a normal gastric mucosa
b intestinal metaplasia
c parasitic infection
d vegetable contaminant

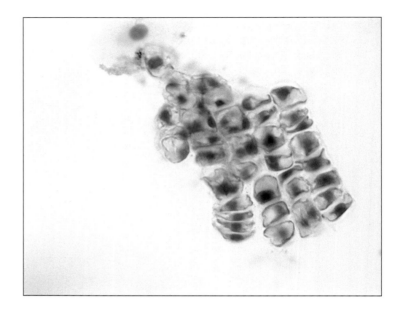

63 These cells were collected from a gastric brush specimen in a patient complaining of GI pain and weight loss. GI bleeding was clinically confirmed. Cytology reveals:

a adenocarcinoma, well differentiated intestinal type
b reactive/reparative
c granulation tissue
d adenocarcinoma, poorly differentiated gastric type

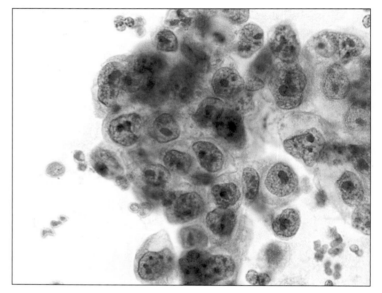

64 A patient receiving corticosteroid therapy for advanced rheumatoid arthritis underwent esophageal brushing. This process reveals:

a rheumatoid granuloma
b *Candida albicans*
c *Geotrichum candidum*
d *Aspergillus* species

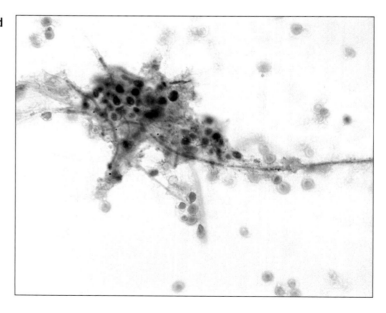

ISBN 978-089189-6357 ©ASCP 2015

65 These cells were collected from a 66-year-old male with a history of hyperplastic gastric polyps. The cytologic pattern represents:

a intestinal metaplasia
b normal gastric mucosa
c pernicious anemia/B$_{12}$ deficiency
d granulation tissue associated with ulceration

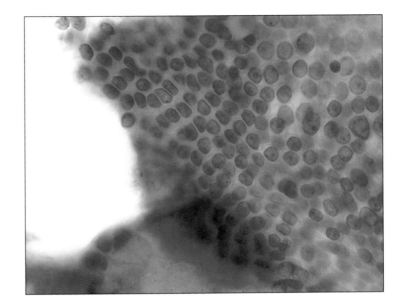

66 A 55-year-old male with a history of giardiasis presents for a colonoscopy. Colonic brushings reveal these cells. These cells are associated with:

a adenocarcinoma, well differentiated
b villous adenoma
c fibroma
d reactive/reparative changes secondary to ulcerative colitis

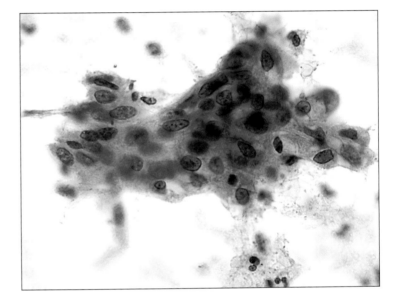

67 A 44-year-old transplant recipient develops multiple sores within the esophagus. An esophageal brushing is performed. The cellular finding is most compatible with:

a pernicious anemia
b Plummer-Vinson syndrome
c herpes
d pemphigus vulgaris

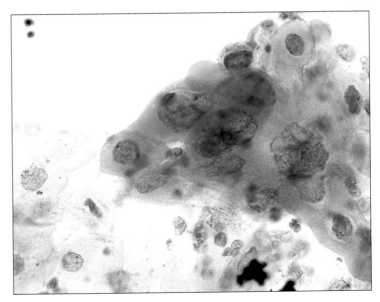

©ASCP 2015   ISBN 978-089189-6357

68 A 42-year-old male had mucosal erosions in his distal esophagus. Esophageal brushing was performed. The best diagnosis is:

   a herpes simplex esophagitis
   b squamous cell carcinoma
   c adenocarcinoma
   d radiation changes

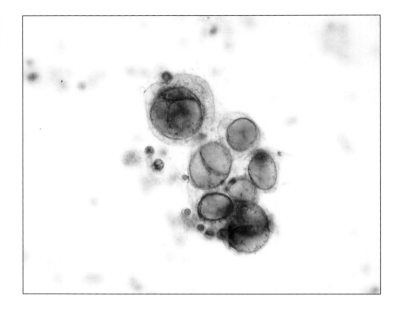

69 Bile duct brushing from a 68-year-old male. What is the diagnosis?

   a positive for adenocarcinoma
   b atypical cells present
   c reactive changes
   d negative for malignancy

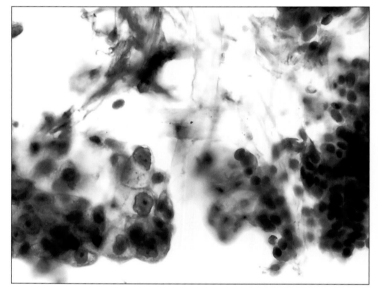

70 A colonic brushing was obtained from this 75-year-old male. What were the colonoscopic findings for this patient?

   a 0.5 cm polyp
   b an ulcerated polypoid 4 cm lesion
   c numerous small ulcers
   d diverticuli

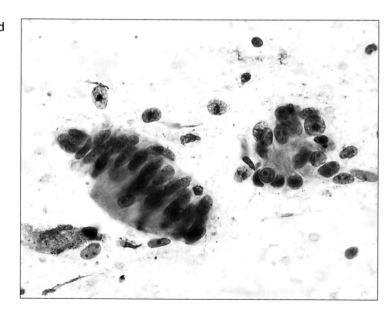

ISBN 978-089189-6357   ©ASCP 2015

71 This is a gastric brushing specimen from a 68-year-old male. What immunocytochemical stain would support the diagnosis?
  a CD117
  b CK20
  c CD31
  d synaptophysin

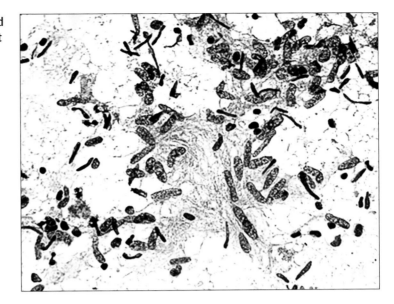

72 A 70-year-old male, receiving immunosuppressive therapy, presented with esophageal ulcers. A brushing of the lesions was obtained. What infectious agent is responsible for this finding?
  a *Candida*
  b cytomegalovirus
  c adenovirus
  d herpesvirus

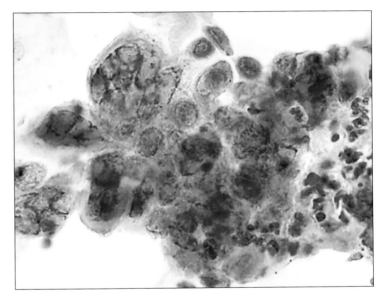

73 A 70-year-old male presented with dysphagia. An esophageal washing was performed. What is the most appropriate diagnosis for these cellular changes?
  a severe reparative reaction
  b Barrett esophagus
  c squamous cell carcinoma
  d herpes esophagitis

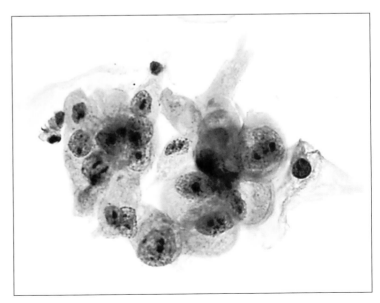

©ASCP 2015 ISBN 978-089189-6357

74 A 27-year-old female with a history of ulcerative colitis (UC) was seen for a routine colonoscopy. A polypoid mass was brushed. What is your diagnosis?

a pernicious anemia
b repair/regeneration
c herpes
d pemphigus vulgaris

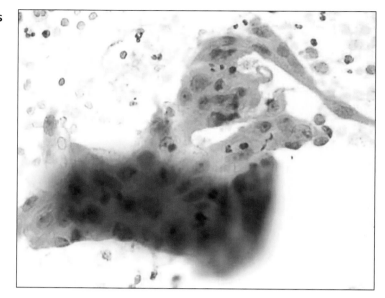

75 A 64-year-old female underwent cholecystectomy 6 months ago. Now she presents with jaundice and signs of an obstruction and biliary stricture. Endoscopic bile duct brushings were obtained. What is your interpretation?

a benign bile duct epithelium
b cholangiocarcinoma
c atypical hyperplasia
d hepatocellular carcinoma

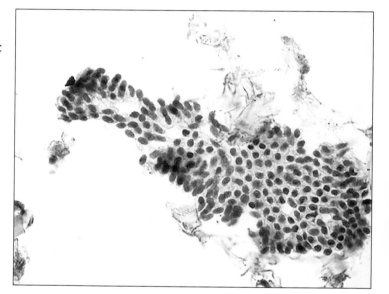

ISBN 978-089189-6357 ©ASCP 2015

Gastrointestinal Tract *Answer Key*

1 a ulcerative colitis

These patients have an increased risk for development of malignant neoplasia. Lesions arising from ulcerative colitis are generally poorly differentiated with multiple foci.

DeMay, A&S 2e. Chronic idiopathic inflammatory bowel disease, p411

2 a counting >10 mitotic figures per high-power field

It may be quite difficult to distinguish leiomyomas from leiomyosarcomas using conventional cytologic morphology. Generally, leiomyosarcomas are more cellular, contain irregular chromatin, and are impressively pleomorphic. However, it is important to count the number of mitotic figures per high power field (HPF) with histopathology to accurately evaluate the aggressiveness of this lesion or determine its malignant nature. Lesions containing <5 mitotic figures per HPF are usually considered benign, those containing between 5 and 10 are borderline, while those possessing over 10 mitoses per HPF are considered malignant.

DeMay, A&S 2e. Leiomyoma and leiomyosarcoma, p110

3 a villous adenoma

Villous adenomas are considered premalignant lesions found within the gastrointestinal tract. The sensitivity of cytologic morphology may be inadequate in distinguishing these lesions from well differentiated adenocarcinomas. It is estimated that 25-75% of villous adenomatous polyps will undergo malignant transformation if surgical resection is not performed. These papillary lesions are also diagnostic within the colon.

DeMay, A&S 2e. Adenoma, p412

4 a PAS

Periodic acid-Schiff (PAS) will stain mucoproteins, mucolipids, and glycoproteins. Cells associated with intestinal metaplasia contain mucin containing "windows." Oil red O stains lipids/fat (choice b), GMS stains fungi (choice c), and Congo red stains amyloid (choice d).

DeMay, A&S 2e. Intestinal metaplasia, p394

5 b reparative/regenerative changes

Reactive/reparative changes seen within the colon are associated with ulcerative colitis, chronic irritation, or trauma. It is imperative to differentiate these conditions from well differentiated adenocarcinomas. Cellular predictability, preserved polarity, hypochromasia, and the absence of nuclear compression are found with repair. Single malignant cells, true tissue fragments, and tall columnar cell morphology containing hyperchromatic nuclei with irregular chromatin are critical for establishing a diagnosis of colonic adenocarcinoma.

DeMay, A&S 2e. Repair/regeneration, p30-31, 394

6 d alcoholic cirrhosis

Carcinoembryonic antigen (CEA) is associated with colonic adenocarcinoma and may prove to be a useful indicator of metastatic carcinoma. There are several conditions, though, that may be falsely positive for CEA, including alcoholic cirrhosis, inflammatory bowel disease, and pancreatitis.

DeMay, A&S 2e. Adenocarcinoma, p412-413

7 d reactive/reparative changes

Reactive/reparative changes seen within the colon are associated with ulcerative colitis, chronic irritation, or trauma. It is imperative to differentiate these conditions from well differentiated adenocarcinomas. Cellular predictability, preserved polarity, hypochromasia, and the absence of nuclear compression are found with repair. Single malignant cells, true tissue fragments, and tall columnar cell morphology containing hyperchromatic nuclei with irregular chromatin are critical for establishing a diagnosis of colonic adenocarcinoma.

DeMay, A&S 2e. Repair/regeneration, p30-31, 394

8 c carcinoid tumor

Carcinoid tumors are the second most common tumor of the duodenum. These argentaffin tumors are neural ectodermal in origin and represent an amine precursor uptake and decarboxylase (APUD) lesion. Their stem cell is the Kulchitsky cell. The diagnosis of carcinoid tumors relies on 2D aggregates of cells with finely granular, regularly distributed chromatin, inconspicuous nucleoli, and abundant granular cytoplasm. Immunocytochemical staining for chromogranin will help elucidate these lesions.

DeMay, A&S 2e. Carcinoid tumors, p245-246, 414

9 b rare

Although most carcinomas of the small bowel are metastatic, primary lesions can include adenocarcinomas, large cell lymphocytic lymphomas, and carcinoid tumors.

DeMay, A&S 2e. Small intestine, p406-409

10 d chronic follicular gastritis

A polymorphic population of small mature lymphocytes, larger immunoblasts, plasma cells, and tingible body macrophages is pathognomonic of pseudolymphoma, chronic follicular gastritis, or benign lymphoreticular hyperplasia. Most cases of chronic follicular gastritis are associated with gastric ulcers and may be concomitantly associated with highly reactive epithelial fragments.

DeMay, A&S 2e. Chronic gastritis, p396

11 b smooth muscle in origin

The presence of smooth muscle cells may be associated with leiomyoma and leiomyosarcoma. It may be quite difficult to distinguish leiomyomas from leiomyosarcomas using conventional cytologic morphology. Generally, leiomyosarcomas are more cellular, contain irregular chromatin, and are impressively pleomorphic. However, it is important to count the number of mitotic figures per high power field (HPF) with histopathology to accurately evaluate the aggressiveness of this lesion or determine its malignant nature. Lesions containing <5 mitotic figures per HPF are usually considered benign, those containing between 5 and 10 are borderline, while those possessing over 10 mitoses per HPF are considered malignant.

DeMay, A&S 2e. Leiomyoma and leiomyosarcoma, p110

12 b *Helicobacter pylori*

These Gram–, spiral shaped flagellated bacteria stain positive with Warthin-Starry, Giemsa, or Dieterle stains. Papanicolaou staining may reveal these bacteria, although often poorly (oil immersion may be required).

DeMay, A&S 2e. The unbelievable story of Helicobacter pylori, p397-398

13 a colorectal adenocarcinoma
Adenocarcinomas arising within the small bowel cytologically recapitulate intestinal type adenocarcinoma. The differential diagnoses include adenocarcinomas of the pancreas, bile duct, and ampulla of Vater.
DeMay, A&S 2e. Adenocarcinoma, p412-413

14 d adenocarcinoma
Colonic adenocarcinomas may be related to benign conditions such as ulcerative colitis, villous adenomas, or familial polyposis. Most adenocarcinomas occur within the rectosigmoid region, are polypoid or ulcerative, and are generally moderately well differentiated at the time of detection.
DeMay, A&S 2e. Adenocarcinoma, p412-413

15 b Fontana
Carcinoid tumors contain argentaffin granules (serotonin), which stain positively with the Fontana stain.
DeMay, A&S 2e. Carcinoid tumors, p245-246

16 a adenocarcinoma
Duodenal adenocarcinomas mimic colonic adenocarcinoma, possessing polypoid growth patterns, and often create stenosis. These lesions are extremely uncommon.
DeMay, A&S 2e. Adenocarcinoma, p412-413

17 b adenocarcinoma, poorly differentiated
Poorly differentiated adenocarcinomas are generally not difficult to establish as malignant due to myriad abnormal features as well as signet ring cells.
DeMay, A&S 2e. Adenocarcinoma, p412-413

18 d *Giardia lamblia*
These protozoa are associated with fatty stools, or steatorrhea, and may be diagnosed cytologically as blue to gray organisms with 4 pairs of flagella. Trophozoites closely resemble those of *Trichomonas* with the exception that *Giardia* are binucleate and have a ventral sucking disk. In addition, they lack an undulating membrane.
DeMay, A&S 2e. Giardia lamblia, p407

19 c intestinal metaplasia
Intestinal metaplasia is a premalignant gastric condition related to chronic atrophic gastritis in which normal columnar epithelial cells are replaced with cells of intestinal type. Cytology reveals sheets of normal glandular epithelium with interspersed goblet cells. Periodic acid-Schiff will stain mucoproteins, mucolipids, and glycoproteins. Cells associated with intestinal metaplasia possess mucin containing "windows." Cytology represents cohesive sheets of mucus neck cells with scattered goblet cells with large signet ring vacuoles.
DeMay, A&S 2e. Intestinal metaplasia, p394

20 c pernicious anemia
Pernicious anemia (PA) occurs as a result of impaired absorption of vitamin B_{12} due to the absence of intrinsic factor. This condition gives rise to atrophic gastritis due to the loss of gastric parietal cells. Cytologically, cells possess enlarged nuclei with karyolytic features and bland nuclear folds. An increase in gastric carcinoma has been associated with PA.
DeMay, A&S 2e. Vitamin deficiency, p383

21 b normal representative findings
Squamous mucosa and nongoblet glandular mucosa (a contaminant from the cardiac region of the stomach) represent normal cytologic findings when brushing the distal third of the esophagus. The absence of goblet cell morphology mitigates against a possible diagnosis of Barrett esophagitis.
DeMay, A&S 2e. The cells, p375-376

22 d squamous carcinoma, keratinizing
90% of primary esophageal tumors are keratinizing squamous cell carcinomas. Generally, these lesions occur in the middle to distal third of the esophagus. Most lesions are polypoid in nature, but may be endophytic or ulcerative. However, the incidence of signet ring adenocarcinomas (choice c) arising from Barrett esophagus is increasing.
DeMay, A&S 2e. Squamous cell carcinoma, p380-381

23 c reparative/regenerative changes
The differential diagnosis between reactive/reparative conditions is imperative in gastrointestinal tract specimens. Reparative/regenerative changes that occur in squamous mucosa of the esophagus resemble those found in the female genital tract. Sheets of cells with well defined cytoplasmic borders, preserved nuclear polarity, predictable nuclear features, fine regular chromatin patterns, micro- to macronucleoli, and characteristic cytoplasmic streaming (squamous) or honeycombing polarity (glandular) are pathognomonic of repair. This process is often associated with ulcerative esophagitis, trauma, reflux, and inflammatory etiology.
DeMay, A&S 2e. Repair/regeneration, p30-31; Reactive/reparative and degenerative changes, p394-395

24 a single cells
Single or isolated malignant cells are extremely important in establishing the diagnosis of gastric adenocarcinoma. These cells possess irregular chromatin, macronucleoli, and hyperchromasia. Should single cells be found from changes secondary to reactive/reparative conditions, they would possess normal chromatin features and be next to or associated with the coexisting reparative sheets.
DeMay, A&S 2e. Adenocarcinoma, p412-413

25 c signet ring cells, single malignant cells
Poorly differentiated adenocarcinoma of the stomach arises from native gastric epithelium—not from intestinal metaplasia. Poorly differentiated adenocarcinomas present as syncytial aggregates or single signet ring cells with nuclear overlapping and compression, increased N:C ratios, pleomorphism, irregular chromatin distribution, and macronucleoli. Malignancies arising from intestinal metaplasia are generally well differentiated.
DeMay, A&S 2e. Gastric type adenocarcinoma, p390, 401-402

ISBN 978-089189-6357 ©ASCP 2015

26 b adenocarcinoma

Predisposition to Barrett metaplasia is often considered an important premalignant change for the subsequent development of adenocarcinoma. Adenocarcinomas of the esophagus must be differentiated from reactive/reparative changes, which generally occur in sheets, not in 2D or 3D clusters with malignant nuclear features as described in this explanation. Reparative/regenerative changes that occur in squamous mucosa of the esophagus resemble those found in the female genital tract. Sheets of cells with well defined cytoplasmic borders, preserved nuclear polarity, predictable nuclear features, fine regular chromatin patterns, micro- to macronucleoli, and characteristic cytoplasmic streaming (squamous) or honeycombing polarity (glandular) are pathognomonic of repair. This process is often associated with ulcerative esophagitis, trauma, reflux, and inflammatory etiology.

DeMay, A&S 2e. Adenocarcinoma, p390, 401-402

27 c parietal cells

Parietal cells are responsible for the production of hydrochloric acid as well as intrinsic factor. The finding of these cells and chief cells (pepsinogen, rennin, gelatinase) in gastric brush specimens is somewhat rare.

DeMay, A&S 2e. Parietal cells, p394

28 d poorly differentiated

Poorly differentiated adenocarcinoma of the stomach arises from native gastric epithelium—not from intestinal metaplasia. Poorly differentiated adenocarcinomas present as syncytial aggregates or single signet ring cells with nuclear overlapping and compression, increased N:C ratios, pleomorphism, irregular chromatin distribution, and macronucleoli. Malignancies arising from intestinal metaplasia are generally well differentiated. Well differentiated gastric adenocarcinomas (WDGAs) arise from areas of intestinal metaplasia but lack the so called signet ring cells.

DeMay, A&S 2e. Gastric type adenocarcinoma, p401-402

29 a have premalignant predisposition

Villous adenomas are considered premalignant lesions found within the gastrointestinal tract. It is estimated that 25-75% of villous adenomatous polyps will undergo malignant transformation if surgical resection is not performed. These papillary lesions are also diagnostic within the colon. The sensitivity of cytologic morphology may be inadequate in distinguishing these lesions from well differentiated adenocarcinomas.

DeMay, A&S 2e. Villous adenoma, p408

30 a pernicious anemia

Pernicious anemia (PA) occurs as a result of impaired absorption of vitamin B_{12} due to the absence of intrinsic factor. This condition gives rise to atrophic gastritis due to the loss of gastric parietal cells. Cytologically, cells possess enlarged nuclei with karyolytic features and bland nuclear folds. An increase in gastric carcinoma has been associated with PA.

DeMay, A&S 2e. Vitamin deficiency, p383

31 b primary lymphoma

The absence of cohesive features, scattered bimorphic single cells without vacuolated cytoplasm, and an absence of true tissue fragments are helpful in discriminating this lesion from one of epithelial nature.

DeMay, A&S 2e. Malignant lymphoma, p409

32 b Plummer-Vinson syndrome

Tobacco smoking, increased ethanol intake, achalasia, hiatal hernia, and Plummer-Vinson syndrome may be predisposing conditions for the subsequent development of esophageal cancer.

DeMay, A&S 2e. Malignant tumors, p408

33 a fungating

90% of primary esophageal tumors are keratinizing squamous cell carcinomas. Generally, these lesions occur in the middle to distal third of the esophagus. Most lesions are polypoid in nature, but may be endophytic or ulcerative.

DeMay, A&S 2e. Squamous cell carcinoma, p388-389

34 b a malignant glandular tumor arising from intestinal metaplasia

Well differentiated gastric adenocarcinomas (WDGAs) arise from areas of intestinal metaplasia but lack the so called signet ring cells associated with poorly differentiated adenocarcinomas.

DeMay, A&S 2e. Intestinal metaplasia, p394

35 c large cell type

Histiocytic or large cell lymphoma is the most common lymphopoietic lesion involving the gastrointestinal tract, including the stomach. These lesions often produce craterlike ulcerations of the gastric mucosa; therefore, a pronounced diathesis may be associated with these malignancies.

DeMay, A&S 2e. Malignant lymphoma, p409

36 d reparative/regenerative cellular changes

Reparative/regenerative changes that occur in the squamous mucosa of the esophagus resemble those found in the female genital tract. Sheets of cells with well defined cytoplasmic borders, preserved nuclear polarity, predictable nuclear features, fine regular chromatin patterns, micro- to macronucleoli, and characteristic cytoplasmic streaming (squamous) or honeycombing polarity (glandular) are pathognomonic of repair. This process is often associated with ulcerative esophagitis, trauma, reflux, and inflammatory etiology.

DeMay, A&S 2e. Repair/regeneration, p30-31, 394

37 b squamous carcinoma, nonkeratinizing

Cell in cell arrangement or cannibalism as seen in single, discohesive cells with the described criteria is suggestive of a poorly differentiated nonkeratinizing squamous carcinoma. These lesions cytologically resemble those poorly differentiated squamous malignancies found elsewhere in the body, often making it difficult to distinguish from adenocarcinoma. Special stains may be needed for confirmation; however, cells negative for mucin do not rule out the possibility of a poorly differentiated adenocarcinoma.

DeMay, A&S 2e. Squamous cell carcinoma, p380-381

38 a intestinal metaplasia
Intestinal type adenocarcinoma is derived from longstanding intestinal metaplasia, a benign condition related to chronic atrophic gastritis. These nonsignet ring cancers may be well to poorly differentiated. Cytology reveals disorderly thick groups in sheets or microacinar structures with columnar or cuboidal shapes. The nucleus has irregular nuclear membranes, pleomorphic shapes, and is hyperchromatic with coarse irregular chromatin and multiple nucleoli. The presence of abnormal single cells is a key diagnostic feature of gastric adenocarcinoma.
DeMay, A&S 2e. Gastric type adenocarcinoma, p401-402

39 c reactive/reparative process
Reparative/reactive conditions, as found in gastrointestinal specimens, are commonly associated with chronic duodenitis, colitis, giardiasis, benign ulcers, and polyposis. It is imperative to differentiate these conditions from well differentiated adenocarcinomas. Cellular predictability, preserved polarity, hypochromasia, and the absence of nuclear compression are found with repair. Single malignant cells, true tissue fragments, and tall columnar cell morphology containing hyperchromatic nuclei with irregular chromatin are critical for establishing a diagnosis of colonic adenocarcinoma.
DeMay, A&S 2e. Reactive/reparative and degeneration changes, p394-395

40 c adenocarcinoma
Duodenal adenocarcinomas mimic colonic adenocarcinoma, possessing polypoid growth patterns, and often create stenosis. These lesions are extremely uncommon.
DeMay, A&S 2e. Adenocarcinoma, p390, 400-402

41 b native gastric epithelium
Poorly differentiated adenocarcinoma of the stomach arises from native gastric epithelium–not from intestinal metaplasia. Poorly differentiated adenocarcinomas present as syncytial aggregates or single signet ring cells with nuclear overlapping and compression, increased N:C ratios, pleomorphism, irregular chromatin distribution, and macronucleoli. Malignancies arising from intestinal metaplasia are generally well differentiated.
DeMay, A&S 2e. Gastric type adenocarcinoma, p401-402

42 a reactive/reparative changes
Sheets of cells with well defined cytoplasmic borders, preserved nuclear polarity, predictable nuclear features, fine regular chromatin patterns, micro- to macronucleoli, and honeycombing polarity (glandular) are pathognomonic of repair.
DeMay, A&S 2e. Reactive/reparative and degeneration changes, p394

43 a adenocarcinoma, well differentiated
Colonic adenocarcinomas may be related to benign conditions such as ulcerative colitis, villous adenomas, or familial polyposis. Most adenocarcinomas occur within the recto/sigmoid region, are polypoid or ulcerative, and are generally moderately well differentiated at the time of detection.
DeMay, A&S 2e. Adenocarcinoma, p390, 400-402

44 d large cell lymphoma
Histiocytic or large cell lymphoma is the most common lymphopoietic lesion involving the gastrointestinal tract, including the stomach. These lesions often produce craterlike ulcerations of the gastric mucosa; therefore, a pronounced diathesis may be associated with these malignancies.
DeMay, A&S 2e. Malignant lymphoma, p403-404

45 c steatorrhea/*Giardia lamblia* infection
This protozoan is associated with fatty stools, or steatorrhea, and may be diagnosed cytologically as blue to gray organisms with 4 pairs of flagella (some of which will not be visible in a single plane). Trophozoites closely resemble those of *Trichomonas* with the exception that *Giardia* are binucleate and have a ventral sucking disk. In addition, they lack an undulating membrane.
DeMay, A&S 2e. Giardia lamblia, p407

46 d carcinoembryonic antigen+
Carcinoembryonic antigen levels may be monitored by radioimmunoassay analysis. Increased serum levels are associated with recurrent or metastatic colonic adenocarcinoma.
DeMay, A&S 2e. Adenocarcinoma, p412-413

47 c Barrett esophagus
Barrett esophagitis/metaplasia is a result of chronic esophageal reflux. The cells must be of goblet cell (signet ring) morphology if the diagnosis is to be established within the distal third of the esophagus because of possible contamination of the esophageal brush from the cardiac region of the stomach. The presence of "cell windows" is helpful in establishing the diagnosis of Barrett esophagus. It is possible to diagnose the condition should intestinal type (goblet) or nonintestinal type gastric epithelium be found in the mid to upper regions of the esophagus. The lesion has been associated with chronic atrophic gastritis and achlorhydria (decreased parietal cells).
DeMay, A&S 2e. Barrett esophagus, p385-387

48 b pseudolymphoma
A polymorphic population of small mature lymphocytes, larger immunoblasts, plasma cells, and tingible body macrophages is pathognomonic of pseudolymphoma, chronic follicular gastritis, or benign lymphoreticular hyperplasia. Most cases of chronic follicular gastritis are associated with gastric ulcers and may be concomitantly associated with highly reactive epithelial fragments.
DeMay, A&S 2e. Pseudolymphoma, p247

49 a adenocarcinoma, well differentiated intestinal type
Intestinal type adenocarcinoma is derived from intestinal metaplasia, a benign condition related to chronic atrophic gastritis. These nonsignet ring cancers may be well to poorly differentiated. Cytology reveals disorderly thick groups in sheets or microacinar structures with columnar or cuboidal shapes. The nucleus has irregular nuclear membranes and pleomorphic shapes, and is hyperchromatic with coarse irregular chromatin and multiple nucleoli. The presence of abnormal single cells is a key diagnostic feature of gastric adenocarcinoma.
DeMay, A&S 2e. Intestinal type adenocarcinoma, p401-402

ISBN 978-089189-6357 ©ASCP 2015

50   c   adenocarcinoma, poorly differentiated
True tissue fragments and columnar cell morphology containing hyperchromatic nuclei with irregular chromatin are anticipated findings in colonic adenocarcinoma.
DeMay, A&S 2e. Adenocarcinoma, p400-401

51   b   herpesvirus
Infection with herpesvirus is generally associated with immunocompromised hosts, including patients affected with concomitant HIV infections, patients receiving therapy for malignant disease, or those with other chronic debilitating disorders. Cytologic identification is based on the finding of multinucleated cells containing ground glass nuclei, karyolytic chromatin, nuclear molding, and eosinophilic Cowdry type A inclusions. Possible contamination from the oral cavity must be considered in the absence of clinically indicated infections.
DeMay, A&S 2e. Herpesvirus, p377, 384

52   d   villous adenoma
Villous adenomas are considered premalignant lesions found within the gastrointestinal tract. The sensitivity of cytologic morphology may be inadequate in distinguishing these lesions from well differentiated adenocarcinomas.
DeMay, A&S 2e. Villous adenoma, p408

53   a   longstanding dysphagia
90% of primary esophageal tumors are keratinizing squamous cell carcinomas. Generally, these lesions occur in the middle to distal third of the organ. Most lesions are polypoid in nature, but may be endophytic or ulcerative.
DeMay, A&S 2e. Squamous cell carcinoma, p388-389

54   a   chronic esophageal reflux
Reparative/regenerative changes that occur in squamous mucosa of the esophagus resemble those found in the female genital tract. Sheets of cells with well defined cytoplasmic borders, preserved nuclear polarity, predictable nuclear features, fine regular chromatin patterns, micro- to macronucleoli, and characteristic cytoplasmic streaming (squamous) or honeycombing polarity (glandular) are pathognomonic of repair. This process is often associated with ulcerative esophagitis, trauma, reflux, and inflammatory etiology.
DeMay, A&S 2e. Esophagitis, p383

55   c   intestinal metaplasia
Periodic acid-Schiff will stain mucoproteins, mucolipids, and glycoproteins. Cells associated with intestinal metaplasia possess mucin containing "windows." Cytology represents cohesive sheets of mucus neck cells with scattered goblet cells with large signet ring vacuoles.
DeMay, A&S 2e. Intestinal metaplasia, p394

56   b   reparative/regenerative changes
Reparative/reactive conditions, as found in gastrointestinal specimens, are commonly associated with chronic duodenitis, colitis, giardiasis, benign ulcers, and polyposis.
DeMay, A&S 2e. Reactive/regenerative cells and degeneration, p394

57   b   food contamination
The finding of striated muscle most often represents meat contamination associated with masticated food.
DeMay, A&S 2e. Other cells, p376

58   d   squamous cell carcinoma, keratinizing
90% of primary esophageal tumors are keratinizing squamous cell carcinomas. Generally, these lesions occur in the middle to distal third of the organ. Most lesions are polypoid in nature, but may be endophytic or ulcerative.
DeMay, A&S 2e. Squamous cell carcinoma, p388-389

59   a   reactive/reparative changes
Reparative/regenerative changes that occur in squamous mucosa of the esophagus resemble those found in the female genital tract. Sheets of cells with well defined cytoplasmic borders, preserved nuclear polarity, predictable nuclear features, fine regular chromatin patterns, micro- to macronucleoli, and characteristic cytoplasmic streaming (squamous) or honeycombing polarity (glandular) are pathognomonic of repair. This process is often associated with ulcerative esophagitis, trauma, reflux, and inflammatory etiology.
DeMay, A&S 2e. Gastroesophageal reflux disease (GERD), p385

60   b   intestinal metaplasia
Periodic acid-Schiff will stain mucoproteins, mucolipids, and glycoproteins. Cells associated with intestinal metaplasia possess mucin containing "windows." Cytology represents cohesive sheets of mucus neck cells with scattered goblet cells with large signet ring vacuoles.
DeMay, A&S 2e. Intestinal metaplasia, p394

61   b   granulomatous esophagitis
Granulomatous esophagitis resembles granulomatous disease elsewhere in the body–characteristic epithelioid histiocytes and foreign body giant cells are detected cytologically. Acid-fast stains would confirm a tuberculosis etiology; however, other diseases such as sarcoid, syphilis, or Crohn disease may also be related.
DeMay, A&S 2e. Granulomatous esophagitis, p385

62   d   vegetable contaminant
Cells with translucent, refractile, squared off cytoplasm containing smudgy nuclei and intracytoplasmic granules indicate vegetable contamination. Caution should be taken not to confuse these cells with indigenous elements such as metaplasia or squamous carcinoma.
DeMay, A&S 2e. Contaminants, p395

63   a   adenocarcinoma, well differentiated intestinal type
Well differentiated gastric adenocarcinomas (WDGAs) arise from areas of intestinal metaplasia but lack the so called signet ring cells. WDGAs must be differentiated from poorly differentiated adenocarcinomas (signet ring type).
DeMay, A&S 2e. Adenocarcinoma, p412-413

64   b   *Candida albicans*
The presence of thin pseudohyphae with interrupted cell walls or spore formations represents *Candida albicans*. The presence of this yeast should be clinically correlated due to its possible representation of oral cavity contamination.
DeMay, A&S 2e. Organisms, p398

65 b normal gastric mucosa

Hyperplastic polyps are composed of normal to reactive glandular cells. The cytologic presence of sheets of glandular cells with honeycombing features or cells with enlarged nuclei and well preserved polarity is characteristic. These lesions have no premalignant association and are often linked to benign inflammatory processes.

DeMay, A&S 2e. Mucous cells, p393-394

66 d reactive/reparative changes secondary to ulcerative colitis

Reactive/reparative changes seen within the colon are associated with ulcerative colitis, chronic irritation, or trauma. It is imperative to differentiate these conditions from well differentiated adenocarcinomas. Cellular predictability, preserved polarity, hypochromasia, and the absence of nuclear compression are found with repair. Single malignant cells, true tissue fragments, and tall columnar cell morphology containing hyperchromatic nuclei with irregular chromatin are critical for establishing a diagnosis of colonic adenocarcinoma.

DeMay, A&S 2e. Reactive cells: repair/regeneration, p410

67 c herpes

Infection with herpesvirus is generally associated with immunocompromised hosts, including patients affected with concomitant HIV infections, patients receiving therapy for malignant disease, or those with other chronic debilitating disorders. Cytologic identification is based on the finding of multinucleated cells containing ground glass nuclei, karyolytic chromatin, nuclear molding, and eosinophilic Cowdry type A inclusions. Possible contamination from the oral cavity must be considered in the absence of clinically indicated infections.

DeMay, A&S 2e. Herpes esophagitis, p384

68 a herpes simplex esophagitis

Herpes simplex infection is characterized by the presence of multinucleated cells with nuclear molding and margination of chromatin. Ground glass nuclei are also a characteristic feature. Intranuclear inclusions are not necessary for diagnosis.

DeMay, A&S 2e. Herpes esophagitis, p384

69 a positive for adenocarcinoma

The left corner of this image contains a 3 dimensional cluster of very pleomorphic glandular cells with vacuolated cytoplasm, irregular nuclear membranes and prominent nucleoli. Note cellular overlapping. Compare this cluster to the normal glandular epithelium on the right.

DeMay, A&S 2e. Adenocarcinoma, p400-401

70 b an ulcerated polypoid 4 cm lesion

The image shows discohesive clusters of malignant epithelial cells. One cluster shows characteristic palisading. The other cluster is composed of less differentiated cells showing marked variation in size, irregularity of nuclear membrane, clearing of chromatin and prominent nucleoli. Notice single malignant cells in the dirty background.

DeMay, A&S 2e. Hyperplastic and serrated colorectal polyps, p412

71 a CD117

This gastrointestinal stromal tumor (GIST) is of the spindle cell type, which comprises 60% of such tumors. The tumor arises from the interstitial intestinal cells that contain a growth factor receptor called c-kit that stains positively with the CD117 antibody.

DeMay, A&S 2e. Gastrointestinal stromal tumor, p405-406

72 d herpesvirus

These multinucleated cells display the typical "ground glass" nuclei with chromatin margination characteristic of herpes infection. Note the nuclear molding. These herpetic cells may also have eosinophilic intranuclear inclusions.

DeMay, A&S 2e. Herpes esophagitis, p384

73 c squamous cell carcinoma

The 2D microtissue fragment present shows too great a degree of anisonucleosis and nuclear chromatin atypia to be considered a benign/reparative process.

DeMay, A&S 2e. Squamous cell carcinoma, p388

74 b repair/regeneration

Ulcerative colitis is a chronic, inflammatory process. These patients can develop dysplasia and adenocarcinomas. However, the cells seen here are arrayed in a flat sheet, with cytoplasmic tails. The nuclei are pale with single prominent nucleoli. These features are characteristic for an inflammatory repairlike process (pseudopolyps). Adenomas would show pencil shaped nuclei. In adenocarcinomas, the cells would have a high N:C ratio with multiple nucleoli and irregular nuclear membranes.

DeMay, A&S 2e. Reactive cells: repair/regeneration, p410

75 a benign bile duct epithelium

Endoscopic bile duct brushing has significant clinical diagnostic utility in the evaluation of bile duct strictures. This image displays typical benign features of bile duct epithelium, which tends to present in flat sheets with a honeycomb arrangement. Cell groups may be, and peripheral cells may show, orderly palisading with basal nuclei. Nuclei are centrally located with minimal variation and lack of prominent nucleoli. Cytoplasm is finely granular cytoplasm. In contrast, malignant cells from cholangiocarcinoma would appear in a more crowded and disorganized fashion with significant nuclear overlap, and display anisonucleosis with nucleoli. Bile duct brushings from malignancies tend to be relatively cellular and contain malignant and benign cells.

Trent V, Khurana KK, Pisharodi LR. Diagnostic accuracy and clinical utility of endoscopic bile duct brushing in evaluation of biliary strictures. Arch Pathol Lab Med 1999;123:712-715 [PMID 10420229]

ISBN 978-089189-6357 ©ASCP 2015

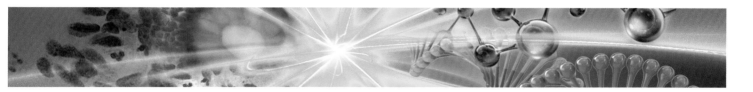

1. A 70-year-old male presents with hypertension and redness of the face, neck and arms. The patient complains of dyspnea and a loss of appetite. The patient has a 30 year history of smoking 2 packs per day. Emphysema was diagnosed 5 years previously. Sputum cytology analysis shows small cells in linear arrays caught in mucus strands with scanty cytoplasm. Hyperchromasia was present as well as a coarse chromatin pattern. Nuclear compression is present and nucleoli are inconspicuous. These cells represent:

   a carcinoid tumor
   b metastatic adenocarcinoma, prostate
   c atypical reserve cells
   d small cell carcinoma, oat cell variety

2. A 42-year-old male with a previous history of malignancy presents with sessile infiltrating growths in the major bronchi. A bronchial brush specimen reveals large cells arranged in nests. The cells possess large nuclei with frankly malignant nuclear features and intranuclear cytoplasmic inclusions. Immunoperoxidase stains with S100 are positive. Based on the preceding criteria, the diagnosis is:

   a melanoma
   b hepatocellular carcinoma
   c adenocarcinoma, bronchogenic
   d mesothelioma

3. Large cells with multinucleation, nuclear molding, chromatin margination, and ground glass nuclei with intranuclear, eosinophilic inclusions found in a sputum specimen are diagnostic of:

   a respiratory syncytial virus
   b herpesvirus
   c molluscum contagiosum
   d cytomegalovirus

4. Cohesive groups and single cells exhibiting uniform polarity, high N:C ratios, cytoplasmic ringing, prominent nucleoli, and coarse irregular chromatin scattered among a necrotic background are diagnostic of:

   a well differentiated squamous cell carcinoma, keratinizing
   b poorly differentiated squamous cell carcinoma
   c bronchogenic adenocarcinoma
   d pulmonary hamartoma

5. All of the following are considered etiologic agents for the development of lung cancer, EXCEPT:

   a radiation
   b tobacco
   c nickel
   d microbacteria

6. A 65-year-old male presents with a 4 × 5 cm focal mass on chest X-ray. Bronchial brushing reveals large numbers of round to oval single cells lying singly and in sheetlike aggregates. The cells have elevated N:C ratios, large nucleoli, and granular to lacy cytoplasmic features. Special stains with mucicarmine are negative. Based on the cytologic features, the diagnosis is:

   a large cell carcinoma
   b adenocarcinoma, bronchogenic
   c squamous cell carcinoma, well differentiated type
   d small cell carcinoma, oat cell type

7. A 66-year-old male on corticosteroid therapy for recent coronary bypass surgery presents with a solitary lesion within the left upper lung. Bronchial brushing reveals hyphaelike structures with dichotomous branching. Large exophytic structures are often found attached to the septa. The diagnosis is:

   a *Actinomyces israelii*
   b *Aspergillus fumigatus*
   c *Nocardia asteroides*
   d *Mucor* species

8   A 32-year-old male presents with pulmonary abscesses, enlargement of the mediastinal nodes, dry hacking cough, low grade fever, and chest pain. A blood streaked sputum cytologically reveals numerous neutrophils as well as large multinucleated histiocytes. Special staining with PAS revealed many single, spherical structures with a thick refractile double contoured cell wall, many of which had attached broad based buds. The diagnosis is most consistent with:

   a *Mycobacterium tuberculosis*
   b *Pneumocystis jiroveci*
   c *Blastomyces dermatitidis*
   d *Cryptococcus neoformans*

9   A bronchial washing of a 2×3 cm mass reveals small, uniform appearing cells lacking cilia or terminal bars. Many of the cells appear in sheets, clusters, cords or nests. Nuclei are uniform and predictable in appearance with salt & pepper chromatin, and nucleoli are inconspicuous. The diagnosis is:

   a reactive bronchial epithelial cells
   b small cell carcinoma, oat cell type
   c reserve cell hyperplasia
   d carcinoid tumor

10 A 55-year-old female presents with a history of tobacco abuse, malaise, and hemoptysis. Based on these clinical symptoms, one may suggest evaluation to rule out:

   a disseminated microbiological infection
   b viral pneumonia
   c atypical squamous metaplasia
   d invasive carcinoma

11 A 2×3 cm bronchial mass discovered in a 62-year-old male with a history of tobacco abuse was brushed using a flexible bronchoscope. The cells were papillary in configuration and possessed vacuolated cytoplasm. The nuclei were oval in shape and often lobulated. Single cells were interspersed among the fragments. The diagnosis is:

   a adenocarcinoma, terminal bronchioloalveolar type
   b adenocarcinoma, bronchogenic type
   c large cell carcinoma, giant cell features
   d mixed adenosquamous carcinoma

12 A 62-year-old female presents with multiple lung lesions in the left and right lung. Abdominal ascites was noted at the time of examination. Bronchial brushing of the lung lesion reveals a large population of cells with hyperchromatic nuclei, fine irregular chromatin, prominent nucleoli, and tall columnar morphology in clusters as well as single cells. The most likely diagnosis/primary site for these cells is:

   a reactive bronchial epithelial cells/lung
   b adenocarcinoma/bronchioloalveolar variety
   c angiosarcoma/breast
   d adenocarcinoma/colon

13 A 56-year-old male with no history of a primary malignancy presents with a 3×4 cm mass in the left lower lobe of the lung. A bronchial washing shows orangeophilic pleomorphic cells with elongated opaque nuclear features and numerous pearl formations. Also present are acinar structures with single distended vacuoles and nuclei with slight hyperchromasia and prominent nucleoli. What diagnosis do you suspect and what special stain might prove useful in your determination?

   a poorly differentiated squamous carcinoma, immunoperoxidase positive for S100
   b large cell carcinoma, mucicarmine negative
   c adenosquamous carcinoma, immunoperoxidase positive for keratin
   d metastatic medullary carcinoma of the thyroid, immunoperoxidase positive for calcitonin

14 A 31-year-old male presents with a spiking temperature and pneumonitis. A bronchioloalveolar lavage reveals a vast population of bronchial epithelial cells with enlarged cleared out nuclei exhibiting chromatinic margination. Large oval intranuclear and occasional small intracytoplasmic basophilic inclusions are seen. The diagnosis is consistent with:

   a metastatic melanoma
   b Hodgkin disease
   c cytomegalovirus
   d hemosiderin laden macrophages

15 A sputum specimen reveals branching organisms with a central mass and peripheral filamentous mycelia. A large population of neutrophils are seen; however, dust cells are absent. Based on these cytologic findings, your recommendation is:

   a repeat sputum, *Actinomyces* species may represent tonsillar contamination
   b recommend removal of lung tissue to prevent further infection by *Aspergillus* species
   c repeat sputum, *Aspergillus* species may represent contamination
   d recommend GMS staining to confirm fungal infection

16 A 43-year-old male shows dense shadows on chest X-ray and diffuse interstitial pneumonia. Cytology reveals a large population of thick walled organisms with a gelatinous capsule. Teardrop budding is frequent. The diagnosis is most consistent with:

   a *Pneumocystis jiroveci*
   b *Histoplasma capsulatum*
   c *Coccidioides immitis*
   d *Cryptococcus neoformans*

ISBN 978-089189-6357   ©ASCP 2015

17 A 38-year-old male presents with difficulty in breathing and an elevated temperature. Chest X-ray reveals multiple nodules in both lungs. Sputum analysis reveals a heterogeneous population of normal lymphocytes, plasma cells, and large binucleate cells with coarse irregular chromatin features and macronucleoli. The diagnosis is:

a plasma cell granulomas
b sclerosing hemangiomas
c chronic follicular bronchitis
d Hodgkin disease

18 A 44-year-old Filipino male presents with a nonproductive cough and constriction and pain in the upper chest. Sputum cytology reveals spherical thick walled structures resembling a pomegranate. Multiple spores are encapsulated within the structures. The diagnosis was confirmed with GMS. The diagnosis is:

a *Coccidioides immitis*
b *Histoplasma capsulatum*
c *Nocardia asteroides*
d *Allescheria boydii*

19 A 49-year-old female with a previous history of a malignant disease presents with multiple lung nodules on chest X-ray. Bronchial brushings revealed small cells in ribbons or cords with hyperchromatic nuclei and frothy, lacy cytoplasm, often with intracytoplasmic alveoli. The diagnosis/primary site may be:

a small cell carcinoma/lung
b carcinoid tumor/lung
c lobular adenocarcinoma/breast
d adenocarcinoma/ovary

20 A 52-year-old male presents with emaciation, leukopenia, and pyrexia. Sputum analysis reveals numerous histiocytes containing intracellular multiple spherules possessing a refractile cell wall. GMS stains are positive. The diagnosis is:

a *Pneumocystis jiroveci*
b *Cryptococcus neoformans*
c *Histoplasma capsulatum*
d *Blastomyces dermatitidis*

21 A 55-year-old male presents with a productive cough and dysphagia. Sputum analysis reveals spindle shaped cells in clusters with orangeophilic staining cytoplasm. The nuclear features are hyperchromatic with irregular nuclear borders, and the chromatin is coarse. Bronchial washings and brushings are negative. The most likely diagnosis/primary site for these cells is:

a squamous cell carcinoma/esophagus
b leiomyosarcoma/colon
c normal squamous metaplasia/lung
d adenocarcinoma/prostate

22 A 61-year-old female presents with chronic obstructive pulmonary disease and pneumonitis. A history of tuberculosis exposure was noted. Sputum analysis revealed small round cells in uniform clusters (20+ cells) exhibiting prominent nuclei with fine, irregular chromatin. Psammoma bodies were also present in a degenerative background. Based on this information, the diagnosis is consistent with:

a adenocarcinoma, poorly differentiated lung
b adenocarcinoma, terminal bronchioloalveolar
c creola bodies
d metastatic breast carcinoma, ductal

23 A 21-year-old AIDS patient presents with a productive cough and purulent sputum. Cytology reveals multiple transparent, thin filamentous branching structures with beaded hyphae. Special stains including acid-fast and Gram stains are positive. The diagnosis represents:

a *Mycobacterium tuberculosis*
b *Nocardia asteroides*
c saprophytic phycomycetes
d *Geotrichum candidum*

24 Cytologic analysis of a bronchial brushing reveals elongated cells, variation in cellular size, refractile/glassy cytoplasm, and opaque India ink nuclei. These cells are arranged singly and in sheets. Orangeophilic whorls are present among a granular amorphous material. The best diagnosis is:

a squamous cell carcinoma, nonkeratinizing
b poorly differentiated squamous cell carcinoma
c well differentiated squamous cell carcinoma, keratinizing
d reparative/regenerative process

25 A sputum specimen from a 70-year-old male with Goodpasture syndrome reveals a population of small cells with eccentrically located nuclei that are reniform in shape. The cytoplasm contains refractile eosinophilic pigment that often occludes the nuclear detail. The most likely diagnosis is:

a a contaminant from the larynx
b malignant melanoma
c Clara cells
d siderophages

26 A 6-year-old child with severe anemia, liver insufficiency, and dyspnea is diagnosed clinically with pulmonary hemosiderosis. Papanicolaou stained bronchoalveolar lavage analysis would reveal histiocytes with:

a brown-black pigment
b distended clear vacuoles
c refractile golden pigment
d green pigment

27 A sputum specimen from a 55-year-old male with a tracheostomy tube reveals a scanty population of small keratinized cells. The nuclei are round to oval and possess fine, regular chromatin. The diagnosis is:
    a keratinizing squamous cell carcinoma
    b atypical squamous metaplasia
    c reserve cell hyperplasia
    d parakeratosis

28 A Papanicolaou stained bronchoalveolar lavage specimen yielded large groups of frothy, eosinophilic mats containing refractile, spherical shaped structures interspersed among alveolar macrophages. These findings would suggest the investigator perform:
    a mucicarmine staining for Cryptococcus neoformans
    b oil red O staining for lipid laden macrophages, suggesting lipoid pneumonia
    c acid-fast stains for confirmation of Nocardia asteroides
    d GMS staining for confirmation of Pneumocystis jiroveci

29 A Saccomanno processed sputum specimen yields small cells with normal N:C ratios and dense cyanophilic cytoplasm. The cells are found in sheets and as single cells. The cytologic findings are considered:
    a pathognomonic of malignancy
    b diagnostic of a benign reparative process
    c suspicious for malignancy
    d bronchial metaplastic cells

30 A sputum specimen reveals a biphasic population of round cells with uniform cell shape and round nuclei possessing fine, regular chromatin. Each of the cells lies singly. The cytologic findings are suggestive of:
    a small cell carcinoma
    b small cell noncleaved lymphoma
    c normal lymphocytes
    d creola bodies

31 In sputum samples, cells demonstrating slight pleomorphism, moderate variation in size, a variable N:C ratio, nuclear hyperchromasia, and finely granular, evenly distributed chromatin are suggestive of:
    a reserve cell hyperplasia
    b large cell undifferentiated carcinoma
    c keratinizing squamous cell carcinoma
    d atypical squamous metaplasia

32 Coiled structures composed of inspissated mucus often associated with bronchial obstruction are:
    a corpora amylacea
    b creola bodies
    c Curschmann spirals
    d calcospherites

33 What epithelia lines the larynx?
    a simple squamous
    b nonkeratinizing stratified squamous
    c simple cuboidal
    d transitional

34 A patient who is a known abuser of nose drops is at risk for developing:
    a lipoid pneumonia
    b Barrett metaplasia
    c sarcoidosis
    d there is no known risk

35 All of the following may yield abundant eosinophils in a pulmonary specimen, EXCEPT:
    a Strongyloides stercoralis
    b Löffler pneumonia
    c asthma
    d inflammatory pseudotumor

36 A 36-year-old male diagnosed as HIV+ presents with an active Mycobacterium tuberculosis infection. Recent sputum analysis shows small cells with scanty cytoplasm and uniform cell size in tight compact sheets. The nuclei are small and dense. These cells represent:
    a small cell carcinoma, oat cell type
    b intermediate cell carcinoma
    c atypical squamous metaplasia, severe
    d reserve cell hyperplasia

37 Cells associated with viral infections and presenting with degenerative qualities and detached cilia represent:
    a reactive bronchial cells
    b creola bodies
    c ciliocytophthoria
    d reserve cell hyperplasia

38 Cells exhibiting eosinophilic cytoplasm containing refractile granules, squared off cytoplasmic borders, and double, translucent, refractile cell walls, and dark/smudged nuclear morphology are diagnostic of:
    a atypical squamous metaplasia
    b keratinizing squamous cell carcinoma
    c plant cells
    d reparative/regenerative cellular changes

39 The findings of creola bodies, Charcot-Leyden crystals, eosinophils, and occasional Curschmann spirals are suggestive of:
    a asthma
    b ciliocytophthoria
    c tuberculosis
    d Wegener granulomatosis

40 A 4-month-old infant presents with difficulty in breathing and chronic vomiting. Chest X-ray reveals a diffuse infiltrate suggestive of pneumonia. A cytologic examination of the regurgitate reveals a large population of bronchial epithelial cells, a population of histiocytes with signet ring formation, and cells with multiple vacuolization. The most likely diagnosis is:
    a Histoplasma capsulatum
    b lipid pneumonia
    c liposarcoma
    d metastatic neuroblastoma

ISBN 978-089189-6357 ©ASCP 2015

41 Which entity is etiologically related to malignant mesothelioma?
    a ferruginous bodies
    b calcospherites
    c *Mycobacterium tuberculosis*
    d *Schistosoma haematobium*

42 A 70-year-old male with a productive cough and a previous negative bronchoscopy presents with a sputum containing cells with large nuclei, corresponding increase in cytoplasm, and multinucleation. The nuclear chromatin is fine and regular. Many of the cells have macronucleoli and terminal bars. These cells are diagnostic of:
    a reactive bronchial epithelial cells
    b atypical squamous metaplasia
    c nonkeratinizing squamous cell carcinoma
    d squamous metaplasia

43 A 44-year-old female with bronchiectasis submits material for sputum analysis. The sample yields cells in 3D fragments, cells in papillary groups, and cells producing mucin and containing nucleoli. The peripheries of the fragments have intact cilia and/or terminal bars. The diagnosis is consistent with:
    a well differentiated bronchogenic adenocarcinoma
    b creola bodies
    c bronchioloalveolar adenocarcinoma
    d carcinoid tumor

44 A common cell type associated with patients diagnosed with anthracosis is:
    a carbon histiocyte
    b beryllium
    c starch
    d hemosiderin laden macrophage

45 A 55-year-old patient with a papillary neoplasm shows structures with concentrically laminated calcifying rings in a sputum specimen. These structures are:
    a corpora amylacea
    b creola bodies
    c Curschmann spirals
    d psammoma bodies

46 The "dysplasia" preceding keratinizing squamous cell carcinoma is:
    a reserve cell hyperplasia
    b atypical bronchial hyperplasia
    c atypical squamous metaplasia
    d atypical reparative processes

47 A 65-year-old female suffers from pulmonary edema. A population of concentrically laminated, noncalcifying structures are found in a sputum specimen prepared using the pick and smear method. These structures represent:
    a Curschmann spirals
    b corpora amylacea
    c calcospherites
    d keratinizing pearl associated with squamous carcinoma

48 Cells from a bronchial washing, prepared using membrane filtration, exhibit nuclear molding/compression, hyperchromatic nuclei, coarsely granular chromatin, and high N:C ratios. The cells are organized into ribbons, nests, and vertebral column formation. The diagnosis is:
    a reserve cell hyperplasia
    b oat cell carcinoma
    c metastatic pancreatic carcinoma
    d bronchioloalveolar adenocarcinoma

49 These cells represent a bronchial brushing obtained from a patient with a 3 cm central pulmonary mass. They are diagnostic of:

a large cell carcinoma
b squamous cell carcinoma
c adenocarcinoma, poorly differentiated
d small cell carcinoma, intermediate cell type

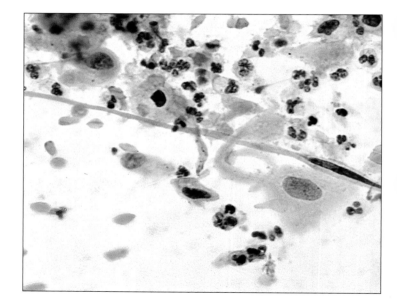

50 A 55-year-old agriculture worker presents with rhinitis and recent weight loss. Sputum cytology reveals these structures. The cellular findings are:

a *Actinomyces israelii*
b phycomycetes
c *Nocardia asteroides*
d *Aspergillus* species

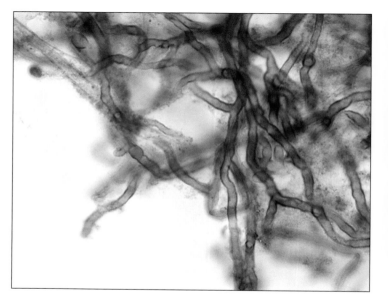

51 These cells found in a sputum sample may be related to:

a bronchioloalveolar adenocarcinoma
b asthma
c well differentiated bronchogenic adenocarcinoma
d metastatic ductal carcinoma of the breast

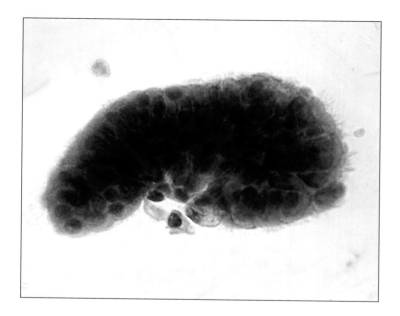

ISBN 978-089189-6357 ©ASCP 2015

52 A 68-year-old male presents with recent weight loss and a history of tobacco use. A coin lesion is observed on chest X-ray. These cells represent a sputum sample. The findings are consistent with:

a squamous cell carcinoma
b neuroendocrine tumor
c malignant lymphoma
d reactive lymphocytes

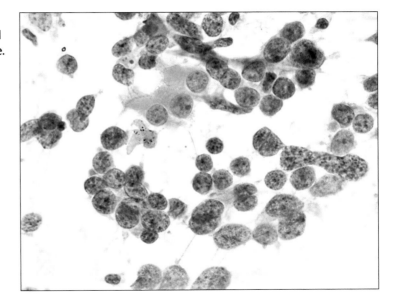

53 These cells were identified in a sputum specimen from a patient with laryngitis and negative bronchoscopic findings. Their most likely origin is:

a lung
b trachea
c pharynx
d oral cavity

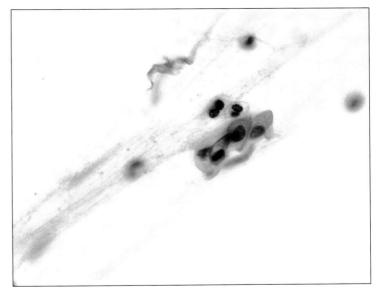

54 A bronchial brushing from a 61-year-old male with a 2 cm coin lesion reveals these cells. The findings are most consistent with:

a large cell lymphoma
b squamous cell carcinoma
c small cell carcinoma
d carcinoid tumor

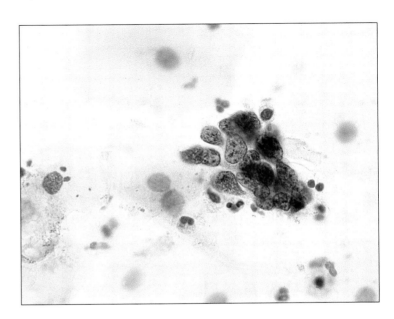

55 A 71-year-old physician recently diagnosed with renal carcinoma, status post excision and post chemotherapy, presents with a pulmonary infiltrate and a 3 cm lesion in the right middle lobe of the lung. A sputum evaluation is performed. These structures are found within alveolar macrophages and fluoresced with auramine O. The findings are:

a *Legionella* species
b *Nocardia asteroides*
c acid-fast bacilli, *Mycobacterium avium-intracellulare*
d *Actinomyces israelii*

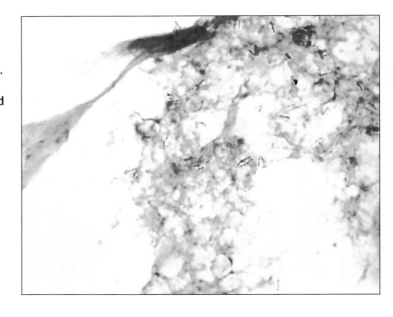

56 An immunosuppressed male with discrete multiple lesions on chest X-ray and a recent diagnosis of a granulomatous pulmonary condition presents for a repeat sputum analysis. The diagnosis is infection with:

a *Strongyloides stercoralis*
b *Echinococcus* species
c *Alternaria* species
d *Paragonimus westermani*

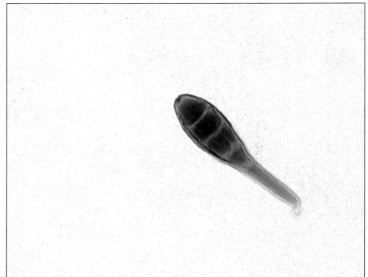

57 A 45-year-old male with a 2×3 cm mass located in the right middle lobe of the lung presents with a spiking fever and recent weight loss. Bronchial brushing reveals these cells, which are diagnostic of:

a small cell carcinoma
b carcinoid tumor
c reactive lymphoid hyperplasia
d non-Hodgkin lymphoma

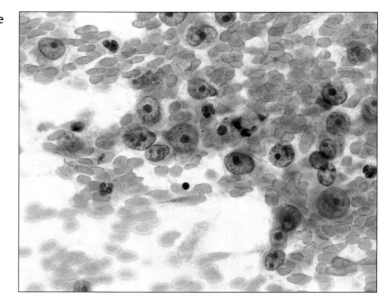

ISBN 978-089189-6357 ©ASCP 2015

58 These cells were obtained from a bronchial brushing from a 44-year-old male with a history of an autoimmune disease. The findings are consistent with:

a squamous cell carcinoma
b sarcoma, not otherwise specified
c epithelioid histiocytes
d microfilaria

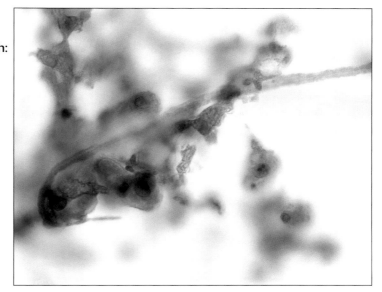

59 These cells were found in a bronchial brushing from a 61-year-old female with a history of tuberculosis now presenting with a peripheral lung mass. These cells:

a are associated with a chronic obstructive disease
b are associated with amine precursor uptake and decarboxylase
c arise from type II pneumocytes
d stain positive with common leukocytic antigen

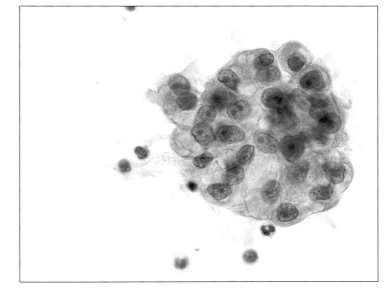

60 A 44-year-old male presents with hemoptysis and enlarged axillary lymph nodes. Sputum analysis reveals these structures. The cytologic pattern depicted is compatible with infection by:

a *Blastomyces dermatitidis*
b *Cryptococcus neoformans*
c *Histoplasma capsulatum*
d *Pneumocystis jiroveci*

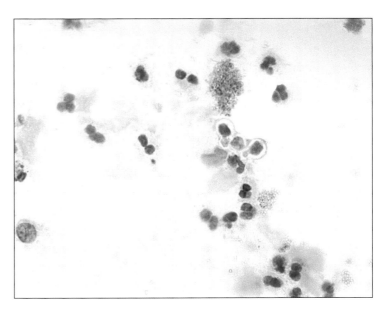

61   The representative cells were found in an
     endobronchial brushing. Which of the following apply?
     a small cell carcinoma; chromogranin–
     b carcinoid tumor; chromogranin+
     c squamous cell carcinoma; parathormone+
     d non-Hodgkin lymphoma; S100+

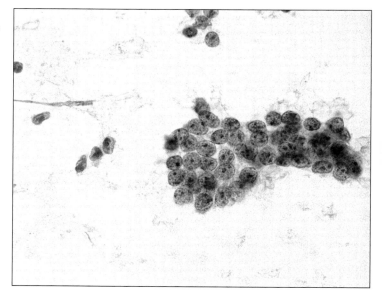

62   A bronchopulmonary washing revealed the following
     cells. What immunocytochemical stain would be
     positive?
     a keratin
     b chromogranin
     c common leukocytic antigen
     d α-fetoprotein

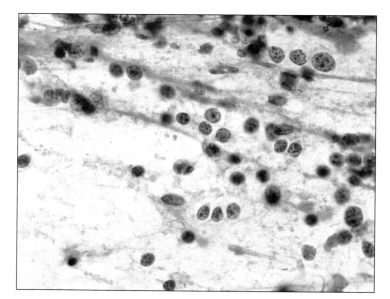

63   These structures contain:
     a glycoproteins (and calcify)
     b glycoproteins (and do not calcify)
     c phosphates (and calcify)
     d phosphates (and do not calcify)

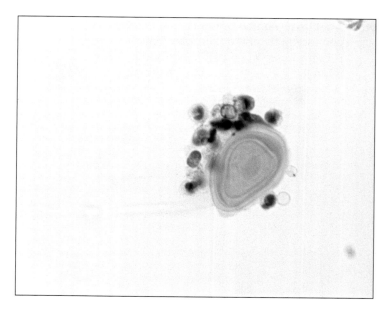

ISBN 978-089189-6357   ©ASCP 2015

64 A 42-year-old male with a history of recurrent generalized infections presents with pneumonia. Laboratory findings include anemia, thrombocytopenia, and an elevated erythrocyte sedimentation rate (>15 mm/h). The diagnosis is:

a cytomegalovirus
b herpes
c respiratory syncytial virus
d parainfluenza virus

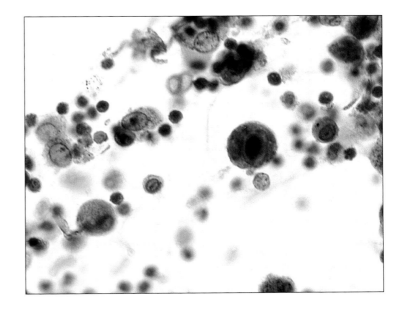

65 A purulent sputum sample from a diabetic patient with pneumonitis reveals these structures. The diagnosis is infection with:

a *Candida* species
b *Actinomyces israelii*
c *Allescheria boydii*
d *Aspergillis* species

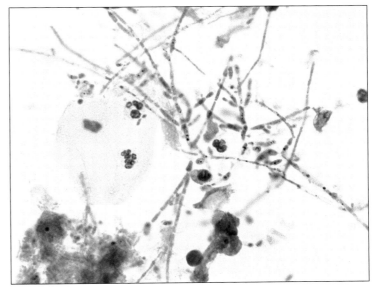

66 An elderly woman presents with pancytopenia, chorioretinitis, and endocarditis. Further examination reveals pneumonia. Sputum samples contain these entities. The cellular findings are:

a *Cryptococcus neoformans*
b *Histoplasma capsulatum*
c *Blastomyces dermatitidis*
d *Toxoplasma gondii*

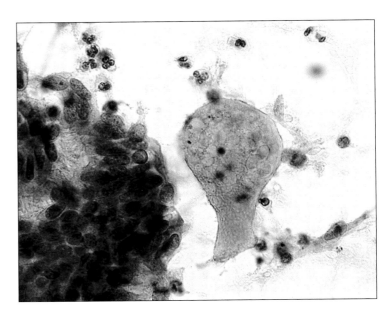

67 A 66-year-old male with a nonproductive cough and shortness of breath produces an induced sputum specimen. The process is consistent with:

a *Histoplasma capsulatum*
b *Pneumocystis jiroveci*
c *Coccidioides immitis*
d *Pseudallescheria boydii*

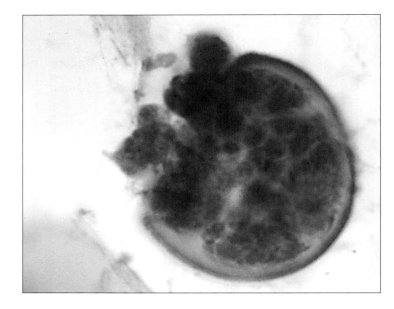

68 A 55-year-old female with a history of endometrial adenocarcinoma presents to her physician complaining of difficulty in breathing. Chest X-ray reveals a diffuse pneumonitis. This bronchial brushing is consistent with:

a metastatic endometrial adenocarcinoma
b large cell undifferentiated carcinoma
c reactive bronchial epithelial cells
d reactive mesothelial cells

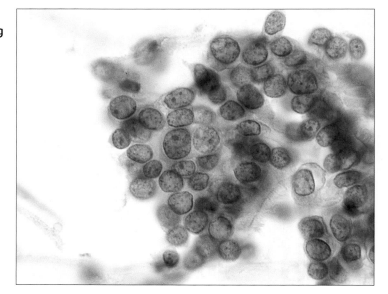

69 A 67-year-old male with advanced carcinoma of the lung presents with recent interstitial pneumonitis. The diagnosis is infection by:

a *Candida* species
b *Actinomyces* species
c *Nocardia asteroides*
d *Aspergillus* species

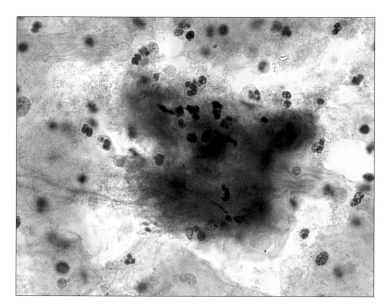

ISBN 978-089189-6357 ©ASCP 2015

70 These cells represent a bronchial brushing from a 55-year-old female. The cellular findings are diagnostic of:

a bronchioloalveolar carcinoma
b poorly differentiated squamous cell carcinoma
c creola bodies associated with asthma
d bronchogenic adenocarcinoma

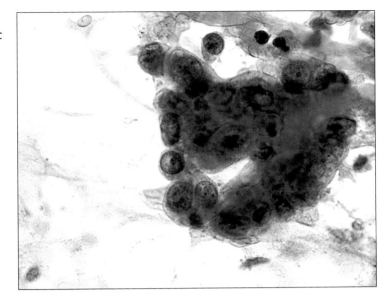

71 These cells were found in a sputum specimen from a patient with a productive purulent cough. The cytologic diagnosis is:

a small cell carcinoma
b carcinoid tumor
c squamous metaplasia
d reserve cell hyperplasia

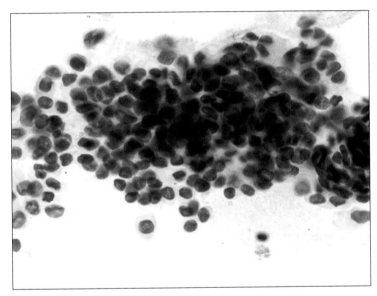

72 The process identified represents a bronchial brushing from a 56-year-old male. The diagnosis is:

a hamartoma
b reactive/reparative changes
c metastatic colonic adenocarcinoma
d granulomatous process

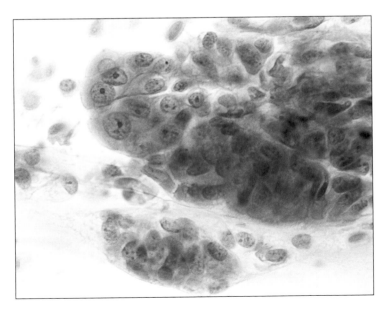

©ASCP 2015   ISBN 978-089189-6357

73 These cells were taken from a 35-year-old male with hemoptysis and a 10 year history of occupational fume inhalation. The cellular findings are most compatible with:

a bronchogenic adenocarcinoma
b atypical histiocytes
c multinucleated bronchial cells
d atypical bronchial cells

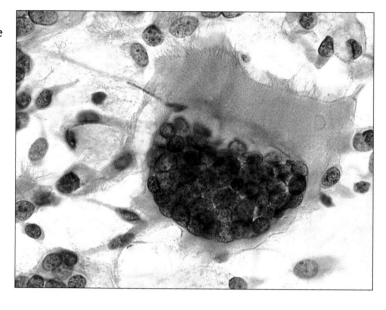

74 These cells were obtained from a sputum sample of an elderly male with recent heart failure. The findings are consistent with:

a melanoma
b bronchioloalveolar adenocarcinoma
c siderophages
d cytomegalovirus

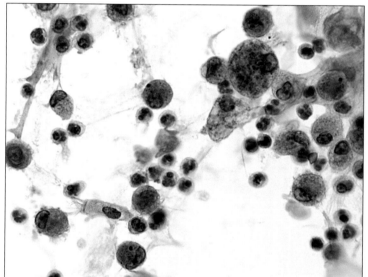

75 When seen in pulmonary specimens, these cells represent:

a atypical metaplastic cells
b normal metaplastic cells
c pneumocytes, type II
d alveolar macrophages

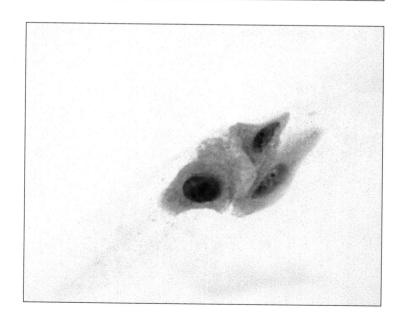

ISBN 978-089189-6357 ©ASCP 2015

76 A special stain often used to help identify these entities is:

a mucicarmine

b oil red O

c Sudan black

d immunocytochemical antibodies against cytomegalovirus (CMV)

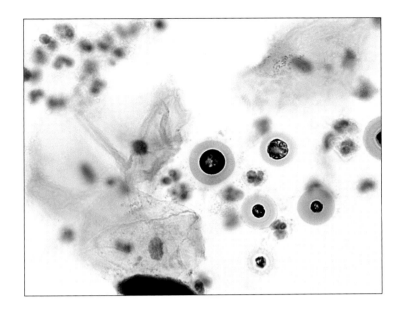

77 The finding depicted in this sputum specimen is often associated with:

a tuberculosis

b tumor diathesis

c contamination

d asthma

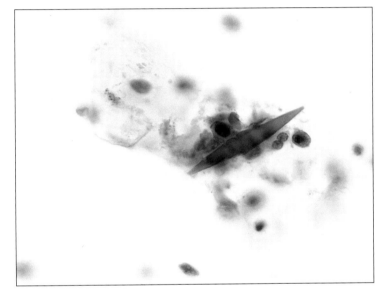

78 These cells originate within:

a granulomas

b bone marrow

c the trachea

d mainstem bronchi

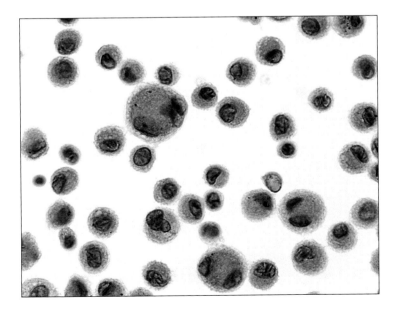

79   A 35-year-old male complains of a dry, nonproductive cough and a 20 pound weight loss. Chest X-ray film reveals interstitial pneumonitis and a disseminated hilar infiltrate. Bronchial brush and alveolar washings are submitted for evaluation. GMS staining reveals:

    a *Histoplasma capsulatum*
    b *Cryptococcus neoformans*
    c degenerated bronchial epithelial cells
    d *Pneumocystis jiroveci*

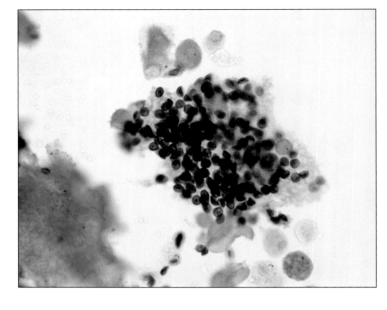

80   A 44-year-old female presents with a productive cough. Sputum analysis reveals these cells. Which of the following clinical histories apply?

    a HIV
    b tuberculosis
    c smoking
    d nose inhalant abuse

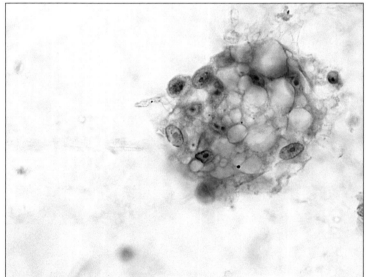

81   A possible clinical explanation for these findings obtained from a sputum specimen is:

    a right upper lobe mass
    b hypersensitivity reaction
    c history of bronchopulmonary silicosis
    d lipoid pneumonia

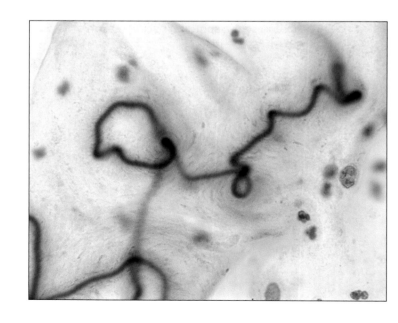

ISBN 978-089189-6357   ©ASCP 2015

82   These cells represent a sputum sample from a
     55-year-old female with a history of smoking. They
     are:
     a lipophages
     b carbon histiocytes
     c siderophages
     d muciphages

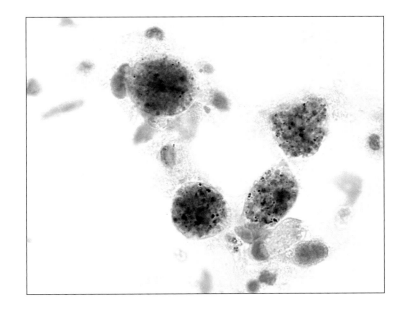

83   A 21-year-old immunocompromised patient presents
     with shortness of breath. Sputum analysis reveals:
     a cytomegalovirus
     b respiratory syncytial virus
     c herpesvirus
     d parainfluenza virus

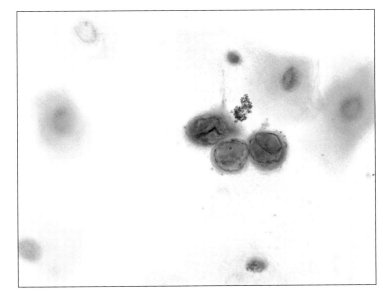

84   These cells represent a sputum specimen from a
     44-year-old male. The diagnosis is consistent with:
     a viral infection
     b carcinoid tumor
     c alveolar proteinosis
     d reserve cell hyperplasia

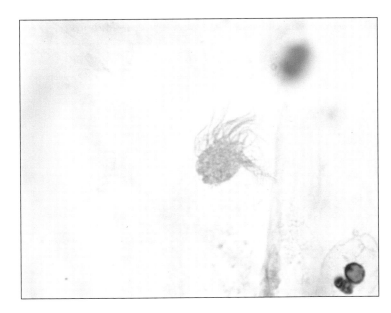

85 A patient who recently underwent surgery for squamous cell carcinoma of the lung presents with a small nodule on chest X-ray in the general area of the original tumor. Bronchial aspiration reveals epithelioid cells, giant cells, and these entities. The findings are most compatible with:

   a starch granulomatosis
   b *Cryptococcus neoformans*
   c *Blastomyces dermatitidis*
   d pollen contamination, suggest repeat bronchoscopy

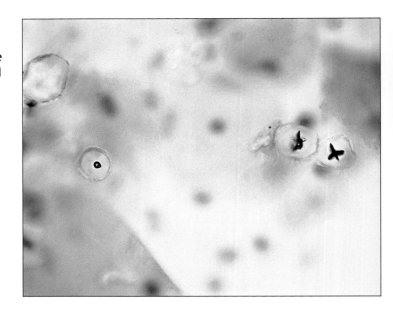

86 A 62-year-old female presents with shortness of breath. A sputum sample is processed for cytology. The diagnosis is consistent with:

   a metastatic spindle cell sarcoma
   b metastatic rhabdomyosarcoma
   c primary neoplasm
   d striated muscle (meat) contamination, repeat sputum

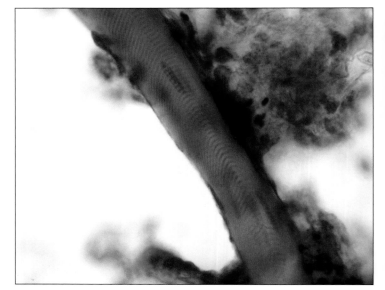

87 These cells represent a cytologic preparation of a sputum sample taken from a 62-year-old female presenting with shortness of breath. The cytologic diagnosis may be related to:

   a large cell lymphoma
   b mesothelioma
   c lipoid pneumonia
   d asthma

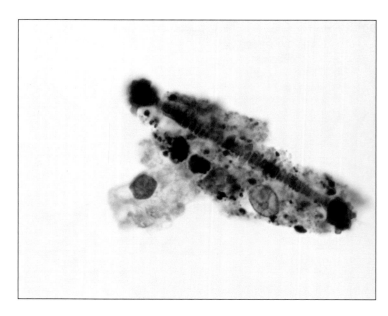

ISBN 978-089189-6357 ©ASCP 2015

88 These cells represent a bronchial brushing obtained from a 63-year-old male with a history of chronic obstructive pulmonary disease. The findings are most consistent with:

a metastatic colonic adenocarcinoma
b carcinoid tumor
c normal bronchial epithelial cells
d nondiagnostic

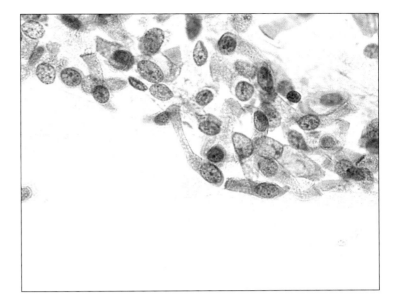

89 A 55-year-old male with a lesion on chest X-ray and a nonproductive cough presents for an early morning induced sputum specimen. These cells are diagnostic of:

a squamous cell carcinoma
b vegetable cells
c atypical squamous metaplasia
d large cell undifferentiated carcinoma

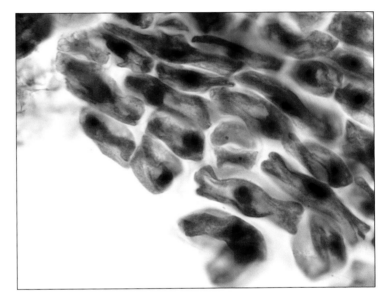

90 These structures found in a sputum specimen represent:

a a primary lung disease
b *Cryptococcus neoformans*
c pollen contamination
d starch

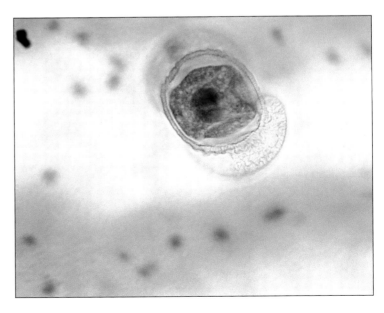

91 This bronchial brushing taken from a 55-year-old male with a history of a pulmonary disorder reveals:

   a adenocarcinoma
   b large cell carcinoma
   c reactive bronchial cells
   d viral infection, not otherwise specified

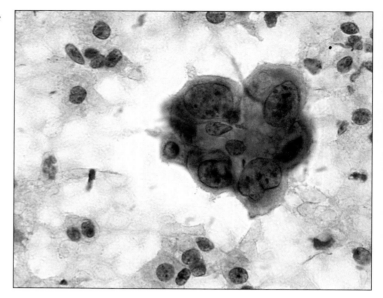

92 The cytologic findings represent a sputum specimen from a 2-week-old premature infant. The diagnosis is:

   a *Cryptococcus neoformans*
   b *Blastomyces dermatitidis*
   c *Pneumocystis jiroveci*
   d none of the above

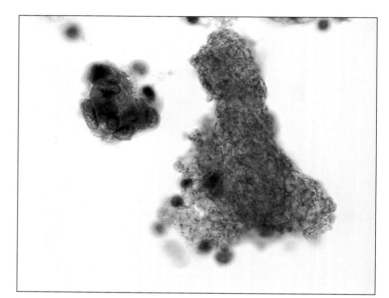

93 A 43-year-old, HIV+ male was seen for fever and a nonproductive cough. A chest X-ray showed nonspecific lung infiltrates. A bronchial washing was performed. The best diagnosis for this liquid based preparation is:

   a zygomycetes
   b *Candida albicans*
   c *Aspergillus* species
   d actinomycosis

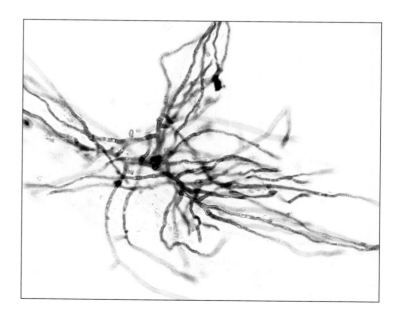

ISBN 978-089189-6357 ©ASCP 2015

94 This bronchial brushing was taken from a 55-year-old male with a bronchial obstruction. What is your diagnosis?

  a intraalveolar histiocytes
  b *Pneumocystis*
  c granular cell tumor
  d granuloma

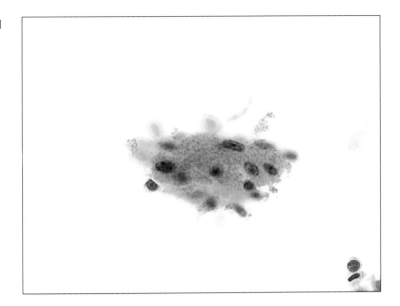

95 This organism was seen in a sputum from a 44-year-old female. What is the recommended course of management?

  a antifungal therapy
  b no treatment necessary
  c HIV testing
  d transbronchial biopsy

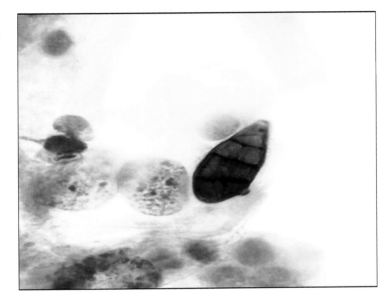

96 A sputum was obtained from a 75-year-old male arriving from Mexico who presented with a cough. What type of organism is present in this image?

  a *Histoplasma*
  b *Coccidioides*
  c *Paracoccidioides*
  d *Blastomyces*

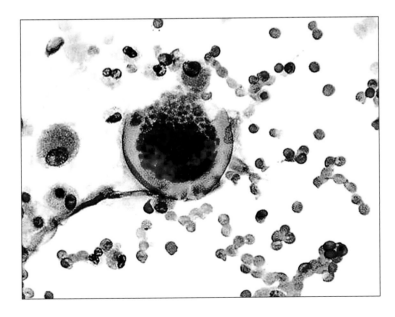

97 A 24-year-old male with history of acute leukemia, who is status post bone marrow transplant, has a BAL specimen submitted. What is the best diagnosis?
a cytomegalovirus
b melanoma
c herpes
d recurrent acute leukemia

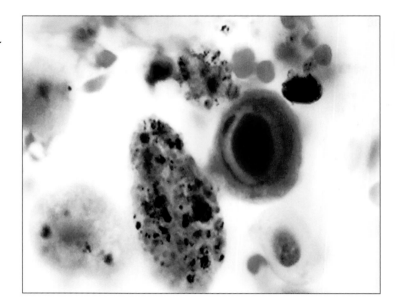

98 This 68-year-old male with pulmonary fibrosis was seen for shortness of breath. A bronchial washing was performed. What is the most appropriate diagnosis?
a Curschmann spirals
b microfilaria
c ferruginous bodies
d alternaria

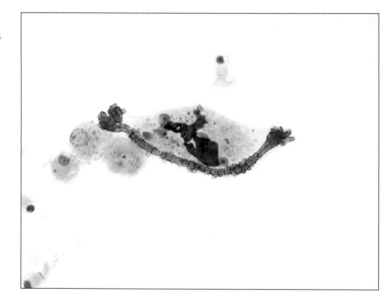

99 This bronchoalveolar lavage was obtained from a 37-year-old female. What might be her underlying disease?
a asthma
b rheumatoid arthritis
c bronchioloalveolar carcinoma
d ovarian mucinous adenocarcinoma

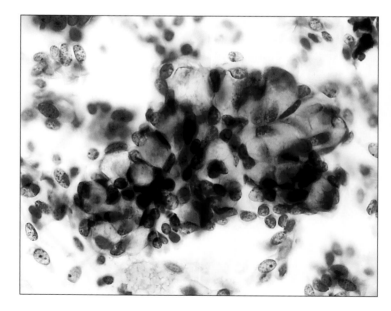

ISBN 978-089189-6357 ©ASCP 2015

100 A 56-year-old male complained of chronic and progressive cough with sputum production. A chest X-ray demonstrated a right perihilar mass. Sputum was submitted for cytologic examination. What is your diagnosis?

a adenocarcinoma
b squamous cell carcinoma, poorly differentiated
c granulomatous inflammation
d small cell carcinoma

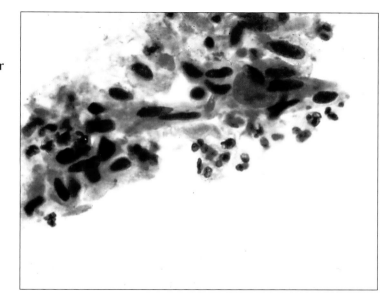

101 This 30-year-old male, HIV+, complained of cough and increasing shortness of breath. A chest film showed diffuse infiltrate in his lungs. A bronchoalveolar lavage was submitted for cytologic examination. What special stain would you order to support interpretation?

a Gram stain
b acid-fast stain
c mucicarmine stain
d GMS stain

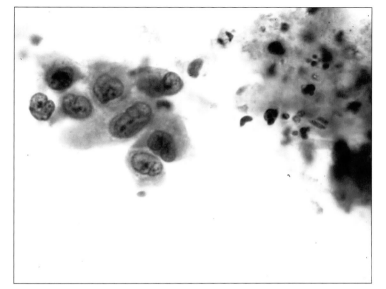

102 A 67-year-old male undergoing immunosuppressive therapy developed a bilateral, hazy pulmonary infiltrate. Bronchial washings were obtained. The best interpretation is:

a cytomegalovirus inclusions present
b herpesvirus inclusions present
c polyomavirus inclusions present
d respiratory adenovirus inclusions present

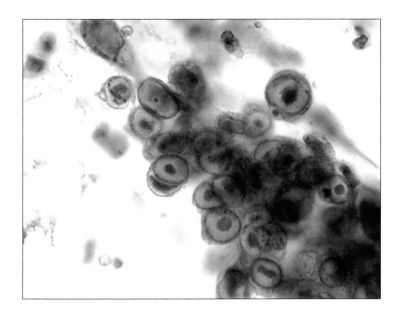

103 A bronchial washing was performed on a 45-year-old female, who is a smoker with a persistent cough. The image suggests a diagnosis of:

   a increased mucus secretion
   b helminth infection
   c contaminant
   d asbestos exposure

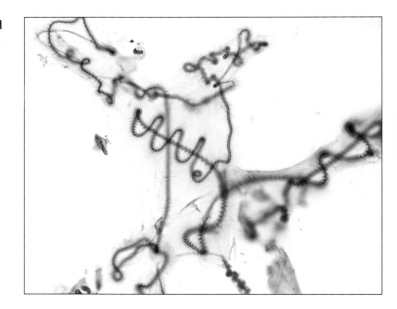

104 Sputum specimen from a 68-year-old male with a 40 year history of cigarette smoking and recent weight loss. What is your diagnosis?

   a benign bronchial epithelium
   b inflammation
   c basal cell hyperplasia
   d small cell carcinoma

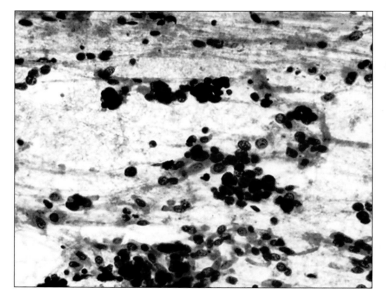

105 A 52-year-old female, nonsmoker, experienced a sudden bout of hemoptysis. Chest X-ray did not demonstrate abnormal findings; however, a mass lesion with superficial erosion of the mucosa was seen in the left upper lobe bronchus at bronchoscopy. Bronchial washings were submitted for cytologic evaluation. What is your best interpretation of the cytology image?

   a carcinoid
   b small cell undifferentiated carcinoma
   c reserve cell hyperplasia
   d bronchoalveolar carcinoma

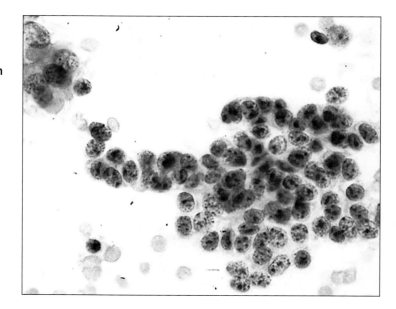

ISBN 978-089189-6357 ©ASCP 2015

106 A bronchial brush specimen from a 56-year-old male, status post chemotherapy for small cell lung carcinoma, reveals these cells. What is the best interpretation?

a recurrent small cell carcinoma
b lymphoid hyperplasia
c lung hamartoma
d reserve cell hyperplasia

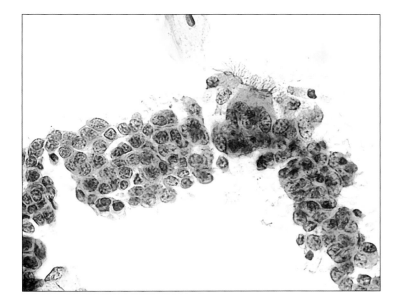

1 **d** small cell carcinoma, oat cell variety

Small cell carcinoma is a highly malignant neuroendocrine neoplasm that is ultrastructurally part of the amine precursor uptake and decarboxylation (APUD) tumors. These cells contain hyperchromatic stippled chromatin, coarse clumping, nuclear molding, scanty cytoplasm, and micronucleoli. They characteristically have vertebral column formation, microbiopsy aggregates, cords, nests, or ribbons. The oat cell type, which may represent a degenerated form of the tumor, typically is found in streams of mucin when evaluating the cells using the pick and smear or crush technique. The Saccomanno technique may not preserve the molding patterns as often. The intermediate cell small cell carcinoma represents both fusiform and polygonal variants, which are typically better preserved with open coarse chromatin patterns and enlarged cell areas. Immunocytochemical staining with chromogranin is helpful in establishing the neurosecretory nature of this tumor.
DeMay, A&S 2e. Oat cell carcinoma, p1182-1185

2 **a** melanoma

Melanoma typically presents in single cells, aggregates, or as spindle cells with bizarre malignant nuclear features, macronucleoli, intranuclear cytoplasmic inclusions, and possibly intracytoplasmic golden-brown pigment. Due to the fact that these diseases may be amelanotic, it may be helpful to confirm this disease process with S100, HMB45, melan A or MITF (microphthalmia associated transcription factor)–all of which preferentially react with melanoma cells.
DeMay, A&S 2e. Metastatic malignancy, p248; Melanoma, p588-590, 1517

3 **b** herpesvirus

Herpesvirus infections may be seen in immunocompromised hosts, including patients affected with concomitant HIV infections, patients receiving therapy for malignant disease, or those with other chronic debilitating disorders. Cytologic identification is based on the findings of multinucleated cells containing ground glass nuclei, karyolytic chromatin, nuclear molding, and eosinophilic Cowdry type A inclusions. Possible contamination from the oral cavity must be considered in the absence of clinically apparent infections.
DeMay, A&S 2e. Viruses, p1467; Viral pneumonia), p1161

4 **b** poorly differentiated squamous cell carcinoma

Cells from poorly differentiated squamous lesions present as single cells and monolayer tissue fragments. Anisocytosis, dense basophilic, hard or waxy cytoplasm often with characteristic cytoplasmic ringing and coarse, irregular chromatin and macronucleoli may be present.
DeMay, A&S 2e. Nonkeratinizing (moderately to poorly differentiated) squamous cell carcinoma, p235-236

5 **d** microbacteria

Tobacco smoke, radiation, radon gas, occupational exposure to certain metals such as nickel and chromate, asbestos, and environmental factors represent some of the etiologic agents associated with bronchogenic carcinoma.
DeMay, A&S 2e. Clinical features of lung cancer, p1171-1173

6 **a** large cell carcinoma

These highly malignant lesions tend to arise within the large bronchi, have idiopathic histogenesis, and are cytologically distinguished as cells arranged in syncytial groupings and in single cell fashion. The absence of true gland formation or the presence of keratinization (including cytoplasmic ringing) make this lesion a diagnosis by exclusion only. The nuclei are hyperchromatic, possessing coarsely granular, irregularly distributed chromatin and multiple irregular macronucleoli, with marked anisonucleosis. The cytoplasm tends to be basophilic and homogeneous. A variant of this lesion is the so called giant cell type, diagnosed primarily based on the macrocytosis.
DeMay, A&S 2e. Large cell carcinoma, p1186-1188

7 **b** *Aspergillus fumigatus*

The cytologic presentation of thick walled hyphae with dichotomous acute angled branching is characteristic of *Aspergillus* species.
DeMay, A&S 2e. Infections, p1161; Fungus, p1470-1473

8 **c** *Blastomyces dermatitidis*

Blastomyces dermatitidis is a yeastlike organism that cytologically presents as single organisms with thick walled refractile cytoplasm. The organism reproduces by single broad based budding, which characteristically differentiates it from *Cryptococcus neoformans.*
DeMay, A&S 2e. Infections, p1161; Fungus, p1470-1473

9 **d** carcinoid tumor

Carcinoid tumors are slow growing neuroendocrine tumors that have association with small cell carcinoma etiology. The polyploid tumors cytologically present as small cells with high N:C ratios and hypochromatic, finely granular, evenly distributed chromatin patterns, with typical oat cell groupings of cords, nests, ribbons, and vertebral column formations. Reactive/reparative cells can be discriminated from these lesions based on the absence of terminal bars and/or cilia with carcinoid tumors. A radiographically detectable lesion and physiological changes are essential elements in diagnosing carcinoid lesions. Immunocytochemical staining with chromogranin will confirm its neuroendocrine origin. Atypical carcinoid tumors, usually associated with the physiological carcinoid syndrome of right sided fibrosis of the heart, cyanotic flushing of the skin, and liver metastasis, generally have classical neuroendocrine malignant features that may be difficult to distinguish from small cell carcinomas.
DeMay, A&S 2e. Carcinoid tumors, p245-246, 586-587; Neuroendocrine carcinomas, p1188-1192

10 **d** invasive carcinoma

The peak incidence of lung cancer occurs at 60 years of age. Signs and symptoms often appear late in the course of the disease with weight loss, dyspnea, weakness, chest pain, hemoptysis, and coughing being most common.
DeMay, A&S 2e. Clinical features of lung cancer, p1171-1173

ISBN 978-089189-6357 ©ASCP 2015

11 b adenocarcinoma, bronchogenic type

Bronchogenic adenocarcinomas cytologically present in 3D acinar clusters, and single cells and have hypochromatic/bland chromatin or, if less well differentiated, hyperchromasia. The presence of central macronucleoli is helpful in establishing this disease process. These true tissue fragments possess frothy cytoplasm, high N:C ratios, and uniform or lobulated nuclei.

DeMay, A&S 2e. Bronchogenic adenocarcinoma, p238-239, 1177-1178

12 d adenocarcinoma/colon

The presence of tall columnar or "cigar shaped" cells in aggregates with frankly malignant nuclear features, granular cytoplasm, or the presence of malignant signet ring cells may suggest a diagnosis of metastatic adenocarcinoma of the colon. Confirmation by surgical pathology of the primary lesion is critical.

DeMay, A&S 2e. Metastases, p1201; Adenocarcinoma, p412-413

13 c adenosquamous carcinoma, immunoperoxidase positive for keratin

The diagnosis of adenosquamous carcinoma depends on the diligence of the cytologist in identifying both epidermal and glandular constituents.

DeMay, A&S 2e. Adenosquamous carcinoma, p1193-1195; Cytokeratin, p1514-1515

14 c cytomegalovirus

Large cells with intranuclear basophilic inclusions surrounded by halos resembling an "owl's eye" are diagnostic of cytomegalovirus.

DeMay, A&S 2e. Viral pneumonia, p227; Infections, p1161; Viruses, p1497

15 a repeat sputum, *Actinomyces* species may represent tonsillar contamination

Actinomyces species, branching diphtheroid saprophytic organisms, produce sulfur granules that contain radiating bacillary fragments. Care must be taken to rule out possible contamination from the oral cavity or tonsils.

DeMay, A&S 2e. Infections, p1161; Bacteria, p1468-1470

16 d *Cryptococcus neoformans*

The presence of single yeastlike structures with mucinous capsules is diagnostic of *Cryptococcus neoformans*. These organisms reproduce by teardrop budding. Special staining with mucicarmine will help elucidate the distinctive mucoid capsule.

DeMay, A&S 2e. Infections, p1161; Fungus, p1470-1473

17 d Hodgkin disease

The presence of a reactive polymorphic inflammatory background composed of eosinophils, neutrophils, plasma cells, and small round lymphocytes, in the presence of large cells with pale cyanophilic cytoplasm, mononuclear and binucleate "mirror image" irregularly lobulated nuclei, coarse irregular chromatin, and macronucleoli, is diagnostic of Reed-Sternberg cells and Hodgkin disease.

DeMay, A&S 2e. Hodgkin disease, p1020-1022

18 a *Coccidioides immitis*

Coccidioides immitis is associated with mild respiratory tract infections. The organisms are cytologically identified as spherical structures containing multiple endospores and revealing a pomegranate appearance.

DeMay, A&S 2e. Infections, p1161; Fungus, p1470-1473

19 c lobular adenocarcinoma/breast

Metastatic lobular carcinoma of the breast typically presents as single bland cells in vertebral column formations, often containing intracytoplasmic or intranuclear inclusions. Immunopositivity with E-cadherin (a cell cohesion protein encoded by a gene on chromosome 16q22.1) may help discriminate between lobular and ductal carcinoma of the breast. Lobular carcinomas lack expression while ductal carcinomas typically express cytoplasmic E-cadherin.

DeMay, A&S 2e. Lobular carcinoma, p1090-1091; Metastases, p1201; Cadherins, p1509

20 c *Histoplasma capsulatum*

Histoplasma capsulatum is a reticuloendothelial organism cytologically presenting as small, thick refractile spherules with endospores that invariably must be identified as intracytoplasmic inclusions within histiocytes. Confirmation with GMS is imperative.

DeMay, A&S 2e. Infections, p1161; Fungus, p1470-1473

21 a squamous cell carcinoma/esophagus

In the absence of a primary lung neoplasm, a diagnosis of metastatic squamous carcinoma should be considered, such as those originating in the oral cavity or esophagus.

DeMay, A&S 2e. Squamous cell carcinoma, p1173-1176; Metastases, p1201;

22 b adenocarcinoma, terminal bronchioloalveolar

Bronchioloalveolar adenocarcinomas present cytologically in large tissue fragments, flower or petal-like acinar clusters with great depth of focus and mucinous or nonmucinous cytoplasm. The cells are typically uniform in size and shape and contain round to oval nuclei. These malignant cells are often accompanied by alveolar macrophages or rare psammoma bodies.

DeMay, A&S 2e. Bronchioloalveolar carcinoma, p239-240, 1178-1180

23 b *Nocardia asteroides*

The diagnosis of *Nocardia asteroides* may be confirmed by identifying the presence of delicate thin, transparent mycelium with beaded hyphae and lacking granule formation. *Nocardia* is a Gram+ organism that may also demonstrate acid-fast positivity should coccal forms be identified.

DeMay, A&S 2e. Infections, p1161; Bacteria, p1468-1470

24 c well differentiated squamous cell carcinoma, keratinizing

Pleomorphic cells with caudate or spindle formations with refractile cytoplasm, anisonucleosis, and opaque India ink nuclei are representative of squamous cell carcinoma. A necrotic background is helpful in establishing this lesion.

DeMay, A&S 2e. Keratinizing (well differentiated) squamous carcinoma, p233-234, 1173-1174

25 d siderophages

The presence of hemosiderin laden (iron positive) macrophages or siderophages is associated with blood within the alveolar septum. These cells may be secondary to hemorrhage, heart failure, necrosis, or pulmonary hemosiderosis.

DeMay, A&S 2e. Alveolar macrophages, p212-213, 1159-1160

26 c refractile golden pigment

Iron stains will help confirm the presence of hemosiderin laden macrophages; however, the diagnosis can only be suggested in light of the clinical findings.

DeMay, A&S 2e. Pneumoconioses, p228, 1165

27 b atypical squamous metaplasia

Parakeratosis, as in the Pap test, may be related to inflammation or precancerous lesions. These cells generally arise from the oral cavity or tracheobronchial tree. Care should be exercised to differentiate these small cells from a more serious process such as squamous cell carcinoma, a lesion with abundant numbers of large pleomorphic cells.

DeMay, A&S 2e. Parakeratosis, p228, 1165

28 d GMS staining for confirmation of *Pneumocystis jiroveci*

Pneumocystis jiroveci, once considered an opportunistic protozoan but now known to be a fungus, often infects patients with acquired immunodeficiency syndrome. Immunocompromised patients and premature infants are considered suitable hosts for infection. Cytologic identification is based on the presence of foamy to frothy casts/mats of eosinophilic material with interspersed "contact lens"–shaped refractile structures containing intranuclear trophozoites (Pap stain). GMS will stain the cell wall of the cyst black with central black dots. In Wright-Giemsa or other Romanowsky based stains, the alveolar casts of *Pneumocystis jiroveci* stain as basophilic masses with the trophozoites appearing as eosinophilic specks within the mass.

DeMay, A&S 2e. Infections, p1161; Fungus, p1470-1473

29 d bronchial metaplastic cells

The replacement of normal bronchial epithelium with a squamous protective epithelium in the lung is consistent with squamous metaplasia. This process may occur in response to a reparative/reactive process secondary to toxic agents such as cigarette smoke, bronchiectasis, tuberculosis, and pneumonia. The cytologic identification is based on the finding of monolayer sheets or single cells with cobblestone pavement configuration and well defined borders, predictable round to oval nuclei, and cyanophilic staining cytoplasm. Differential diagnoses include those of atypical nature.

DeMay, A&S 2e. Squamous metaplasia, p220

30 c normal lymphocytes

Lymphocytes are small, round, single cells without cohesive cytoplasmic features. The presence of lymphogranular bodies distributed throughout the background (best visualized with air dried preparations; see Chapter 8, Fine Needle Aspiration) may also help in confirming the lymphoid origin of these cells.

DeMay, A&S 2e. Inflammatory cells, p214-215

31 d atypical squamous metaplasia

Atypical squamous metaplasia or squamous dysplasia is an antecedent for squamous cell carcinoma of the lung. The finding of small cells in sheets and as single cells with slight pleomorphism, hyperchromatic nuclei, moderate N:C ratios, finely granular regularly distributed chromatin staining cyanophilic to orangeophilic is diagnostic of this process.

DeMay, A&S 2e. Differential diagnosis of squamous metaplasia, low grade dysplasia, high grade dysplasia, and cancer, p236

32 c Curschmann spirals

Curschmann spirals are casts of inspissated mucus created by occluded or stenotic bronchi. The association of these structures with hypersensitivity reactions such as asthma as well as other mucus producing pulmonary disorders is common.

DeMay, A&S 2e. Curschmann spirals, p215

33 b nonkeratinizing stratified squamous

The presence of nonkeratinizing epithelium in respiratory specimens may represent cells from the oral cavity, epiglottis, vocal cords, oropharynx, and the pharynx.

DeMay, A&S 2e. Squamous cells, p208

34 a lipoid pneumonia

The finding of lipid laden histiocytes or lipophages may be seen in patients who chronically abuse lipid solvent nose inhalants, in patients who have aspirated food material, or in lipoid pneumonia. Cytologic changes associated with pneumonia are common. These macrophages contain abundant intracytoplasmic clear to granular vacuoles. Confirmation with oil red O or Sudan black is helpful in establishing the presence of lipid due to the fact that the alcoholic Papanicolaou stain dissolves these products.

DeMay, A&S 2e. Lipophages, p213; Lipid pneumonia, p1164

35 d inflammatory pseudotumor

The finding of eosinophils is more likely to be associated with parasitic infections and hypersensitivity reactions.

DeMay, A&S 2e. Charcot-Leyden crystals, p216; Inflammatory pseudotumor, p225

36 d reserve cell hyperplasia

Subcolumnar cells with uniform features, scanty cytoplasm, and dark nuclei, found in sheets, as single cells, or attached to mature bronchial cells, are consistent with reserve cell hyperplasia (RCH). RCH may be related to an assortment of bronchial disorders including pneumonia, fungal infections, viral infections, or tuberculosis. Caution must be exercised to differentiate these benign entities from small cell carcinoma.

DeMay, A&S 2e. Reserve cell hyperplasia, p219; t2.9 Differential diagnosis of reserve cell hyperplasia vs small cell carcinoma, p242; Bronchial cells, p1160

ISBN 978-089189-6357 ©ASCP 2015

37 c ciliocytophthoria

Viral infections such as adenovirus, measles, and parainfluenza, often with less specific cytomorphologic criteria, may have associated ciliocytophthoria (CCP). The cytology shows degenerative nuclear changes (karyorrhexis) and pinched off ciliated tufts with eosinophilic nonspecific intracytoplasmic inclusions. Other causes of CCP include nonspecific injury, air pollution, and hot or dry air.

DeMay, A&S 2e. Ciliocytophthoria, p211

38 c plant cells

Cells with double cell walls, squared off cytoplasm containing smudgy nuclei, and intracytoplasmic granules are diagnostic of vegetable contaminant. Care should be taken not to diagnose these as metaplasia or squamous carcinoma.

DeMay, A&S 2e. Plant cells/food, p218-219

39 a asthma

Bronchial hyperplasia is often found in patients with asthma. The presence of papillary 3D clusters of cells with well defined cytoplasmic interior borders, along with the presence of terminal bars and/or cilia, is diagnostic of "creola" bodies. These groupings may easily be differentiated from well differentiated bronchogenic adenocarcinoma due to the presence of cilia and/or terminal bars. Curschmann spirals are casts of inspissated mucus created by occluded or stenotic bronchi. The association of these structures with hypersensitivity reactions such as asthma as well as other mucus producing pulmonary disorders is common. Small crystalline structures with sharp, pointed ends represent Charcot-Leyden crystals, often associated with asthma. These structures, in addition to creola bodies, Curschmann spirals, and eosinophils, are nonspecific findings of this hypersensitivity reaction.

DeMay, A&S 2e. Asthma, p228

40 b lipid pneumonia

Aspiration pneumonia (milk) can be confirmed with oil red O staining by the presence of lipid laden macrophages.

DeMay, A&S 2e. Lipophages, p213; Lipid pneumonia, p1164

41 a ferruginous bodies

Ferruginous bodies are hemosiderin coated fibers and may be detected in the respiratory samples of patients who have inhaled any one of a variety of mineral fibers, most notably asbestos. They may be identified by the presence of rod or dumbbell shaped golden-brown structures with an iron protein matrix. Their association with mesothelioma has been established, and a role in the carcinogenesis of the lung has been suggested.

DeMay, A&S 2e. Ferruginous (asbestos) bodies, p216

42 a reactive bronchial epithelial cells

Multinucleated bronchial cells are associated with a variety of pulmonary conditions, including viral pneumonitis, previous bronchoscopy, bronchiectasis, or fume inhalation. Their presence indicates a reactive process. Cells with typical reactive criteria reveal nuclear pleomorphism with finely granular, evenly distributed chromatin, prominent nucleoli, and well preserved cytoplasmic borders (often with terminal bars and/or cilia).

DeMay, A&S 2e. Inflammation, p223; Repair/regeneration, p593

43 b creola bodies

Bronchial hyperplasia is often found in patients with asthma. The presence of papillary 3D clusters of cells with well defined cytoplasmic interior borders, along with the presence of terminal bars and/or cilia, is diagnostic of these "creola" bodies. These groupings may easily be differentiated from well differentiated bronchogenic adenocarcinoma due to the presence of cilia and/or terminal bars.

DeMay, A&S 2e. Bronchial hyperplasia and creola bodies, p220

44 a carbon histiocyte

The presence of abundant carbon laden histiocytes is commonly associated with anthracosis, a pneumoconiosis (dust disease) related to carbon inhalation.

DeMay, A&S 2e. Pneumoconiosis, p228-231; Miscellaneous benign conditions, p1165-1166

45 d psammoma bodies

Psammoma bodies (calcospherites) are composed of calcifying concentric rings of phosphate, iron, and magnesium. These eosinophilic structures may be associated with bronchioloalveolar adenocarcinomas, metastatic papillary carcinoma, tuberculosis, and less common conditions such as pulmonary lithiasis.

DeMay, A&S 2e. Calcospherites and psammoma bodies, p217; Psammoma bodies, p592

46 c atypical squamous metaplasia

Atypical squamous metaplasia or squamous dysplasia is an antecedent for squamous cell carcinoma of the lung. The finding of small cells in sheets and as single cells with slight pleomorphism, hyperchromatic nuclei, moderate N:C ratios, finely granular, regularly distributed chromatin, and cytoplasm staining cyanophilic to orangeophilic is diagnostic of this process.

DeMay, A&S 2e. Squamous metaplasia, p219-220

47 b corpora amylacea

Corpora amylacea are condensed glycoproteins associated with heart failure, pulmonary infarction, or bronchitis. The cytologic finding of these round masses may be differentiated from psammoma bodies by their lack of calcification; however, they are birefringent.

DeMay, A&S 2e. Corpora amylacea, p217

48 b oat cell carcinoma

Small cell carcinoma is a highly malignant neuroendocrine neoplasm that is ultrastructurally part of amine precursor uptake and decarboxylation (APUD) tumors. These cells contain hyperchromatic stippled chromatin, coarse clumping, nuclear molding, scanty cytoplasm, and micronucleoli. They characteristically have vertebral column formation, microbiopsy aggregates, cords, nests, or ribbons. The oat cell type, which may represent a degenerated form of the tumor, typically is found in streams of mucin when evaluating the cells using the pick and smear or crush technique. The Saccomanno technique may not preserve the molding patterns. The intermediate cell small cell carcinoma represents both fusiform and polygonal variants, which are typically better preserved cells with open coarse chromatin patterns and enlarged cell areas. Immunocytochemical staining with chromogranin is helpful in establishing the neurosecretory nature of this tumor.

DeMay, A&S 2e. Oat cell carcinoma, p241-242; Small cell carcinoma, p1182-1185

49 b squamous cell carcinoma

Cells from poorly differentiated squamous lesions present as single cells and monolayer tissue fragments. Anisocytosis, dense basophilic, hard or waxy cytoplasm often with characteristic cytoplasmic ringing and coarse, irregular chromatin and macronucleoli may be present.

DeMay, A&S 2e. Nonkeratinizing (moderately to poorly differentiated) squamous cell carcinoma, p235-236; Squamous cell carcinoma, p1174-1176

50 d *Aspergillus* species

The cytologic presentation of thick walled hyphae with dichotomous acute angled branching is characteristic of *Aspergillus* species.

DeMay, A&S 2e. Fungus, p1470-1473

51 b asthma

Bronchial hyperplasia is often found in patients with asthma. The presence of papillary 3D clusters of cells with well defined cytoplasmic interior borders, along with the presence of terminal bars and/or cilia, is diagnostic of "creola" bodies. These groupings may easily be differentiated from well differentiated bronchogenic adenocarcinoma due to the presence of cilia and/or terminal bars.

DeMay, A&S 2e. Bronchial hyperplasia and creola bodies, p220; Asthma, p228

52 b neuroendocrine tumor

Small cell carcinoma is a highly malignant neuroendocrine neoplasm that is ultrastructurally part of the amine precursor uptake and decarboxylation (APUD) tumors. These cells contain hyperchromatic stippled chromatin, coarse clumping, nuclear molding, scanty cytoplasm, and micronucleoli. They characteristically have vertebral column formation and microbiopsy aggregates, and are grouped as cords, nests, or ribbons. The oat cell type, which may represent a degenerated form of the tumor, typically is found in streams of mucin when evaluating the cells using the pick and smear or crush technique. The Saccomanno technique may not preserve the molding patterns as often. The intermediate cell small cell carcinoma represents both fusiform and polygonal variants, which are typically better preserved with open coarse chromatin patterns and enlarged cell areas. Immunocytochemical staining with chromogranin is helpful in establishing the neurosecretory nature of this tumor.

DeMay, A&S 2e. Small cell carcinoma, p241-244; Neuroendocrine carcinomas, p1188-1189

53 c pharynx

Small regular elliptical eosinophilic or orangeophilic single cells with degenerated nuclei and parakeratotic features may represent nonpulmonary cells such as those from the pharynx or upper respiratory tract ("Pap cells").

DeMay, A&S 2e. Pap cells, p220

54 c small cell carcinoma

These cells contain hyperchromatic stippled chromatin, coarse clumping, nuclear molding, scanty cytoplasm, and micronucleoli. They characteristically have vertebral column formation, microbiopsy aggregates, cords, nests, or ribbons. The oat cell type, which may represent a degenerated form of the tumor, typically is found in streams of mucin when evaluating the cells using the pick and smear or crush technique. The Saccomanno technique may not preserve the molding patterns as often. The intermediate cell small cell carcinoma represents both fusiform and polygonal variants, which are typically better preserved with open coarse chromatin patterns and enlarged cell areas. Immunocytochemical staining with chromogranin is helpful in establishing the neurosecretory nature of this tumor.

DeMay, A&S 2e. Small cell carcinoma, p241-244, 1182-1185

55 c acid-fast bacilli, *Mycobacterium avium-intracellulare*

Mycobacterium avium-intracellulare may be seen within macrophages using Kinyoun or Ziehl-Neelsen stain, where it appears as rod shaped bacilli.

DeMay, A&S 2e. Tuberculosis, p225-226; Bacteria, p1468-1470

56 c *Alternaria* species

Alternaria species are cytologically identified as dark brown conidia in chains often resembling "snow shoes."

DeMay, A&S 2e. Fungus, p1470-1473

57 d non-Hodgkin lymphoma

Large cell cleaved lymphomas typically present with a predominant population (80%) of large cleaved lymphocytes with coarse irregular chromatin and prominent nucleoli. A smaller population of small round or cleaved lymphocytes completes the cytologic picture.

DeMay, A&S 2e. Malignant neoplasms, p233; Malignant lymphoma, p572-574

58 c epithelioid histiocytes

Elongated, round, or oval cells presenting singly or in syncytial aggregates with oval/reniform nuclei containing finely granular, evenly distributed chromatin and micronucleoli are diagnostic of epithelioid histiocytes. These cells are part of the spectrum of granulomatous inflammation. Other cells associated with granulomatous inflammation include multinucleated histiocytes, fibroblasts, and assorted white blood cells.

DeMay, A&S 2e. Granulomatous inflammation, p223; Granular cells, p584-585; Granulomas, p1162

59 c arise from type II pneumocytes

Bronchioloalveolar adenocarcinomas present cytologically in large tissue fragments, flower or petal-like acinar clusters with great depth of focus, and mucinous or nonmucinous cytoplasm. The cells are typically uniform in size and shape and contain round to oval nuclei. These malignant cells are often accompanied by alveolar macrophages or rare psammoma bodies.

DeMay, A&S 2e. Bronchioloalveolar carcinoma, p239-241, 1178-1181

ISBN 978-089189-6357 ©ASCP 2015

60 a *Blastomyces dermatitidis*

Blastomyces dermatitidis is a yeastlike organism that cytologically presents as single organisms with thick walled refractile cytoplasm. The organism reproduces by single broad based budding, which characteristically differentiates it from *Cryptococcus neoformans*.
DeMay, A&S 2e. Fungus, p1470-1473

61 b carcinoid tumor; chromogranin+

Carcinoid tumors are slow growing neuroendocrine tumors that have association with small cell carcinoma etiology. The polyploid tumors cytologically present as small cells with high N:C ratios and hypochromatic, finely granular, evenly distributed chromatin patterns, with typical oat cell grouping of cords, nests, ribbons, and vertebral column formations. Reactive/reparative cells can be discriminated from these lesions based on the absence of terminal bars and/or cilia with carcinoid tumors. A radiographically detectable lesion and physiological changes are essential elements in diagnosing carcinoid lesions. Immunocytochemical staining with chromogranin will confirm neuroendocrine origin. Atypical carcinoid, usually associated with the physiological carcinoid syndrome of right sided fibrosis of the heart, cyanotic flushing of the skin, and liver metastasis, generally has classical neuroendocrine malignant features that may be difficult to distinguish from small cell carcinomas.
DeMay, A&S 2e. Carcinoid tumors, p245-246, 586-587; Neuroendocrine carcinomas, p1188-1192

62 c common leukocytic antigen

The image represents a hypercellular population of polymorphic cells diagnostic of normal/reactive lymphocytes. Lymphocytes present as small, round, single cells without cohesive cytoplasmic features. The presence of lymphogranular bodies distributed throughout the background (best visualized with air dried preparations; see Chapter 8, Fine Needle Aspiration) may also help in confirming the lymphoid origin of these cells.
DeMay, A&S 2e. Lymphocytes, p215

63 b glycoproteins (and do not calcify)

Corpora amylacea are condensed glycoproteins associated with heart failure, pulmonary infarction, or bronchitis. The cytologic finding of these round masses may be differentiated from psammoma bodies by their lack of calcification; however, they are birefringent.
DeMay, A&S 2e. Corpora amylacea, p217

64 a cytomegalovirus

Large cells with intranuclear basophilic inclusions surrounded by halos resembling an "owl's eye" are diagnostic of cytomegalovirus.
DeMay, A&S 2e. Viruses, p1466-1468

65 a *Candida* species

The presence of thin pseudohyphae with interrupted cell walls ("sticks") or spore formations ("stones") represents *Candida albicans*. Oral cavity contamination must be ruled out.
DeMay, A&S 2e. Fungus, p1470-1473

66 b *Histoplasma capsulatum*

Histoplasma capsulatum is a reticuloendothelial organism cytologically presenting as small, thick refractile spherules with endospores that invariably must be identified as intracytoplasmic inclusions within histiocytes. Confirmation with GMS is imperative.
DeMay, A&S 2e. Fungus, p1470-1473

67 c *Coccidioides immitis*

Coccidioides immitis is associated with mild respiratory tract infections. The organisms are cytologically identified as spherical structures containing multiple endospores and revealing a pomegranate appearance.
DeMay, A&S 2e. Fungus, p1470-1473

68 c reactive bronchial epithelial cells

Reactive/reparative bronchial cells may be secondary to granulomatous disease, pneumonitis, or bronchitis. Cells with typical reactive criteria including enlarged hypochromatic nuclei with finely granular, evenly distributed chromatin, prominent nucleoli, and well preserved cytoplasmic borders are characteristic of these benign cellular changes.
DeMay, A&S 2e. Repair/regeneration, p210-211, 593

69 b *Actinomyces* species

Actinomyces species, branching diphtheroid saprophytic organisms, produce sulfur granules that contain radiating bacillary fragments. Care must be taken to rule out possible contamination from the oral cavity or tonsils.
DeMay, A&S 2e. Bacteria, p1468-1470

70 d bronchogenic adenocarcinoma

Bronchogenic adenocarcinomas, cytologically present in 3D acinar clusters and single cells, have hypochromatic/bland chromatin or, if less well differentiated, hyperchromasia. The presence of central macronucleoli is helpful in establishing this disease process. These true tissue fragments possess frothy cytoplasm, high N:C ratios, and uniform or lobulated nuclei.
DeMay, A&S 2e. Bronchogenic adenocarcinoma, p1177-1178

71 d reserve cell hyperplasia

Subcolumnar cells with uniform features, scanty cytoplasm and dark nuclei, found in sheets, as single cells, or attached to mature bronchial cells, are consistent with reserve cell hyperplasia (RCH). RCH may be related to an assortment of bronchial disorders including pneumonia, fungal infections, viral infections, or tuberculosis. Caution must be exercised to differentiate these benign entities from small cell carcinoma.
DeMay, A&S 2e. Reserve cell hyperplasia, p219; t2.9 Differential diagnosis of reserve cell hyperplasia vs small cell carcinoma, p242; Bronchial cells, p1160

72 b reactive/reparative changes

Reactive/reparative bronchial cells may be secondary to granulomatous disease, pneumonitis, or bronchitis. Cells with typical reactive criteria including enlarged hypochromatic nuclei with finely granular, evenly distributed chromatin, prominent nucleoli, and well preserved cytoplasmic borders are characteristic of these benign cellular changes.
DeMay, A&S 2e. Repair/regeneration, p210-211, 593

73   **c**   **multinucleated bronchial cells**

Multinucleated bronchial cells are associated with a variety of pulmonary conditions, including viral pneumonitis, previous bronchoscopy, bronchiectasis, or fume inhalation. Their presence indicates a reactive process.

DeMay, A&S 2e. Multinucleation, p210

74   **c**   **siderophages**

The presence of hemosiderin laden (iron positive) macrophages or siderophages is associated with blood within the alveolar septum. These cells may be secondary to hemorrhage, heart failure, necrosis, or pulmonary hemosiderosis.

DeMay, A&S 2e. Siderophages, p213

75   **b**   **normal metaplastic cells**

The replacement of normal bronchial epithelium with a squamous protective epithelium in the lung is consistent with squamous metaplasia. This process may occur in response to a reparative/reactive process secondary to toxic agents such as cigarette smoke, bronchiectasis, tuberculosis, and pneumonia. The cytologic identification is based on the finding of monolayer sheets or single cells with cobblestone pavement configuration and well defined borders, predictable round to oval nuclei, and cyanophilic-staining cytoplasm. Differential diagnoses include those of atypical nature.

DeMay, A&S 2e. Squamous metaplasia, p219-220

76   **a**   **mucicarmine**

The presence of single yeastlike structures with mucinous capsules is diagnostic of *Cryptococcus neoformans*. These organisms reproduce by teardrop budding. Special staining with mucicarmine will help elucidate the distinctive mucoid capsule.

DeMay, A&S 2e. Infections, p1161; Fungus, p1470-1473

77   **d**   **asthma**

Small crystalline structures with sharp, pointed ends represent Charcot-Leyden crystals, often associated with asthma. These structures, in addition to creola bodies, Curschmann spirals, and eosinophils, are nonspecific findings of this hypersensitivity reaction.

DeMay, A&S 2e. Charcot-Leyden crystals, p216; Asthma, p228

78   **b**   **bone marrow**

The pulmonary macrophage is a bone marrow derived cell that has an eccentrically located round, oval or reniform shaped nucleus with or without nucleoli.

DeMay, A&S 2e. Alveolar macrophages, p212-214

79   **d**   *Pneumocystis jiroveci*

Pneumocystis jiroveci, once considered an opportunistic protozoan but now known to be a fungus, often infects patients with acquired immunodeficiency syndrome. Immunocompromised patients and premature infants are considered suitable hosts for infection. Cytologic identification is based on the presence of foamy to frothy casts/mats of eosinophilic material with interspersed "contact lens" shaped refractile structures containing intranuclear trophozoites (Pap stain). GMS will stain the cell wall of the cyst black with central black dots. In Wright-Giemsa or other Romanowsky based stains, the alveolar casts of *P jiroveci* stain as basophilic masses with the trophozoites appearing as eosinophilic specks within the mass.

DeMay, A&S 2e. Infections, p1161; Fungus, p1470-1473

80   **d**   **nose inhalant abuse**

The finding of lipid laden histiocytes or lipophages may be seen in patients who chronically abuse lipid solvent nose inhalants, in patients who have aspirated food material, or in lipoid pneumonia. These macrophages contain abundant intracytoplasmic clear to granular vacuoles. Confirmation with oil red O or Sudan black is helpful in establishing the presence of lipid due to the fact that the alcoholic Papanicolaou stain dissolves these products.

DeMay, A&S 2e. Lipophages, p213

81   **b**   **hypersensitivity reaction**

Curschmann spirals are casts of inspissated mucus created by occluded or stenotic bronchi. The association of these structures with hypersensitivity reactions such as asthma as well as other mucus producing pulmonary disorders is common.

DeMay, A&S 2e. Curschmann spirals, p215

82   **b**   **carbon histiocytes**

The pulmonary macrophage is a bone marrow derived cell that has an eccentrically located round, oval or reniform shaped nucleus with or without nucleoli. Pulmonary macrophages with engulfed intracytoplasmic carbonaceous inclusions are referred to as "dust cells." The presence of dust cells is essential in establishing the adequacy of a satisfactory deep sputum specimen.

DeMay, A&S 2e. Carbon histiocytes, p215

83   **c**   **herpesvirus**

Herpesvirus infections may be seen in immunocompromised hosts, including patients affected with concomitant HIV infections, patients receiving therapy for malignant disease, or those with other chronic debilitating disorders. Cytologic identification is based on the findings of cells containing ground glass nuclei, karyolytic chromatin, nuclear molding, and eosinophilic Cowdry type A inclusions. Possible contamination from the oral cavity must be considered in the absence of clinically apparent pulmonary infections.

DeMay, A&S 2e. Viruses, p1466-1468; Infections, p1161

ISBN 978-089189-6357 ©ASCP 2015

84 a viral infection

Viral infections such as adenovirus, measles, and parainfluenza, often with less specific cytomorphologic criteria, may have associated ciliocytophthoria (CCP). The cytology shows degenerative nuclear changes (karyorrhexis) and pinched off ciliated tufts with eosinophilic nonspecific intracytoplasmic inclusions. Other causes of CCP include nonspecific injury, air pollution, and hot or dry air.

DeMay, A&S 2e. Viruses, p1466-1468

85 a starch granulomatosis

The structures with characteristic Maltese cross formations are associated with starch contamination. Their presence may be associated with a granulomatous response.

DeMay, A&S 2e. Contaminants, p1478

86 d striated muscle (meat) contamination, repeat sputum

The finding of striated muscle within sputum cytology most often represents meat contamination associated with masticated food.

DeMay, A&S 2e. Contaminants, p218, 1478

87 b mesothelioma

Ferruginous bodies are hemosiderin coated fibers that may be detected in the respiratory samples of patients who have inhaled any one of a variety of mineral fibers, most notably asbestos. These structures are identified by the presence of a rod or dumbbell shaped golden-brown structure with an iron protein matrix. Their association with mesothelioma has been established, and a role in the carcinogenesis of the lung has been suggested.

DeMay, A&S 2e. Ferruginous (asbestos) bodies, p216

88 c normal bronchial epithelial cells

The presence of columnar to prismatic shaped cells with centrally to basally located nuclei and finely granular, regularly distributed chromatin, often containing micronucleoli, is diagnostic of normal bronchial mucosa. Terminal bars and/or cilia also help confirm the normality of these cells.

DeMay, A&S 2e. Glandular cells, p213-214

89 b vegetable cells

Cells with double cell walls, squared off cytoplasm containing smudgy nuclei, and intracytoplasmic granules are diagnostic of vegetable contaminant. Caution should be given not to overdiagnose these cells as true indigenous processes such as metaplasia or squamous carcinoma.

DeMay, A&S 2e. Contaminants, p218, 1478

90 c pollen contamination

Small symmetrical structures with centrally located pores and spiky surfaces are indicative of pollen contamination. These structures should be differentiated from fungal infections such as *Blastomyces dermatitidis* or *Cryptococcus neoformans*.

DeMay, A&S 2e. Contaminants, p218, 1478; Fungus, p1470-1473

91 c reactive bronchial cells

Reactive/reparative bronchial cells may be secondary to granulomatous disease, pneumonitis, or bronchitis. Cells, arranged singly or in clusters, with typical reactive criteria including enlarged hypochromatic nuclei with finely granular, evenly distributed chromatin, prominent nucleoli, and well preserved cytoplasmic borders are characteristic of these benign cellular changes. Cells secondary to pulmonary infarct may exhibit "atypical features," but on close examination terminal bars or cilia are often found.

DeMay, A&S 2e. Repair/regeneration, p210-211, 593

92 c *Pneumocystis jiroveci*

Pneumocystis jiroveci, once considered an opportunistic protozoan but now known to be a fungus, often infects patients with acquired immunodeficiency syndrome. Immunocompromised patients and premature infants are considered suitable hosts for infection. Cytologic identification is based on the presence of foamy to frothy casts/mats of eosinophilic material with interspersed "contact lens" shaped refractile structures containing intranuclear trophozoites (Pap stain). GMS will stain the cell wall of the cyst black with central black dots. In Wright-Giemsa or other Romanowsky based stains, the alveolar casts of *P jiroveci* stain as basophilic masses with the trophozoites appearing as eosinophilic specks within the mass.

DeMay, A&S 2e. Infections, p1161; Fungus, p1470-1473

93 c *Aspergillus* species

This specimen shows septate fungal hyphae with 45° angle branching. Although not seen in this particular image, calcium oxalate crystals may be an associated finding.

DeMay, A&S 2e. Fungus, p1470-1473

94 c granular cell tumor

This specimen shows an aggregate of cells with abundant granular cytoplasm and indistinct cell borders. The nuclei are oval, with small but distinct nucleoli. Granular cell tumors, although most commonly presenting as subcutaneous masses, or in the oral cavity, have been described in multiple anatomic locations, including the lung.

DeMay, A&S 2e. Granular cell tumor, p232; Granular cells, p584-585; Granulomas, p1162

95 b no treatment necessary

This image shows *Alternaria* displaying a snowshoelike appearance. *Alternaria* is usually present as a contaminant.

DeMay, A&S 2e. Alternaria, p1470

96 b *Coccidioides*

This image shows a disrupted spherule containing nonbudding endospores that is characteristic for coccidioidomycosis.

DeMay, A&S 2e. Fungus, p1470-1473

97 a cytomegalovirus

This image shows a cell infected with cytomegalovirus showing classic large intranuclear inclusion surrounded by halo. There is also a faint, small basophilic cytoplasmic inclusion around the 6 o'clock position in the cell.

DeMay, A&S 2e. Viruses, p1466-1468

98 c ferruginous bodies

This image shows a ferruginous body often associated with asbestos exposure. Asbestos exposure is common in certain construction, shipbuilding and industrial workers. The inhaled uncoated fibers are translucent and scarcely visible. In the lung, they become coated with protein and iron, giving these fibers the characteristic golden-brown, segmented or beaded bamboo shape with knobbed or bulbous ends.

DeMay, A&S 2e. Ferruginous (asbestos) bodies, p216

99 a asthma

The image shows a cluster of benign bronchial epithelium with mucinous metaplasia. These findings are commonly seen in patients with asthma, chronic bronchitis, bronchiectasis and allergic conditions.

DeMay, A&S 2e. Asthma, p228

100 b squamous cell carcinoma, poorly differentiated

The image shows a relatively flat sheet of cells with enlarged very hyperchromatic nuclei. The cytoplasm is easily visible and hard where well preserved but frayed at the edges of several cells, indicating tumor degeneration and necrosis. Some tumor cells show cytoplasmic orangeophilia, which is a characteristic for squamous cell carcinoma.

DeMay, A&S 2e. Squamous cell carcinoma, p233-237, 1173-1176

101 b acid-fast stain

Some of the macrophages have a striated appearance to the cytoplasm that is straight or slightly curved and narrow lines in the cytoplasm that do not stain, so called "negative images." These negative staining areas represent intracytoplasmic bacilli of mycobacterial organisms. This is a cytologic pattern that one can observe in the severely immunocompromised patient, usually suffering from AIDS. An acid-fast stain will demonstrate large numbers of positive intracytoplasmic organisms, many more than is apparent on the Pap stain.

DeMay, A&S 2e. Mycobacteria, p1469

102 b herpesvirus inclusions present

There are multiple cells with intranuclear inclusion bodies. There is 1 cell at the top of the image with ground glass nuclear change. The presence of many inclusions, their size and the identification of the ground glass nuclear change are what is seen in the cytology of herpesvirus infection. The differential interpretation includes, most prominently, cytomegalovirus inclusions. However, they are much fewer in number, even in immunocompromised patients. They are also much larger with a rather narrow rim of clearing between the inclusion and the nuclear membrane. Cytomegalovirus does not exhibit the ground glass nuclear change that is typical for herpesvirus infection.

DeMay, A&S 2e. Viruses, p1466-1468

103 a increased mucus secretion

This liquid based specimen shows Curschmann spirals, which are casts of inspissated mucus. These spirals have a dark central axis and a translucent periphery. They are caused by increased mucus production due to chronic bronchitis, asthma, goblet cell hyperplasia or metaplasia.

DeMay, A&S 2e. Curschmann spirals, p215

104 d small cell carcinoma

The image shows small cohesive clusters of tightly packed small cells consistent with small cell carcinoma. Notice numerous apoptotic bodies in the background.

DeMay, A&S 2e. Small cell carcinoma, p241-244, 1182-1185

105 a carcinoid

The cytology shows relatively tight clusters of small cells that have round uniform nuclei and scant or absent cytoplasm. The nuclear chromatin is coarsely granular and speckled. Small nucleoli are visible. The cells gather in a nesting pattern. These cytologic features are those of a low grade neuroendocrine neoplasm, carcinoid tumor. The preferred terminology is low grade neuroendocrine neoplasm, since, while generally benign in behavior, if resected, some of these tumors can produce recurrence and metastasis.

DeMay, A&S 2e. Carcinoid tumors, p245-246, 586-587, 1188-1192

106 d reserve cell hyperplasia

Tight and cohesive fragments of small, bland and uniform cells are seen, with overlying ciliated bronchial epithelium. Mitoses and karyorrhexis and other features of small cell carcinoma are absent.

DeMay, A&S 2e. Reserve cell hyperplasia, p219; t2.9 Differential diagnosis of reserve cell hyperplasia vs small cell carcinoma, p242

ISBN 978-089189-6357 ©ASCP 2015

Chapter 6

Breast Secretions/Aspirations

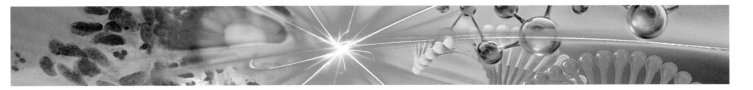

1. A well demarcated lesion presents cytologically as a large population of cells predominantly in syncytia, few glandular formations, and abundant single cells all possessing large nuclei with coarse, irregular chromatin and macronucleoli. The background contains numerous lymphocytes and plasma cells. The diagnosis is:
   a. poorly differentiated ductal carcinoma
   b. colloid carcinoma
   c. medullary carcinoma
   d. lobular carcinoma

2. FNA reveals apocrine cells with cellular crowding, slightly enlarged nuclei, fine chromatin, smooth nuclear borders, and prominent nucleoli, as well as naked bipolar nuclei. Based on these findings, the cells most likely represent:
   a. fibroadenoma
   b. comedocarcinoma
   c. reactive apocrine cells
   d. apocrine carcinoma

3. Which of the following lesions are more likely to be estrogen receptor positive by immunocytochemistry?
   a. colloid carcinoma
   b. medullary carcinoma
   c. ductal comedocarcinoma
   d. anaplastic carcinoma

4. Malignant breast tumors that clinically present as red, edematous lesions and have dermal lymphatic involvement are termed:
   a. sclerosing adenosis
   b. comedocarcinoma
   c. inflammatory carcinoma
   d. scirrhous carcinoma

5. Which of the following diagnoses may possibly be clinically managed using ductal lavage cytology?
   a. apocrine metaplasia
   b. fibrocystic disease
   c. ductal carcinoma in situ
   d. atypical ductal hyperplasia

6. A 68-year-old female presents with a bilateral breast tumor. FNA reveals a hypocellular sample of small cells attached to fibrocollagenous tissue with scanty cytoplasm and little pleomorphism. Single cells with intracytoplasmic lumens are also seen. The diagnosis is:
   a. lobular carcinoma
   b. tubular carcinoma
   c. carcinoid tumor
   d. adenoid cystic carcinoma of the breast

7. A 2 cm circumscribed mass was identified in the right upper outer quadrant of the breast of a 17-year-old female. FNA cytology reveals a clear fluid containing cells with central nuclei and eosinophilic granular cytoplasm in papillary groups, cells with foamy cytoplasm, a marked population of cells in sheets with uniform polarity, and naked bipolar nuclei. The diagnosis is:
   a. poorly differentiated ductal adenocarcinoma
   b. fibrocystic disease
   c. juvenile papillomatosis
   d. well differentiated ductal adenocarcinoma

8. The FNA of a breast mass yields a hypercellular population of monotonous, bland cells obtained from an elderly woman. Based on this, these findings are:
   a. consistent with a benign neoplasm
   b. diagnostic of ductal hyperplasia
   c. suggestive of an in situ carcinoma
   d. suspicious for malignancy

9. A 64-year-old female presented with a 3 cm mass in the right breast. FNA reveals a hypercellular smear containing large fragments of cells in a papillary grouping with dense fibrous cores, elongated pleomorphic nuclei with hyperchromasia and irregular nuclear membranes, and a background of necrosis. The diagnosis suggests:
   a. metastatic melanoma
   b. papillary neoplasm, rule out carcinoma
   c. spindle cell sarcoma
   d. Paget disease

10 The structures that are formed by the terminal ducts and ductules in the nonlactating breast are known as:
   a myoepithelial layers
   b fibroadipose tissue
   c nipples
   d lobules

11 FNA of nonpalpable mammographically detected microcalcifications in a 52-year-old patient reveals obvious malignant cells. Lymph node biopsies are negative. Which of the following may represent the cellular findings?
   a ductal carcinoma in situ
   b apocrine carcinoma
   c mucinous carcinoma
   d Paget disease

12 A bulky tumor of the breast that cytologically presents as monomorphic cells appearing singly or in clusters floating in islands of mucin as well as transverse branching capillaries is diagnostic of:
   a adenoid cystic carcinoma
   b papillary carcinoma
   c Paget disease
   d colloid carcinoma

13 FNA of a 3 cm breast mass yields a hypercellular population of small, uniform, basaloid cells arranged around balls of pink homogeneous globules. A mucinous background is identified as metachromatic with the Romanowsky stain. The diagnosis is:
   a adenoid cystic carcinoma
   b comedocarcinoma
   c medullary carcinoma
   d ductal carcinoma

14 A 50-year-old female with a firm, gritty mass in the left breast is evaluated with FNA. Cytology reveals a highly cellular population of disorganized and overlapping cell clusters, microacini, and single cells. Pleomorphic nuclei, prominent nucleoli, irregular nuclear membranes, and chromatin clumping are noted. The diagnosis is:
   a ductal adenocarcinoma
   b mucinous adenocarcinoma
   c lobular carcinoma
   d comedocarcinoma

15 An infiltrating ductal carcinoma that invades the epidermis of the breast is termed:
   a Paget disease
   b adenoid cystic carcinoma
   c papillary carcinoma
   d scirrhous carcinoma

16 A 55-year-old male with a history of estrogen treatment for prostate cancer presents with bilateral breast enlargement. FNA cytology reveals a large population of cells in sheets, some forming papillary fragments, surrounded by loose connective tissue. The diagnosis is:
   a ductal adenocarcinoma
   b metastatic prostatic adenocarcinoma
   c gynecomastia
   d idiopathic

17 A 67-year-old female presents to the clinician with multiple bilateral breast masses. FNA reveals an abundant population of pleomorphic cells with India ink elongated nuclei. Orangeophilic pearls were scattered across the slide. The most likely diagnosis is:
   a squamous carcinoma, breast primary
   b metastatic carcinoma, lung primary
   c fibromatosis
   d metastatic spindle cell melanoma

18 Benign mononucleate and multinucleated cells possessing frothy cytoplasm in nipple discharges are diagnostic of:
   a apocrine cells
   b foam cells
   c ductal cells
   d lipophages

19 A 52-year-old female presents with a bloody nipple discharge of 3 months' duration. Cytology of the breast smear reveals many 3D papillary groupings. The nuclei were oval with irregular nuclear membranes, anisonucleosis, and anisocytosis. Chromatin was finely granular with irregular distribution and macronucleoli were noted in most cells. A necrotic background is identified. These findings suggest:
   a micropapillomatosis
   b papillary apocrine metaplasia
   c atypical ductal cells
   d adenocarcinoma

20 A 6 cm breast mass was detected by a 33-year-old female. Cytology reveals a large population of fibromyxoid stroma and sheets of cells with honeycomb configuration. The lesion was removed. Grossly, the tumor, removed with wide excision, contained slitlike structures across the surface. The diagnosis is:
   a metaplastic carcinoma
   b primary breast sarcoma
   c fibroadenoma
   d phyllodes tumor

ISBN 978-089189-6357 ©ASCP 2015

21 A 45-year-old female presents with a bloody breast discharge and a subareolar nodule in her right breast. Cytology reveals 3D clusters of cells with smooth or scalloped cohesive borders and containing predictable nuclei that maintain polarity throughout the fragment. The diagnosis is:
a ductal adenocarcinoma
b ductal carcinoma in situ
c papilloma, neoplasm not excluded
d apocrine metaplasia

22 A 32-year-old female presents with a solid 2×3 cm mass in the upper outer quadrant of the right breast. Cytology reveals a hypercellular sample of cells in sheets with honeycombing characteristics, and cigar shaped bipolar cells. A fibromyxoid background is present. The diagnosis is:
a fibrocystic disease
b fibroadenoma
c fat necrosis
d lipoma

23 Benign nipple discharges are most often related to:
a ductal dilatation
b granulomatous disease
c cystosarcoma phyllodes
d lipoma

24 A 68-year-old female presents with thelitis, edematous areola, and nipple discharge. Cytology reveals large cells with abundant cytoplasm containing large nucleoli. Chromatin is fine and irregular in distribution. The diagnosis is:
a Paget disease
b foam cells
c papillomatosis
d medullary carcinoma

25 In the breast, an initial insult of periductal mastitis followed by scarring, stasis of ducts, and ductal dilatation forming macrocysts and fibrosis is considered to be:
a tuberculomas
b fibrocystic disease
c mammary adenocarcinoma
d apocrine papillomatosis

26 A 32-year-old postpartum patient with a painful thick breast discharge reveals abundant neutrophils and round to oval cells with fine regular chromatin, smooth nuclear membranes, and macronucleoli. A necrotic background is noted. The diagnosis is:
a cystic disease
b fibroadenoma
c lactating adenoma
d mastitis

27 A 42-year-old female presents with a 1 cm firm left breast mass after jogging 3 days earlier. FNA aspiration shows a yellow, thick substance cytologically containing amorphous debris, hemosiderin laden macrophages, multinucleated giant cells, as well as a population of cells in honeycomb configuration with enlarged nuclei. The diagnosis is:
a fibroadenoma
b mastitis
c fat necrosis
d fibrocystic disease

28 A 58-year-old female presents with a nipple discharge. Cytology reveals a monotonous population of cells with intracytoplasmic vacuoles, high N:C ratios, and hyperchromasia. Cellular configuration reveals a slightly cohesive population of cells forming a "stack of coins" or vertebral column. The diagnosis is:
a degenerative ductal cells
b ductal adenocarcinoma
c carcinoid tumor of the breast
d lobular carcinoma

29 Which is not associated with breast disease in pregnancy?
a lactating adenoma
b fibroadenoma
c fibrocystic disease
d physiologic nipple discharge without a mass

30 A 29-year-old pregnant woman in her second trimester presents with a 1.5 cm mass. Cytology presents a dirty background staining positive with PAS. A large population of cells in sheets with good polarity is present, as well as naked oval shaped cells. The diagnosis is:
a lactating adenoma
b fibrocystic disease
c ductal adenocarcinoma
d mucinous adenocarcinoma

31 A 33-year-old female presents with a 4 cm mass in the left breast. FNA reveals a colorless material cytologically presenting in an equal population of clusters of enlarged cells with prominent nucleoli and eosinophilic granular cytoplasm, cells with honeycomb appearance, foamy histiocytes, and blood. The diagnosis is:
a fibroadenoma
b ductal adenocarcinoma
c medullary carcinoma
d fibrocystic disease

32 What is considered the premalignant disease of the breast?
a fibrocystic disease
b fibroadenoma
c lactating adenoma
d lipoma

©ASCP 2015 ISBN 978-089189-6357

33 Sheets of small epithelial cells with smooth nuclear
    membranes and prominent cell borders found in nipple
    secretions are diagnostic of:
    a ductal lining cells
    b apocrine cells
    c foam cells
    d mastitis

34 An FNA specimen of a 2 cm soft nodular mass in the
    left breast of a woman presents cytologically as cells
    in sheets, producing a "chicken wire" appearance with
    crisscrossing capillaries. The diagnosis is:
    a fat necrosis
    b fibrocystic disease
    c fibroadenoma
    d lipoma

35 Cuboidal cells with centrally placed nuclei and
    eosinophilic granular cytoplasm found in nipple
    secretions are diagnostic of:
    a intraductal papilloma
    b foam cells
    c apocrine cells
    d lipocytes

ISBN 978-089189-6357 ©ASCP 2015

36 FNA of a 2 cm, bulky, gelatinous breast mass yields thick bloody material and malignant cells. What special stain will help confirm the diagnosis?

  a Congo red/medullary carcinoma
  b oil red O/ductal carcinoma
  c keratin/lobular carcinoma
  d alcian blue/colloid carcinoma

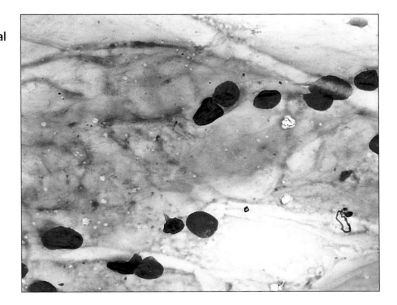

37 A 0.75 cm nonpalpable mammographically detected breast lesion is found in a 55-year-old female. FNA performed with a 22 gauge needle yields these cells. The diagnosis is:

  a mucinous carcinoma
  b tubular carcinoma
  c comedocarcinoma
  d medullary carcinoma

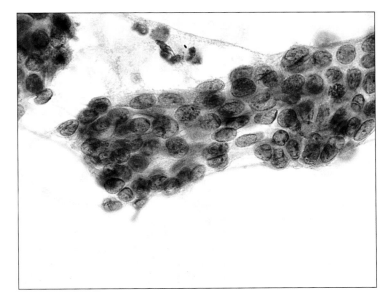

38 A 77-year-old male with a firm 4 cm lesion of the left breast presents for FNA. Cytology reveals:

  a ductal adenocarcinoma
  b gynecomastia
  c fat necrosis
  d mastitis

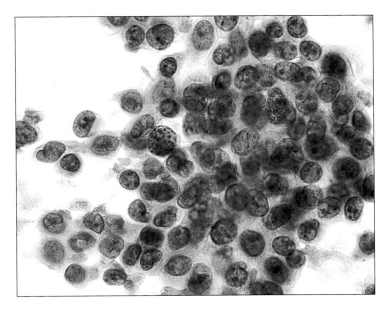

39 A 45-year-old female with a 4 cm lesion identified on mammography undergoes FNA evaluation. Aspiration of a soft fleshy mass yields copious blood and these cells. The cellular findings are diagnostic of:

   a ductal carcinoma
   b colloid carcinoma
   c medullary carcinoma
   d scirrhous carcinoma

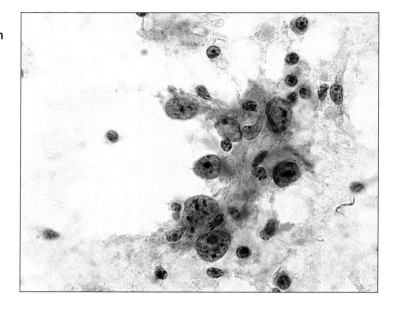

40 A 32-year-old female in her third trimester presents with a firm 3 cm lesion that had not been present 3 months earlier. The aspirated lesion reveals:

   a lactating adenoma
   b fibrocystic disease
   c ductal adenocarcinoma
   d Paget disease

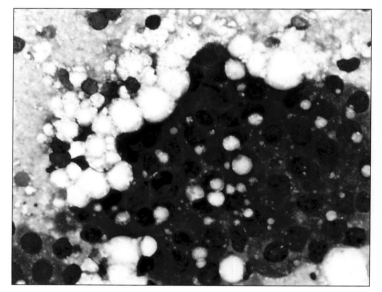

41 A 66-year-old female presents with an eczematous lesion of the breast and itching. Clinical examination reveals a 1 cm palpable mass. FNA reveals these cells. A positive reaction with which special stain will help confirm the diagnosis?

   a HMB45/melanoma
   b chromogranin/infiltrating ductal carcinoma
   c S100/lobular carcinoma
   d mucicarmine/Paget disease

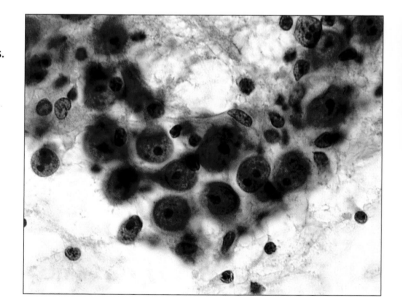

ISBN 978-089189-6357 ©ASCP 2015

42 A 32-year-old female with silicone breast implants presents with a pea sized lesion located in the left breast. The cellular findings from an FNA specimen with a 22 gauge needle represent:

    a chronic mastitis
    b inflammatory carcinoma
    c non-Hodgkin lymphoma
    d granulomatous mastitis

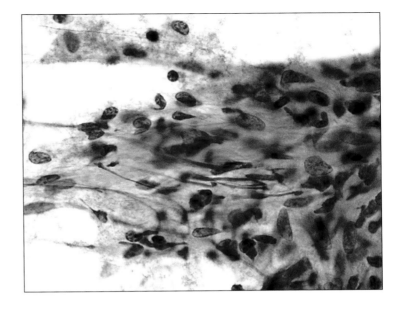

43 A 62-year-old female with a 3 cm nonmovable nodule in the upper outer quadrant of the left breast and dimpling of the nipple undergoes FNA. These cells are diagnostic of:

    a lobular carcinoma
    b fibroadenoma, tubular adenoma variant
    c mucinous adenocarcinoma
    d infiltrating ductal carcinoma

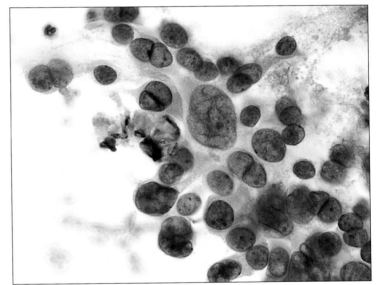

44 A firm 2 cm lesion of the breast is identified in a 22-year-old female athlete. Retraction of the nipple is evident. FNA of a gritty nodule reveals a yellow pasty material. Cytology reveals:

    a comedocarcinoma
    b colloid carcinoma
    c fibroadenoma
    d fat necrosis

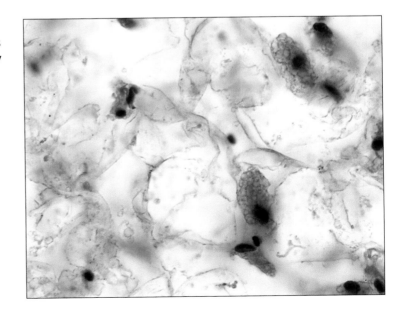

45 A 44-year-old female with periductal inflammation presents with a cystic mass in the left upper outer quadrant of the breast. Fine needle aspiration (FNA) reveals a cystic fluid. These cells represent:

   a fibroadenoma, juvenile variant
   b mastitis
   c fat necrosis
   d simple fibrocystic disease

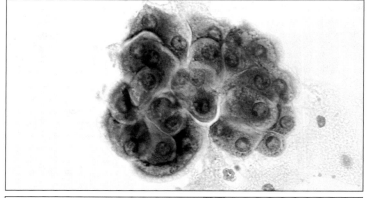

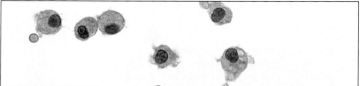

46 This group of cells is observed in a bloody nipple secretion from a 44-year-old female with no history of malignancy. Cytology reveals:

   a multinucleated foam cells
   b papillary ductal adenocarcinoma
   c papillary apocrine metaplasia
   d papillary clusters, neoplasm not excluded

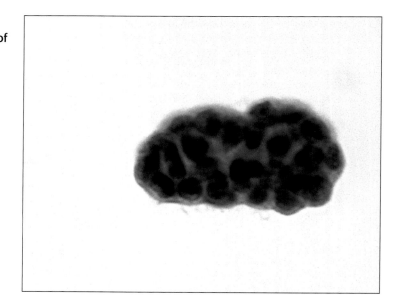

47 When found in nipple discharges, these cells represent holocrine secretion. These findings are consistent with:

   a foam cells
   b apocrine cells
   c ductal lining cells
   d mastitis

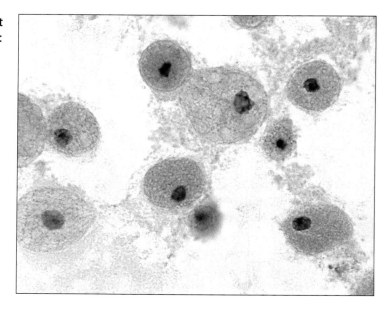

ISBN 978-089189-6357 ©ASCP 2015

48 A 2 cm, freely mobile mass aspirated from a
28-year-old female yields these cells upon FNA. The
cytologic findings are diagnostic of:
   a fibrocystic disease
   b lipoma
   c ductal carcinoma
   d fibroadenoma

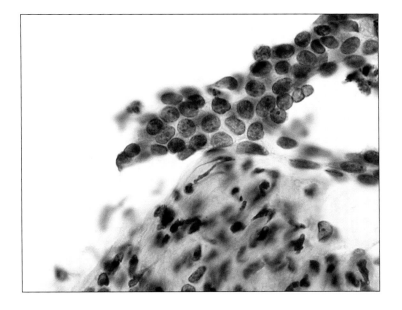

49 An aspiration of a gritty, 2 cm lesion from the left
breast of a 50-year-old postmenopausal woman yields
little material. These cells, identified upon cytologic
evaluation, are diagnostic of:
   a lobular carcinoma
   b ductal carcinoma
   c non-Hodgkin lymphoma
   d colloid carcinoma

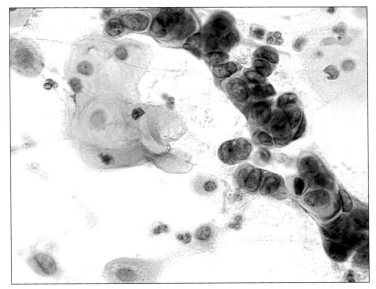

50 A yellowish nipple secretion yields these cells. The
cytologic pattern depicted is:
   a papilloma
   b apocrine metaplastic cells
   c ductal lining cells
   d foam cells

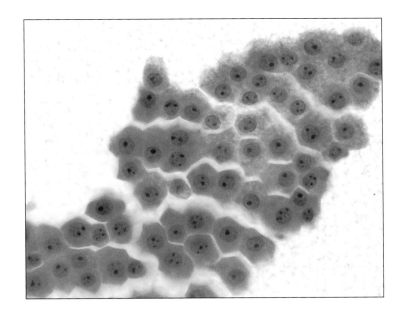

51 A firm, 5 cm mass is identified in the right breast of a 44-year-old female. FNA reveals the cells shown. These cells represent:

a fibrocystic disease
b medullary carcinoma
c tuberculoma
d phyllodes tumor

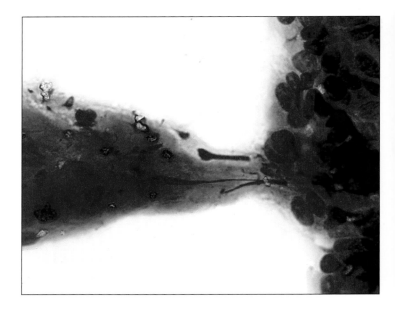

52 A 55-year-old male with cirrhosis of the liver presents with painful bilateral breast enlargement. FNA yields these cells. The diagnosis is:

a ductal carcinoma
b gynecomastia
c fat necrosis
d mastitis

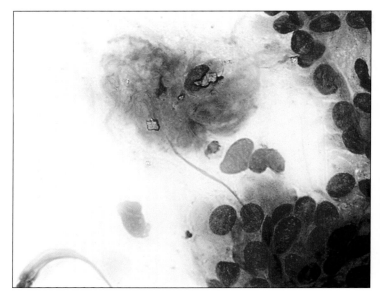

53 This smear from a breast mass FNA in a 50-year-old female with recent augmentation surgery demonstrates which of the following?

a coccidioidomycosis
b mucinous carcinoma
c myospherulosis
d silicone granuloma

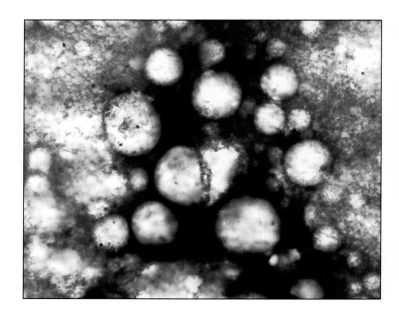

ISBN 978-089189-6357 ©ASCP 2015

54 This smear from a breast mass FNA in a 40-year-old female shows features most characteristic of which of the following?
- **a** papillary neoplasm
- **b** tubular carcinoma
- **c** lobular carcinoma
- **d** benign breast ducts

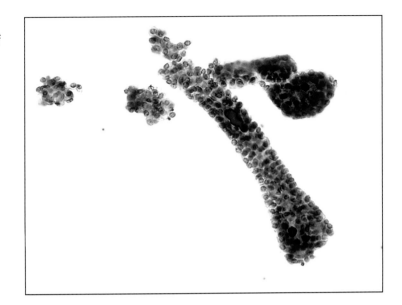

55 This breast FNA from a firm irregular mass with skin retraction in a 45-year-old female probably represents which of the following?
- **a** benign ductal cells
- **b** myoepithelial cells
- **c** macrophages
- **d** granular cell tumor

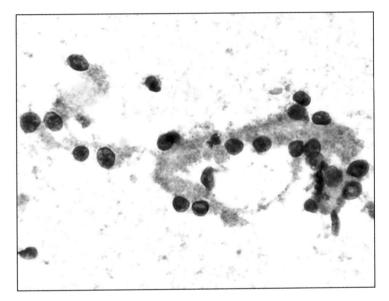

56 The darker staining nuclei in this benign breast FNA most likely represent:
- **a** apocrine cells
- **b** myoepithelial cells
- **c** macrophages
- **d** lymphocytes

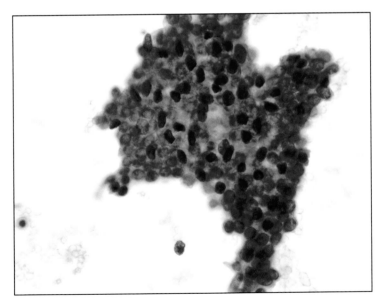

57 The large tissue fragment on the left in this FNA of a clinically suspicious breast mass most likely represents:

 a benign terminal duct lobular unit
 b fibroadenoma
 c ductal carcinoma in situ
 d papillary carcinoma

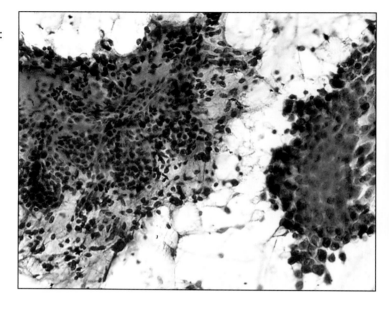

58 Breast FNA of a 2 cm soft round and mobile nodule clinically thought to be a fibroadenoma from a 54-year-old female reveals these cells. What is the most likely interpretation?

 a mucocele
 b nipple adenoma with ectasia
 c mucinous metaplasia in a fibroadenoma
 d colloid (mucinous) carcinoma

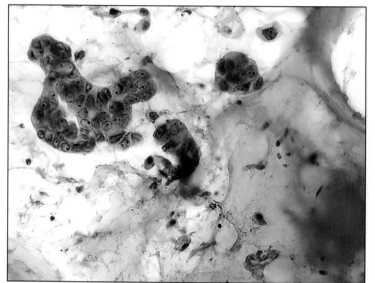

59 The most appropriate recommendation for this breast mass fine needle aspirate in a 50-year-old female is:

 a routine clinical follow-up with exams and mammography
 b flow cytometry
 c tissue sampling
 d repeat aspiration in 6-12 months

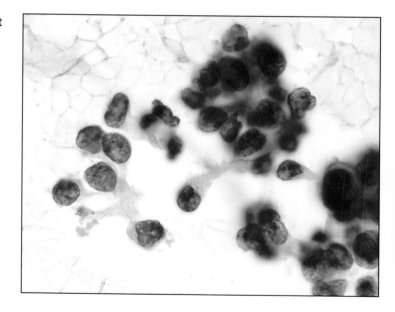

ISBN 978-089189-6357 ©ASCP 2015

60 This image from an aspirate of a 2 cm breast mass in a 75-year-old female depicts:

a mucinous (colloid) carcinoma
b metaplastic carcinoma
c apocrine carcinoma
d fat necrosis

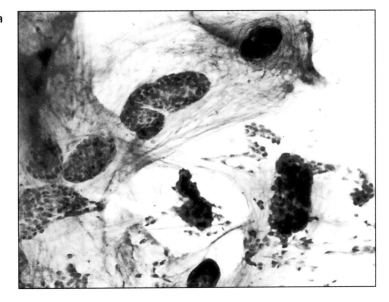

Breast Secretions/Aspirations *Answer Key*

1 c medullary carcinoma

These classic malignant features, as well as abnormal mitotic figures in conjunction with a background composed of lymphocytes, plasma cells, and histiocytes, identify this lesion as medullary carcinoma. Care should be exercised to differentiate the benign lymphocytes from lymphoma. Medullary carcinoma is mucin negative.

DeMay, A&S 2e. Medullary carcinoma, p1093-1094

2 c reactive apocrine cells

The appearance of "atypical" apocrine morphology is often associated with benign cystic changes. The described morphology suggests a reactive variant; furthermore, the presence of bipolar naked nuclei helps confirm the benign nature of the aspirate. The finding of apocrine cells, regardless of slightly atypical changes, is generally indicative of a benign process. True apocrine carcinoma is rare and often has concomitant ductal carcinoma.

DeMay, A&S 2e. Atypical apocrine cells, p1059-1060

3 a colloid carcinoma

Estrogen receptor (ER) status has become an important determinant in the therapeutic evaluation of patients with breast cancer. These steroid receptors may be identified with immunocytochemical techniques using antireceptor antibodies. Microscopically, ER positivity can be semiquantitated by the number and intensity of the cells staining. ER positive lesions are generally found in older, postmenopausal patients rather than premenopausal females. Small, well differentiated lesions, such as papillary and colloid carcinoma, are more likely to be ER positive, whereas large, undifferentiated lesions exhibiting aneuploidy are usually ER negative. In addition, tumors that exhibit necrosis or chronic inflammation are typically ER negative.

DeMay, A&S 2e. Hormone receptors, p1083

4 c inflammatory carcinoma

Inflammatory carcinomas are underlying carcinomas (usually ductal) which have spread to the dermal lymphatics; thus, the clinical presentation is that of inflammation and mastitis. This diagnosis carries a poor prognosis.

DeMay, A&S 2e. Inflammatory carcinoma, p1103

5 d atypical ductal hyperplasia

Women with a cytologic diagnosis of ductal atypia (atypical ductal hyperplasia) from ductal lavage or nipple aspirate fluid specimens are at a 4.9× greater risk for developing breast cancer compared with women without cellular atypia. Moreover, the risk of breast cancer increases 18 fold in women with confirmed cellular atypia (via ductal lavage) coupled with a family history of breast carcinoma.

DeMay, A&S 2e. Proliferative breast disease with atypia, p1116

6 a lobular carcinoma

Lobular carcinomas present as moderate cellular specimens composed of small, monomorphic epithelial cells with minimal nuclear deviation or pleomorphism. The cells possess scanty cytoplasm, often with signet ring morphology or intracytoplasmic lumens. Nuclear overlapping and eccentric nuclei may be noted on high power. Rare vertebral column formation may be noted. Fibrocollagenous tissue may be interspersed amongst the groups of epithelial cells. Mucin positivity is usually noted. Immunopositivity with E-cadherin (a cell cohesion protein encoded by a gene on chromosome 16q22.1) may help discriminate between lobular and ductal carcinoma of the breast. Lobular carcinomas lack expression while ductal carcinomas typically express cytoplasmic E-cadherin.

DeMay, A&S 2e. Lobular carcinoma, p1090-1091

7 c juvenile papillomatosis

The diagnosis of juvenile papillomatosis mirrors the cytologic findings seen with fibroadenoma. The diagnosis is predominately a clinical one; that is, it must be established in adolescent females. In juvenile papillomatosis, both the patient and the mother are at an increased risk for the subsequent development of breast cancer. Fibroadenomas cytologically present as hypercellular specimens containing sheets or clusters of ductal epithelium and abundant fibroconnective tissue (metachromatic with Romanowsky stain). The background contains copious single, naked, oval nuclei (often myoepithelial in origin) that are spindle or "cigar" shaped with bipolar features.

DeMay, A&S 2e. Juvenile papillomatosis, p1111-1112

8 d suspicious for malignancy

FNA of breast masses from elderly females should be carefully evaluated should the smears reveal a hypercellular population of monomorphic cells. These cells may represent infiltrating ductal carcinoma, mimicking the minimal deviation cytopathy also seen in lobular and colloid carcinoma. Ductal carcinomas found in elderly patients do not resemble their counterparts identified in younger patients. These lesions show little evidence of the classic malignant features detailed in younger females, appearing as monotonous sheets of ductal cells. Despite these cytologic findings, the vast majority of these lesions are histologically malignant; therefore, tissue evaluation must be performed even with the most innocuous appearing cytomorphology.

DeMay, A&S 2e. FNA biopsy of breast cancer, p1083-1084

ISBN 978-089189-6357 ©ASCP 2015

9   b   papillary neoplasm, rule out carcinoma

Papillary carcinoma resembles benign papillomas in its architectural patterns, presenting as hypercellular populations of 3D true tissue clusters with smooth borders and central fibrovascular interiors. Overlapping nuclei and nuclear atypia may be observed. Variation in number of cell types is a key in discriminating these malignancies from benign papillomas. Malignant papillary neoplasms are composed of a monotypic population of cells, whereas benign papillomas typically have polytypic populations that include apocrine cells, foam cells, and hemosiderin laden macrophages in addition to the papillary epithelial fragments. Papillary neoplasms presenting in older females are more likely to be malignant. Together, these minimal deviations may preclude an outright diagnosis of malignancy; therefore, the diagnosis of papillary neoplasm is recommended. Tissue biopsy must be performed to rule out invasion.

DeMay, A&S 2e. Papillary neoplasms, p1100-1102

10   d   lobules

The breast is composed of 15-25 radially arranged lobes that drain from separate ducts and terminate at the nipple. The ducts are composed of epithelial cells and surrounded by a myoepithelial layer. The lobes are subdivided into lobules that, in the nonlactating breast, result from the terminal ducts and ductules, collectively termed the terminal duct lobular unit.

DeMay, A&S 2e. Anatomy, embryology, and physiology of the breast, p1056-1057

11   a   ductal carcinoma in situ

Microductal carcinoma in situ (DCIS) may be detected on mammography but is usually nonpalpable. Axillary lymph nodes are disease free. The histologic presentation of these intraductal carcinomas shows a confinement to their basement membrane. The cytologic diagnosis cannot distinguish DCIS from frankly invasive ductal carcinoma. A variant of DCIS, comedo DCIS, presents cytologically as malignant ductal cells among a necrotic background– virtually indistinguishable from its malignant counterpart.

DeMay, A&S 2e. Carcinoma in situ, p1088-1090

12   d   colloid carcinoma

Colloid or mucinous carcinomas of the breast present as a monomorphic population of cells presenting in balls, acini, sheets, or as single cells scattered amongst a richly mucinous background ("sea of mucin"). The mucin is demonstrated as metachromatic with the Romanowsky stain or pale blue to pink with the Papanicolaou stain. These cells demonstrate few nuclear abnormalities with only slight anisokaryosis. The presence of anatomizing capillaries often accompanies the monotonous epithelial cells. Special stains with alcian blue or PAS will verify the mucinous nature of the background. Differentiation is important to distinguish these neoplasms from benign papillomas and mucocelelike lesions; however, colloid carcinomas generally occur in older patients and cytologically present with more abundant epithelial cells and irregular groupings.

DeMay, A&S 2e. Mucinous (colloid) carcinoma, p1094-1095

13   a   adenoid cystic carcinoma

Adenoid cystic carcinoma of the breast cytologically presents with metachromatic eosinophilic globules, either free within the background of the smear or contained within central lumens surrounded by acinar cellular formations, resembling "gumballs." The cytologic diagnosis of adenoid cystic carcinoma mimics those lesions arising within the salivary glands.

DeMay, A&S 2e. Adenoid cystic carcinoma, p1104

14   a   ductal adenocarcinoma

FNA cytomorphology of infiltrating ductal carcinoma of the breast presents as hypercellular epithelial cells arranged in sheets, cords, well formed microacini, and single cells. Pleomorphic nuclei, nuclear crowding and overlapping, hyperchromasia, irregular nuclear membranes, irregular chromatin, and prominent nucleoli make up the malignant nuclear characteristics. Special emphasis should be given to the identification of single cells and intracytoplasmic lumens (often mucin or lipid) with the above mentioned malignant criteria. Necrosis is exhibited in 60% of the cases.

DeMay, A&S 2e. Infiltrating ductal carcinoma, p1087-1088

15   a   Paget disease

Paget disease of the breast is a ductal carcinoma (arising within the lactiferous duct) which has eroded to the surface of the breast, often involving the nipple. Palpable lesions associated with this disease are usually malignant; conversely, nonpalpable lesions may represent an in situ carcinoma. Cytologic criteria mirror a typical ductal carcinoma. Differential diagnosis includes melanoma, a rare disease of the nipple. S100 and HMB45 may stain positive for both Paget disease and melanoma; however, the mucin positivity associated with Paget disease excludes melanoma.

DeMay, A&S 2e. Paget disease of the nipple, p1103

16   c   gynecomastia

Gynecomastia affects 50% of middle aged men. This disease may be related to an increase in endogenous or exogenous estrogen, illicit drugs, germ cell tumors, cirrhosis, and estrogen therapy for prostate cancer. The cellular findings associated with gynecomastia are similar to those found in fibroadenoma. Fibroadenomas cytologically present as hypercellular specimens containing sheets or clusters of ductal epithelium and abundant fibroconnective tissue (metachromatic with Romanowsky stain). The background contains copious single, naked, oval nuclei (often myoepithelial in origin) that are spindle or "cigar" shaped with bipolar features.

DeMay, A&S 2e. Gynecomastia, p1112-1113

17 b metastatic carcinoma, lung primary

The described cells represent a keratinizing squamous cell carcinoma, most likely metastatic from the lung. Due to the presence of multiple bilateral masses, a metastatic lesion would be favored over a primary SCC. Primary SCC of the breast is extremely rare and usually has an associated population of malignant ductal cells upon close microscopic examination, thus representing a metaplastic adenosquamous carcinoma. Metastatic malignancies account for <5% of all breast tumors. Other metastatic tumors may include melanoma, ovarian carcinoma, lymphoma, and genitourinary malignancies. Prostatic carcinoma should be considered when differentiating malignant breast tumors arising within men. In such cases, special staining with prostate specific antigen is useful.

DeMay, A&S 2e. Squamous cell carcinoma, p1099

18 b foam cells

Foam cells represent histiocytic cells that are often associated with physiologic nipple discharges. Their abundant frothy cytoplasm is easily visualized in cytology, and their nuclei are typically round to oval. At times, these cells are multinucleated.

DeMay, A&S 2e. The cells (foam cells), p294

19 d adenocarcinoma

FNA cytomorphology of infiltrating ductal carcinoma of the breast presents as hypercellular epithelial cells arranged in sheets, cords, well formed microacini, and single cells. Pleomorphic nuclei, nuclear crowding and overlapping, hyperchromasia, irregular nuclear membranes, irregular chromatin, and prominent nucleoli make up the malignant nuclear characteristics. Special emphasis should be given to the identification of single cells and intracytoplasmic lumens (often mucin or lipid) with the above mentioned malignant criteria. Necrosis is exhibited in 60% of the cases.

DeMay, A&S 2e. Infiltrating ductal carcinoma, p1087-1078

20 d phyllodes tumor

Phyllodes tumors cytologically mimic their counterpart fibroadenoma with the exception that these lesions typically present with greater cellularity. The presence of sheets and clusters (often atypical) of epithelial cells and abundant fibroconnective tissue (generally greater than that of fibroadenoma) with associated capillaries is helpful in establishing the diagnosis. Care should be exercised not to overestimate the atypia within the epithelial sheets. The prominent stroma and the lack of single abnormal cells should help to differentiate this neoplasm from ductal carcinoma of the breast. Conversely, malignant phyllodes tumors show abundant stromal overgrowth in sheets, poorly cohesive clusters, and single cells. The stromal cells exhibit nuclear atypia consisting of irregular nuclear membranes, irregular chromatin, multiple nucleoli, and, sometimes, intranuclear cytoplasmic inclusions. In malignant phyllodes tumors, osteosarcoma, chondrosarcoma, liposarcoma, angiosarcoma, or neurofibrosarcoma may represent the sarcomatous neoplasm.

DeMay, A&S 2e. Phyllodes tumors, p1077-1078

21 c papilloma, neoplasm not excluded

3D glandular fragments with smooth or scalloped cohesive borders and containing predictable nuclei that maintain polarity throughout the fragment are diagnostic of an intraductal papilloma (IP). These fragments may be associated with bloody discharges; thus hemosiderin laden macrophages may be present. Most papillomas and subareolar ductal lesions are generally of benign origin, often secondary to mastitis. This central breast lesion should not be confused with papillomatosis (also known as epithelial hyperplasia and epitheliosis), a peripheral breast lesion associated with ductal epithelial proliferation and fibrocystic disease. Fibrocystic disease is considered a "dysplasia," which places the patient at an increased risk for subsequent development of carcinoma of the breast. Although IP is a common benign disease, its exclusion from papillary carcinoma cannot be assumed, due to their shared cytomorphology. The diagnosis, "papillary clusters, neoplasm is not possible, excluded" is preferred until tissue biopsy or ductal excision is performed.

DeMay, A&S 2e. Papillary neoplasms, p1100-1102

22 b fibroadenoma

Fibroadenomas cytologically present as hypercellular specimens containing sheets or clusters of ductal epithelium and abundant fibroconnective tissue (metachromatic with Romanowsky stain). The background contains copious single, naked, oval nuclei (often myoepithelial in origin) that are spindle or "cigar" shaped with bipolar features. Naked oval nuclei are a necessary component in establishing the benign nature of this neoplasm. Care should be taken not to overestimate the importance of rare atypical cells that may sometimes be seen in conjunction with the cellular findings.

DeMay, A&S 2e. Fibroadenoma, p1073-1074

23 a ductal dilatation

Ductal dilatation secondary to fibrocystic disease, papillomas, or mastitis may create unilateral nipple discharges. Bilateral discharges may be subsequent to physiologic or endocrine disturbances.

DeMay, A&S 2e. Nipple discharge, p293-294

24 a Paget disease

Paget disease represents a ductal carcinoma (arising within the lactiferous duct) that has eroded to the surface of the breast, often involving the nipple and creating a "peau d'orange." Palpable lesions associated with this disease are usually malignant; conversely, nonpalpable lesions may represent an in situ carcinoma. Cytologic criteria mirror a typical ductal carcinoma. Differential diagnosis includes melanoma, a rare disease of the nipple. S100 and HMB45 may stain positive for both Paget disease and melanoma; however, the mucin positivity associated with Paget disease excludes melanoma.

DeMay, A&S 2e. Paget disease of the nipple, p1103

ISBN 978-089189-6357 ©ASCP 2015

25 b fibrocystic disease

Fibrocystic disease (FCD) is a result of initial periductal mastitis that in time produces scarring, ductal stasis with retrograde dilatation, and macrocystic lesions. FNA cytology reveals mastitis, foam cells, adipose tissue, clusters of normal appearing ductal epithelium, and apocrine metaplastic cells with their characteristic granular cytoplasm as well as prominent nucleoli. Certain variants of FCD, namely epithelial proliferation predominant, place the patient at an increased risk for subsequent development of carcinoma. FCD is seen as a triad consisting of cysts (fluid), fibrosis (acellular), or epithelial proliferation (papillomas).

DeMay, A&S 2e. Fibrocystic disease of the breast, p1068-1069

26 d mastitis

FNA specimens representing acute mastitis reveal acute inflammatory components rich in polymorphonuclear neutrophils and granulomatous tissue (epithelioid histiocytes and/or multinucleated giant cells). Reactive epithelial and mesenchymal cells may complement the cellular findings. Care should be exercised not to overcall these cells–clinical history and the benign nuclear features (smooth nuclear membranes, fine even chromatin) help discriminate these inflammatory lesions from a malignant process.

DeMay, A&S 2e. Acute mastitis and breast abscess, p1062

27 c fat necrosis

Smears with rich inflammatory components, including neutrophils, lipid laden histiocytes, multinucleated giant cells (with normal nuclear features), hemosiderin laden macrophages, and hypocellular populations of ductal epithelial cells found in association with a bubbly appearing lipid laden background are characteristic of fat necrosis. Reactive histiocytes and fibroblasts suggest mesenchymal repair. Although atypical nuclear features may be detected in mesenchymal cells, these changes should be treated with skepticism in light of the above benign cytologic findings. Furthermore, a clinical history of trauma and a recently appearing mass help support an acute diagnosis.

DeMay, A&S 2e. Fat necrosis, p1065

28 d lobular carcinoma

Lobular carcinomas present as moderate cellular specimens composed of small, monomorphic epithelial cells with minimal nuclear deviation or pleomorphism. The cells possess scanty cytoplasm, often with signet ring morphology or intracytoplasmic lumens. Nuclear overlapping and eccentric nuclei may be noted on high power. Rare vertebral column formation may be noted. Fibrocollagenous tissue may be interspersed amongst the groups of epithelial cells. Mucin positivity is usually noted. Immunopositivity with E-cadherin (a cell cohesion protein encoded by a gene on chromosome 16q22.1) may help discriminate between lobular and ductal carcinoma of the breast. Lobular carcinomas lack expression while ductal carcinomas typically express cytoplasmic E-cadherin.

DeMay, A&S 2e. Lobular carcinoma, p1090-1091

29 c fibrocystic disease

Fibrocystic disease (FCD) is a result of initial periductal mastitis that in time produces scarring, ductal stasis with retrograde dilatation, and macrocystic lesions. FNA cytology reveals mastitis, foam cells, adipose tissue, clusters of normal appearing ductal epithelium, and apocrine metaplastic cells with their characteristic granular cytoplasm as well as prominent nucleoli. Certain variants of FCD, namely epithelial proliferation predominant, place the patient at an increased risk for subsequent development of carcinoma. FCD is seen as a triad consisting of cysts (fluid), fibrosis (acellular), or epithelial proliferation (papillomas).

DeMay, A&S 2e. Fibrocystic disease (change) of the breast, p1068-1070

30 a lactating adenoma

These benign lesions are related to hypersecretory activity of the breast. FNA reveals true acinar cells with foamy cytoplasm that, when smeared, create a proteinaceous background due to the disruption of the intracytoplasmic secretory products. Tight lobules and sheets of ductal epithelium are typically found and may exhibit active nuclear criteria. The presence of bare nuclei that are uniform in size but may contain prominent nucleoli (related to reactivity) may be confused with a true neoplastic process. Slight anisokaryosis may be identified in rare cells. The clinical history of pregnancy should safeguard against the possibility of rendering a malignant diagnosis. Special staining with oil red O or PAS will help elucidate the proteinaceous nature of the background.

DeMay, A&S 2e. Lactational nodule (lactating adenoma), p1067

31 d fibrocystic disease

Fibrocystic disease (FCD) is a result of initial periductal mastitis that in time produces scarring, ductal stasis with retrograde dilatation, and macrocystic lesions. FNA cytology reveals mastitis, foam cells, adipose tissue, clusters of normal appearing ductal epithelium, and apocrine metaplastic cells with their characteristic granular cytoplasm as well as prominent nucleoli. Certain variants of FCD, namely epithelial proliferation predominant, place the patient at an increased risk for subsequent development of carcinoma. FCD is seen as a triad consisting of cysts (fluid), fibrosis (acellular), or epithelial proliferation (papillomas).

DeMay, A&S 2e. Fibrocystic disease of the breast, p1068-1070

32 a fibrocystic disease

Fibrocystic disease (FCD) is a result of initial periductal mastitis that in time produces scarring, ductal stasis with retrograde dilatation, and macrocystic lesions. FNA cytology reveals mastitis, foam cells, adipose tissue, clusters of normal appearing ductal epithelium, and apocrine metaplastic cells with their characteristic granular cytoplasm as well as prominent nucleoli. Certain variants of FCD, namely epithelial proliferation predominant, places the patient at an increased risk for subsequent development of carcinoma. FCD is seen as a triad consisting of cysts (fluid), fibrosis (acellular), or epithelial proliferation (papillomas).

DeMay, A&S 2e. Fibrocystic disease of the breast, p1068-1070

33 a ductal lining cells

Ductal epithelium presents in 2D sheets or clusters with normal polarity or often with honeycombing features, scanty cytoplasm, and round to oval dense appearing nuclei with micronucleoli. Moderate crowding may be seen (often related to hyperplasia). Should these cells contain secretory mucin, carcinoma should be considered.

DeMay, A&S 2e. Ductal cells, p1058

34 d lipoma

Lipomas represent benign neoplasms consisting of soft nodular collections of fat between septa. Capillaries and scanty connective tissue elements may also be seen. Differential diagnoses include fat necrosis or an inadequate sample due to an improperly sampled lesion.

DeMay, A&S 2e. Miscellaneous, p1060-1061

35 c apocrine cells

Apocrine cells are metaplastic ductal cells that resemble oncocytes of the salivary gland or thyroid. These cells present in polygonal forms arranged in sheets and clusters, or found as single cells. The cytoplasm is characteristically coarsely granular, containing central nuclei and often prominent nucleoli. DPAS+ glycolipid deposits may be present (Lendrum granules).

DeMay, A&S 2e. Apocrine cells, p1059

36 d alcian blue/colloid carcinoma

Colloid or mucinous carcinomas of the breast present as a monomorphic population of cells presenting in balls, acini, sheets, or as single cells scattered amongst a richly mucinous background ("sea of mucin"). The mucin is demonstrated as metachromatic with the Romanowsky stain or pale blue to pink with the Papanicolaou stain. These cells demonstrate few nuclear abnormalities with only slight anisokaryosis. The presence of anatomizing capillaries often accompanies the monotonous epithelial cells. Special stains with alcian blue or PAS will verify the mucinous nature of the background. Differentiation is important to distinguish these neoplasms from benign papillomas and mucocelelike lesions; however, colloid carcinomas generally occur in older patients and cytologically present with more abundant epithelial cells and irregular groupings.

DeMay, A&S 2e. Mucinous (colloid) carcinoma, p1094-1095

37 b tubular carcinoma

Tubular carcinomas may represent a stage in the development of ductal carcinoma, such as carcinoma in situ (DCIS). Cytology reveals cohesive clusters, single cells with intracytoplasmic lumens, tubular "garden hose" structures with central lumens, and glands with arrowheadlike outlines. The nuclei have fine, regular chromatin, and micronucleoli. Irregular nuclear membranes help support a malignant diagnosis. Differential diagnosis includes benign adenosis; however, this condition possesses grapelike glandular morphology.

DeMay, A&S 2e. Tubular carcinoma, p1092-1093

38 a ductal adenocarcinoma

Most breast cancers in men represent ductal carcinomas that recapitulate infiltrating ductal carcinoma arising within the female breast. FNA cytomorphology of infiltrating ductal carcinoma of the breast presents as hypercellular epithelial cells arranged in sheets, cords, well formed microacini, and single cells. Pleomorphic nuclei, nuclear crowding and overlapping, hyperchromasia, irregular nuclear membranes, irregular chromatin, and prominent nucleoli make up the malignant nuclear characteristics. Special emphasis should be given to the identification of single cells and intracytoplasmic lumens (often mucin or lipid) with the above mentioned malignant criteria. Necrosis is exhibited in 60% of the cases.

DeMay, A&S 2e. Cancer of the male breast, p1113-1114

39 c medullary carcinoma

This plate shows large anaplastic cells in sheets, clusters, and as single cells. These classic malignant features, as well as abnormal mitotic figures in conjunction with a background composed of lymphocytes, plasma cells, and histiocytes, identify this lesion as medullary carcinoma. Care should be exercised to differentiate the benign lymphocytes from lymphoma. Medullary carcinoma is mucin negative.

DeMay, A&S 2e. Medullary carcinoma, p1093

40 a lactating adenoma

These benign lesions are related to hypersecretory activity of the breast. FNA reveals true acinar cells with foamy cytoplasm that, when smeared, create a proteinaceous background due to the disruption of the intracytoplasmic secretory products. Tight lobules and sheets of ductal epithelium are typical and may exhibit active nuclear criteria. The presence of bare nuclei that are uniform in size but may contain prominent nucleoli (related to reactivity) may be confused with a true neoplastic process. Slight anisokaryosis may be identified in rare cells. The clinical history of pregnancy should safeguard against the possibility of rendering a malignant diagnosis. Special staining with oil red O or PAS will help elucidate the proteinaceous nature of the background.

DeMay, A&S 2e. Lactational nodule (lactating adenoma), p1067

41 d mucicarmine/Paget disease

Paget disease of the breast is a ductal carcinoma (arising within the lactiferous duct) that has eroded to the surface of the breast, often involving the nipple. Palpable lesions associated with this disease are usually malignant; conversely, nonpalpable lesions may represent an in situ carcinoma. Cytologic criteria mirror a typical ductal carcinoma. Differential diagnosis includes melanoma; a rare disease of the nipple. S100 and HMB45 may stain positive for both Paget disease and melanoma; however, the mucin positivity associated with Paget disease excludes melanoma.

DeMay, A&S 2e. Paget disease of the nipple, p1103

ISBN 978-089189-6357 ©ASCP 2015

42 d granulomatous mastitis

Leaky silicone implants have been associated with granulomatous mastitis, a disease that may clinically mimic infiltrating breast carcinoma. Cytologically, the presence of multinucleated giant cells with asteroid body inclusions, epithelioid histiocytes, and assorted inflammatory cells will be seen amongst a yellow or blue homogeneous, refractile/nonbirefringent background; however, silicone may dissolve in the staining process, leaving a background containing clear empty spaces.

DeMay, A&S 2e. Granulomatous mastitis, p1064

43 d infiltrating ductal carcinoma

FNA cytomorphology of infiltrating ductal carcinoma of the breast presents as hypercellular epithelial cells arranged in sheets, cords, well formed microacini, and single cells. Pleomorphic nuclei, nuclear crowding and overlapping, hyperchromasia, irregular nuclear membranes, irregular chromatin, and prominent nucleoli make up the malignant nuclear characteristics. Special emphasis should be given to the identification of single cells and intracytoplasmic lumens (often mucin or lipid) with the above mentioned malignant criteria. Necrosis is exhibited in 60% of the cases.

DeMay, A&S 2e. Infiltrating ductal carcinoma, p1087-1088

44 d fat necrosis

Smears with rich inflammatory components including neutrophils, lipid laden histiocytes, multinucleated giant cells (with normal nuclear features), hemosiderin laden macrophages, and hypocellular populations of ductal epithelial cells found in association with a bubbly appearing, lipid laden background are characteristic of fat necrosis. Reactive histiocytes and fibroblasts suggest mesenchymal repair. Although atypical nuclear features may be detected in mesenchymal cells, these changes should be treated with skepticism in light of the above benign cytologic findings. Furthermore, a clinical history of trauma and a recently appearing mass helps support an acute diagnosis.

DeMay, A&S 2e. Fat necrosis, p1065-1066

45 d simple fibrocystic disease

Fibrocystic disease (FCD) is a result of initial periductal mastitis, which in time produces scarring, ductal stasis with retrograde dilatation, and macrocystic lesions. FNA cytology reveals mastitis, foam cells, adipose tissue, clusters of normal appearing ductal epithelium, and apocrine metaplastic cells with their characteristic granular cytoplasm as well as prominent nucleoli. Certain variants of FCD, namely epithelial proliferation predominant, places the patient at an increased risk for subsequent development of carcinoma. FCD is seen as a triad consisting of cysts (fluid), fibrosis (acellular), or epithelial proliferation (papillomas). Simple FCD, such as that illustrated in these images, is composed of cysts and fibrosis.

DeMay, A&S 2e. Fibrocystic disease of the breast, p1068-1069

46 d papillary clusters, neoplasm not excluded

3D glandular fragments with smooth or scalloped cohesive borders, containing predictable nuclei that maintain polarity throughout the fragment are diagnostic of an intraductal papilloma (IP). These fragments may be associated with bloody discharges, thus hemosiderin laden macrophages may be present. Most papillomas and subareolar ductal lesions are generally of benign origin, often secondary to mastitis. This central breast lesion should not be confused with papillomatosis (also known as epithelial hyperplasia and epitheliosis), a peripheral breast lesion associated with ductal epithelial proliferation and fibrocystic disease. Fibrocystic disease is considered a "dysplasia," which places the patient at an increased risk for subsequent development of carcinoma of the breast. Although IP is a common benign disease, its exclusion from papillary carcinoma is not possible, due to their shared cytomorphology. The diagnosis "papillary clusters, neoplasm cannot be excluded" is preferred until tissue biopsy or ductal excision is performed.

DeMay, A&S 2e. Papillary neoplasms, p1100-1102

47 a foam cells

Foam cells represent histiocytic cells that are often associated with physiologic nipple discharges. Their abundant frothy cytoplasm is easily visualized in cytology, and their nuclei are typically round to oval. At times, these cells are multinucleated.

DeMay, A&S 2e. Foam cells, p1059

48 d fibroadenoma

Fibroadenomas cytologically present as hypercellular specimens containing sheets or clusters of ductal epithelium and abundant fibroconnective tissue (metachromatic with Romanowsky stain). The background contains copious single, naked, oval nuclei (often myoepithelial in origin) that are spindle or "cigar" shaped with bipolar features. Naked oval nuclei are a necessary component in establishing the benign nature of this neoplasm. Care should be taken not to overestimate the importance of rare atypical cells that may sometimes be seen in conjunction with the cellular findings.

DeMay, A&S 2e. Fibroadenoma, p1073-1074

49 a lobular carcinoma

Lobular carcinomas present as moderate cellular specimens composed of small, monomorphic epithelial cells with minimal nuclear deviation or pleomorphism. The cells possess scanty cytoplasm, often with signet ring morphology or intracytoplasmic lumens. Nuclear overlapping and eccentric nuclei may be noted on high power. Rare vertebral column formation may be noted. Fibrocollagenous tissue may be interspersed amongst the groups of epithelial cells. Mucin positivity is usually noted. Immunopositivity with E-cadherin (a cell cohesion protein encoded by a gene on chromosome 16q22.1) may help discriminate between lobular and ductal carcinoma of the breast. Lobular carcinomas lack expression while ductal carcinomas typically express cytoplasmic E-cadherin.

DeMay, A&S 2e. Lobular carcinoma, p1090-1091

50 b apocrine metaplastic cells

Apocrine cells are metaplastic ductal cells that resemble oncocytes of the salivary gland or thyroid. These cells present in polygonal forms arranged in sheets and clusters, or found as single cells. The cytoplasm is characteristically coarsely granular, containing central nuclei and often prominent nucleoli. DPAS+ glycolipid deposits may be present (Lendrum granules).

DeMay, A&S 2e. Apocrine carcinoma, p1096-1097

51 d phyllodes tumor

Phyllodes tumors cytologically mimic their counterpart fibroadenoma, with the exception that these lesions typically present with greater cellularity. The presence of sheets and clusters (often atypical) of epithelial cells and abundant fibroconnective tissue (generally greater than that of fibroadenoma) with associated capillaries is helpful in establishing the diagnosis. Care should be exercised not to overestimate the atypia within the epithelial sheets. The prominent stroma and the lack of single abnormal cells should help to differentiate this neoplasm from ductal carcinoma of the breast. Conversely, malignant phyllodes tumors show abundant stromal overgrowth in sheets, poorly cohesive clusters, and single cells. The stromal cells exhibit nuclear atypia consisting of irregular nuclear membranes, irregular chromatin, multiple nucleoli, and, sometimes, intranuclear cytoplasmic inclusions. In malignant phyllodes tumors, osteosarcoma, chondrosarcoma, liposarcoma, angiosarcoma, or neurofibrosarcoma may represent the sarcomatous neoplasm.

DeMay, A&S 2e. Phyllodes tumors, p1077-1079

52 b gynecomastia

The cellular findings associated with gynecomastia are similar to those found in fibroadenoma. Fibroadenomas cytologically present as hypercellular specimens containing sheets or clusters of ductal epithelium and abundant fibroconnective tissue (metachromatic with Romanowsky stain). The background contains copious single naked oval nuclei (often myoepithelial in origin) that are spindle or "cigar" shaped with bipolar features. Naked oval nuclei are a necessary component in establishing the benign nature of this neoplasm.

DeMay, A&S 2e. Gynecomastia, p1112

53 c myospherulosis

Myospherulosis represents the interaction of lipids and red blood cells, most often seen in aspirates of fatty sites, such as the breast. It is an incidental finding that by itself does not explain the presence of a mass.

DeMay, A&S 2e. Myospherulosis, p1062

54 b tubular carcinoma

The findings that support the diagnosis include rigid open tubular structures ("garden hose"), mild nuclear atypia, and lack of myoepithelial cells.

DeMay, A&S 2e. Tubular carcinoma, p1092

55 d granular cell tumor

The findings are characteristic of granular cell tumor, a usually benign mesenchymal neoplasm of probable Schwann cell origin (PAS+, CK–, S100+), which may clinically mimic carcinoma in the breast. The cells show abundant cytoplasm with prominent coarse granules, which may disperse in the background due to cellular fragility. Single cells and bare nuclei may be present. The nuclei are usually uniform, round to oval, and lack malignant features.

DeMay, A&S 2e. Granular cell tumor, p1092

56 b myoepithelial cells

The image demonstrates a sheet of benign ductal cells with a second layer of myoepithelial cells in a slightly different plane of focus. They are less regularly distributed than the ductal cells, have dark, often ovoid (bipolar) nuclei and inconspicuous cytoplasm. They may dangle from the edge of ductal groups or be dispersed as naked nuclei in the background. They are characteristic of benign lesions.

DeMay, A&S 2e. Myoepithelioma, p1105

57 a benign terminal duct lobular unit

The image demonstrates an intact lobular unit on the left, which contrasts sharply with a group of malignant ductal cells on the right. Intact lobular units are an uncommon benign nonspecific finding, which may be more commonly seen in aspirates of pregnant or lactating women.

DeMay, A&S 2e. The cells, p1058-1060

58 d colloid (mucinous) carcinoma

Abundant background mucin with cytologically malignant breast ductal epithelium, characteristic of a colloid (mucinous) carcinoma.

DeMay, A&S 2e. Mucinous (colloid) carcinoma, p1094-1095

59 c tissue sampling

Aspirates of ductal carcinoma show dispersed single malignant appearing cells. Such aspirates, whether diagnostic or suspicious, should have rapid follow-up with either additional biopsy material or resection depending on the clinical parameters.

DeMay, A&S 2e. Infiltrating ductal carcinoma, p1087-1090

60 a mucinous (colloid) carcinoma

Mucinous (colloid) carcinoma of the breast is characterized by cohesive groups of mildly atypical ductal epithelium in a background of mucin. Since the atypia can be slight, excision of mucinous lesions of the breast is usually recommended for a definitive diagnosis. Metaplastic carcinomas show striking atypia with a variety of stromas. Apocrine carcinoma consists of larger more atypical cells, often with a necrotic background. Fat necrosis usually shows macrophages and giant cells admixed with scanty, but mildly atypical ductal epithelium.

DeMay, A&S 2e. Mucinous (colloid) carcinoma, p1094-1095

ISBN 978-089189-6357 ©ASCP 2015

Chapter 7

Urinary Tract

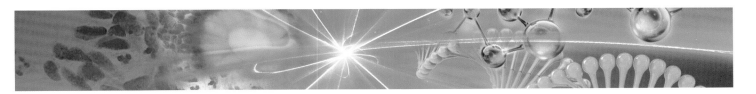

1   When evaluating papillary clusters in a urine specimen, what is imperative?
    a   knowledge of specimen color/texture
    b   knowledge of specimen collection method
    c   knowledge of a history of prostatic carcinoma
    d   knowledge of a history of prostatic hyperplasia

2   A voided urine specimen from a 68-year-old female reveals a large population of cells with cohesive features, tall columnar morphology, and palisading hyperchromatic nuclei with irregular nuclear membranes and irregular chromatin. A bloody, granular, "dirty" background is noted. What clinical finding would explain these cells?
    a   cystitis
    b   calculi
    c   rectovesical fistula shedding colonic adenocarcinoma
    d   nonpapillary urothelial carcinoma

3   A 60-year-old male, status post radical prostatectomy 2 years, presents with microhematuria and dysuria. Cytologic examination reveals abundant polymorphonuclear leukocytes, red blood cells, and a granular "dirty" background. Scattered degenerated and few well preserved single and clustered epithelial cells presenting with enlarged smudgy nuclei, irregular nuclear membranes, and macronucleoli are present. The cytoplasm, usually absent, is poorly preserved and vacuolated when present. The cytoplasm is often invaded with neutrophils. The cytologic findings are consistent with:
    a   cystitis related changes
    b   malakoplakia
    c   heavy metal related poisoning
    d   urothelial carcinoma, grade III

4   Cells presenting in loose clusters or papilla, with increased N:C ratios, enlarged hyperchromatic nuclear features, micronucleoli, and irregular chromatin from a voided urine are diagnostic of:
    a   renal cell carcinoma, grade I
    b   reactive urothelial cells
    c   papilloma
    d   urothelial carcinoma, low grade

5   A 66-year-old male presents with microhematuria and dysuria. Cystoscopy reveals red velvety focal patches on the bladder wall. A voided urine reveals papillary structures with irregular borders, crowded nuclei, and nuclear atypia. The chromatin is coarse and demonstrates clearing. The diagnosis is:
    a   urothelial carcinoma in situ
    b   papilloma
    c   low grade papillary urothelial carcinoma, grade I
    d   normal urothelial cells

6   A voided urine specimen from a 42-year-old female reveals an abundance of squamous cells among a mild inflammatory background. Your interpretation is:
    a   bilharzia
    b   squamous cell carcinoma, well differentiated
    c   unsatisfactory: contamination
    d   pathognomonic of bladder diverticula

7   A malignancy that may be derived from Brunn nests or cystitis glandularis is:
    a   squamous carcinoma
    b   adenocarcinoma
    c   renal cell carcinoma
    d   urothelial carcinoma

8   Bilharzia is associated with an increased risk of developing:
    a   squamous carcinoma of the bladder
    b   adenocarcinoma of the bladder
    c   urothelial carcinoma
    d   renal cell carcinoma

9   A bladder washing from a 55-year-old female showed many flat sheets of polyhedral cells with increased cellular and nuclear size. Cystoscopy was normal. The findings indicate:
    a   urothelial carcinoma, grade I
    b   benign papilloma
    c   normal cellular findings
    d   atypical hyperplasia

10 Adenocarcinomas arising within the urinary bladder cytologically resemble:
    a   reactive urothelial cells
    b   renal cell carcinoma
    c   colonic adenocarcinoma
    d   pancreatic adenocarcinoma

11 In the United States, bladder cancer is more common in:
    a   Caucasian women
    b   Caucasian men
    c   African American women
    d   African American men

12 A post prostatic massage urine specimen reveals round, concentric, noncalcifying structures in a population of columnar cells. These structures are identified as:
    a   psammoma bodies
    b   corpora amylacea
    c   cytomegalovirus
    d   nonspecific degeneration

13 Carcinoma of the bladder is common than carcinoma of the renal pelvis?
    a   more
    b   less
    c   bladder and renal cancer are similar in incidence
    d   the incidence of bladder and renal cancer are exactly the same

14 A catheterized urine specimen contains a sparse population of cells presenting in clusters with scalloping knobby borders and enlarged nuclei with central micronucleoli. A large population of normal urothelial cells is also present. The diagnosis is:
    a   reactive urothelial cells associated with catheterization
    b   urothelial carcinoma, grade I
    c   papilloma
    d   adenocarcinoma of the kidney

15 Cells from a voided urine specimen have abundant vacuolated cytoplasm and large nuclei with macronucleoli. Oil red O stains are positive. The diagnosis is:
    a   renal cell carcinoma
    b   melanoma
    c   metastatic colonic carcinoma
    d   hepatocellular carcinoma

16 A catheterized urine reveals single cells with coarse, irregular chromatin and irregular nuclear membranes in a bloody, necrotic background. The diagnosis is:
    a   urothelial carcinoma, grade III
    b   urothelial carcinoma, grade I
    c   squamous cell carcinoma
    d   adenocarcinoma

17 A 55-year-old female with dysuria undergoes a negative cystoscopy. Cytology of a voided urine specimen reveals many single cells with high N:C ratios, hyperchromasia, and macronucleoli. The diagnosis is:
    a   urothelial carcinoma, grade III
    b   papillary urothelial carcinoma
    c   reactive urothelial cells
    d   carcinoma in situ

18 A voided urine specimen contains papillary structures with fibrovascular cores and well preserved vesicular nuclear features. The best cytologic diagnosis is:
    a   benign papilloma
    b   papillary urothelial neoplasm of low malignant potential (PUNLMP)
    c   urothelial carcinoma, grade II
    d   renal cell carcinoma

19 A 4-year-old male presents with hematuria and flank pain. Cytology of a voided urine specimen reveals a mixed population of small, round cells with scanty cytoplasm and hyperchromasia as well as a rare population of spindle cells. The diagnosis is consistent with:
    a   Ewing sarcoma
    b   neuroblastoma
    c   Wilms tumor
    d   embryonal rhabdomyosarcoma

20 A mucosal neoplasm measuring 2 cm in diameter is found in the urinary bladder of a 61-year-old female. Cytology of a voided urine specimen reveals a population of small cells occurring singly and clustered with nuclear molding. Nuclear chromatin is coarse and irregular, and micronucleoli are identified. The patient has no previous history of malignancy. Which of the following may represent the findings?
    a   urothelial carcinoma, low grade
    b   Wilms tumor
    c   primary lymphoma
    d   small cell carcinoma, rule out bladder primary

21 A 57-year-old female presents to the clinician with flank pain, microhematuria, longstanding fatigue, and mental confusion. Serum analysis reveals hypercalcemia and abnormal liver function. Cytologic examination of a voided urine specimen reveals abundant degenerated cells found singly or in small groups with large, round, eccentrically located hyperchromatic nuclei and prominent macronucleoli. The cytoplasm, although sparse, is wispy or frothy. Special stains with oil red O, using fresh unfixed urine, reveal rare positive cells. The diagnosis is most suggestive of:
    a   prostatic adenocarcinoma
    b   renal cell carcinoma
    c   melanoma
    d   urothelial carcinoma

22 Keratinizing pearls were found along with a population of malignant urothelial cells in a voided urine specimen taken from a 51-year-old female. A hemorrhagic lesion is identified on the anterior wall of the bladder. Your diagnosis is:
    a   metastatic squamous carcinoma
    b   normal constituents of the trigone
    c   trigone hyperplasia
    d   squamous differentiated urothelial carcinoma

ISBN 978-089189-6357   ©ASCP 2015

23 Which of the following is associated with urothelial carcinoma of the urinary bladder?
   a aniline dye exposure
   b asbestos
   c neuroendocrine conditions
   d radium

24 The observation of isolated cells displaying variation in size and shape; cyanophilic cytoplasm; some cells with intracytoplasmic eosinophilic granules; fine, regular chromatin patterns; micronucleoli; and some multinucleated cells is diagnostic of:
   a transitional epithelial cells
   b squamous cell contaminant
   c navicular cells
   d renal tubule cells

25 A urine sample containing abundant degenerated columnar cells in a highly cellular inflammatory exudate is most often derived from which of the following collection types?
   a catheterized urine
   b voided "clean catch" urine
   c ileal conduit urine
   d bladder washing

26 Michaelis-Gutmann bodies are associated with:
   a malakoplakia
   b polyomavirus
   c sulfonamides
   d cholesterol plaques

27 A cystic condition involving the Brunn nests is termed:
   a cystitis
   b urethritis
   c barbotage
   d cystitis glandularis

28 Cystoscopy reveals glistening yellow plaques on the bladder mucosa. A voided urine specimen contains a few cyanophilic macrophages with laminated, calcified, intracytoplasmic, PAS+ structures. The diagnosis is:
   a Schistosoma infection
   b lithiasis
   c transitional hyperplasia
   d malakoplakia

29 Large numbers of cells in groups and clusters, numerous multinucleated cells, vesicular and degenerative nuclear features, and slight anisonucleosis are characteristic of which collection method?
   a voided
   b catheterized
   c post prostatic massage
   d ileal conduit

30 A patient receiving estrogen therapy for prostatic cancer submits a voided urine specimen for evaluation. Many cells with elongated cytoplasm, low N:C ratios, round to oval nuclei, and finely granular chromatin represent:
   a squamous metaplasia
   b renal tubule cells
   c seminal vesicle cells
   d prostatic adenocarcinoma

31 An HIV+ patient with complaints of fever and petechiae submits a voided urine specimen for cytologic analysis. Cells with large nuclei and basophilic intranuclear inclusions that demonstrate a clear zone between the inclusions and the nuclear rim are identified. These cells are associated with:
   a cytomegalovirus
   b urothelial carcinoma
   c polyomavirus
   d lithiasis

32 Colorless flat platelike structures with cut out corners in 9 "stairsteps" configuration found in a voided urine are diagnostic of:
   a bilirubin
   b sulfa
   c ammonium urate
   d cholesterol

33 Nuclear degeneration, necrosis, large numbers of erythrocytes, lymphocytes, and neutrophils among a scattered population of renal tubular cells are associated with:
   a chemotherapy associated changes
   b renal parenchymal disease
   c malakoplakia
   d urothelial carcinoma

34 What organism possesses a midlateral spine and is often associated with gastrointestinal disease?
   a *Schistosoma haematobium*
   b *Schistosoma mansoni*
   c *Schistosoma japonicum*
   d *Schistosoma egyptii*

35 A 60-year-old male presents with ureteral obstruction, hematuria, and flank pain. Cytology reveals rare cells with large nuclei, large multiple nucleoli, and abundant clear/vacuolated cytoplasm. Which stain might aid in the diagnosis?
   a alcian blue-hyaluronidase
   b Gomori methenamine silver
   c Wright-Giemsa
   d Sudan black

36 A 44-year-old male on corticosteroid therapy presents with urinary stasis. A catheterized urine reveals small cells with elongated/stretched cytoplasm and degenerative smudged nuclei. These cells may represent:
a urothelial carcinoma, grade III
b hypernephroma
c polyomavirus infection
d cytomegalovirus infection

37 A 50-year-old male being evaluated for prostatic hyperplasia submits a urine specimen for evaluation. Seen are cuboidal to bizarre cells with large, irregular, hyperchromatic nuclei and micronucleoli in single forms and clusters. Cyanophilic cytoplasm with golden-orange granules are found. These cells represent:
a urothelial carcinoma, grade III
b seminal vesicle cells
c prostatic adenocarcinoma
d renal cell carcinoma

38 The presence of intracytoplasmic eosinophilic inclusions composed of mucopolysaccharide is diagnostic of:
a degeneration
b lithiasis
c polyomavirus infection
d herpesvirus infection

39 A 44-year-old airline flight attendant presents with spiking fever. Urine cytology reveals abundant binucleate single cells with eosinophilic refractile intracytoplasmic granules. Also found were multiple large oval structures with a terminal spinelike structure. Cytology is consistent with a diagnosis of:
a idiopathic eosinophilia
b *Schistosoma haematobium*
c calculus
d malakoplakia

40 A 42-year-old male with a history of urothelial carcinoma is treated intravesicularly with triethylenethiophosphoramide (thiotepa). Cytology reveals many large cells with abundant cytoplasm and proportionately enlarged nuclei. Many cells demonstrate normochromasia and others reveal smudgy nuclear features. Multinucleation is common. Based on the following, these cells are:
a recurrent urothelial carcinoma
b renal cell carcinoma
c chemotherapy associated changes
d urothelial carcinoma in situ

41 Crystalline structures that are described as fine silky needles in sheaves or rosettes are:
a cystine
b calcium carbonate
c calcium oxalate
d tyrosine

42 Areas of mucus secreting glandular epithelium may represent:
a heavy metal exposure
b cystitis cystica
c fecal contaminant
d pyelogram effect

43 Acid-fast intranuclear inclusions staining eosinophilic with the Papanicolaou stain are found within the cytoplasm of cells of a voided urine specimen. The specimen was taken from a 4-year-old child with abdominal pain. The diagnosis is:
a polyomavirus infection
b degenerative changes
c infectious mononucleosis
d lead poisoning

44 A voided urine specimen from an immunosuppressed patient reveals cells with large basophilic intranuclear inclusions obliterating the nucleus. Electron microscopy indicates many nonencapsulated virions arranged in a crystalline fashion. The diagnosis is:
a herpesvirus
b cytomegalovirus
c human polyomavirus
d human papillomavirus

ISBN 978-089189-6357 ©ASCP 2015

45 The cytologic findings represent a voided urine specimen from a 55-year-old Egyptian immigrant. These cells represent:

   a squamous cell carcinoma, bladder primary
   b metastatic squamous cell carcinoma
   c squamous dysplasia
   d normal contaminant from the uterine corpus

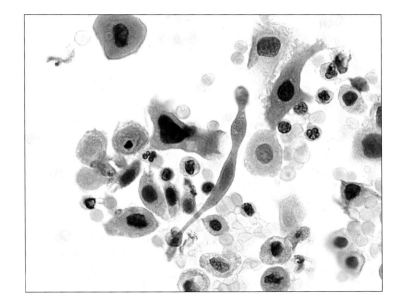

46 A 66-year-old female with a history of urinary stones presents with these structures in a voided urine specimen. They represent:

   a uric acid crystals
   b triple phosphate crystals
   c calcium phosphate crystals
   d calcium carbonate crystals

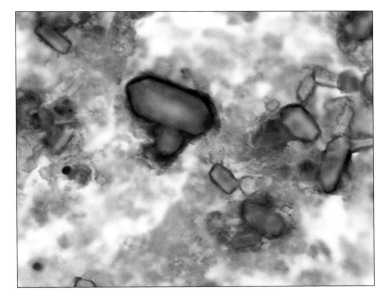

47 A 26-year-old female being treated for a gynecologic infection with broad spectrum antibiotics presents with cystitis and microhematuria. The cytologic findings suggest an infection by:

   a *Blastomyces* species
   b *Aspergillus* species
   c *Candida* species
   d *Nocardia* species

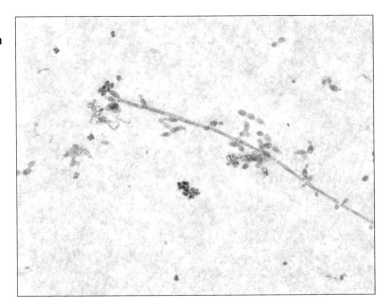

48 A catheterized urine specimen is collected from a 44-year-old female with urinary obstruction. The findings suggest:

   a lithiasis, cholesterol crystals
   b lithiasis, calcium phosphate crystals
   c lithiasis, calcium oxalate crystals
   d lithiasis, calcium carbonate crystals

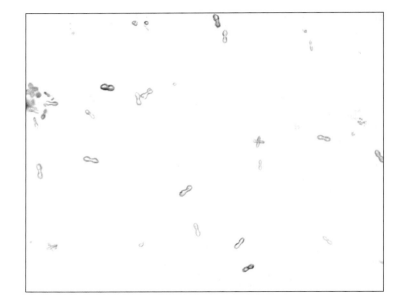

49 A voided urine specimen from a patient with a negative cystoscopic test result yields these cells for analysis. Their presence suggests:

   a urothelial carcinoma, grade III
   b urothelial carcinoma in situ
   c papillary urothelial carcinoma, grade I
   d degenerating transitional epithelial cells

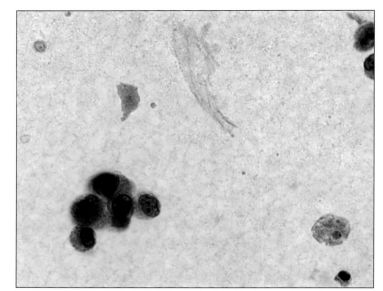

50 A voided urine specimen from a 55-year-old male yields these cells. The best diagnosis is:

   a benign papilloma
   b papillary neoplasm, rule out urothelial carcinoma
   c urothelial carcinoma in situ
   d reactive/reparative cellular changes

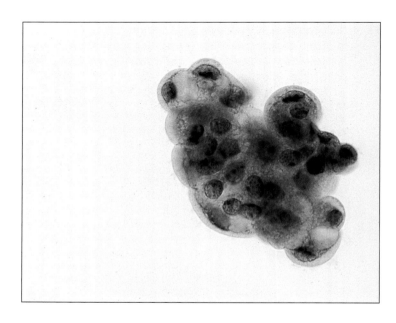

ISBN 978-089189-6357 ©ASCP 2015

51 A 67-year-old male with urethral obstruction and elevated alkaline phosphatase levels yields a catheterized urine specimen. The cytologic pattern represents:

a urothelial carcinoma
b renal cell carcinoma
c squamous cell carcinoma
d prostate adenocarcinoma

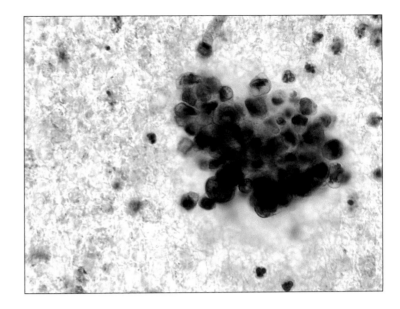

52 These cells are identified in a voided urine specimen in a 45-year-old female with flank pain and microhematuria. A 3 cm lesion is identified within the renal calyces. What stain will help confirm the diagnosis?

a mucicarmine
b oil red O
c alcian blue
d Warthin-Starry

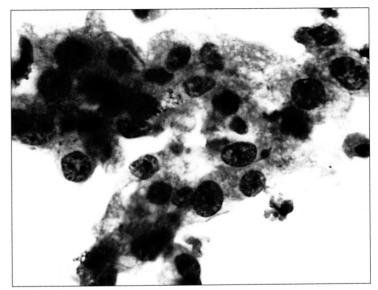

53 These cells were identified in a catheterized urine specimen from a 69-year-old male with an ulcerative lesion and microhematuria. The diagnosis is consistent with:

a urothelial carcinoma, grade I
b renal cell carcinoma
c urothelial carcinoma, grade III
d adenocarcinoma arising from cystitis glandularis

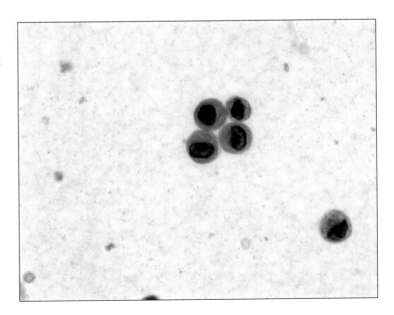

54 These cells in a voided urine specimen are from a 44-year-old female with hematuria. Their presence is most likely related to:

  a well differentiated squamous carcinoma
  b vaginal contamination
  c lead poisoning
  d lithiasis

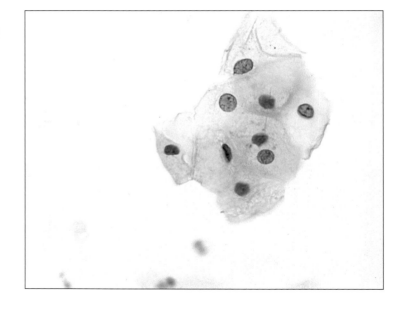

55 This catheterized urine specimen from a 44-year-old female with cystitis shows:

  a normal catheterized urothelial changes
  b *Escherichia coli*
  c human polyomavirus
  d urothelial carcinoma, grade I

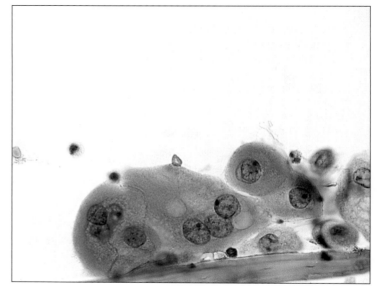

56 These cells in a voided urine specimen may arise from:

  a malakoplakia
  b vulva
  c bladder dome
  d nephron

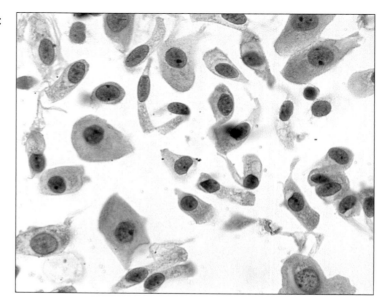

ISBN 978-089189-6357 ©ASCP 2015

57 An alkaline urine sample reveals these structures. They are suggestive of:

a uric acid crystals
b triple phosphate crystals
c calcium phosphate crystals
d calcium carbonate crystals

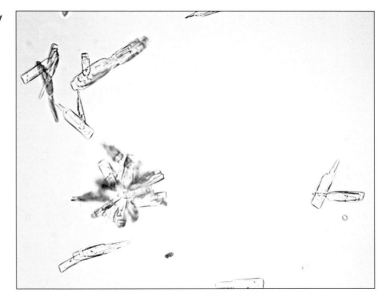

58 These structures identified in a post prostate massage specimen are suggestive of:

a psammoma body
b corpora amylacea
c navicular cell
d metastatic adenocarcinoma

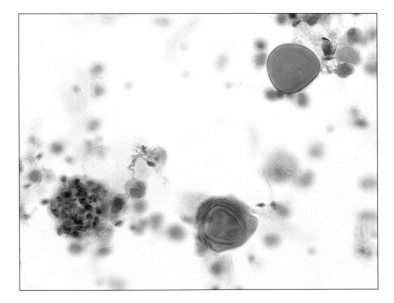

59 This structure is found in a 55-year-old female. Which of the following statements is most applicable?

a the findings are consistent with malignant renal cell carcinoma
b the patient has a history of schistosomiasis exposure
c the patient has a history of malakoplakia
d this cell is infected with the human polyomavirus

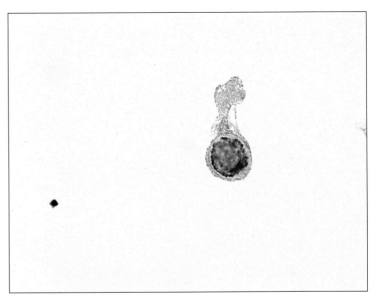

60 These structures are associated with:
  a urinary calculi
  b malakoplakia
  c *Escherichia coli* infection
  d carcinoma of the bladder

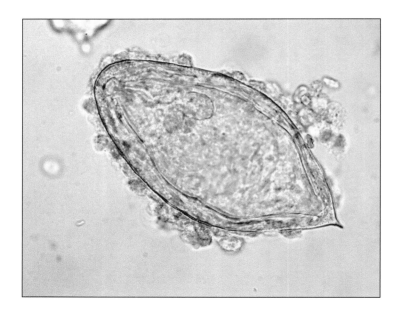

61 A febrile 2-year-old female is unable to urinate. A catheterized urine sample reveals these cells. They represent:
  a herpesvirus
  b cytomegalovirus
  c polyomavirus
  d nonspecific cellular findings

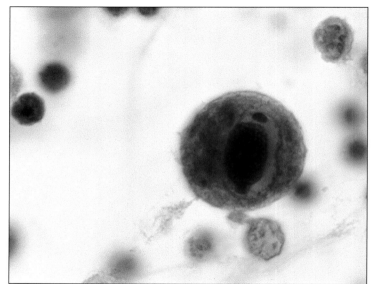

62 A 55-year-old diabetic male who recently underwent kidney transplantation presents with microhematuria and flank pain. A voided urine specimen reveals these structures. They are:
  a renal casts
  b columnar urothelial cells
  c prostatic cells
  d glomeruli

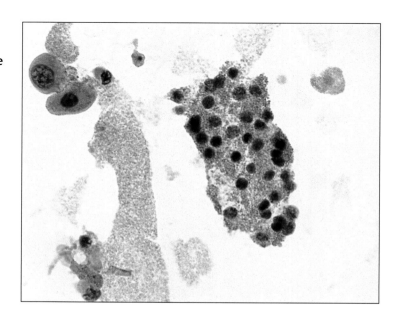

ISBN 978-089189-6357 ©ASCP 2015

63 A voided urine specimen from a 55-year-old male with a recent urinary obstruction reveals these cells. The diagnosis is:

  a prostatic adenocarcinoma
  b benign prostatic hypertrophy
  c normal urothelial cells
  d human polyomavirus infection

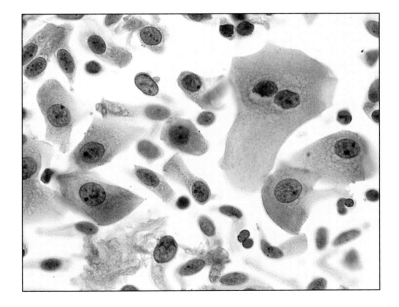

64 This voided urine shows changes compatible with a diagnosis of:

  a high grade urothelial carcinoma
  b polyomavirus
  c cytomegalovirus
  d treatment effect

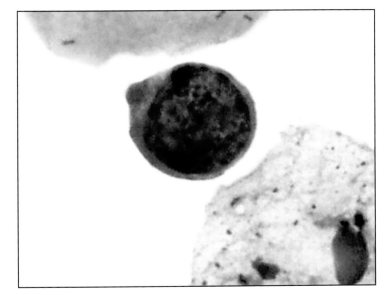

65 This bladder washing, obtained at cystoscopy from a 60-year-old patient with hematuria who is status post bone marrow transplant, shows:

  a adenocarcinoma
  b herpes infection
  c umbrella cells
  d high grade urothelial cell carcinoma

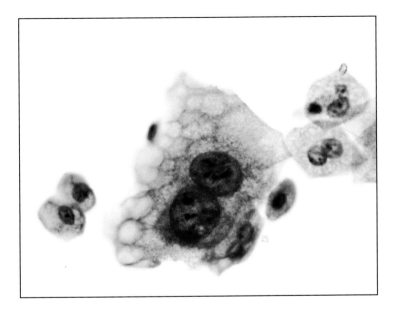

66 This bladder washing is from a 73-year-old male with a history of a urothelial carcinoma in situ. What is the apppropriate interpretation of this cell group?

 a persistant carcinoma in situ
 b invasive urothelial carcinoma
 c granulomatous cystitis
 d eosinophilic cystitis

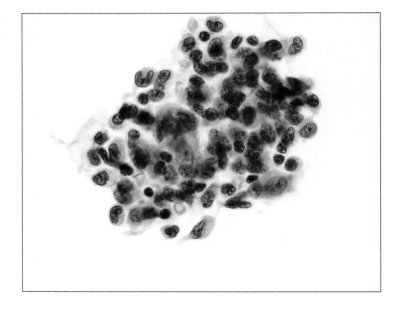

67 This voided urine from a 65-year-old male with hematuria shows:

 a low grade urothelial carcinoma
 b treatment effect
 c prostatic adenocarcinoma
 d polyomavirus

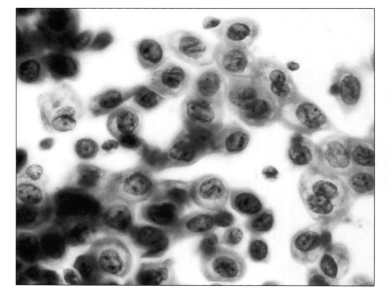

68 This 56-year-old female presented with hematuria and left flank pain. A voided urine submitted for cytologic evaluation favors which disease process?

 a nephrolithiasis
 b osmotic nephrosis
 c urothelial carcinoma, high grade
 d chromophobe carcinoma

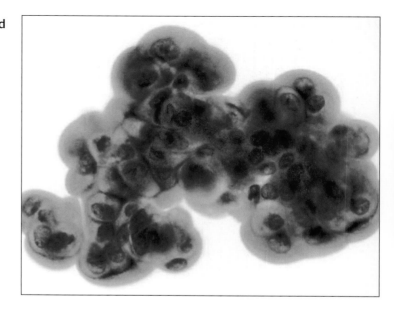

ISBN 978-089189-6357 ©ASCP 2015

69 This urine specimen was obtained from:

   a 34-year-old female with microscopic hematuria
   b 73-year-old male with history of a T3 stage bladder cancer
   c 64-year-old female with a T1 stage bladder cancer
   d 53-year-old female with colon cancer

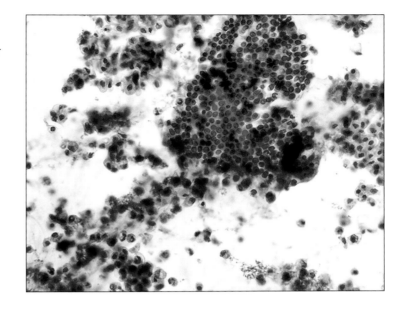

70 Voided urine from a 45-year-old male with microhematuria. What would be the favored diagnosis?

   a urothelial carcinoma, high grade
   b urothelial carcinoma, low grade
   c prostatic adenocarcinoma
   d nephrolithiasis

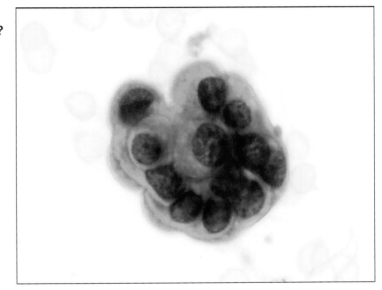

71 Voided urine from a 67-year-old male with a history of urothelial carcinoma. What is your diagnosis?

   a low grade urothelial carcinoma
   b high grade urothelial carcinoma
   c seminal vesicle cell
   d polyomavirus infected cell

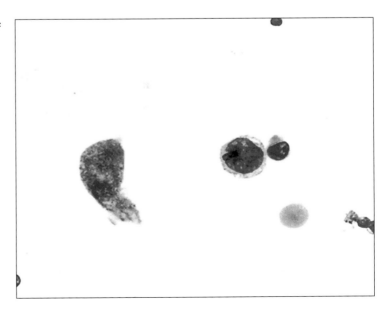

72   What type of a specimen is depicted in the image?
   a   voided urine
   b   ileal conduit
   c   bladder washing
   d   kidney FNA

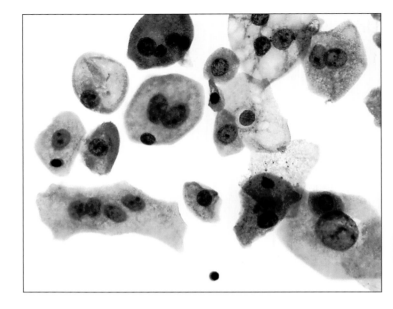

ISBN 978-089189-6357 ©ASCP 2015

Urinary Tract *Answer Key*

1   **b**   **knowledge of specimen collection method**

Normal catheterized urine specimens contain a hypercellular and heterogeneous population of normal urothelial cells that includes dome or superficial cells, sheets of oval intermediate type urothelial cells, squamous cells, and occasional columnar cells, usually from the Brunn nests. The urothelial cells contain round, hypochromatic or degenerative nuclei and granular cytoplasm. Reactive nuclear changes may be detected by the observation of slightly enlarged nuclei and prominent nucleoli; however, normal N:C ratios and benign chromatin patterns detected in well preserved urothelial cells establish their benignity. Careful attention should be given to the differentiation of pseudoclusters (associated with catheterization) from true papillary groupings (such as those found with low grade papillary neoplasms).

DeMay, A&S 2e. Catheterized urine, p448

2   **c**   **rectovesical fistula shedding colonic adenocarcinoma**

Colonic adenocarcinomas extending into the bladder present with columnar morphology, apical cytoplasmic densities ("terminal barlike"), and palisading nuclei with classic malignant nuclear criteria. Due to its direct invasion, a granular, necrotic diathesis is also present (most metastatic lesions appear in a clean background unless they have seeded). Clinical history is important in establishing any metastatic lesion.

DeMay, A&S 2e. Other metastases, p476

3   **a**   **cystitis related changes**

Cystitis is a common finding in women (due to the short nature of the urethra), often secondary to fecal contamination (infection by *Escherichia coli, Proteus, Klebsiella, Enterobacter, Streptococcus, Pseudomonas*) and in patients who have had genitourinary surgery (such as transurethral resection of the prostate or prostatectomy). Degenerative cells are common, although the preserved urothelial cells will often have alarming features, including hyperchromatic nuclei and coarse chromatin with clearing. Malignancy, though, is generally associated with increased necrosis and less inflammation (unless ulcerative), and is usually composed of well preserved cells with crisp, distinct nuclei and typical malignant features (coarsely granular, irregularly distributed chromatin). Other infectious agents which may be cytologically detected in urinary specimens include trichomonads, amebae, and schistosomes. Cellular changes secondary to tuberculosis may also create mild to severe reactive epithelial atypia.

DeMay, A&S 2e. Cystitis, p450-454

4   **d**   **urothelial carcinoma, low grade**

Loosely cohesive groups and papillae with frankly malignant criteria are diagnostic of urothelial carcinoma, grade II (low grade). The presence of abnormal nuclear features, including enlarged nuclei and irregular chromatin distribution represent key features of urothelial cell malignancies. Suspicion should be raised if the background contains a population of small pyknotic urothelial cells.

DeMay, A&S 2e. Low grade urothelial carcinoma, p402

5   **c**   **low grade papillary urothelial cell carcinoma, grade I**

The presence of true papillary clusters identified in urinary specimens is suggestive of a low grade papillary neoplasm. These lesions cannot be excluded from grade I urothelial carcinoma. In the absence of classic malignant nuclear morphology, the diagnosis of carcinoma remains. These cells present with uniform cell borders, micronucleoli and finely granular, regularly distributed chromatin (when visible). Differentiating these low grade neoplasms in catheterized specimens may prove difficult; however, the presence of true cohesive smooth borders will help confirm a neoplastic process.

DeMay, A&S 2e. Low grade papillary urothelial carcinoma, p462-463

6   **c**   **unsatisfactory: contamination**

Vaginal contamination may preclude the possibility of a satisfactory diagnosis in voided urine specimens. Voided urine specimens normally contain a hypocellular population of urothelial cells. Squamous contamination may easily obscure urothelial cells or be the sole representative population in unsatisfactory urine specimens.

DeMay, A&S 2e. Squamous cells and squamous metaplasia, p444, 472-473

7   **b**   **adenocarcinoma**

2 varieties of adenocarcinoma may arise within the bladder. The first type resembles colonic adenocarcinoma (mucin+), while the second variety is a signet ring carcinoma (also mucin+).

DeMay, A&S 2e. Adenocarcinoma, p407-408

8   **a**   **squamous carcinoma of the bladder**

Schistosoma haematobium is a parasitic fluke found in Africa and the Middle East that embeds within the bladder mucosa, eventually creating squamous metaplasia and squamous cell carcinoma. The cytology reveals transparent ova with a terminal spine. Schistosomiasis is also referred to as bilharzia. Differential diagnosis is the lemon drop form of uric acid crystals.

DeMay, A&S 2e. Schistosomiasis, p451

9   **c**   **normal cellular findings**

Bladder washings or barbotage yield hypercellular specimens consisting of sheets of urothelial cells, pseudopapillary fragments, and single cells. Cells from the deeper regions of the transitional epithelium are small and hypochromatic, and exhibit macronucleoli. Reactive nuclear changes may necessitate the differential diagnosis of neoplasia.

DeMay, A&S 2e. Bladder washings, p448-449

10   **c**   **colonic adenocarcinoma**

2 varieties of adenocarcinoma may arise within the bladder. The first type resembles colonic adenocarcinoma (mucin+), while the second variety is a signet ring carcinoma (also mucin+).

DeMay, A&S 2e. Adenocarcinoma, p473

11   **b**   **Caucasian men**

Bladder cancer is 3× more common in men than women, and 2× as common in Caucasians than African Americans.

DeMay, A&S 2e. Urinary tract cancer, p460

12 b corpora amylacea

Corpora amylacea are basophilic, condensed, concentrically laminated, glycogenated, noncalcifying structures originating from the prostate.

DeMay, A&S 2e. Corpora amylacea, p446

13 a more

In the United States, there are 50,000 new cases of bladder cancer annually and 11,000 deaths, representing ~2% of all cancer related mortalities. Bladder cancer is 10-20× more common than carcinoma of the renal pelvis and ureter and is increasing in incidence. The average age of patients is between 65 and 70 years (rare before age 40).

DeMay, A&S 2e. Urinary tract cancer, p460

14 a reactive urothelial cells associated with catheterization

Normal catheterized urine specimens contain a hypercellular and heterogeneous population of normal urothelial cells that includes dome or superficial cells, sheets of oval intermediate type urothelial cells, squamous cells, and occasional columnar cells, usually from the Brunn nests. The urothelial cells contain round, hypochromatic or degenerative nuclei and granular cytoplasm. Reactive nuclear changes may be detected by the observation of slightly enlarged nuclei and prominent nucleoli; however, normal N:C ratios and benign chromatin patterns detected in well preserved urothelial cells establish their benignity. Careful attention should be given to the differentiation of pseudoclusters (associated with catheterization) from true papillary groupings (found with low grade papillary neoplasms).

DeMay, A&S 2e. Catheterized urine, p448

15 a renal cell carcinoma

Renal cell adenocarcinomas cytologically present with large nuclei, prominent nucleoli, and abundant vacuolated neutral lipid laden cytoplasm. Special staining with oil red O or Sudan black must be performed with air dried preparations due to the dissolution of fat in the alcoholic Papanicolaou stain. Primary adenocarcinoma of the bladder generally arises within the Brunn nest as a result of cystitis cystica and presents cytologically with classic malignant mucinous glandular morphology, often resembling colonic adenocarcinoma.

DeMay, A&S 2e. Renal cell carcinoma, p475-476

16 a urothelial carcinoma, grade III

Grade III urothelial carcinomas yield a hypercellular population of single cells with few clusters, anisokaryosis and pleomorphism, coarsely granular, irregularly distributed chromatin, and macronucleoli. An adverse host response and necrotic diathesis are found within the background. These cells are easily recognized as malignant; however, in the absence of a necrotic background (a "clean" background), the diagnosis of carcinoma in situ might be entertained due to its frequency of exfoliation and mimicking cytomorphology.

DeMay, A&S 2e. High grade urothelial carcinoma, p462

17 d carcinoma in situ

Carcinoma in situ recapitulates grade III nonpapillary urothelial carcinoma, with the exception that these preinvasive lesions present with a clean background and a negative or "cystitis mimicking" red transitional mucosa. The cytologic diagnosis may be of great importance in high risk groups (industrial or aniline dye workers and patients with previously resected carcinoma).

DeMay, A&S 2e. Dysplasia and carcinoma in situ, p468-469

18 b papillary urothelial neoplasm of low malignant potential (PUNLMP)

The presence of true papillary clusters identified in urinary specimens is suggestive of a low grade papillary neoplasm. These lesions cannot be excluded from grade I urothelial carcinoma. In the absence of classic malignant nuclear morphology, the diagnosis of carcinoma remains. These cells present with uniform cell borders, micronucleoli and finely granular, regularly distributed chromatin (when visible). Differentiating these low grade neoplasms in catheterized specimens may prove difficult; however, the presence of true cohesive smooth borders is helpful.

DeMay, A&S 2e. Papillary urothelial neoplasm of low malignant potential (PUNLMP), p462

19 c Wilms tumor

Wilms tumors cytologically present as small cells with anaplastic features and infrequent spindle cells, often mimicking neuroblastoma of the adrenal gland as well as other "small blue cell tumors." Clinical history is extremely important in establishing this disease process.

DeMay, A&S 2e. Wilms tumor, p476

20 d small cell carcinoma, rule out bladder primary

Although rare, small cell carcinomas resemble their diagnostic counterparts in the lung. The cells contain hyperchromatic stippled chromatin, coarse clumping, nuclear molding, scanty cytoplasm, and micronucleoli. They characteristically have vertebral column formation, microbiopsy aggregates, and cords, nests, or ribbons. The oat cell type, which may represent a degenerated form of the tumor, typically is found in streams of mucin.

DeMay, A&S 2e. Small cell carcinoma, p474

21 b renal cell carcinoma

Renal cell carcinoma may be diagnosed in urine specimens; however, the cells are generally not shed until the latter stages of the disease; therefore, the early detection of this disease by cytologic examination has limited practical utility. Degenerated cells may accompany the cytologic findings detailed in the question. The identification of neutral lipid by special stains may aid in the confirmation of a kidney primary; however, a negative reaction does not mitigate against the diagnosis of a less well differentiated lesion. Conversely, false positive lipid reactions may be associated with lithiasis, transplant rejection, bladder outlet obstruction, and metastatic carcinoma.

DeMay, A&S 2e. Renal cell carcinoma, p475

22 d squamous differentiated urothelial carcinoma

The concomitant finding of squamous cell carcinoma and urothelial carcinoma indicates a squamous differentiation of urothelial carcinoma. These coexisting findings, which are quite common, suggest a high grade neoplasm.

DeMay, A&S 2e. Squamous cell carcinoma, p474

ISBN 978-089189-6357 ©ASCP 2015

23 a aniline dye exposure

Other "high risk" groups include textile workers, painters, and occupations that involve work with metal and rubber. Exposure to naphthylamine derivatives (aniline dye) has been shown to have a carcinogenic effect. By far, cigarette smoking is the greatest risk factor for the subsequent development of urothelial cancer–accounting for >40% of all lesions.

DeMay, A&S 2e. Urinary tract cancer, p460

24 a transitional epithelial cells

Normal voided urine specimens are hypocellular, containing predominantly superficial/dome/umbrella/caplike urothelial cells. Urothelial cells contain dense granular cytoplasm with homogeneous texture. Urothelial nuclei may be round and slightly enlarged and possess finely granular, evenly distributed chromatin patterns and micronucleoli. The N:C ratios of urothelial cells are low. Scattered squamous cells, either indigenous or contamination from the vaginal mucosa, and rare columnar cells from the renal tubules, Brunn nests, or glands of Littre may be observed. Inflammatory exudate is typically mild unless an inflammatory process exists.

DeMay, A&S 2e. Urothelial cells, p441-442

25 c ileal conduit urine

Normal urine from ileal conduit bladders will contain abundant degenerative columnar cells, necrotic debris, and a background containing bacteria and mucus.

DeMay, A&S 2e. Ileal conduit urine, p470

26 a malakoplakia

This granulomatous disease grossly appears as yellow plaques in place of the bladder mucosa. Cytology reveals rare histiocytes and giant cells (von Hansemann histiocytes) containing granular intracytoplasmic inclusions representing bacteria, as well as macrophages with intracytoplasmic, cyanophilic, spherical, laminated calcospherites, referred to as Michaelis-Gutmann bodies.

DeMay, A&S 2e. Malakoplakia, p454-455

27 d cystitis glandularis

Brunn nests are areas of columnar epithelium in which urothelial cells extend into the lamina propria, separate, and form mucus producing nests (cystitis glandularis). These cystic nests are lined by normal colonic type mucosal cells.

DeMay, A&S 2e. Brunn nests, cystitis cystica, and cystitis glandularis, p449

28 d malakoplakia

This granulomatous disease grossly appears as yellow plaques in place of the bladder mucosa. Cytology reveals rare histiocytes and giant cells (von Hansemann histiocytes) containing granular intracytoplasmic inclusions representing bacteria, as well as macrophages with intracytoplasmic, cyanophilic, spherical, laminated calcospherites, referred to as Michaelis-Gutmann bodies.

DeMay, A&S 2e. Malakoplakia, p454-455

29 b catheterized

Normal catheterized urine specimens contain a hypercellular and heterogeneous population of normal urothelial cells that includes dome or superficial cells, sheets of oval intermediate type urothelial cells, squamous cells, and occasional columnar cells, usually from the Brunn

nests. The urothelial cells contain round, hypochromatic or degenerative nuclei and granular cytoplasm. Reactive nuclear changes may be detected by the observation of slightly enlarged nuclei and prominent nucleoli; however, normal N:C ratios and benign chromatin patterns detected in well preserved urothelial cells establish their benignity. Careful attention should be given to the differentiation of pseudoclusters (associated with catheterization) from true papillary groupings (such as those found with low grade papillary neoplasms).

DeMay, A&S 2e. Catheterized urine, p448

30 a squamous metaplasia

Squamous metaplasia resembling "navicular" cells is often identified in urinary specimens from females, representing a progesterone stimulated epithelium, such as that found within the vaginal mucosa in pregnant patients. In men, their presence may represent squamous metaplastic cells of the prostatic ducts secondary to estrogen therapy for prostatic adenocarcinoma.

DeMay, A&S 2e. Squamous cells and squamous metaplasia, p444

31 a cytomegalovirus

Cytomegalovirus may be identified in immunosuppressed patients such as those infected with HIV, patients with cancer, or renal transplant recipients. Large renal tubular cells with intranuclear basophilic inclusions surrounded by halos resembling an "owl's eye" are diagnostic of cytomegalovirus.

DeMay, A&S 2e. Cytomegalovirus, p452

32 d cholesterol

Cholesterol crystals abnormally appear as colorless structures in urine specimens.

DeMay, A&S 2e. Cholesterol crystals, p218

33 b renal parenchymal disease

Renal tubular cells, oval cells with granular cytoplasm and eccentrically located nuclei, or polygonal cells occurring singly or in clusters are found in patients with renal parenchymal diseases, such as glomerulonephritis or pyelonephritis. Other associated changes include cellular casts, necrosis, and erythrocytes.

DeMay, A&S 2e. Renal tubular cells, p443-444

34 b *Schistosoma mansoni*

The location of the spine differentiates this species from *Schistosoma haematobium* (which possesses a terminal spine).

DeMay, A&S 2e. Schistosomiasis, p457

35 d Sudan black

Renal cell carcinomas cytologically present with large nuclei, prominent nucleoli, and abundant vacuolated neutral lipid laden cytoplasm. Special staining with oil red O or Sudan black must be performed with air dried preparations due to the dissolution of fat in the alcoholic Papanicolaou stain. Primary adenocarcinoma of the bladder generally arises within the Brunn nest as a result of cystitis cystica and presents cytologically with classic malignant mucinous glandular morphology, often resembling colonic adenocarcinoma.

DeMay, A&S 2e. Renal cell carcinoma, p475

36 c polyomavirus infection

Polyomavirus infections present in urine cytology with enlarged, degenerated, karyopyknotic, eccentrically located nuclei with trailing cytoplasmic tails, often described as decoy (mimicking CIS) or "comet cells" (long cytoplasmic tails). Basophilic intranuclear inclusions are necessary to establish this diagnosis. Care should be exercised to differentiate these benign infections from true neoplastic cells.

DeMay, A&S 2e. human polyomavirus, p452

37 b seminal vesicle cells

Cells originating from the seminal vesicles in males cytologically appear as single cuboidal cells with intracytoplasmic yellow lipofuscin granules. The nuclei of these cells may appear quite abnormal; however, the cytoplasmic pigment should indicate the benignity of these cells.

DeMay, A&S 2e. Seminal vesicle cells, p444

38 a degeneration

Eosinophilic (or cyanophilic) intracytoplasmic inclusions in urothelial cells commonly represent nonspecific mucopolysaccharide degeneration, or giant lysosomes. These cells are not associated with urinary pathology and care should be exercised when interpreting the significance of their presence.

DeMay, A&S 2e. Metastatic malignancy, p248

39 b *Schistosoma haematobium*

Schistosoma haematobium is a parasitic fluke found in Africa and the Middle East that embeds within the bladder mucosa, eventually creating squamous metaplasia and squamous cell carcinoma. The cytology reveals transparent ova with a terminal spine. Schistosomiasis is also referred to as bilharzia. Differential diagnosis is the lemon drop form of uric acid crystals.

DeMay, A&S 2e. Schistosomiasis, p457

40 c chemotherapy associated changes

The presence of large cells with elevated N:C ratios, degenerated nuclear features, and chromatic margination (associated with degeneration) in single cells is related to therapeutic changes secondary to treatment of malignant disease. More "atypical" cytologic changes may be seen with Cytoxan or busulfan therapy, whereas the administration of thiotepa usually creates more reactive urothelial changes. The differential diagnosis of chemotherapy associated changes includes high grade urothelial carcinoma, carcinoma in situ, and polyomavirus infection; however, the absence of single cells with well preserved, classic malignant nuclear morphology should mitigate against the possibility of a neoplastic process.

DeMay, A&S 2e. Chemotherapy, p457-458

41 d tyrosine

Tyrosine crystals are typically found in urine from patients with hepatitis, cirrhosis, or trauma to the liver.

DeMay, A&S 2e. Miscellaneous, p446

42 b cystitis cystica

Columnar cells identified in urinary specimens are most commonly derived from the bladder dome or Brunn nests, areas in which columnar mucosa extends into the lamina propria. Other sources include cystitis glandularis, gland os, lacunae of Morgagni, female genital system, prostate, and renal tubules.

DeMay, A&S 2e. Columnar cells, p442

43 d lead poisoning

Cellular changes secondary to lead poisoning are often found in children who consume paint or water high in lead content.

DeMay, A&S 2e. Other inclusions, p446

44 c human polyomavirus

Polyomavirus infections present in urine cytology with enlarged, degenerated, karyopyknotic, eccentric nuclei with trailing cytoplasmic tails, often described as decoy (mimicking CIS) or "comet" cells (long cytoplasmic tails). Basophilic intranuclear inclusions are necessary to establish this diagnosis. Care should be exercised to differentiate these benign infections from true neoplastic cells.

DeMay, A&S 2e. human polyomavirus, p452

45 a squamous cell carcinoma, bladder primary

Schistosoma haematobium is a parasitic fluke found in Africa and the Middle East that embeds within the bladder mucosa, eventually creating squamous metaplasia and squamous cell carcinoma. Squamous cell carcinoma of the bladder (secondary to bilharzia) presents with typical pleomorphic keratinizing morphology identical to that found in other primary sites. These lesions may be very well differentiated; therefore, extreme caution should be exercised when discriminating these lesions from normal squamous cells.

DeMay, A&S 2e. Squamous cell carcinoma, p474

46 b triple phosphate crystals

Triple phosphate crystals generally present with "coffin lid" or prism morphology in urinary tract specimens.

DeMay, A&S 2e. Miscellaneous, p446

47 c *Candida* species

Immunocompetent individuals taking broad spectrum antibiotics are at an increased risk for isolated fungal infections; however, immunocompromised patients (such as diabetics) are more commonly at risk. The photomicrograph illustrates an infection by *Candida* species, demonstrated by the presence of pseudohyphae or elongated yeast with attached buds (resembling "balloon dogs") as well as scattered budding yeast (often collectively referred to as "sticks and stones"). Other fungal infections, such as *Blastomyces* species, *Cryptococcus* species, and *Aspergillus* species, may also be seen in urine specimens as a part of a local or systemic infection.

DeMay, A&S 2e. Fungal infections, p451

ISBN 978-089189-6357 ©ASCP 2015

48 d   lithiasis, calcium carbonate crystals

Calcium carbonate crystals are easily identified in urinary specimens as dumbbell and granule structures. Their presence may be associated with the overconsumption of vegetables.

DeMay, A&S 2e. Miscellaneous, p446

49 b   urothelial carcinoma in situ

Carcinoma in situ recapitulates high grade urothelial carcinoma, with the exception that these preinvasive lesions present with a clean background and a negative or "cystitis-mimicking" red transitional mucosa. The cytologic diagnosis may be of great importance in high risk groups (industrial or aniline dye workers and patients with previously resected carcinoma).

DeMay, A&S 2e. Dysplasia and carcinoma in situ, p468-469

50 b   papillary neoplasm, rule out urothelial carcinoma

The presence of true papillary clusters identified in urinary specimens is suggestive of a low grade papillary neoplasm. These lesions cannot be excluded from papillary urothelial neoplasm of low malignant potential. In the absence of classic malignant nuclear morphology, the diagnosis of carcinoma remains. These cells present with uniform cell borders, micronucleoli, and finely granular, regularly distributed chromatin (when visible). Differentiating these low grade neoplasms in catheterized specimens may prove difficult; however, the presence of true cohesive smooth borders will help confirm a neoplastic process.

DeMay, A&S 2e. Low grade papillary urothelial carcinoma, p462-463

51 d   prostate adenocarcinoma

Prostatic adenocarcinomas cytologically appear in repeating microacinar structures and syncytial groupings with anisonucleosis, crowding nuclear features, finely granular chromatin, and irregular macronucleoli within every cell. The positivity with immunocytochemistry for prostate specific antigen is helpful in distinguishing these lesions from those from bladder or renal primary sites.

DeMay, A&S 2e. Prostatic adenocarcinoma, p476

52 b   oil red O

Renal cell adenocarcinomas cytologically present with large nuclei, prominent nucleoli, and abundant, faintly vacuolated, lipid laden cytoplasm. Special staining with oil red O or Sudan black must be performed with air dried preparations due to the dissolution of fat in the alcoholic Papanicolaou stain. Primary adenocarcinoma of the bladder generally arises within the Brunn nest as a result of cystitis cystica and presents cytologically with classic malignant mucinous glandular morphology, often resembling colonic adenocarcinoma.

DeMay, A&S 2e. Renal cell carcinoma, p475

53 c   urothelial carcinoma, grade III

High grade urothelial carcinomas yield a hypercellular population of single cells with few clusters, anisokaryosis and pleomorphism, coarsely granular, irregularly distributed chromatin, and macronucleoli. An adverse host response and necrotic diathesis are found within the background.

These cells are easily recognized as malignant; however, in the absence of a necrotic background (a "clean" background), the diagnosis of carcinoma in situ might be entertained due to its frequency of exfoliation and mimicking cytomorphology.

DeMay, A&S 2e. High grade urothelial carcinoma, p462

54 b   vaginal contamination

The most common source of squamous cells in urine specimens is vaginal contamination. The urethra and the bladder trigone are also possible sources of squamous mucosa.

DeMay, A&S 2e. Squamous cells and squamous metaplasia, p390

55 a   normal catheterized urothelial changes

Normal catheterized urine specimens contain a hypercellular and heterogeneous population of normal urothelial cells, including dome or superficial cells, sheets of oval intermediate type urothelial cells, squamous cells, and occasional columnar cells, usually from the Brunn nests. The urothelial cells contain round, hypochromatic or degenerative nuclei and granular cytoplasm. Reactive nuclear changes may be detected by the observation of slightly enlarged nuclei and prominent nucleoli; however, normal N:C ratios and benign chromatin patterns detected in well preserved urothelial cells establish their benignity. Careful attention should be given to the differentiation of pseudoclusters (associated with catheterization) from true papillary groupings (found with low grade papillary neoplasms).

DeMay, A&S 2e. Catheterized urine, p448

56 c   bladder dome

Columnar cells identified in urinary specimens are most commonly derived from the bladder dome or Brunn nests, areas in which the columnar mucosa extends into the lamina propria. Other sources include cystitis glandularis, gland of Littre, lacunae of Morgagni, female genital system, prostate, and renal tubules.

DeMay, A&S 2e. Columnar cells, p442

57 c   calcium phosphate crystals

These transparent crystals cytologically present as wedge shaped prisms or irregular platelike structures.

DeMay, A&S 2e. Miscellaneous, p446

58 b   corpora amylacea

Corpora amylacea are basophilic, condensed, concentrically laminated, glycogenated, noncalcifying structures, originating from the prostate.

DeMay, A&S 2e. Corpora amylacea, p446

59 d   this cell is infected with the human polyomavirus

Polyomavirus infections present in urine cytology with enlarged, degenerated, karyopyknotic, eccentrically located nuclei with trailing cytoplasmic tails, often described as decoy (mimicking CIS) or "comet" cells (long cytoplasmic tails). Basophilic intranuclear inclusions are necessary to establish this diagnosis. Care should be exercised to differentiate these benign infections from true neoplastic cells.

DeMay, A&S 2e. human polyomavirus, p452

60 d carcinoma of the bladder
Schistosoma haematobium is a parasitic fluke found in Africa and the Middle East that embeds within the bladder mucosa, eventually creating squamous metaplasia and squamous cell carcinoma. The cytology reveals transparent ova with a terminal spine. Schistosomiasis is also referred to as bilharzia. Differential diagnosis is the lemon drop form of uric acid crystals.
DeMay, A&S 2e. Schistosomiasis, p451-452

61 b cytomegalovirus
Cytomegalovirus may be identified in immunosuppressed patients, such as those infected with HIV, patients with cancer, or renal transplant recipients. Large renal tubular cells with intranuclear basophilic inclusions surrounded by halos resembling an "owl's eye" are diagnostic of cytomegalovirus.
DeMay, A&S 2e. Cytomegalovirus, p452

62 a renal casts
The presence of renal casts may be associated with kidney rejection or other renal pathology, although their presence may not indicate pathology (depending upon the type of cast).
DeMay, A&S 2e. Miscellaneous, p446

63 c normal urothelial cells
Normal voided urine specimens are hypocellular, containing predominantly superficial/dome/umbrella/caplike urothelial cells. Urothelial cells contain dense granular cytoplasm with homogeneous texture. Urothelial nuclei may be round and slightly enlarged, and possess finely granular, evenly distributed chromatin patterns and micronucleoli. The N:C ratios of urothelial cells are low. Scattered squamous cells, either indigenous or contamination from the vaginal mucosa, and rare columnar cells from the renal tubules, Brunn nests, or glands of Littre may be observed. Inflammatory exudate is typically mild unless a pathologic process exists.
DeMay, A&S 2e. Urothelial cells, p441-442

64 b polyomavirus
The cell presented on this image shows a large round nucleus with the chromatin arranged in a "netlike" fashion, characteristic for this infection. The lack of significant nuclear irregularity is against the diagnosis of high grade urothelial carcinoma.
DeMay, A&S 2e. human polyomavirus, p452

65 c umbrella cells
This image shows multinucleated umbrella cells. Notice scalloped cellular borders, normal nuclear cytoplasmic ratio, normal chromatin distribution and smooth nuclear contours.
DeMay, A&S 2e. Superficial cells (umbrella cells), p441-442

66 c granulomatous cystitis
The image shows a granuloma composed of epithelioid histiocytes and lymphocytes. BCG, the mainstay treatment of CIS, induces a granulomatous reaction with formation of granulomas in the lamina propria. If urothelium is ulcerated, a forceful washing may dislodge granulomas into urine.
DeMay, A&S 2e. Benign urinary tract diseases and conditions, p449

67 a low grade papillary urothelial carcinoma
Low grade papillary urothelial carcinoma is characterized by clusters of urothelial cells with mild nuclear hyperchromasia, irregular nuclear membranes, and mildly increased N:C ratios.
DeMay, A&S 2e. Low grade papillary urothelial carcinoma, p462

68 a nephrolithiasis
The abrasive nature of renal calculi may produce epithelial cell changes ranging from unremarkable to pronounced, and in some instances indistinguishable from that of a low grade papillary urothelial carcinoma. In many cases, though, changes such as seen in this case, in light of clinical history, are reliably predictive of nephrolithiasis. These changes include cohesive clusters of urothelial cells with rounded borders, abundant cytoplasm with only slightly increased cellular N:C ratios, round nuclei with uniform nuclear contours, fine chromatin and prominent nucleoli.
DeMay, A&S 2e. Lithiasis i5.23, p480

69 b 73-year-old male with history of a T3 stage bladder cancer
The image represents an ileal conduit type of specimen. Notice the flat sheet of benign intestinal epithelium and numerous degenerated cells and histiocytes. Usually, patients with a deep muscle invasion (stage T2/T3) undergo cystectomy and a portion of the ilium is used to create a conduit or a neobladder.
DeMay, A&S 2e. Ileal conduit and neobladder urine, p470

70 d nephrolithiasis
This image shows a single cluster of benign urothelial cells with abundant cytoplasm, centrally located nuclei with smooth nuclear membranes and a fine chromatin pattern. Notice a "cytoplasmic collar" around the nuclei, usually indicating a reactive process. The cell cluster is therefore best interpreted as reactive urothelial hyperplasia associated with nephrolithiasis.
DeMay, A&S 2e. Lithiasis i5.23, p480

71 b high grade urothelial carcinoma
The image shows a single malignant urothelial cell with a high N:C ratio, eccentric placement of the nucleus, and irregular nuclear membrane. Chromatin is irregularly distributed.
DeMay, A&S 2e. High grade urothelial carcinoma, p462-463

72 c bladder washing
The image shows numerous single umbrella cells with abundant cytoplasm and centrally located nuclei. Notice that umbrella cells can have single, double, or multiple nuclei. Presence of numerous umbrella cells indicates a forceful sampling characteristic of washing.
DeMay, A&S 2e. Superficial cells (umbrella cells), p441-442

ISBN 978-089189-6357 ©ASCP 2015

Chapter 8

Fine Needle Aspiration

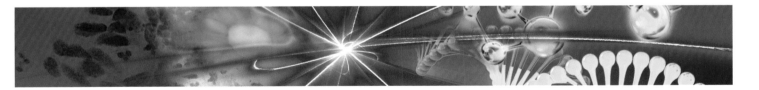

1 A 51-year-old female presents with an enlarged thyroid. Staining the FNA material with May-Grunwald-Giemsa reveals small uniform cells in monolayers and sheets with honeycombing patterns, circular groups with central material, hemosiderin laden macrophages, and blood, contained in a background of abundant amorphous material. These cells are diagnostic of:
   a follicular neoplasm
   b Hashimoto thyroiditis
   c colloid goiter
   d papillary carcinoma

2 A good rule of thumb for identifying an adequate thyroid specimen is the presence of:
   a colloid
   b a single follicular cell in every slide
   c at least 6 clusters of 10 cells over 2 slides
   d at least 2 clusters on 1 of the slides

3 A 65-year-old male with a history of alcohol abuse and cirrhosis of the liver presents with jaundice. A 2 cm lesion is identified within the liver. FNA reveals a malignant group of glandular cells. ANA staining for bile canaliculi is positive within the malignant cell population. The diagnosis is:
   a cholangiocarcinoma
   b hepatocellular carcinoma
   c metastatic colonic adenocarcinoma
   d metastatic pancreatic adenocarcinoma

4 HIV+ patients may suffer from which of the following salivary gland lesions?
   a basal cell adenomas
   b benign lymphoepithelial cyst
   c lipomas
   d hemangiomas

5 A thyroid aspirate reveals a hypercellular population of follicular cells in acinar formation with enlarged, hyperchromatic nuclei and coarse, irregular chromatin. Macronucleoli are noted. The findings suggest:
   a follicular adenoma
   b follicular carcinoma
   c Hashimoto thyroiditis
   d papillary carcinoma

6 A 55-year-old male with a history of previous excision of a pleomorphic adenoma presents with a recurrent parotid tumor. FNA reveals sheets and clusters of cells with frothy cytoplasm and hyperchromatic nuclei, irregular chromatin, and macronucleoli. The background could be characterized as proteinaceous and watery. The diagnosis is:
   a mucoepidermoid carcinoma
   b polymorphous low grade adenocarcinoma
   c acinic cell carcinoma
   d malignant mixed tumor

7 FNA of a parotid tumor from a 55-year-old male yields a brown doughy substance. Cytology reveals a large population of polygonal cells with eosinophilic granular cytoplasm, central or eccentric nuclei, and prominent nucleoli. The background contains a lymphocytic infiltrate and proteinaceous necrotic debris. The diagnosis is:
   a pleomorphic adenoma
   b oncocytoma
   c Warthin tumor
   d monomorphic adenoma

8 A 35-year-old male with a 3 cm parotid mass evaluated by FNA cytologically presents with a mixture of round cells with foamy cytoplasm, hyperchromatic nuclei, irregular chromatin, and nucleoli. Another smaller cellular component yields cells with dense cytoplasm, pleomorphic cell forms and opaque/India ink nuclear features. A watery background is present. These cells are diagnostic of:
   a mucoepidermoid carcinoma, well differentiated
   b mucoepidermoid carcinoma, poorly differentiated
   c acinic cell carcinoma, well differentiated
   d acinic cell carcinoma, poorly differentiated

©ASCP 2015 ISBN 978-089189-6357

9 A malignant minor salivary gland lesion is characterized cytologically as clusters or papillary structures of bland appearing cuboidal to elongated cells with central lumens containing small nuclei, micronucleoli, and vacuolated cytoplasm. Tyrosine rich crystals are seen. The diagnosis suggests:
 a polymorphous low grade primary adenocarcinoma
 b adenoid cystic carcinoma
 c poorly differentiated mucoepidermoid carcinoma
 d malignant mixed tumor, "benign" metastasizing mixed tumor variant

10 Should FNA suggest a Warthin tumor but lack the characteristic lymphocytic infiltrate, the diagnosis suggests:
 a monomorphic adenoma
 b acinic cell carcinoma
 c adenoid cystic carcinoma
 d oncocytoma

11 A 51-year-old female with a painful submaxillary tumor presents for FNA. Cytology reveals a highly cellular smear with bland cells appearing in nests or rosette clusters with central hyaline basement membrane "pink gumball-like" inclusions. Nucleoli are small and inconspicuous. PAS stains are negative. The diagnosis is:
 a pleomorphic adenoma
 b monomorphic adenoma
 c acinic cell carcinoma
 d adenoid cystic carcinoma

12 A 5-year-old male presents with an enlarged parotid gland. A 2 cm lesion is noted upon examination. FNA reveals a bloody fluid composed of bland spindle cells. The diagnosis is:
 a malignant lymphoma
 b hamartoma
 c sarcoma
 d hemangioma

13 A 60-year-old female presents with a 2 cm lesion within the minor salivary glands. FNA reveals cohesive clusters of small cells with round to oval dark nuclear features without nucleoli, but with high N:C ratios. These cells are diagnostic of:
 a adenoid cystic carcinoma
 b pleomorphic adenoma
 c monomorphic adenoma
 d Mikulicz associated sialadenitis

14 The most common tumor of the liver is:
 a hepatocellular carcinoma
 b bile duct carcinoma
 c malignant lymphoma
 d metastatic carcinoma

15 Patients suffering from α1-antitrypsin deficiency often contain which of the following cytomorphologic features in hepatocytes?
 a neutral triglycerides
 b hyaline globules
 c Mallory bodies
 d melanin

16 FNA of a parotid mass reveals a cellular sample containing sheets and clusters of cells with clear to basophilic foamy cytoplasm with PAS+ granules. Nuclei are uniform with finely granular chromatin. This diagnosis is:
 a adenoid cystic carcinoma
 b acinic cell carcinoma
 c malignant mixed tumor
 d mucoepidermoid carcinoma

17 To diagnose follicular carcinoma, which of the following may be helpful?
 a coarse chromatin
 b vascular or capsular invasion as determined histologically
 c clusters of follicular cells
 d nucleoli

18 The most common malignancy that often occurs secondary to benign lymphoepithelial lesions or Sjögren syndrome and arises within intraparotid lymph nodes is:
 a Hodgkin lymphoma
 b lymphangioma
 c adenoid cystic carcinoma
 d non-Hodgkin lymphoma

19 Which thyroid tumor arises from parafollicular cells?
 a medullary carcinoma
 b follicular carcinoma
 c papillary carcinoma
 d Hürthle cell carcinoma

20 A liver aspirate composed of a hypercellular population of bile ductal cells and scattered endothelial cells, fibromyxoid stroma, and adipose tissue is diagnostic of:
 a cells indigenous to Glisson capsule
 b fatty metamorphosis
 c liver cell adenoma
 d hamartoma

21 FNA revealed cells in monolayer sheets and single cells with nuclei showing anisonucleosis, irregular membranes, washed out chromatin, and nuclear grooves. Intranuclear cytoplasmic invaginations were noted in many cells. Occasional psammoma bodies were also seen. The diagnosis is:
 a medullary carcinoma
 b Hashimoto thyroiditis
 c papillary carcinoma
 d follicular neoplasm

ISBN 978-089189-6357 ©ASCP 2015

22 A 55-year-old male presents with a 2 × 3 cm nodule in the upper pole of the thyroid. FNA reveals numerous spindle to oval cells with fibrillar cytoplasm with dendritic processes. Enlarged eccentric nuclei, multinucleation, and salt & pepper chromatin are noted. Intranuclear cytoplasmic invaginations are noted in many of the cells. Macronucleoli are apparent in a large majority of the cells. Amorphous sheets of eosinophilic material are exhibited with the Papanicolaou stain. Immunoperoxidase staining for calcitonin is positive. The diagnosis is:
   a papillary carcinoma
   b follicular carcinoma
   c anaplastic carcinoma
   d medullary carcinoma

23 A thyroid aspirate reveals large polygonal cells with central and eccentric nuclei, prominent nucleoli, and granular cytoplasm as well as a numerous population of lymphocytes. The diagnosis is:
   a Hürthle cell adenoma
   b Hashimoto thyroiditis
   c follicular neoplasm
   d nodular goiter

24 A thyroid aspiration from a 34-year-old female with a recent history of mumps consists of small degenerated follicular cells, large multinucleated giant cells surrounding and engulfing colloid, lymphocytes, and epithelioid histiocytes. The diagnosis is:
   a Hashimoto thyroiditis
   b follicular neoplasm
   c Hürthle cell adenoma
   d granulomatous thyroiditis (de Quervain)

25 The most reliable criterion for discriminating liver cell dysplasia from nontrabecular hepatocellular carcinoma by FNA cytology is:
   a monolayer hepatocytes with random atypical cells are found with liver cell dysplasia
   b monolayer hepatocytes with random atypical cells are found with hepatocellular carcinoma
   c absence of atypia in liver cell dysplasia
   d poorly differentiated anaplastic cells are generally found in hepatocellular carcinoma

26 A 35-year-old female with a history of long term birth control pill use with a 10 cm liver nodule presents for FNA. No previous history of malignancy is noted. Cytology reveals a hypercellular population of polygonal cells arranged in a monolayers with well defined cytoplasm. The nuclei are often binucleate, intranuclear inclusions are noted, and chromatin is fine and regular. A low N:C ratio is present. PAS stains are positive. These cells are diagnostic of:
   a liver cell adenoma
   b hepatocellular carcinoma
   c cholangiocarcinoma
   d metastatic melanoma

27 An aspiration of a paramidline neck mass yielded an amorphous fluid containing abundant squamous epithelial cells. The diagnosis is:
   a thyroglossal duct cysts
   b parathyroid cyst
   c epidermoid cysts
   d carotid body tumor

28 A 41-year-old female presents with a cold 2 cm thyroid nodule. FNA reveals sheets and clusters of small cells with round, uniform nuclei and macronucleoli. Colloid is scarce. These cells are diagnostic of:
   a papillary carcinoma
   b goiter
   c clear cell carcinoma
   d follicular neoplasm

29 Elongated ropy hyaline intracytoplasmic inclusions surrounding the nucleus in hepatocytes associated with alcoholic cirrhosis are called:
   a Councilman bodies
   b Mallory bodies
   c bile
   d lipofuscin

30 A hypercellular population of polygonal cells with eosinophilic granular cytoplasm, round to oval nuclei, and macronucleoli are identified in a thyroid FNA. The background is clean. The diagnosis is:
   a Hashimoto thyroiditis
   b Hürthle cell neoplasm
   c hyalinizing trabecular adenoma
   d Hürthle cell thyroiditis

31 A 77-year-old female with a large thyroid mass is evaluated with FNA. Cytology shows a highly cellular population of pleomorphic cells with hyperchromasia, irregular chromatin, macronucleoli, and a necrotic background. Giant tumor cells are noted. Immunostaining for keratin, epithelial membrane antigen, thyroglobulin, and thyrocalcitonin are all negative. These cells are diagnostic of:
   a squamous cell carcinoma
   b medullary carcinoma
   c papillary carcinoma
   d anaplastic carcinoma

32 The aspiration of a cystic liver is contraindicated because of the possibility of anaphylaxis when dealing with:
   a *Echinococcus germinosis*
   b *Echinococcus hydatidosis*
   c *Echinococcus cestodosis*
   d *Echinococcus granulosus*

©ASCP 2015   ISBN 978-089189-6357

33 CT scan reveals a large nodular lesion in the liver. FNA reveals a hypercellular population of polygonal cells with anisocytosis, binucleation, macronucleoli, intranuclear cytoplasmic invaginations, and numerous bile ductal cells. Mixed chronic inflammation is present. Intracytoplasmic greenish-black globules are identified with Giemsa staining. These findings are suggestive of:
   a hepatocellular carcinoma
   b cholangiocarcinoma
   c cirrhosis
   d metastatic carcinoma

34 FNA biopsy of which of the following lung lesions is considered to be contraindicated?
   a central lesions
   b vascular lesions
   c peripherally located nodules
   d inflammatory lesions

35 A pulmonary aspiration of an upper left lobe peripheral mass shows 3D cell clusters with 20 or more cells, tall columnar in shape, with bland basally located nuclei, increased N:C ratios, and fine, irregular chromatin patterns with large, round, often irregular, centrally located macronucleoli. Intracytoplasmic lumens and occasional intranuclear cytoplasmic invaginations are noted. These cells are diagnostic of:
   a creola bodies
   b pulmonary infarct
   c bronchogenic adenocarcinoma
   d bronchioloalveolar adenocarcinoma

36 A 5 cm lesion extending from the major bronchi to the periphery of the left lower lobe of the lung is examined by fine needle aspiration. Many isolated cells, as well as cells in syncytia with nuclear overlapping, anisocytosis, cyanophilic cytoplasm with little polarity and indistinct borders, and coarse, irregular chromatin, parachromatin clearing, and irregular macronucleoli, are found in a necrotic background. This presentation best describes a diagnosis of:
   a large cell carcinoma
   b well differentiated squamous carcinoma
   c chronic interstitial pneumonitis
   d small cell carcinoma, intermediate cell type

37 If one suspects a hematopoietic pathological process, which of the following stains is best for cytologic identification?
   a Romanowsky
   b hematoxylin and eosin
   c oil red O
   d PAS

38 FNA of a central solitary lesion from a 51-year-old female shows isolated monotonous cells in sheets, nests, ribbons, and cords. The cells are oval to columnar with basophilic cytoplasm and no evidence of terminal bars and/or cilia, and possess uniform nuclei with moderately high N:C ratios containing finely granular, evenly distributed chromatin with inconspicuous nucleoli. These cells are diagnostic of:
   a malignant lymphoma
   b small cell carcinoma
   c chronic follicular bronchitis
   d carcinoid tumor

39 A 66-year-old male presents with a solitary coin lesion measuring 2 cm on chest X-ray. FNA reveals isolated cells in syncytial-like aggregates with nuclear molding. The cytoplasm is scanty, and the nuclei are hyperchromatic with coarse, regular chromatin. The background shows crush artifact, cell ghosts, and necrotic debris. The diagnosis is:
   a pulmonary lymphocytic infiltrates
   b poorly differentiated non-small cell carcinoma
   c bronchial carcinoid
   d small cell carcinoma

40 FNA of the lung reveals sheets of monotonous cells with finely granular, evenly distributed chromatin, cells with a spindle appearance and oval nuclei with micronucleoli, and large well circumscribed structures with eccentrically located nuclei and capillaries. These cells are diagnostic of:
   a normal pulmonary constituents
   b metastatic hepatocellular carcinoma
   c bronchogenic adenocarcinoma
   d squamous cell carcinoma

41 Which of the following may be associated with a false negative fine needle aspiration?
   a aspiration of necrotic center
   b soft nodules
   c pencil point needles
   d Chiba needles

42 FNA of a 4 cm mass reveals snakelike pleomorphic cells, cells with concentric ringing, ink dot nuclear features, and ghost cells. The diagnosis is:
   a spindle cell sarcoma
   b leiomyosarcoma
   c squamous carcinoma
   d large cell carcinoma

43 A population of small cells, as well as loose acinar structures with hyperchromasia and prominent nucleoli, were found in an FNA of a lung nodule from a 70-year-old male. Immunostaining for PSA was positive. The diagnosis is:
   a small cell carcinoma
   b adenocarcinoma, kidney
   c transitional cell carcinoma
   d adenocarcinoma, prostate

ISBN 978-089189-6357 ©ASCP 2015

44 A 44-year-old female with a known malignancy presents with multiple lung nodules. FNA reveals round to oval cells with eccentric nuclei, anisocytosis, and prominent nucleoli with intranuclear cytoplasmic invaginations and intracytoplasmic brownish refractile granules. Staining with HMB45 is positive. The diagnosis is:
a metastatic hepatocellular carcinoma
b hemosiderin laden macrophages
c dust cells
d metastatic melanoma

45 What mediastinal tumor is most common?
a lipoma
b neural sheath tumors
c parathyroid tumors
d lymphangioma

46 A thyroid aspirate yields a hypercellular population of polygonal cells containing eccentric nuclei, prominent nucleoli, and granular cytoplasm accompanied by numerous lymphocytes. These cellular findings are diagnostic of:
a Hashimoto thyroiditis
b follicular neoplasm
c colloid goiter
d lymphocytic lymphoma

47 FNA of a diffuse lung nodule from an immunocompromised patient reveals GMS+ structures presenting in "contact lens" shapes, 4-6 mm in diameter with central basophilic intranuclear inclusions among mats of frothy material. The diagnosis is:
a Mycobacterium tuberculosis
b Histoplasma capsulatum
c Pneumocystis jiroveci
d Cryptococcus neoformans

48 A 55-year-old smoker with emphysema presents with a mediastinal shadow on the right lower lobe on chest X-ray. FNA of the area reveals a large inflammatory infiltrate composed of neutrophils, lymphocytes, necrotic detritus, fibrin, macrophages, and blood. The diagnosis is:
a osteomyelitis
b abscess
c granulomatous disease
d teratoma

49 What mediastinal lesion is considered common in infants?
a mesenchymal tumors
b lymphatic cysts
c gastroenteric cysts
d seminoma

50 A 58-year-old male with multicentric lung nodules shows a monomorphic population of cells lying singly containing round cleaved nuclei and coarse chromatin on FNA evaluation. Leu M5 staining was positive. These cells are diagnostic of:
a atypical carcinoid
b malignant lymphoma
c small cell carcinoma, intermediate cell type
d normal mesothelial cells

51 The most common complication associated with pulmonary needle aspirations is:
a needle tract tumor seeding
b infection
c pneumothorax
d air embolus

52 A 44-year-old female presents with a single nodule in the left upper lobe of the lung. FNA reveals sheets of columnar cells with preserved cellular polarity, cells with large vacuoles with associated capillaries, and cells with eosinophilic cytoplasm, multiple nuclei, and central lacunae. A stringy background is identified. These cells are diagnostic of:
a lipoma
b hamartoma
c leiomyosarcoma
d liposarcoma

53 A 44-year-old male with a history of malignancy presents with multiple lung nodules and a concomitant pleural effusion. FNA of the lung shows a monotonous population of small round to oval cells without cohesion, nuclear grooves, and cleaving with coarse chromatin and frequent nucleoli. These cells are diagnostic of:
a small cell carcinoma, oat cell type
b carcinoid tumor
c small cell carcinoma, intermediate cell type
d malignant lymphoma

54 A 55-year-old male with a 3 × 4 cm coin lesion presents for FNA evaluation. Cytology reveals a heterogeneous population of cells including large cells with multiple nuclei and fine regular chromatin with frothy cytoplasm, spindle appearing cells with oval nuclei and fine chromatin, and lymphocytes. These cells are diagnostic of:
a giant cell carcinoma
b poorly differentiated adenocarcinoma
c poorly differentiated squamous cell carcinoma
d granuloma

55 A 45-year-old female presents with a painless, 3 cm salivary gland mass and complaint of dry eyes and mouth. FNA cytology reveals lymphocytes, plasma cells, and degenerated acinar structures as well as multinucleated giant cells and epithelioid histiocytes. What etiology is associated with the cytologic findings?
a Sjögren syndrome
b tuberculoma
c Hashimoto disease
d sarcoidosis

©ASCP 2015 ISBN 978-089189-6357

56 A fine needle aspiration of a 2 × 3 cm lung mass proved difficult due to a strong desmoplastic response surrounding the tumor. An 18 gauge needle yielded a heterogeneous population of cells in 3D groups with mucin positivity. Acinar structures were common. Chromatin was irregular and macronucleoli were present in almost every cell. Based on these findings, the diagnosis is:
    a bronchogenic adenocarcinoma
    b large cell carcinoma
    c squamous cell carcinoma
    d carcinoid tumor

57 A benign salivary disorder, often related to *Staphylococcus aureus,* presenting as lithiasis and acute inflammation and exhibiting the clinical symptom of painful swelling, is referred to as:
    a mucocele
    b sialadenitis
    c pleomorphic adenoma
    d Warthin tumor

58 A small population of single cells with nuclear molding and coarse chromatin were found in an aspirate from a peripheral lung nodule. Special stains with leukocyte common antigen (LCA) will be:
    a positive
    b negative
    c indeterminate
    d peripherally positive

59 A middle mediastinal tumor composed of single cells with hyperchromatic eccentric nuclei and coarse clock faced peripheral chromatin and binucleate and bizarre multinucleated giant cells is diagnostic of:
    a malignant lymphoma, small cell cleaved
    b malignant lymphoma, large cell noncleaved
    c plasmacytoma
    d small cell carcinoma, intermediate cell type

60 A malignant anterior mediastinal tumor, often associated with paraneoplastic syndromes that presents cytologically as a biphasic cell pattern of cortical epithelial cells and lymphoid components is:
    a invasive thymoma
    b cystic hygroma
    c neurofibroma
    d schwannoma

61 The most common benign salivary gland neoplasm is:
    a Warthin tumor
    b oxyphilic adenoma
    c pleomorphic adenoma
    d basal cell adenoma

62 A 44-year-old female presents with a painless, freely movable mass of the parotid. FNA reveals sheets of cells and clusters with well defined cell borders as well as elongated cells with attenuated ends. A basophilic background is seen with Papanicolaou staining. These cells are diagnostic of:
    a granuloma
    b monomorphic adenoma
    c Warthin tumor
    d pleomorphic adenoma

63 When performing FNA, what recommendation would be suggested for evaluating excessive bloody aspirates?
    a discard and repuncture identical area
    b prepare as is with cell block technique
    c treat with 100% glacial acetic acid
    d treat with Carnoy fixative

64 A multifocal lesion is found in the right lung of a 66-year-old male who has a history of extra-pulmonary cancer. FNA of the nodules reveals large columnar cells in cigar shapes and granular cytoplasm with loss of polarity. The nuclei contain hyperchromatic, fine irregular chromatin with jagged macronucleoli. These cells best describe:
    a metastatic pancreatic carcinoma
    b metastatic squamous carcinoma
    c metastatic colonic adenocarcinoma
    d viral pneumonitis

65 Which of the following is considered a posterior mediastinal malignant lesion?
    a malignant schwannoma
    b thymoma
    c hemangioma
    d parathyroid adenoma

66 A 55-year-old female with a history of radiation and busulfan therapy for bronchogenic adenocarcinoma is evaluated by FNA due to a shadow seen on chest X-ray. Macrocytes with large, dark nuclei and good cell to cell recognition are found. Cellular crowding with terminal bars is seen in the presence of a clean background. The diagnosis is:
    a recurrent bronchogenic adenocarcinoma
    b terminal bronchioloalveolar carcinoma
    c reactive bronchial cells
    d hamartoma

67 In comparison with other pulmonary specimen collection techniques, fine needle aspiration biopsy is most useful for the diagnosis of:
    a central lesions
    b hilar lesions
    c peripheral lesions
    d necrotic lesions

ISBN 978-089189-6357 ©ASCP 2015

68 A 32-year-old male presents with a nodule located within the vertebral column. FNA reveals multinucleated giant cells (some up to 20 nuclei per cell); spindle cells with predictable cellular features, monomorphic small cells with well defined borders, granular cytoplasm, and round, eccentric nuclei; and fragments of mature bone in a metachromatic fibrous and bloody background. The diagnosis is:
  a osteosarcoma
  b chondroblastoma
  c osteoblastoma
  d chondrosarcoma

69 FNA of a lung lesion reveals large cells with dense cytoplasm, thick refractile cell walls, and smudgy, greasy appearing nuclear features, with intracytoplasmic basophilic inclusions. The diagnosis is:
  a creola bodies
  b aspiration pneumonia, plant material
  c squamous cell carcinoma
  d atypical squamous metaplasia

70 A benign lesion occurring in the epiphysis of the long bones cytologically presents as polygonal cells with dense, glassy cytoplasm and round to oval nuclei containing grooves. Many cells present with binucleate eccentric features. Multinucleated osteoclasts are found in addition to dense eosinophilic background. These cells are diagnostic of:
  a osteoblastoma
  b chondrosarcoma
  c chondroblastoma
  d giant cell tumor of the bone

71 A 67-year-old female presents with a 2 cm liver nodule located with nuclear magnetic resonance. A history of intrahepatic lithiasis is noted. FNA reveals a hypercellular population containing sheets and microacinar formation, large cells with irregular nuclear membranes, disorderly growth, mild nuclear enlargement, and nuclear crowding. Immunocytochemical analysis shows CEA positivity and α-fetoprotein negativity. Based on the following, the diagnosis is:
  a hepatocellular carcinoma, well differentiated
  b reactive hepatocytes
  c cholangiocarcinoma, well differentiated
  d normal bile ductal epithelium

72 A cartilaginous tumor affecting individuals between the ages of 40 and 60, occurring within the pelvis or femur, and cytologically composed of anaplastic chondrocytes, chondroblasts, and epithelioid cells among a bright metachromatic myxoid background is diagnostic of:
  a giant cell tumor
  b villonodular synovitis
  c chondroblastoma
  d chondrosarcoma

73 A 14-year-old male presents with femur pain. FNA reveals slightly cohesive small round cells with granular cytoplasm, coarse chromatin, and rare nucleoli, with cell size about twice that of a lymphocyte. Rosettes are often noted. Which special stain and what diagnosis would confirm your suspicions?
  a PAS–/osteogenic sarcoma
  b PAS+/Ewing sarcoma
  c neuron specific enolase+/osteosarcoma
  d leukocyte common antigen+/small round cell lymphoma

74 A 63-year-old female with a history of a total hysterectomy without bilateral salpingo-oophorectomy presents with a golf ball size tumor involving the left ovary. FNA reveals a scanty population of predictable thin spindle shaped cells with fine regular chromatin. The diagnosis is consistent with:
  a Sertoli cell tumor
  b fibroma
  c interstitial cell tumor
  d granulosa cell tumor

75 FNA of a retroperitoneal tumor consists of pleomorphic vacuolated cells with eccentric nuclei, small round cells, and elongated, spindle shaped, vacuolated cells. A population of multinucleated giant cells containing irregular chromatin and prominent nucleoli with granular cytoplasm arranged in clusters and lacking polarity is also seen. The diagnosis is:
  a proliferative myositis
  b liposarcoma
  c angiosarcoma
  d granulomatous disease

76 Cells in sheets with abundant granular to foamy cyanophilic cytoplasm containing fine yellowish pigment and small eccentric round nuclei with prominent nucleoli in a bloody background when seen in ovarian aspirations are diagnostic of:
  a follicular cyst
  b luteal cyst
  c parovarian cyst
  d Brenner tumor

77 FNA is performed on a 6 cm well circumscribed kidney mass from an elderly male presenting with hematuria and abdominal pain. Cytology reveals a monotonous population consisting purely of large polygonal cells with abundant granular cytoplasm in loose clusters and as single cells. The cells have small central and eccentrically located nuclei with fine regular chromatin and micronucleoli. The diagnosis is consistent with a:
  a renal cell carcinoma
  b papillary carcinoma
  c collecting duct carcinoma
  d oncocytic neoplasm

78 A 19-year-old male with a lesion contained within the metaphyseal portion of the distal femur presents for FNA. Cytology reveals a predominant population of cells with plasmacytoid appearance and hyperchromatic nuclei, irregular chromatin, and nucleoli. In addition, multinucleated cells with metachromatic cytoplasmic granules, and central hyaline fibrillar material surrounded by pleomorphic spindle cells are present. The diagnosis is:
a osteoblastoma
b osteosarcoma
c osteoid osteoma
d osteochondroma

79 A lesion comprised of pleomorphic endothelial cells with coarse irregular chromatin and macronucleoli, associated epithelioid cells, and "erythrophagocytosis" best describes:
a myositis ossificans
b benign fibrous histiocytoma
c malignant fibrous histiosarcoma
d angiosarcoma

80 Which lesion may commonly present with accompanying granulomatous disease?
a seminoma
b asthma
c encephalitis
d choroid plexus papillomas

81 FNA of a 5 cm ovarian mass reveals abundant squamous and adnexal material contained within a granular background. These cells are diagnostic of:
a Sertoli-Leydig cell tumor
b granulosa cell tumor
c mature cystic teratoma
d dysgerminoma

82 An FNA of an ileum mass from a 18-year-old male reveals a hypercellular population of eosinophils and cells with granular to dense cytoplasm with eccentric nuclei and prominent nuclear grooves. Foreign body giant cells, foamy histiocytes, and mature inflammatory components are also identified. The diagnosis is consistent with a(n):
a callus
b eosinophilic granuloma
c aneurysmal bone cyst
d hemangioma

83 Which statement regarding the FNA of pheochromocytomas is correct?
a cytology cannot distinguish pheochromocytoma from adrenal cortical adenoma
b aspiration may precipitate a hypertensive crisis
c they are associated with decreased urinary catecholamines
d they are associated with decreased vanillylmandelic acid

84 FNA of an ovarian mass reveals sheets of cells with large overlapping nuclei, coarse, irregular chromatin, prominent nucleoli, clear, lacy cytoplasm with punched out vacuoles, naked nuclei, and scattered lymphocytes. Epithelioid and multinucleated histiocytes are noted. A tiger-striped background pattern is demonstrated with Diff-Quik. Staining is positive for PAS but negative for α-fetoprotein and common leukocyte antigen. The diagnosis is:
a dysgerminoma
b lymphoma
c yolk sac tumors
d embryonal carcinoma

85 A recent kidney transplant patient presents with a solitary lesion of the lung. FNA evaluation reveals a hypercellular population of cells with large nuclei, macronucleoli, and cilia. Another population of cells shows large nuclei containing intranuclear basophilic inclusions surrounded by halos and chromatic margination. Nuclear molding is absent. These cells are diagnostic of:
a herpesvirus
b bronchogenic adenocarcinoma
c metastatic renal cell carcinoma
d cytomegalovirus

86 If a Diff-Quik stained FNA specimen of the lung is negative for malignancy, one should:
a restain in case of faulty staining technique
b reaspirate due to faulty sampling technique
c perform cultures for identification of possible inflammatory process
d suggest no need for further evaluation

87 A 44-year-old female presents with a raised pigmented cutaneous lesion on the thigh. FNA reveals well defined, slender, elongated cells with notched ends and fine regular chromatin, cells with foamy cytoplasm and eccentrically located reniform nuclei, and long slender anatomizing processes containing flattened, peripherally arranged, elongated nuclei. This best describes:
a hemangioma
b liposarcoma
c benign fibrous histiocytoma
d pleomorphic fibrosarcoma

88 The most common nonneoplastic ovarian cyst is:
a luteal
b parovarian
c endometriotic
d follicular

ISBN 978-089189-6357 ©ASCP 2015

89 A 34-year-old female with an enlarged ovary presents for FNA. Cuboidal cells arranged in clusters as well as monolayered sheets with scanty cytoplasm are seen in conjunction with a population of ciliated cells. Papillary groupings and psammoma bodies are also seen. The diagnosis is:
   a mucinous cystadenoma
   b serous cystadenoma
   c mucinous cystadenocarcinoma
   d serous cystadenocarcinoma

90 FNA of a left ovarian mass yields a sticky mucoid material. Cytology reveals a hypercellular sample with endocervical cell morphology, irregular clusters, single cells, and malignant nuclear features. Deep, basophilic wispy material is demonstrated in the background with Diff-Quik stain. The diagnosis is:
   a endometriod carcinoma
   b mucinous cystadenocarcinoma
   c dysgerminoma
   d yolk sac tumor

91 FNA of a visceral pleural lung mass from a patient, status post resection for stage II bronchogenic adenocarcinoma, postirradiation therapy, reveals scarce well defined sheets of cells with spindle shaped morphology and cytoplasmic streaming, binucleation, and moderate to low N:C ratios. These cells are diagnostic of:
   a recurrent bronchogenic adenocarcinoma
   b granulomatous process
   c spindle cell sarcoma
   d mesenchymal repair

92 An ovarian aspirate from a 32-year-old patient consists of cells with foamy cytoplasm with refractile red pigment and cells with cuboidal morphology, demonstrating regular chromatin arranged in balls and loose clusters. The background consists of fresh and old blood. The diagnosis suggests:
   a luteal cyst
   b sex cord stromal tumor
   c endometriotic cyst
   d mucinous cystadenoma

93 A 44-year-old female with a 3 cm lesion located by ultrasound submits for FNA. Cytology reveals sheets of cells with abundant cytoplasm and uniform nuclei containing grooves appearing morphologically as "coffee beans." Many cells are arranged in islands with central eosinophilic globules. The diagnosis is:
   a Sertoli-Leydig cell tumor
   b teratoma
   c germinoma
   d Brenner tumor

94 A testicular mass was aspirated from a 22-year-old patient and revealed numerous poorly cohesive large cells with frankly malignant nuclei found in the presence of an interwoven PAS+ tigroid background. What other cellular population is helpful in establishing which diagnosis?
   a lymphohistiocytic bodies, histiocytic lymphoma
   b benign lymphocytic population, seminoma
   c malignant lymphocytic population, anaplastic seminoma
   d Sertoli cells, benign hydrocele fluid

95 FNA of an enlarged 2 × 3 cm lymphoid mass reveals multiple intracytoplasmic histiocytic inclusions. Special staining with Giemsa is positive but negative with GMS. Which organism is represented?
   a Leishmania
   b Histoplasma capsulatum
   c Pneumocystis jiroveci
   d Coccidioides immitis

96 An ovarian aspirate reveals single cells and clusters with rounded smooth and folded bean shaped nuclei and scanty foamy cytoplasm contained within a proteinaceous background. An intact ovum is surrounded by these cells. Carcinoembryonic antigen and α-fetoprotein serum levels are minimal. The diagnosis is:
   a follicular cyst
   b luteal cyst
   c serous cystadenoma
   d mucinous cystadenoma

97 FNA of a pelvic lymph node reveals terminal barlike densities on the apical cytoplasmic borders of the malignant cells. Which of the following may represent a possible primary site/diagnosis?
   a adrenal/pheochromocytoma
   b pancreas/serous cystadenocarcinoma
   c kidney/oncocytic neoplasm
   d colorectal/carcinoma

98 A 44-year-old female with endometrial hyperplasia presents with an ovarian tumor. FNA of the ovary reveals a hypercellular population of uniform cells in sheets and rosettes surrounding amorphous metachromatic structures. The nuclei are round and have fine regular chromatin and micronucleoli. The background is clean. These cells are diagnostic of:
   a fibroma
   b germinoma
   c serous cystadenocarcinoma
   d granulosa cell tumor

99 Pancreatic FNA reveals cells in loose sheets with flat sheets with well defined cell borders, honeycomb appearance, fine regular chromatin, micronucleoli, smooth nuclear membranes, and pale, finely vacuolated cytoplasm. These cells best describe:
   a acinar cells
   b pancreatic adenocarcinoma, well differentiated
   c normal biliary duct
   d pancreatic pseudocyst

100 A gallbladder aspirate reveals sheets of ductal cells with enlarged overlapping nuclei and prominent nucleoli. Few single cells are identified. These cells are diagnostic of:
   a normal gallbladder epithelium
   b acute cholecystitis
   c adenocarcinoma
   d xanthogranulomatous cholecystitis

101 Which criteria are reliable for distinguishing well differentiated trabecular hepatocellular carcinomas (HCCs) from the fibrolamellar variant of HCC?
   a bile ducts are intermingled with the tumor cells in well differentiated trabecular HCC
   b the cells of the fibrolamellar variant of HCC are larger and more dispersed, with fewer trabeculae
   c the cells of well differentiated trabecular HCC possess oncocytic cytoplasm with well defined homogeneous intracytoplasmic pale bodies
   d the cells of the fibrolamellar variant of HCC are morphologically similar to "small blue cell tumors," ie, there is a uniform population of small, round to oval anaplastic cells with high N:C ratios

102 A 55-year-old female presents with abdominal pain and high levels of serum amylase. FNA of the pancreas reveals neutrophils and small clusters of cells with abundant granular cytoplasm, round nuclei, and chromatinic margination. These cells are diagnostic of:
   a microcystic adenoma
   b mucinous cystadenoma
   c papillary epithelial neoplasm
   d pancreatitis

103 Tall columnar mucinous secreting cells (mucicarmine+) as well as signet ring cells with low N:C ratios and stromal cells were identified in a 4 cm mass located in the pancreas of a 44-year-old female. The background contains abundant metachromatic fibrillary material on Diff-Quik. The diagnosis/method of treatment is:
   a poorly differentiated mucinous adenocarcinoma/surgical resection
   b papillary epithelial carcinoma/no resection required
   c mucinous cystic tumor/surgical resection
   d microcystic adenoma/no resection required

104 A prostatic aspiration yields a hypercellular population of uniform cells in irregular sheets with well defined cytoplasmic borders. Microacinar complexes are not identified. No nucleoli are found. These cells are diagnostic of:
   a prostatic adenocarcinoma, well differentiated
   b prostatic adenocarcinoma, poorly differentiated
   c seminal vesicle cells
   d prostatic hyperplasia

105 Pancreatic pseudocysts are a result of:
   a pancreatitis
   b calcification of pancreatic parenchyma
   c granulation tissue scarring
   d fatty metamorphosis

106 What is the correct order for normal lymphocytic differentiation?
   a cleaved→large noncleaved→immunoblastic→plasma cell
   b small round cells→small cleaved→large cleaved→small noncleaved→large noncleaved→immunoblastic→plasma cell
   c small cleaved→large noncleaved→large cleaved→small noncleaved→immunoblastic→plasma cell
   d plasma cell→small noncleaved→small cleaved→large cleaved→immunoblasts

107 Lymphogranular bodies as seen in the FNA of lymph nodes suggest which process?
   a lymphoid
   b malignant
   c metastatic
   d granulomatous

108 A 3 cm mass located in the tail of the pancreas is found to contain a hypercellular population of single cells with round nuclei, coarse chromatin, multiple nucleoli, and increased mitotic figures, with a large population of multinucleated giant malignant cells containing irregular chromatin and irregular nuclear membranes. The diagnosis is:
   a metastatic giant cell carcinoma, lung
   b nonmucus producing adenocarcinoma, pancreas
   c spindle cell sarcoma
   d anaplastic carcinoma, pancreas

109 A 67-year-old male presenting for a routine annual examination has an elevated serum prostate specific antigen analysis. FNA is performed on a hard, gritty, pea sized lesion of the prostate. Cytology reveals numerous cells arranged in repeated microacinar formations with small round nuclei, high N:C ratios, and prominent nucleoli. The diagnosis is:
   a malacoplakia
   b well differentiated adenocarcinoma
   c prostatitis
   d benign prostatic hyperplasia

110 The presence of lymphohistiocytic aggregates in the FNA of lymphadenopathy is usually indicative of:
   a lymphoma
   b metastatic carcinoma
   c reactive condition
   d cat scratch disease

111 The cytomorphologic diagnosis of small round cell lymphoma may be aided by immunocytochemical staining for:
   a common acute lymphocytic leukemia antigen (CALLA/CD10)
   b T cell and pan B cell surface antigens (Leu/CD5)
   c T cell surface antigens only
   d B cell surface antigens only

ISBN 978-089189-6357 ©ASCP 2015

112 The most common benign differential diagnosis of immunoblastic lymphoma is:
 a early reactive lymph node hyperplasia
 b midphase reactive lymph node hyperplasia
 c end stage lymph node hyperplasia
 d recurrent lymph node hyperplasia

113 A 66-year-old female with a previously diagnosed malignancy presents with multiple liver nodules. FNA cytology reveals many single cells with well defined intracytoplasmic eosinophilic inclusions giving the nucleus a targetoid appearance on Diff-Quik stain. Some cells are cohesive with vertebral column formation, contain hyperchromatic nuclei with nucleoli, and have frothy cytoplasm. The background was thick and eosinophilic with interspersed fat vacuoles and small fibrous stromal elements. The diagnosis is:
 a colonic adenocarcinoma
 b pancreatic carcinoma
 c ovarian adenocarcinoma
 d breast adenocarcinoma

114 What cell types predominate in late stage lymph node hyperplasia?
 a small round lymphocytes, small cleaved lymphocytes, plasma cells
 b large cleaved and large noncleaved lymphocytes
 c immunoblasts, large cleaved and large noncleaved lymphocytes
 d plasma cells, large cleaved and small cleaved lymphocytes

115 The predominant cellular population(s) found in the diagnosis of reactive lymph node hyperplasia is (are):
 a small round and small cleaved lymphocytes over large cleaved and noncleaved lymphocytes, lymphohistiocytic aggregates
 b large cleaved and noncleaved lymphocytes over small cleaved and noncleaved lymphocytes, lymphohistiocytic aggregates
 c immunoblasts and plasma cells over small cleaved and large noncleaved lymphocytes
 d immunoblasts and large cleaved lymphocytes over plasma cells and small cleaved lymphocytes

116 A 62-year-old male with dysuria presents for prostatic aspiration. Many pleomorphic cells in loose cohesive clusters with macronucleoli are found. The cytoplasm contains coarse golden-brown pigment on Papanicolaou and dark blue-green on Diff-Quik stain. Sperm is noted within the background. These cells are diagnostic of:
 a well differentiated adenocarcinoma, prostate
 b poorly differentiated adenocarcinoma, prostate
 c a benign cellular component
 d renal cell carcinoma

117 The FNA diagnosis of an axillary lymph node reveals a hypercellular population representing predominantly large single cells with smooth uniform nuclear borders, fine open chromatin patterns, up to 3 nucleoli per cell, and a scarce population of small cleaved and small round cells with coarse, dense to moderately open chromatin patterns. Lymphogranular bodies are noted. This process is usually:
 a CALLA/CD10+
 b Leu1/CD5+
 c of monoclonal B cell origin
 d of monoclonal T cell origin

118 Which is true regarding soft tissue tumors?
 a malignant tumors are more common than benign lesions
 b benign lesions are more common than malignant tumors
 c most needle aspirates require the use of 14 gauge needles
 d primary sarcomas of soft tissue are more common than metastatic carcinomas

119 A 72-year-old female with abdominal pain, weight loss, and jaundice presents with a 10 cm mass located in the head of the pancreas. FNA reveals a hypocellular sample of small clusters of cells with abundant clear cytoplasm. The nuclei are round with fine, regular chromatin. Staining is PAS+, PAS-D−, and mucicarmine−. The diagnosis is:
 a pancreatitis
 b microcystic adenoma
 c mucinous cystic neoplasm
 d pancreatic adenocarcinoma

120 In reactive lymph node hyperplasia, which of the following are seen?
 a a polynuclear population of immature lymphoid cells
 b a population of immunoblasts only
 c a polymorphic population of lymphoid cells
 d a single population of immature lymphocytes

121 The most common subtype of Hodgkin disease found in young adults associated with the cytologic diagnosis of mononucleate, nonclassical Reed-Sternberg cells is:
 a lymphocyte predominant type
 b lymphocyte depleted type
 c nodular sclerosing type
 d mixed cellularity type

122 A lymph node aspirate reveals a hypercellular sample that includes neutrophils, debris, histiocytes, and small round lymphocytes. What may be responsible for the cytologic findings?
 a viral infection
 b bacterial infection
 c diffuse immunoblastic hyperplasia
 d granulomatous lymphodermitis

123 A 55-year-old African American male with lymphadenopathy and an enlarged jaw presents for FNA. Small single cells with deep blue, finely vacuolated lipid+ cytoplasm are observed in the aspirate. Mitotic figures are present in many of the cells. A monoclonal B cell lesion with IgM κ surface markers is demonstrated with flow cytometry. The diagnosis is:
a immunoblastic lymphoma
b lymphoblastic lymphoma
c small round cell lymphoma
d Burkitt lymphoma

124 An FNA biopsy of a pancreatic mass from a 70-year-old male with mental weakness, fatigue, and a recent onset of convulsions reveals a monomorphic population of cells with salt & pepper chromatin and prominent nucleoli. Intracytoplasmic granules are demonstrated with Diff-Quik, and immunocytochemical staining for chromogranin and insulin is positive. Amyloid is noted within the background. These cells are diagnostic of:
a islet cell tumor of the pancreas, α cell predominance
b islet cell tumor of the pancreas, β cell predominance
c islet cell tumor of the pancreas, G cell predominance
d islet cell tumor of the pancreas, VIP cell predominance

125 What is considered a primary lymphoid granulomatous disease without necrosis?
a tuberculosis
b anthrax
c *Blastomyces dermatitidis*
d sarcoidosis

126 When confirming the diagnosis of mixed cell lymphoma (MCL) over that of reactive lymph node hyperplasia (RLNH), which cytologic criteria and flow cytometric techniques are helpful?
a there is an increase in small round cells and immunoblasts in MCL; MCL is polyclonal for light chains
b there is a lack of small round cells and immunoblasts in MCL; MCL is monoclonal for light chains
c there is an increase in small round cells and tingible body macrophages in MCL; MCL coexpresses T & B cell surface antigens
d there is an increase in immunoblasts, tingible body macrophages, and plasma cells in MCL; flow cytometry is not useful in the discrimination of MCL from other lymphomas

127 An FNA of an enlarged cervical lymph node from a 12-year-old male with fever, unexplained rashes, and recent unexplained weight loss reveals single binucleate cells with large irregular nucleoli. Abundant small round lymphocytes and epithelioid cells are found. These cells are diagnostic of:
a mixed cell lymphoma
b large cell noncleaved lymphoma
c immunoblastic lymphoma
d Hodgkin disease

128 A good indicator for the diagnosis of well differentiated mucus producing adenocarcinomas of pancreatic ductal origin is:
a fine chromatin with macronucleoli
b drunken honeycombs and goblet cells
c irregular chromatin and pleomorphism
d PAS-D negativity

129 A pancreatic mass was analyzed using FNA. Cytology reveals a hypercellular population of polygonal cells with granular cytoplasm, eccentric nuclei, irregular chromatin, macronucleoli, and a necrotic background. Serum analysis indicates an increase in amine/peptide products. Staining with neuron specific enolase was positive. These cells are diagnostic of:
a oncocytic neuroendocrine carcinoma of the pancreas
b mucinous cystadenoma
c pancreatic ductal adenocarcinoma
d pseudocyst

130 The predominant cell populations seen in the early reactive stages of lymph node hyperplasia are (in descending number):
a large cleaved lymphocytes, small round lymphocytes, immunoblasts
b plasma cells, large cleaved lymphocytes, small round lymphocytes
c large noncleaved lymphocytes, immunoblasts, plasma cells
d small round lymphocytes, small cleaved lymphocytes, large cleaved lymphocytes, large noncleaved lymphocytes, immunoblasts, plasma cells

131 A 33-year-old female with axillary lymphadenopathy associated with lymphodermatitis and erythematous papules at the site of the trauma and cytologically seen as epithelioid cells, giant cells, small round lymphocytes and necrosis is associated with a diagnosis of:
a lipophagic granuloma
b eosinophilic granuloma
c cat scratch disease
d toxoplasmosis

132 What lymphoma is characterized histologically as having a "starry sky" pattern?
a small cell cleaved lymphoma
b Burkitt lymphoma
c large cell cleaved lymphoma
d immunoblastic lymphoma

133 A 58-year-old female presents with abdominal pain and an 8 cm lesion in the upper pole of the kidney. FNA reveals a hypercellular population of tall columnar cells with wispy, granular to frothy cytoplasm staining gossamer blue and floral groups with radiating petal-like projections with a central core. The cells contain large nuclei with fine pale chromatin and cherry-red "stop sign" macronucleoli. Special staining with oil red O is positive. The diagnosis is:
a oncocytoma
b metastatic ovarian adenocarcinoma
c clear cell renal cell carcinoma
d sarcomatoid renal cell carcinoma

ISBN 978-089189-6357 ©ASCP 2015

134 A 67-year-old female with multiple liver nodules presents for FNA. Cytology reveals a slightly cohesive monotonous population of single cells attached to fibrocollagenous tissue. The cells have scanty cytoplasm, intracytoplasmic lumens, high N:C ratios, and hyperchromasia. The cellular configuration reveals cells forming a "stack of coins." Special stains reveal the cells are negative for neuron specific enolase and positive for mucicarmine. Which of the following may represent the cytologic findings?
   a metastatic breast carcinoma
   b metastatic kidney carcinoma
   c metastatic colon carcinoma
   d metastatic gastrointestinal leiomyosarcoma

135 The peak incidence of papillary carcinoma of the thyroid occurs:
   a <20 years of age
   b 20s-40s
   c 50s-70s
   d >80 years of age

136 A 62-year-old female with a previously established malignancy presents with an increased serum level of carcinoembryonic antigen and multiple liver nodules as demonstrated by CAT scan. FNA of the liver reveals cells with columnar morphology, vacuolated cytoplasm, signet rings, and polar nuclei with coarse, granular chromatin and multiple nucleoli. An extensive necrosis is identified in the background. The diagnosis is most suggestive of:
   a hepatocellular carcinoma
   b metastatic colonic carcinoma
   c metastatic breast carcinoma
   d metastatic small cell undifferentiated carcinoma of the lung

137 A 2-year-old male presents with an 2 cm well circumscribed solitary liver mass. Serum analysis for α-fetoprotein is markedly elevated. FNA of the liver reveals a uniform population of small, round, loosely cohesive cells with scanty cytoplasm and high N:C ratios. The chromatin is fine to coarse with micronucleoli. The cellular pattern is suggestive of:
   a metastatic neuroblastoma
   b adenomatous hyperplasia
   c hepatocellular carcinoma
   d hepatoblastoma

138 A 55-year-old male with a 4 cm minor salivary gland nodule undergoes FNA. These cells represent a highly cellular aspirate. They are diagnostic of:
  a acinic cell carcinoma
  b adenoid cystic carcinoma
  c basal cell adenoma
  d pleomorphic adenoma

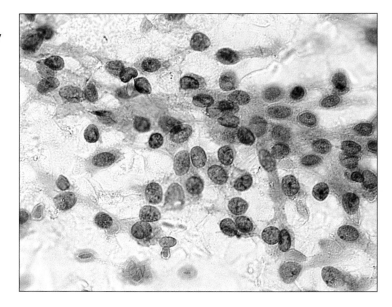

139 An FNA of the thyroid reveals these cells. They are:
  a follicular cells
  b parafollicular cells
  c Hürthle cells
  d macrophages

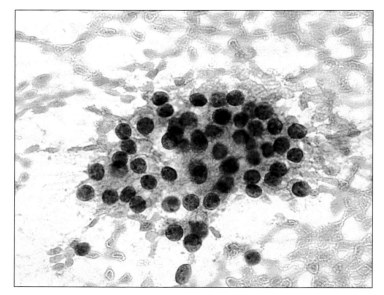

140 A 39-year-old female with a palpable thyroid nodule undergoes FNA. The depicted cellular process suggests:
  a medullary carcinoma
  b anaplastic carcinoma
  c follicular neoplasm
  d papillary carcinoma

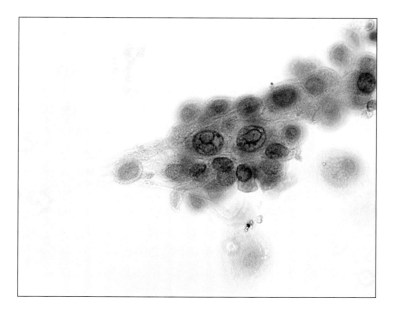

ISBN 978-089189-6357   ©ASCP 2015

141 Represented is a fine needle aspirate from a 42-year-old female presenting with a 3 cm parotid mass. These cellular findings represent:

    a mucoepidermoid carcinoma
    b acinic cell carcinoma
    c adenoid cystic carcinoma
    d pleomorphic adenoma

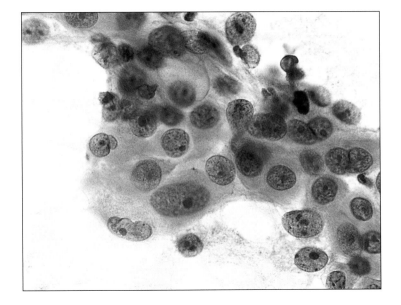

142 These cells are from a 60-year-old female with a history of thyroiditis. They are:

    a follicular cells
    b parafollicular cells
    c Hürthle cells
    d epithelioid histiocytes

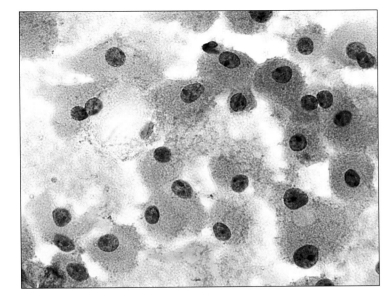

143 This cellular pattern is from a 35-year-old male presenting with painless cervical lymphadenopathy and complaining of a low grade fever and night sweats. Upon examination, hepatosplenomegaly is noted. FNA of the spleen suggests a diagnosis of:

    a lymphoreticular hyperplasia
    b metastatic sarcoma
    c signet ring adenocarcinoma
    d Hodgkin disease

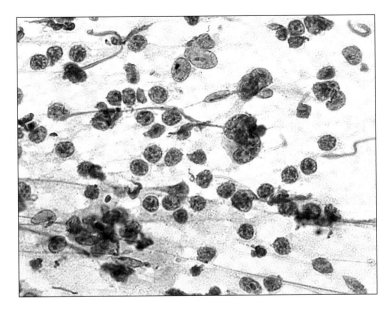

144   A thyroid aspirate from a 56-year-old female yields these cells. The diagnosis is:

    a   de Quervain thyroiditis
    b   Hashimoto thyroiditis
    c   oncocytoma
    d   colloid goiter

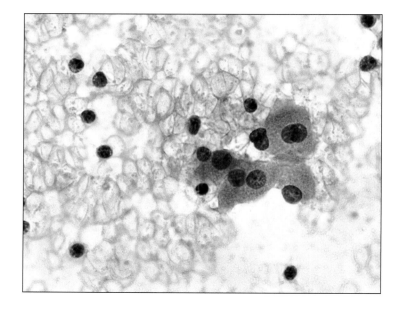

145   A 50-year-old female with a submandibular mass presents for FNA evaluation. The patient complains of a severe pain during the aspiration procedure. Cytologic findings are suggestive of:

    a   acinic cell carcinoma
    b   adenoid cystic carcinoma
    c   pleomorphic adenoma
    d   basal cell adenoma

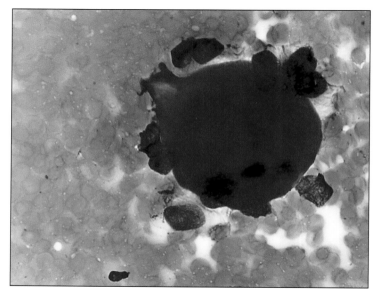

146   FNA of a 4 cm nodule in the cervical region of the neck from a 55-year-old male reveals these cells. These cells were positive for microphthalmia associated transcription factor (MITF). The cytologic pattern represents:

    a   malignant fibrous histiocytoma
    b   osteosarcoma
    c   metastatic large cell undifferentiated carcinoma
    d   metastatic melanoma

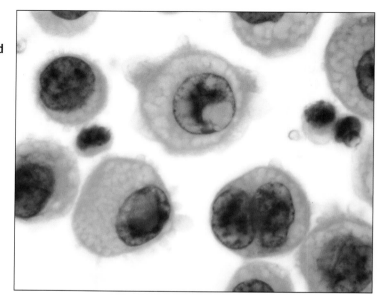

ISBN 978-089189-6357 ©ASCP 2015

147   A 56-year-old female with an enlarged palpable thyroid mass that actively takes up radioactive iodine undergoes FNA. The cellular findings are diagnostic of:
   a   follicular neoplasm
   b   papillary carcinoma
   c   nodular goiter
   d   medullary carcinoma

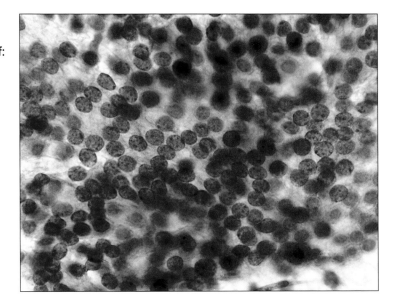

148   A 45-year-old female presents with an enlarged thyroid. FNA is performed on the mass and yields these cells. The cell at center represents:
   a   colloid goiter
   b   thyrotoxic goiter
   c   giant cell thyroiditis
   d   medullary carcinoma

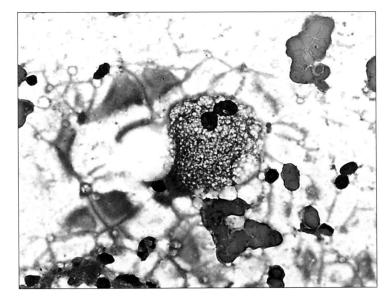

149   A 55-year-old female presents with bilateral parotid masses. Aspiration cytology confirms the presence of PAS(+) granules within the cytoplasm. The cellular findings are diagnostic of:
   a   acinic cell carcinoma
   b   monomorphic adenoma
   c   adenoid cystic carcinoma
   d   lymphoma

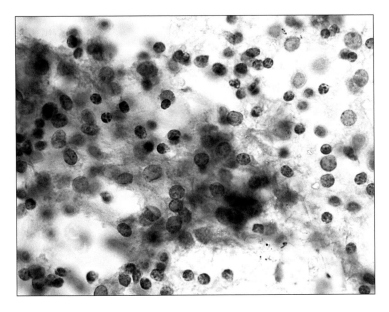

150 A 67-year-old patient who recently underwent lymphangiography presents with an abdominal lymphoid nodule. The cytologic pattern depicted is:
a sinus histiocytosis
b large cell cleaved lymphoma
c end stage lymphoid hyperplasia
d lipophagic granuloma

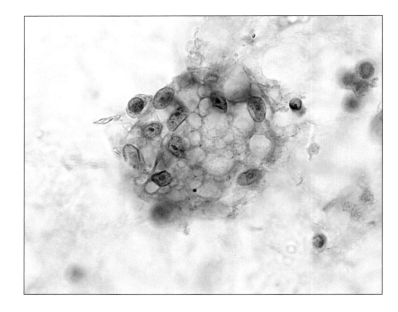

151 A cervical lymphoid nodule in a 65-year-old female with an established diagnosis of extralymphatic cancer is evaluated by FNA. The cytologic pattern depicted may represent which of the following?
a metastatic melanoma
b metastatic squamous cell carcinoma
c metastatic adenocarcinoma, breast
d granulomatous lymphadenopathy

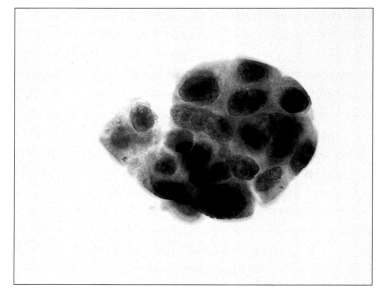

152 An enlarged thyroid from a 67-year-old male is evaluated with FNA. The cytologic pattern depicted is consistent with:
a Hashimoto thyroiditis
b Hürthle cell adenoma
c de Quervain thyroiditis
d lymphoma

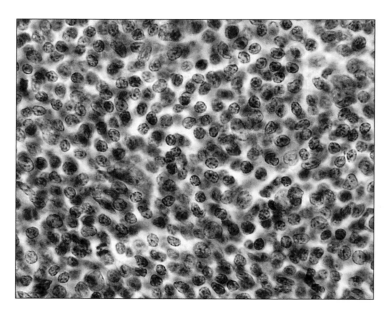

ISBN 978-089189-6357 ©ASCP 2015

153 A 16-year-old female with confirmed viral mononucleosis presents with an enlarged pelvic lymph node. These cells, obtained by FNA, represent:
a immunoblastic hyperplasia
b follicular hyperplasia
c lymphoblastic lymphoma
d Hodgkin disease

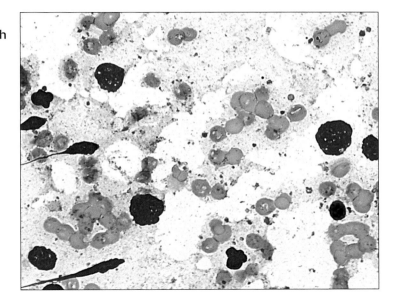

154 Which thyroid lesion is associated with the findings in this photomicrograph?
a follicular neoplasm
b papillary carcinoma
c medullary carcinoma
d metastatic melanoma

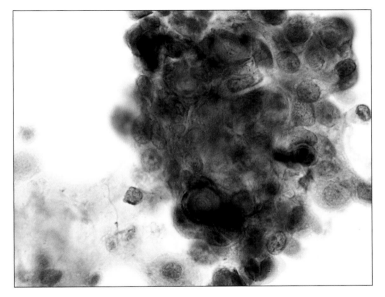

155 These cells were aspirated from a large painful thyroid mass in an elderly woman. Staining is negative for thyroglobulin and calcitonin, and positive for epithelial membrane antigen. Based on cellular findings and special staining, the diagnosis is:
a follicular carcinoma
b giant cell anaplastic carcinoma
c medullary carcinoma
d papillary carcinoma

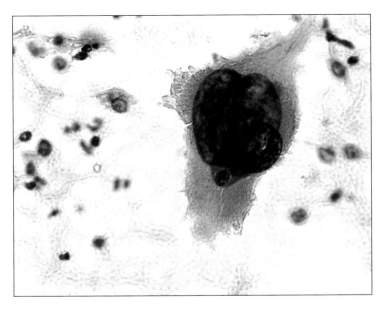

156 The best interpretation of this 2 cm painful parotid mass from a 42-year-old male is (FNA):
   a acinic cell carcinoma
   b pleomorphic adenoma
   c mucoepidermoid carcinoma
   d adenoid cystic carcinoma

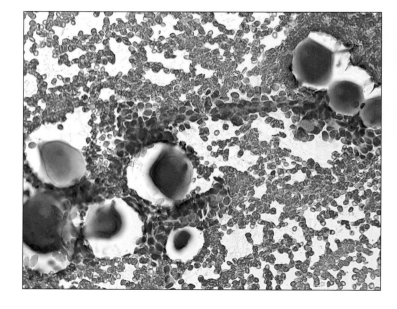

157 These cells are from a cervical lymph node aspirate from a patient with tuberculosis. They are diagnostic of:
   a small cell cleaved lymphoma
   b granulomatous lymphadenitis
   c Burkitt lymphoma
   d midphase lymphoid hyperplasia

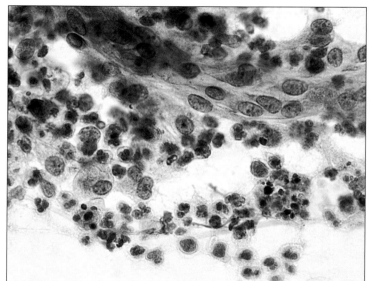

158 A 68-year-old male with an elevated prostate specific antigen (PSA) level presents for FNA evaluation of the prostate. The cytologic pattern depicted is:
   a adenocarcinoma
   b seminal vesicle cells
   c transitional cell carcinoma
   d benign prostatic hyperplasia

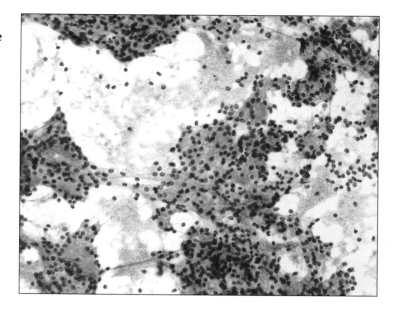

ISBN 978-089189-6357 ©ASCP 2015

159 These cells are identified in an inguinal lymph node aspirate from a 52-year-old male. Flow cytometry reveals monoclonal serum immunoglobulin. Cytologic correlation suggests:
a mycosis fungoides
b large cell lymphoma
c plasma cell myeloma
d diffuse immunoblastic hyperplasia

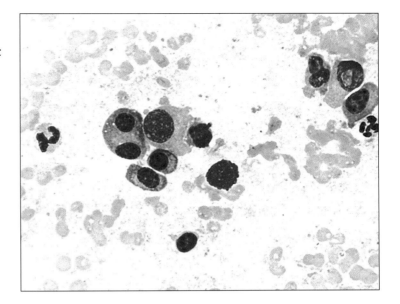

160 A 57-year-old female with a supraclavicular lymph node enlargement presents for FNA. These cells are identified in the cytologic preparation. The diagnosis is:
a immunoblastic lymphoma
b large cell cleaved lymphoma
c lymphoblastic lymphoma
d end stage lymph node reaction with recurrent antigenic stimulation

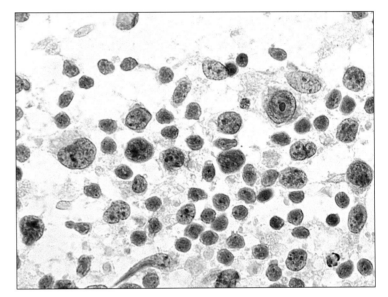

161 A 32-year-old male presents with an enlarged axillary lymph node. FNA reveals:
a follicular (reactive) hyperplasia
b granulomatous hyperplasia
c cat scratch disease
d toxoplasmosis

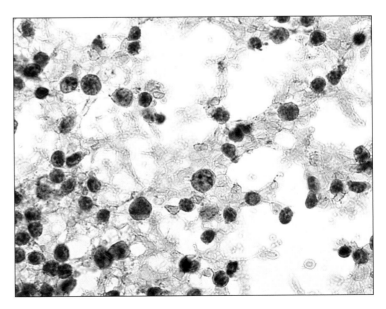

162 A 44-year-old patient presents with an enlarged inguinal lymph node. Microabscess formation and suppurative necrosis are identified. Which diagnosis is associated with the depicted cellular findings?
  a toxoplasmosis granulomatosis
  b cat scratch disease
  c sarcoidosis
  d large cell cleaved lymphoma

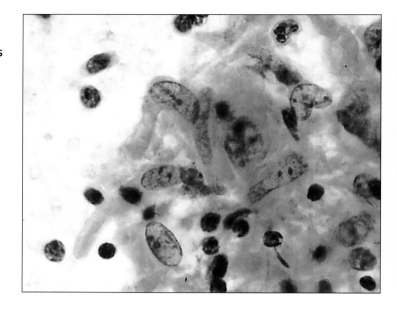

163 A lesion found within the proximal tibia of a 15-year-old male is evaluated with FNA. The cytologic pattern depicted is:
  a osteosarcoma
  b callus
  c giant cell tumor of the bone
  d osteoblastoma

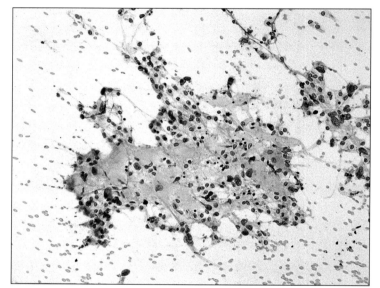

164 A 55-year-old African American male presents with a markedly enlarged lymph node within the jaw. An FNA specimen is prepared for cytology as well as flow cytometry, which indicates a monoclonal B cell neoplasm. These cells represent what process?
  a small round cell lymphoma
  b lymphoblastic lymphoma
  c diffuse immunoblastic hyperplasia
  d Burkitt lymphoma

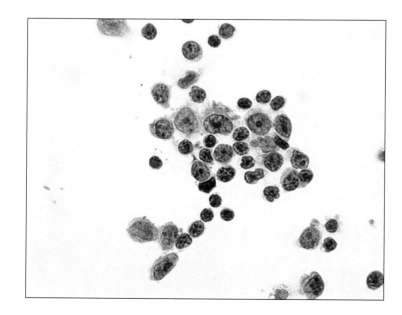

ISBN 978-089189-6357 ©ASCP 2015

165 A 52-year-old female presents with an enlarged
cervical lymph node. Based on the cellular findings,
the diagnosis is:
  a small cell noncleaved lymphoma
  b signet ring cell lymphomas
  c follicular hyperplasia
  d mixed small cleaved, large cell lymphoma

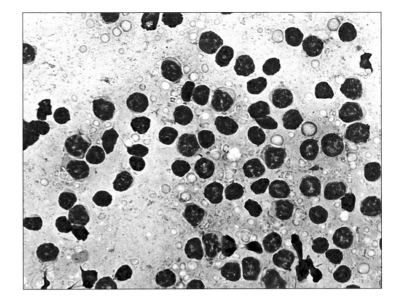

166 A 55-year-old male with a retroperitoneal soft-
tissue mass presents for fine needle aspiration (FNA)
evaluation. The cells shown are diagnostic of:
  a liposarcoma
  b angiosarcoma
  c malignant fibrous histiocytoma
  d hemangioma

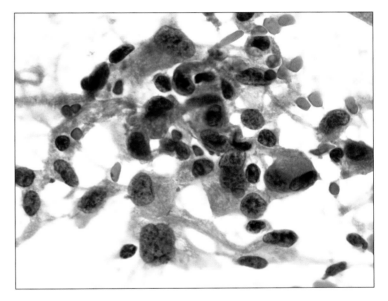

167 A 16-year-old male with a history of a testicular tumor
presents with a peritoneal lesion. FNA of the pelvic
mass reveals these cells. The diagnosis is:
  a choriocarcinoma
  b seminoma
  c embryonal cell carcinoma
  d endodermal sinus tumor

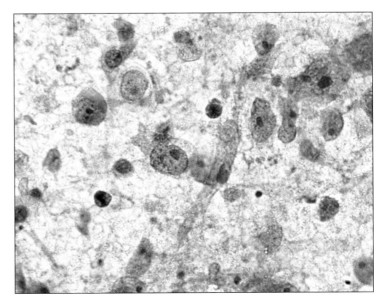

168 A 55-year-old male with a history of multiple lipomas presents with a firm, nontender nodule in the left thigh (an area resected 5 years earlier). These cells were found in a hypercellular aspirate. The cytologic findings represent:

  a lipoma
  b liposarcoma
  c reactive lymphadenopathy
  d metastatic sarcoma

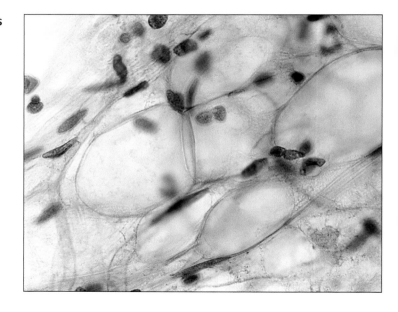

169 A coin lesion of the lung was identified in a 65-year-old male with a history of smoking. FNA cytology reveals:

  a normal bronchial cells
  b metastatic melanoma
  c hemosiderin laden macrophages
  d hepatocytes, suggest reaspiration

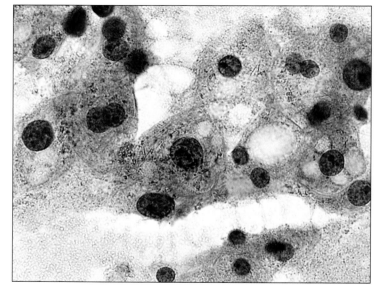

170 Shown is an FNA of a pulmonary lesion, which, when aspirated, may yield a false negative diagnosis because of:

  a contaminants
  b poor staining quality
  c faulty technique–aspiration of necrotic center
  d vascular nature of the lesion

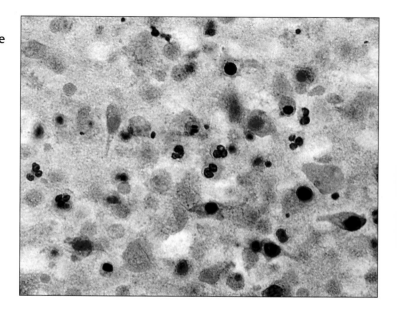

ISBN 978-089189-6357 ©ASCP 2015

171 This image from an aspirate from a 4 cm cavitary mass of the right middle lobe of a 75-year-old male displays:

    a histoplasmosis
    b cryptococcus
    c pollen
    d coccidioidomycosis

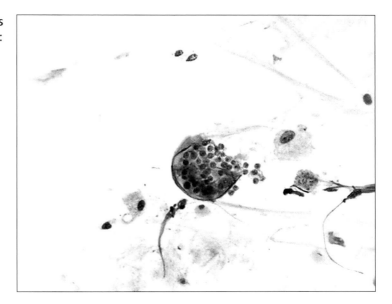

172 The cells in the center of the photomicrograph could arise from:

    a hepatocellular carcinoma
    b melanoma
    c papillary neoplasm of the thyroid
    d any of the above

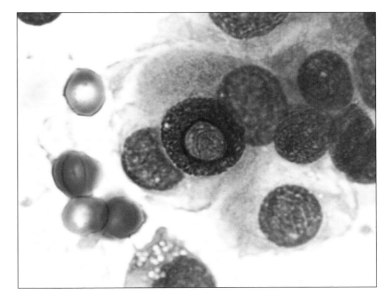

173 What special stain is helpful in establishing the pancreatic islet cell origin of these cells?

    a α-fetoprotein
    b S100
    c chromogranin
    d vimentin

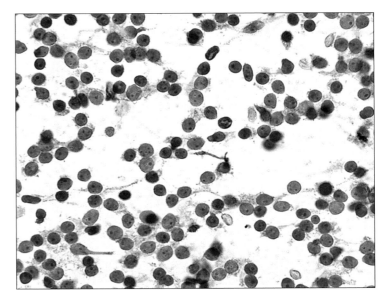

174 A patient develops anaphylaxis when a 3 cm cystic nodule is aspirated. The aspirated material is gritty in nature. This finding is suggestive of:

- **a** *Strongyloides stercoralis*
- **b** *Echinococcus granulosis*
- **c** *Entamoeba histolytica*
- **d** *Schistosoma mansoni*

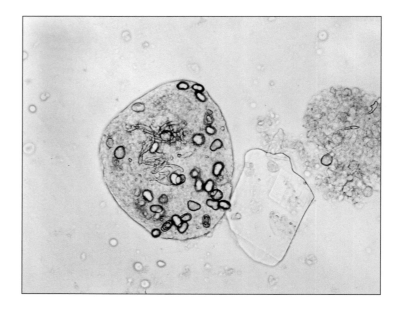

175 A 55-year-old female with a 4 cm nodule in the head of the pancreas presents for FNA evaluation. Clinical symptoms include jaundice, weight loss, and deep radiating back pain. The cellular findings are diagnostic of:

- **a** ductal adenocarcinoma
- **b** microcystic adenoma
- **c** pancreatitis
- **d** anaplastic pancreatic carcinoma

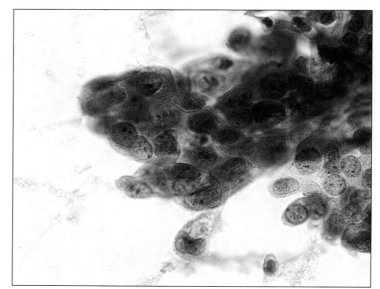

176 A 55-year-old female with history of pancreatic carcinoma presents with a 1 cm liver nodule. These cells were obtained via aspiration with a 22 gauge needle. Which immunocytochemical results will help establish a diagnosis of metastatic pancreatic carcinoma by differentiating it from primary trabecular hepatocellular carcinoma?

- **a** α-fetoprotein–, keratin+
- **b** α-fetoprotein+, keratin–
- **c** α-fetoprotein–, keratin–
- **d** α-fetoprotein+, keratin+

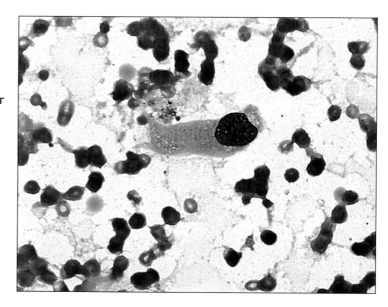

ISBN 978-089189-6357   ©ASCP 2015

177　A 33-year-old AIDS patient presents with multiple pigmented erythematous cutaneous lesions of the face and legs. Aspiration cytology of one of the leg lesions reveals these cells. The diagnosis is:

a　squamous cell carcinoma
b　Kaposi sarcoma
c　melanoma
d　basal cell carcinoma

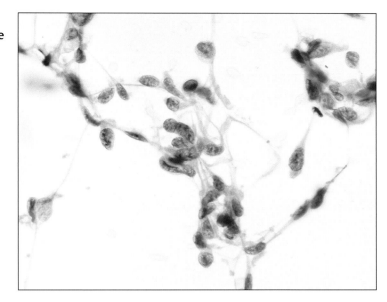

178　These cells are identified in an aspirate of a 3 cm liver nodule in a 71-year-old male with a history of intrahepatic lithiasis. Immunocytochemical staining for α-fetoprotein is negative. The depicted cells represent:

a　hepatocellular carcinoma
b　cholangiocarcinoma
c　liver cell dysplasia
d　reactive hepatocytes, secondary to lithiasis

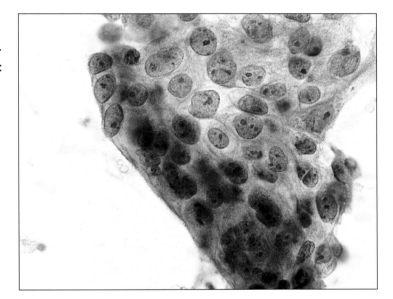

179　Depicted is an FNA specimen of a 3×4 cm coin lesion in the left upper lobe of the lung. The patient is a 65-year-old male with a 120 pack/year, 20 year history of smoking. He presents with obstructive pneumonitis and atelectasis. The diagnosis should include:

a　*Aspergillus species*, rule out secondary malignancy by reaspirating from various areas of the mass
b　*Geotrichum candidum,* treat patient for fungal infection
c　Actinomyces species, rule out secondary malignancy by reaspirating from various areas of the mass
d　saprophytic phycomycetes, treat patient for fungal infection

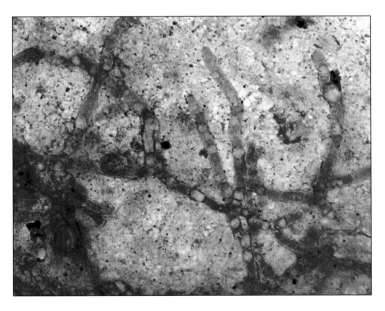

180 What special stain will positively confirm the interpretation of these aspirated cells from a solitary lung nodule?
  a chromogranin
  b HMB45
  c α-fetoprotein
  d periodic acid-Schiff

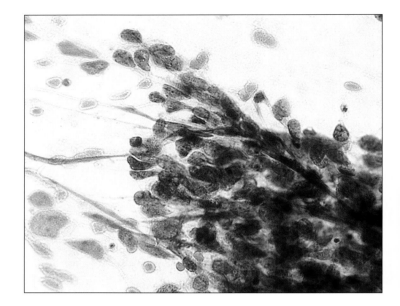

181 These cells in a purulent supraclavicular lymph node aspirate located near the mandible, are diagnostic of:
  a diffuse immunoblastic lymphoma
  b follicular hyperplasia
  c acute lymphadenitis
  d sinus histiocytosis

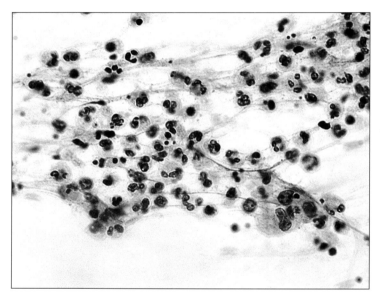

182 These cells represent an FNA specimen from a patient with no history of a primary tumor but currently presenting with a 4 cm liver lesion and seropositivity for hepatitis B. The diagnosis is:
  a reactive hepatocytes
  b reactive bile ductal cells
  c cholangiocarcinoma
  d hepatocellular carcinoma

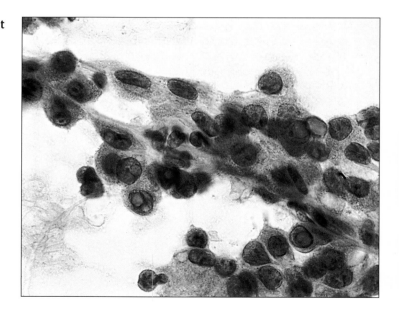

ISBN 978-089189-6357 ©ASCP 2015

183 These cells from pulmonary aspirations are:
- **a** bronchial cells
- **b** mesothelial cells
- **c** fat cells
- **d** diagnostic of hamartoma

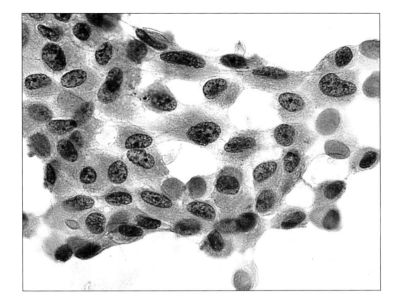

184 A 23-year-old male with a previously confirmed case of small cell cleaved lymphoma, status post chemotherapy and postirradiation, presents with pneumonitis. FNA is performed to rule out metastatic disease. A GMS stain is performed. The cytologic findings suggest:
- **a** metastatic lymphoma
- **b** *Pneumocystis jiroveci*
- **c** *Histoplasma capsulatum*
- **d** nondiagnostic, suggest repeat aspiration

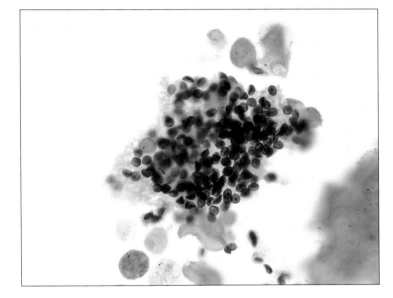

185 A 66-year-old alcoholic patient with multiple liver nodules undergoes FNA. The depicted cells represent what type of process?
- **a** reactive
- **b** malignant primary
- **c** metastatic
- **d** hamartomatous

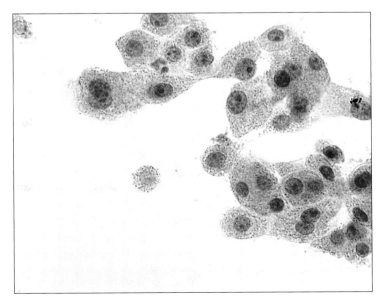

186 A 44-year-old male with a 3 cm lesion of the parotid gland undergoes FNA. A soft mass yields a brownish watery substance. These cells represent:

a Warthin tumor
b oxyphilic adenoma
c pleomorphic adenoma
d acinic cell carcinoma

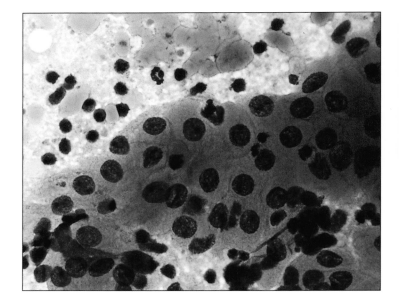

187 These cells from a 5 cm nodule located in the parotid gland suggest a diagnosis of:

a oncocytoma
b adenoid cystic carcinoma
c mucoepidermoid carcinoma
d pleomorphic adenoma

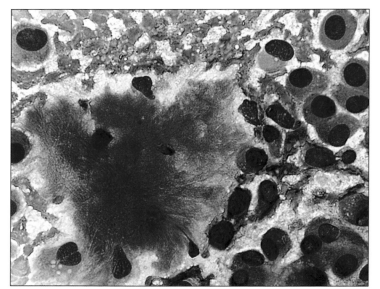

188 These cells represent a transbronchial aspirate from a peripheral 2 cm mass. The cellular findings suggest:

a adenocarcinoma, poorly differentiated
b large cell undifferentiated carcinoma
c squamous cell carcinoma, poorly differentiated
d adenosquamous carcinoma

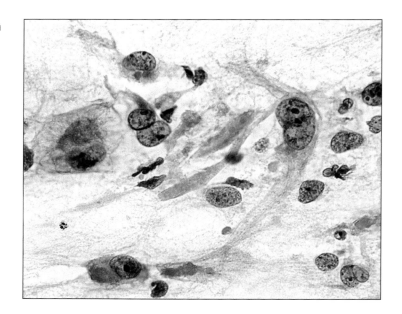

ISBN 978-089189-6357 ©ASCP 2015

189 A 72-year-old patient with a history of a primary esophageal malignancy presents with multiple solid neck masses. An FNA specimen revealed these cells. The diagnosis is:

a metastatic squamous cell carcinoma
b branchial cleft cyst
c epidermal inclusion cyst
d follicular carcinoma, metastatic from the thyroid

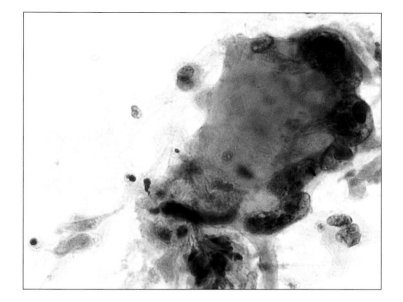

190 These cells are identified in a pancreatic aspirate from a 65-year-old female with jaundice and Trousseau syndrome. A dilated common bile duct and gallbladder is demonstrated by endoscopic retrograde cholangiopancreatography. Based on the cellular findings, what is the primary diagnosis?

a secretory ductal carcinoma, pancreas
b nonsecretory ductal carcinoma, pancreas
c oncocytic neoplasm, pancreas
d pancreatoblastoma

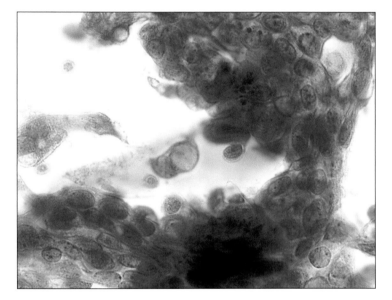

191 A 55-year-old female with shortness of breath and dyspnea presents with a central cavitating lung lesion as demonstrated by computed tomography. Radiographically guided transbronchial aspiration reveals these cells. Based on the cytologic findings, the diagnosis is:

a metastatic leiomyosarcoma
b atypical squamous metaplasia
c large cell undifferentiated carcinoma
d squamous carcinoma

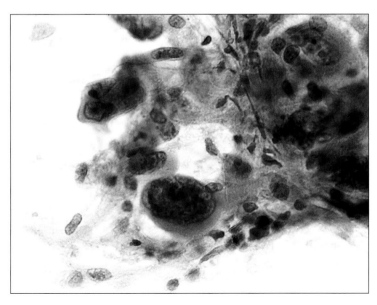

192 A 42-year-old male clinically diagnosed with HIV presents with a 2 cm liver lesion. FNA is performed using a 22 gauge needle. These cells represent:
  a granuloma
  b fat necrosis
  c adenoma
  d liver cell dysplasia

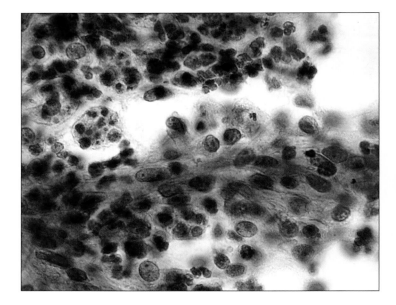

193 These cells from a parotid aspirate are diagnostic of:
  a monomorphic adenoma
  b Warthin tumor
  c oxyphilic adenoma
  d normal parenchyma

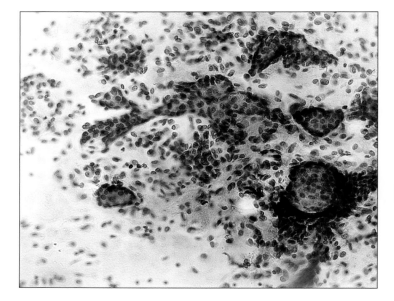

194 A 42-year-old female with a history of gallstones presents with a cystic pancreas and increased serum amylase levels. FNA evaluation of the pancreas reveals these cells. The diagnosis is:
  a islet cell neoplasm
  b acute pancreatitis
  c microcystic adenoma
  d ductal adenocarcinoma

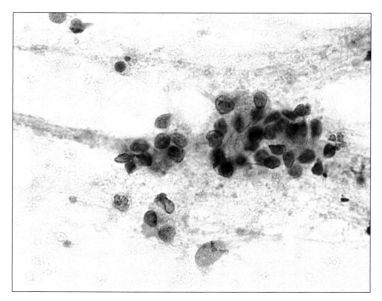

ISBN 978-089189-6357 ©ASCP 2015

195 Which of the following immunostains will help confirm the morphologic diagnosis of this adrenal aspirate?

   a melan A
   b CD10
   c chromogranin
   d TTF1

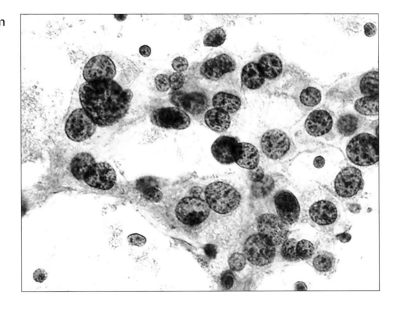

196 Which of the following immunostains will help confirm the morphologic diagnosis of this adrenal aspirate?

   a HepPar1
   b CD10
   c inhibin
   d chromogranin

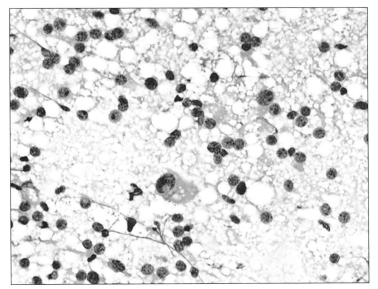

197 This 77-year-old male presented with a solitary peripheral lung nodule. An FNA of the lung mass was performed. What is your diagnosis?

   a bronchioloalveolar carcinoma
   b creola bodies
   c mesothelioma
   d reactive pneumocytes

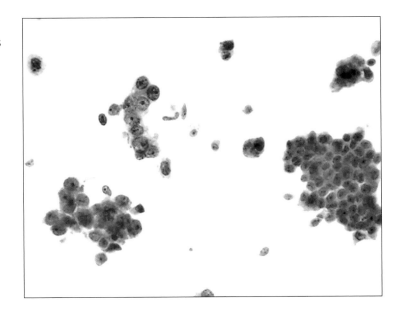

198 Which of the following blood tests is most likely
elevated in a patient with this thyroid aspirate?
a parathyroid hormone
b thyroglobulin
c antithyroid peroxidase antibodies
d calcitonin

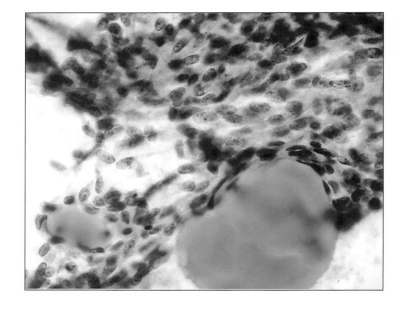

199 A 60-year-old male presents with a 2 cm kidney mass.
A difficult aspirate yielded the material shown in the
image. The best interpretation is:
a renal cell carcinoma
b angiosarcoma
c glomerulus structure
d papillary renal cell carcinoma

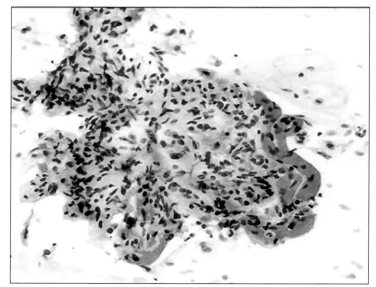

200 A 60-year-old male presents with a left supraclavicular
enlarged lymph node. The most likely diagnosis of the
aspirated material of this node is:
a metastatic renal cell carcinoma
b metastatic signet ring cell carcinoma
c malignant lymphoma
d sinus histiocytosis

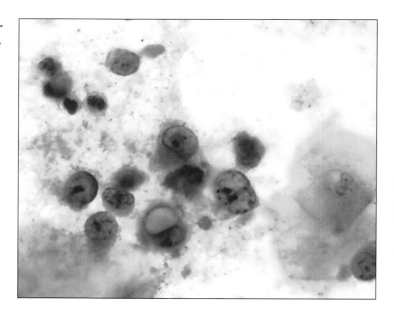

ISBN 978-089189-6357   ©ASCP 2015

201 Which pattern of immunostains from this aspirate of a 5 cm mass in the right kidney of a 72-year-old female be expected for this neoplasm?

a CD10+, CK7–
b CK7+/CK20+, CD10–
c CD10–, CK7–
d CD10+, CK7+

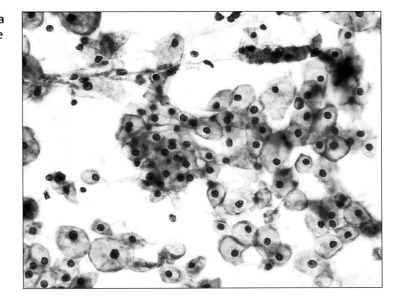

202 Which of the following blood tests is most likely elevated in a patient with this thyroid aspirate?

a parathyroid hormone
b thyroglobulin
c antithyroid peroxidase antibodies
d calcitonin

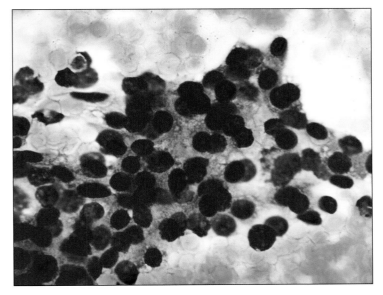

203 This aspirate from a 70-year-old female with elevated blood calcium and lytic lesion of T10 depicts:

a metastatic carcinoma of the breast
b multiple myeloma
c osteoid osteoma
d chronic osteomyelitis

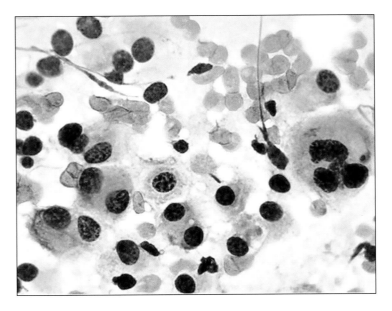

204 The image depicted from an EUS aspirate performed on a 72-year-old male with a pancreatic mass and elevated blood glucose represents:

a pancreatic acinar tissue
b pancreatic islet cell neoplasm
c benign gastric tissue
d pancreatic adenocarcinoma

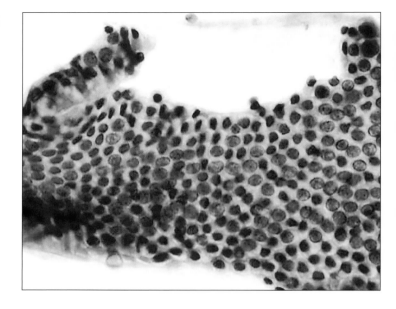

205 This image of a fine needle aspirate from a 2 cm left cervical mass in a 65-year-old male depicts:

a metastatic squamous cell carcinoma
b branchial cleft cyst
c Hodgkin disease
d granulomatous lymphadenitis

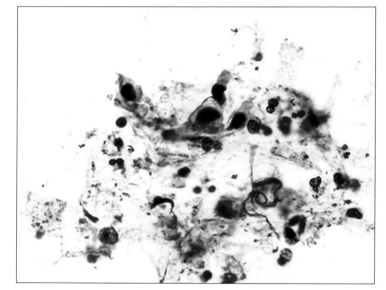

206 This fine needle aspirate is from a 30-year-old male with a 2 month history of a 3 cm mass in his forearm most likely represents:

a rheumatoid nodule
b nodular fasciitis
c pilomatrixoma
d metastatic melanoma

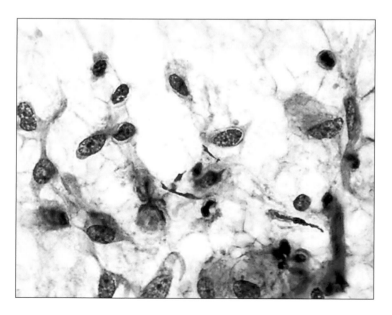

ISBN 978-089189-6357   ©ASCP 2015

207 This image from a fine needle aspirate from a 45-year-old female with a 3 cm mass in her right thyroid depicts:

a colloid nodule
b papillary carcinoma
c medullary carcinoma
d follicular neoplasm

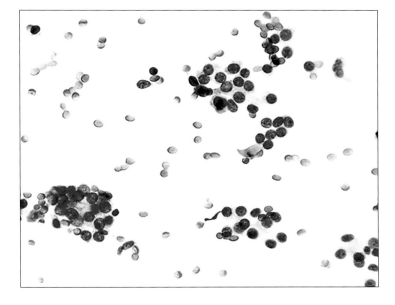

208 This fine needle aspirate from a 22-year-old female with a 3 month history of a 2 cm midline thyroid mass most likely represents:

a colloid nodule
b thyroglossal duct cyst
c cystic papillary carcinoma
d metastatic squamous cell carcinoma

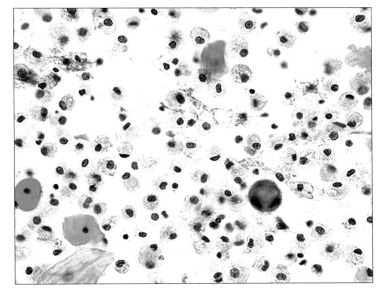

209 This image from a fine needle aspirate of a necrotic 4 cm left upper lobe mass depicts:

a squamous cell carcinoma
b aspergillosis
c small cell carcinoma
d metastatic colonic adenocarcinoma

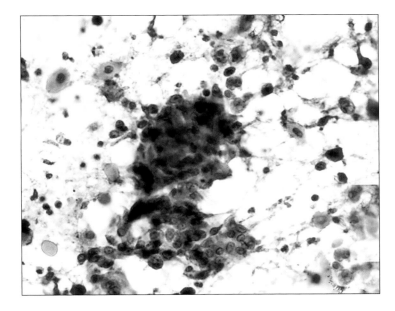

210 This image from a fine needle aspirate performed on a 45-year-old female with a 4 cm mass of her left 6th rib represents:

  a myeloma
  b metastatic adenocarcinoma
  c low grade chondrosarcoma
  d artifactual foreign material

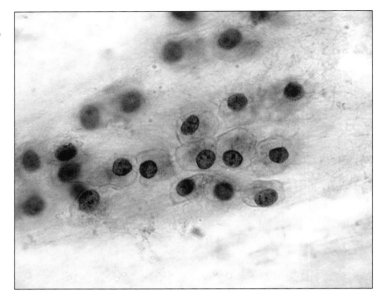

211 The most appropriate diagnosis for this EUS FNA of a pancreatic body mass in an 83-year-old male is:

  a chronic pancreatitis
  b benign enteric contamination
  c ductal adenocarcinoma
  d pancreatic endocrine neoplasm

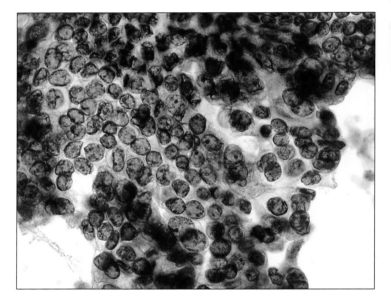

212 The most appropriate diagnosis for this transgastric EUS FNA of a pancreatic body mass in a 55-year-old male is:

  a pancreatic acinar cells
  b benign gastric mucosal cells
  c ductal adenocarcinoma
  d pancreatic endocrine neoplasm

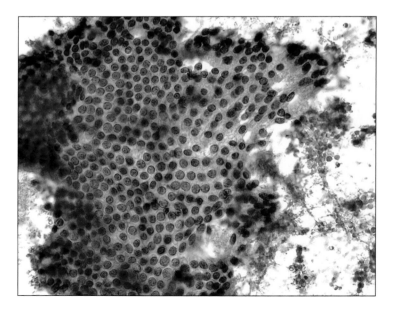

ISBN 978-089189-6357 ©ASCP 2015

213 A 54-year-old male was evaluated for increasing cough, sometimes with hemoptysis. He was a 2 pack a day smoker for many years. He had also recently begun to loose weight. Evaluation by chest film showed a large perihilar mass on the right. CT scan of the abdomen showed several liver nodules. Fine needle aspiration biopsy was performed on one of the liver nodules. What is your interpretation of the cytologic findings?

a large cell neuroendocrine carcinoma
b malignant lymphoma
c metastatic small cell carcinoma
d low grade neuroendocrine carcinoma

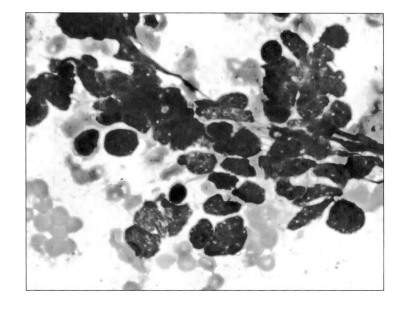

214 This 55-year-old female with a 3 cm pancreatic tail mass is most likely suffering from:

a ductal adenocarcinoma
b pancreatic endocrine neoplasm
c benign acinar cells
d plasma cell neoplasm

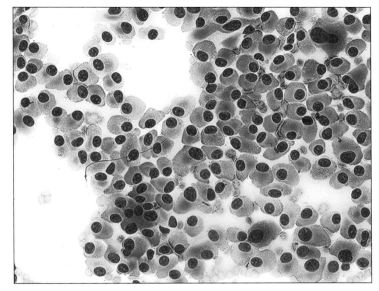

215 FNA from a suspected thyroid nodule in an 18-year-old female revealed these cells. What is the most likely interpretation?

a medullary thyroid carcinoma
b papillary thyroid carcinoma
c parathyroid tissue
d lymphocytic thyroiditis

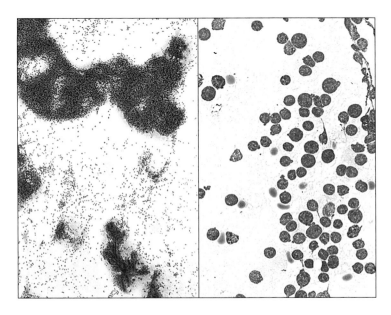

216 A transgastric, ultrasound guided endoscopic FNA of a pancreatic neck/body mass from a 40-year-old male showed this morphology. What would be the next step in confirming the diagnosis?

a serum CA19-9
b flow cytometry
c immunostaining for synaptophysin and chromogranin
d chest CT scan

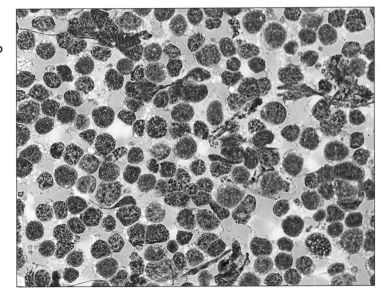

217 While assisting at a pancreatic mass FNA, the clinician inquires as to the adequacy of the current EUS FNA specimen. Your interpretation of these cells would lead you to indicate:

a these cells are nondiagnostic (gastric contamination)
b these cells represent benign ductal cells
c these cells are diagnostic, and adequacy of the FNA is complete
d ancillary techniques will be required

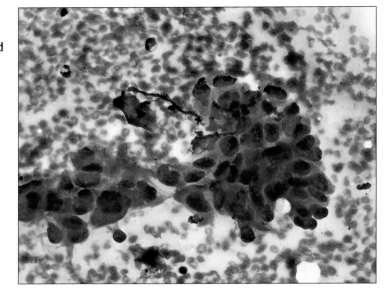

218 The most appropriate diagnosis for this EUS FNA of a partially cystic pancreatic body mass in a 30-year-old female is:

a acinar carcinoma
b solid pseudopapillary tumor
c ductal adenocarcinoma
d pancreatic endocrine neoplasm

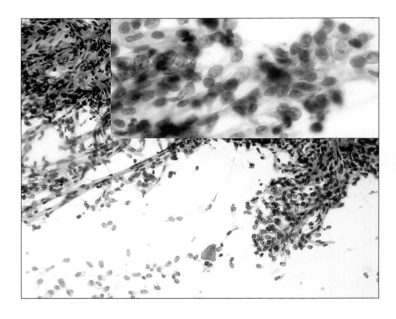

ISBN 978-089189-6357 ©ASCP 2015

219 A peripancreatic mass is sampled in an 84-year-old male, who has a history of jaundice and abdominal pain. Your interpretation of these cells is:
   a positive for malignancy, ductal adenocarcinoma
   b suspicious for malignancy, neuroendocrine differentiation
   c cells consistent with peripheral ganglion sampling
   d positive for malignancy, metastatic renal cell carcinoma

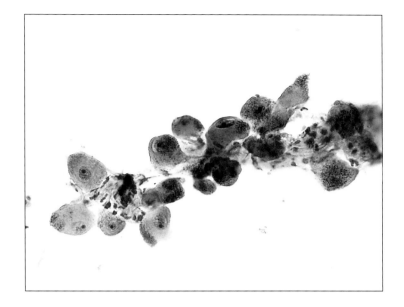

220 An 18-year-old male complained of pain in his lower back and some pain when defecating. This had progressed over several months from the time that he first noted the pain. An X-ray revealed a large but circumscribed lesion of the sacrum. A needle core biopsy and aspiration were performed. The best interpretation of the image shown is:
   a malignant cells of osteosarcoma
   b no malignant cells, aneurysmal bone cyst
   c giant cell tumor of bone
   d malignant cells of small round blue cell tumor

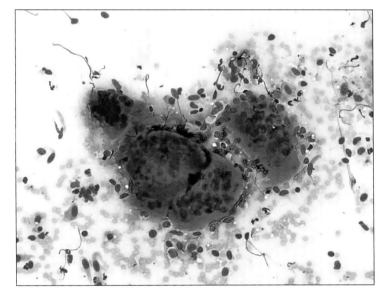

221 A 69-year-old male had a nephrectomy 2 years previously for conventional renal cell carcinoma. He recently noticed a mass in the subcutaneous tissue around his left elbow. Though not painful, the mass seemed to be enlarging over the past several weeks. What is your interpretation?
   a plasmacytoma of soft tissue
   b alveolar soft part sarcoma
   c metastatic renal cell carcinoma
   d rhabdomyosarcoma

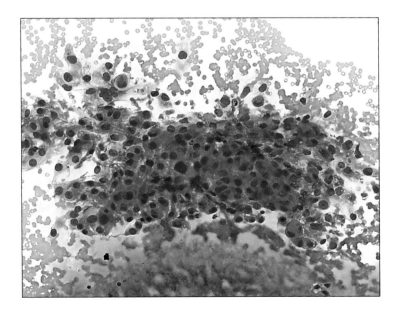

222 FNA of a 3 cm solitary round peripheral lung nodule in a 48-year-old female revealed these cells. What is the most likely diagnosis?
  a mucinous adenocarcinoma with desmoplasia
  b metastatic chondrosarcoma
  c pulmonary hamartoma
  d spindle cell carcinoid

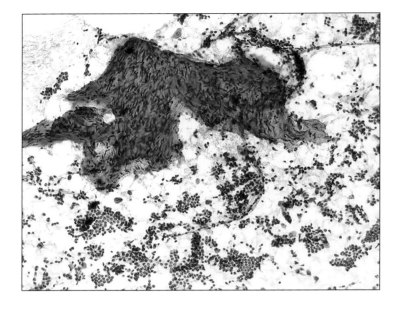

223 A 67-year-old female presents with a 5 cm hard cervical lymph node. FNA revealed these cells. What is the most probable source of these cells?
  a Hodgkin lymphoma
  b anaplastic lymphoma
  c metastatic melanoma
  d reactive immunoblasts

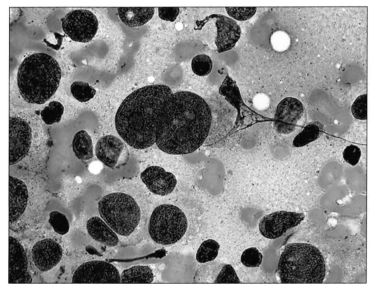

224 Transthoracic FNA of a solitary lung lesion in a 53-year-old female showed extensive necrosis and clusters of cells, as shown here. She had a skin lesion resected from her face a year ago. What is the most likely diagnosis?
  a metastatic Merkel cell carcinoma
  b metastatic melanoma
  c malignant lymphoma
  d granulomatous inflammation

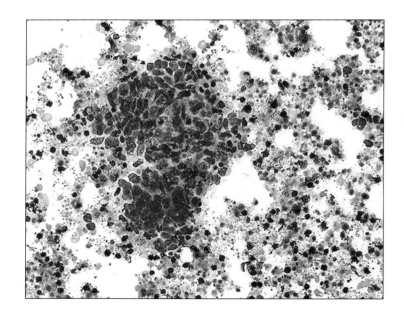

ISBN 978-089189-6357   ©ASCP 2015

225 Which of the following blood tests is most likely elevated in a patient with this thyroid aspirate?

 a parathyroid hormone
 b thyroglobulin
 c antithyroid peroxidase antibodies
 d calcitonin

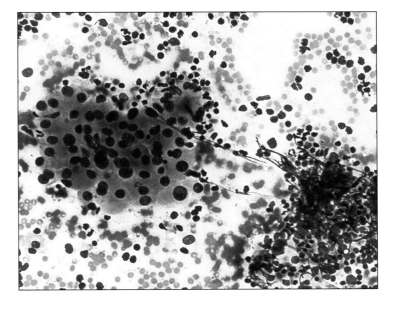

226 This 75-year-old female presented with multiple lung nodules. A fine needle aspiration was performed. What is the most likely site of the primary tumor?

 a breast
 b colon
 c kidney
 d ovary

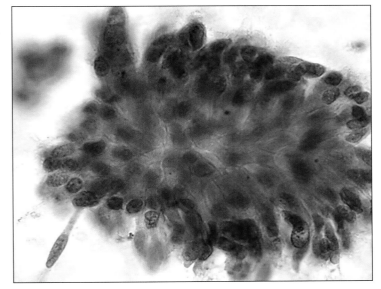

227 What recommendation is best during on site evaluation of this endoscopic ultrasound guided fine needle aspirate of a stomach wall mass in a 40-year-old female?

 a obtain material for a core biopsy or cell block to perform immunohistochemical stains
 b obtain core biopsy or cellular rinse material for flow cytometry
 c adequate material for definitive diagnosis
 d benign tissue; repeat fine needle aspirate

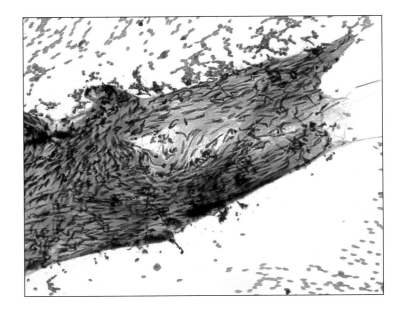

228 A pineal gland stereotactic biopsy in a 35-year-old
male revealed these cells. What is the most probable
immune profile of this lesion based on the illustrated
cytomorphology?
a PLAP+, CK–
b CK+, LCA–
c GFAP+, CK+
d HMB45+, CK–

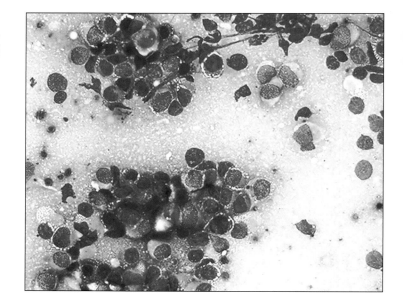

229 A 68-year-old female presented with a rapidly
enlarging right sided neck mass. Past history was
significant for thymic radiation as a child. She is most
likely suffering from:
a foreign body giant cell reaction
b anaplastic thyroid carcinoma, giant cell variant
c metastatic squamous cell carcinoma
d ruptured branchial cleft cyst

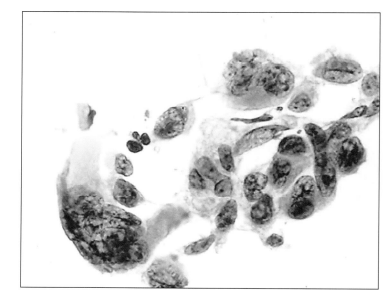

230 Which of the following immunostains will help confirm
the morphologic diagnosis of this adrenal aspirate:
a HepPar1
b CD117 (c-kit)
c inhibin
d chromogranin

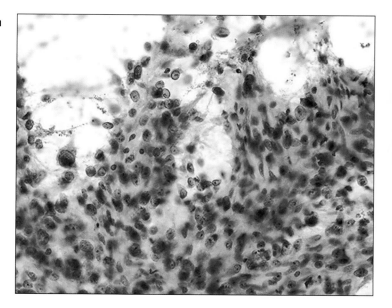

ISBN 978-089189-6357 ©ASCP 2015

231 This aspirate is from a painful, lytic lesion in the distal femur in an 18-year-old male. What is your diagnosis?
  a Ewing sarcoma
  b malignant lymphoma
  c osteosarcoma
  d giant cell tumor of the bone

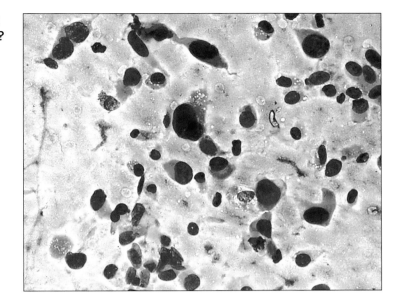

232 This liver fine needle aspirate from a 55-year-old HCV+ woman shows a poorly differentiated malignancy. What is the most likely immunoprofile of this tumor?
  a cytokeratin AE1/AE3+
  b CDX2+
  c CAM5.2+
  d CEA+ (monoclonal)

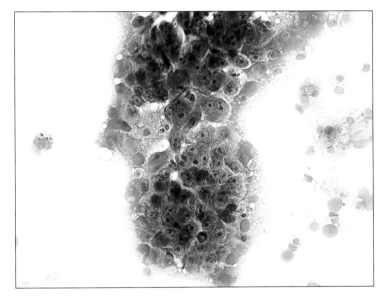

233 The most serious complication of the lesion depicted in the fine needle aspirate of a liver mass in this 28-year-old female is:
  a intraperitoneal hemorrhage
  b metastases
  c tumor seeding of the needle tract
  d malignant hypertension

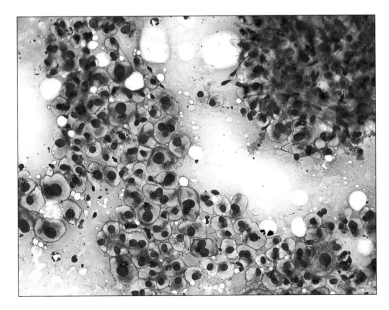

234 The most likely diagnosis in this fine needle aspirate from a 38-year-old male with a longstanding history of primary sclerosing cholangitis is:

   a cholangiocarcinoma
   b reactive biliary epithelium
   c hepatocellular carcinoma
   d regenerative nodule

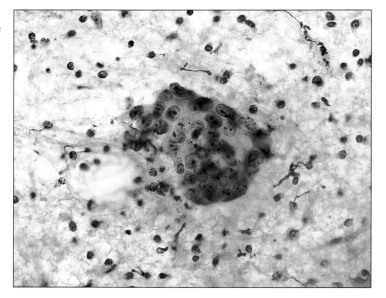

235 This fine needle aspirate was obtained from a 2 cm intraoral ulcerated lesion of a 54-year-old female with a history of breast carcinoma. She is suffering from:

   a polymorphous low grade adenocarcinoma
   b metastatic breast carcinoma
   c basaloid squamous cell carcinoma
   d ameloblastoma

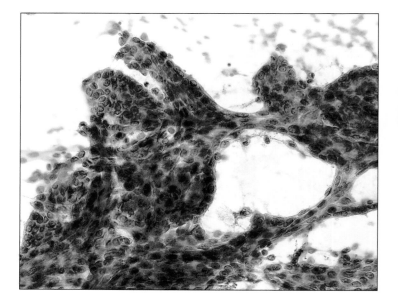

236 The best next diagnostic step for this fine needle aspirate of a parotid tail mass in a 18-year-old male is:

   a flow cytometry
   b immunostaining with 013 (CD99)
   c in situ staining for EBV
   d karyotyping for t(11,22)

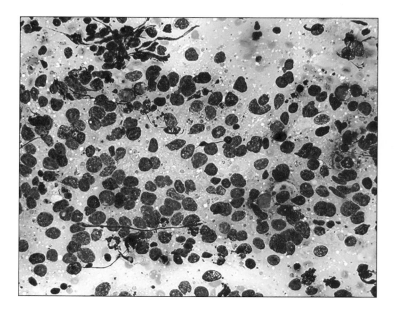

ISBN 978-089189-6357 ©ASCP 2015

Fine Needle Aspiration *Answer Key*

1 **c** colloid goiter

Benign follicular cells in monolayer or honeycombing sheets in the presence of abundant colloid, appearing as ropy amorphous background material, and associated hemosiderin laden macrophages and fibroblasts are typical findings associated with the FNA of benign colloid nodules.

DeMay, A&S 2e. Goiter, p881-882, t12.12

2 **c** at least 6 clusters of 10 cells over 2 slides

Thyroid aspirates are hypocellular in nature, containing abundant colloid and blood. The presence of follicular epithelium is necessary to establish the diagnosis of a satisfactory specimen.

DeMay, A&S 2e. FNA biopsy: The gold standard, p849-856

3 **a** cholangiocarcinoma

Well differentiated cholangiocarcinomas present cytologically as hypercellular specimens containing sheets of cells with slightly enlarged, overlapping nuclei and micronucleoli. Their resemblance to normal ductal cells may cause difficulty in establishing a malignant diagnosis. Careful attention should be given to mild nuclear deviations in light of a radiographically identified neoplasm. Cholangiocarcinomas are negative for α-fetoprotein and positive for CEA, whereas hepatocellular carcinomas are positive and negative, respectively.

DeMay, A&S 2e. Cholangiocarcinoma, p1272-1274

4 **b** benign lymphoepithelial cyst

Cystic parotid glands are common findings in patients infected with HIV. The cytologic identification of these lesions is based on the finding of a polymorphic population of lymphocytes, tingible body macrophages, and rare keratinizing and nonkeratinizing epithelial cells. Absent from these lesions are oncocytes, therefore, the diagnosis of Warthin tumor may be excluded.

DeMay, A&S 2e. Benign lymphoepithelial cysts in HIV infection, p791-792

5 **b** follicular carcinoma

Cells with follicular morphology, possessing numerous classic malignant nuclear features, may suggest follicular carcinoma. Follicular neoplasms cytologically present as a hypercellular population of overlapping follicular cells with cohesive microfollicular or trabecular groupings. Colloid is scanty to absent. The diagnosis of follicular neoplasm is given to those samples in which definitive atypical nuclear features are absent. Follicular adenoma should be reserved for histologic diagnosis only due to the possibility of capsular invasion by these benign appearing cells and the lack of distinguishable cytologic criteria necessary to differentiate these lesions from well differentiated carcinomas.

DeMay, A&S 2e. Follicular neoplasms, p882-891

6 **d** malignant mixed tumor

These malignant neoplasms may be related to the recurrence of an incompletely excised pleomorphic adenoma; hence it is appropriately named carcinoma ex pleomorphic adenoma. These lesions represent epithelial malignancies arising from pleomorphic adenomas. Cytologically, they present as pure populations of either poorly differentiated adenocarcinoma (most common), squamous cell carcinoma, or adenoid cystic carcinoma.

DeMay, A&S 2e. Malignant mixed tumors (carcinoma ex pleomorphic adenoma), p680-681

7 **c** Warthin tumor

Warthin tumor (papillary cystadenoma lymphomatosum) cytologically presents with reactive lymphoid populations and oxyphilic/oncocytic epithelial cells. Oncocytes, cytologically presenting as cuboidal cells with eosinophilic granular cytoplasm and central or eccentric nuclei with prominent nucleoli, are suspended within a watery, proteinaceous, or dirty background. The concomitant finding of a lymphocytic infiltrate (representing a germinal center) alongside the oncocytic population excludes the diagnosis of pure oncocytoma or oxyphilic adenoma. Atypical squamous metaplasia (elongated caudate shaped cells) may be present if the lesion is infarcted or infected; therefore, exercise caution to prevent overinterpretation of these lesions as squamous cell carcinoma.

DeMay, A&S 2e. Warthin tumor, p798-800

8 **a** mucoepidermoid carcinoma, well differentiated

Mucus producing columnar cells containing bland nuclei, foamy cytoplasm, and a population of benign polygonal intermediate cells define low grade mucoepidermoid carcinomas of the salivary gland. High grade lesions present with predominant populations of malignant squamous cells revealing keratinizing features. Differential diagnosis includes a pure keratinizing squamous cell carcinoma, which diagnosis may be preferred in the presence of pearl formations.

DeMay, A&S 2e. Mucoepidermoid carcinoma, p926-927

9 **a** polymorphous low grade primary adenocarcinoma

These terminal duct neoplasms are rare minor salivary gland lesions that cytologically present as well differentiated adenocarcinomas. They generally recapitulate gastrointestinal tract neoplasms but rarely metastasize.

DeMay, A&S 2e. Adenocarcinomas, p810

10 **d** oncocytoma

The cellular evidence of a pure population of oncocytes devoid of a lymphocytic background (as seen in Warthin tumor) is diagnostic of oncocytoma. The cellular groupings, like Warthin tumors, are generally single; however, occasionally 3D microacinar groupings may be seen. Although a lymphocytic infiltrate is not part of the diagnostic spectrum, a few mature lymphocytes may be seen. These lesions are considered rare tumors, usually involving elderly patients.

DeMay, A&S 2e. Oncocytoma (and oncocytic carcinoma), p801

11　d　adenoid cystic carcinoma

Adenoid cystic carcinomas are frequent submaxillary and minor salivary gland neoplasms arising from the intercalated ducts. These lesions often present as painful lesions due to perineural invasion. Adenoid cystic carcinomas are cytologically identified by the presence of small round epithelial cells in clusters, acinar formations, and 3D tissue fragments in balls or cylinders containing central, eosinophilic, hyaline/homogeneous, fibrillar basement membrane material.

DeMay, A&S 2e. Adenoid cystic carcinoma, p802-804

12　d　hemangioma

These benign vascular lesions are the most common parotid gland neoplasm in children.

DeMay, A&S 2e. Hemangioma, p678-679

13　c　monomorphic adenoma

Basal cell adenomas are cytologically composed of a pure population of epithelial cells. Small, cohesive basaloid cells in cords, aggregates, or irregular clusters with high N:C ratios and predictable nuclear features lacking atypia in the presence of copious amounts of metachromatic basement membrane and fibrous stroma are seen in the FNA smears. The absence of neural symptoms may help differentiate these lesions from adenoid cystic carcinomas.

DeMay, A&S 2e. Basal cell adenoma, p796-797

14　d　metastatic carcinoma

Metastatic carcinomas represent 90% of the liver malignancies. The most common metastatic neoplasms of the liver include colon, stomach, pancreas, breast, lung, and kidney.

DeMay, A&S 2e. Metastases, p1277-1279

15　b　hyaline globules

These eosinophilic intracytoplasmic inclusions may stain PAS+ or PAS−. They may also be found in cirrhosis, regeneration, or hepatocellular carcinoma.

DeMay, A&S 2e. Hyaline globules, p1251

16　b　acinic cell carcinoma

Acinic cell carcinomas are considered rare lesions predominantly arising within parotid gland. Cytologically, these lesions may be difficult to interpret except for the lack of typical lobular architecture, their increased cellular size, and the presence of PAS+ granules within the cytoplasm. However, the presence of a pure population of acinic cells and no recognizable ducts suggests the diagnosis of acinic cell carcinoma. Chronic inflammation may accompany the acinic cells.

DeMay, A&S 2e. Acinic cell carcinoma, p807-808

17　b　vascular or capsular invasion as determined histologically

Although histology is considered the gold standard for determining whether follicular neoplasms have capsular or vascular invasion, up to 3/4 of follicular carcinomas are misdiagnosed in tissue due to interobserver variability. Follicular neoplasms cytologically present as a hypercellular population of overlapping follicular cells with cohesive microfollicular or trabecular groupings. Colloid is scanty to absent. The diagnosis of follicular neoplasm is given to those samples in which definitive atypical nuclear features are absent. The diagnosis of follicular adenoma should be reserved for histologic diagnosis only due to the possibility of capsular invasion by these benign appearing cells and the lack of distinguishable cytologic criteria necessary to differentiate these lesions from well differentiated carcinomas.

DeMay, A&S 2e. Follicular neoplasms, p858-859

18　d　non-Hodgkin lymphoma

Lymphomas arising within the salivary gland are of large cell or small cell cleaved B cell lineage and reveal light chain clonality. Cytology reveals a monotypic population of neoplastic lymphocytes.

DeMay, A&S 2e. Malignant lymphoma, p573-575

19　a　medullary carcinoma

These rare neuroendocrine thyroid lesions that arise from parafollicular or "C" cells actively secrete calcitonin. A familial predilection has been established, related to multiple endocrine neoplasia syndrome. Hypercellular aspirates consist of pleomorphic spindle appearing cells (often containing intranuclear intracytoplasmic inclusions), lympho/plasmacytoid cells, and Hürthle cells. These cells are suspended within an eosinophilic amorphous background consisting of amyloid, demonstrated by positive apple green birefringence and positive with Congo red. In addition, the tumor cells are immunocytochemically positive for thyrocalcitonin.

DeMay, A&S 2e. Medullary thyroid carcinoma, p910-915

20　d　hamartoma

Bile ductal hamartomas or Meyenburg complexes are composed of embryological bile duct cells and connective tissue constituents. Hepatocytes are absent.

DeMay, A&S 2e. Bile duct proliferations: adenomas and hamartomas, p1259

21　c　papillary carcinoma

Papillary carcinoma generally presents in monolayer sheets or in papillary groupings with fibrovascular cores. The cells contain irregular nuclear membranes with bland chromatin features, nuclear grooves, and intranuclear intracytoplasmic inclusions representing cytoplasmic intranuclear invaginations or nuclear pseudoinclusions. Colloid, foreign body giant cells, and psammoma bodies may accompany these findings. Intranuclear cytoplasmic invaginations (INCIs), or pseudoinclusions, are often found within papillary carcinoma of the thyroid, melanomas, and hepatocellular carcinomas.

DeMay, A&S 2e. Papillary thyroid carcinoma, p892-905

ISBN 978-089189-6357　©ASCP 2015

22 d medullary carcinoma

These rare neuroendocrine thyroid lesions that arise from parafollicular or "C" cells actively secrete calcitonin. A familial predilection has been established, related to multiple endocrine neoplasia syndrome. Hypercellular aspirates consist of pleomorphic spindle appearing cells (often containing intranuclear intracytoplasmic inclusions), lympho/plasmacytoid cells, and Hürthle cells. These cells are suspended within an eosinophilic amorphous background consisting of amyloid, demonstrated by positive apple green birefringence and positive with Congo red. In addition, the tumor cells are immunocytochemically positive for thyrocalcitonin.

DeMay, A&S 2e. Medullary thyroid carcinoma, p910-915

23 b Hashimoto thyroiditis

A predominantly rich heterogeneous population of lymphocytes and follicular center cells with associated Hürthle cells are diagnostic of Hashimoto thyroiditis. Colloid, if present, is scanty.

DeMay, A&S 2e. Hashimoto thyroiditis, p874-879

24 d granulomatous thyroiditis (de Quervain)

Although of unknown cause, it is postulated that these lesions are linked to systemic viral infections, such as the mumps virus. This lesion is rarely aspirated due to the clinical history; however, it represents one of the most common causes of a painful thyroid.

DeMay, A&S 2e. Granulomatous thyroiditis (de Quervain or subacute thyroiditis), p869-872

25 a monolayer hepatocytes with random atypical cells are found with liver cell dysplasia

Nontrabecular hepatocellular carcinomas (HCCs) present with numerous cells containing more pronounced nuclear abnormalities and classic malignant features (irregular chromatin with prominent macronucleoli). Although the cellular findings in liver cell dysplasia (LCD) closely resemble those seen in nontrabecular hepatocellular carcinomas, the cytology of LCD shows only random tumor cells, rather than numerous tumor cells. Furthermore, the presence of lipofuscin, iron, or chronic inflammation suggests LCD rather than HCC.

DeMay, A&S 2e. Cirrhotic nodules: adenomatous hyperplasia, dysplasia, and HCC, p1254-1256

26 a liver cell adenoma

The finding of normal hepatocytes possessing normal appearing nuclear features in concert with abundant clear (lipid/glycogen+) cytoplasm allows for differentiation of this benign tumor from well differentiated hepatocellular carcinoma. Bile duct cells are not identified.

DeMay, A&S 2e. Liver cell adenoma, p1258-1259

27 c epidermoid cysts

These cysts are composed of a pure population of squamous epithelial cells; however, secondary granulomatous changes may be present.

DeMay, A&S 2e. Dermoid and epidermoid cysts, p1442

28 d follicular neoplasm

Follicular neoplasms cytologically present as a hypercellular population of overlapping follicular cells with cohesive microfollicular or trabecular groupings. Colloid is scanty to absent. The diagnosis of follicular neoplasm is given to those samples in which definitive atypical nuclear features are absent. The diagnosis of follicular adenoma should be reserved for histologic diagnosis only due to the possibility of capsular invasion by these benign appearing cells and the lack of distinguishable cytologic criteria necessary to differentiate these lesions from well differentiated carcinomas.

DeMay, A&S 2e. Follicular neoplasms, p858-859

29 b Mallory bodies

These cytoplasmic inclusions may be associated with alcoholic cirrhosis and hepatocellular carcinoma.

DeMay, A&S 2e. Mallory bodies, p1251

30 b Hürthle cell neoplasm

The presence of a pure population of Hürthle cells lacking a lymphocytic infiltrate (Hashimoto thyroiditis) is suggestive of a Hürthle cell neoplasm. As with other follicular neoplasms, the absence of classic malignant nuclear criteria does not preclude the possibility of a well differentiated carcinoma. Therefore, the diagnosis of "neoplasm" is preferred until histologic confirmation can determine capsular or vascular involvement. Hürthle cells represent mitochondria rich follicular cells found singly and in clusters, containing abundant, eosinophilic, granular cytoplasm. The nuclei are round to oval and often possess prominent nucleoli. Hürthle cells are also found in Hashimoto thyroiditis, Hürthle cell neoplasms, and benign goiters.

DeMay, A&S 2e. Hürthle cell neoplasms, p920-922

31 d anaplastic carcinoma

Giant (anaplastic) cell carcinomas of the thyroid are highly anaplastic lesions that comprise between 5% and 10% of thyroid neoplasms.

DeMay, A&S 2e. Anaplastic (undifferentiated) carcinoma, p907-909

32 d *Echinococcus granulosus*

Hydatid sand is composed of scoleces and hooklets derived from *Echinococcus granulosus*. Aspiration of cystic liver nodules is generally contraindicated due to the possibility of anaphylaxis.

DeMay, A&S 2e. Hydatid cysts, p1256

33 c cirrhosis

Polygonal cells arranged in rows or trabeculae with dense, granular cytoplasm, enlarged central placed bi- or multinucleated cells with smooth nuclear membranes, prominent nucleoli, intranuclear cytoplasmic invaginations, and intracytoplasmic bile pigmentation are diagnostic of reactive hepatocytes. These changes are commonly associated with conditions such as alcoholic cirrhosis or viral hepatitis. Bile duct cells, fibrous connective tissue, and numerous lymphocytes represent concomitant cytologic findings.

DeMay, A&S 2e. Cirrhosis, p1254-1255

34 **b** **vascular lesions**

Vascular lesions, bleeding abnormalities, pulmonary hypertension, uncooperative or debilitated patients, patients with contralateral pneumonectomy, and patients with chronic obstructive pulmonary disease represent some of the possible contraindications for performing pulmonary aspirations.

DeMay, A&S 2e. Vascular tumors, p678-679

35 **d** **bronchioloalveolar adenocarcinoma**

The mucinous variant of bronchioloalveolar adenocarcinoma (BAC) presents cytologically as large tissue fragments with a greater depth of focus than bronchogenic adenocarcinoma. The cells are typically uniform in size and shape and contain round to oval nuclei. Nonmucinous (nm) BAC is cytologically represented in monolayered sheets and pleomorphic nuclei, with large intranuclear cytoplasmic invaginations. In addition, the cells from nm BAC may be accompanied by alveolar macrophages or psammoma bodies.

DeMay, A&S 2e. Bronchioloalveolar carcinoma, p1178-1181

36 **a** **large cell carcinoma**

These highly malignant lesions tend to arise within the large bronchi, representing a poorly differentiated non-small cell tumor. Although described as undifferentiated, this diagnosis is reserved for those lesions that, under light microscopy, show neither glandular nor squamous differentiation. However, ultrascopically, these lesions usually show gland formation. Cytologically, these cells are arranged in syncytial-like groupings and lie singly. Nuclei are hyperchromatic, possess coarsely granular, irregularly distributed chromatin, multiple irregular macronucleoli, with marked anisonucleosis. The cytoplasm tends to be basophilic and homogeneous. A variant of this lesion is the so called giant cell type, which exhibits macrocytic and multinucleated malignant tumor giant cells.

DeMay, A&S 2e. Large cell undifferentiated carcinoma, p1186

37 **a** **Romanowsky**

If one suspects a hematopoietic neoplasm, the staining of choice may be the Romanowsky, Giemsa, or the modified Wright (Diff-Quik) stain. Because these procedures require air dried smears, cellular ballooning and gigantism will be accentuated; however, nuclear detail is often lost. Therefore, nuclear criteria utilized for interpreting alcohol fixed specimens should not be followed.

DeMay, A&S 2e. Romanowsky stain, p1505

38 **d** **carcinoid tumor**

Carcinoid tumors are slow growing neuroendocrine tumors which have association with a Kulchitsky (K) cell etiology. These polypoid tumors cytologically present as small cells with N:C ratios and hypochromatic, finely granular, evenly distributed chromatin patterns, with typical oat cell grouping of cords, nest, ribbons, and vertebral column formations. Reactive/reparative cells can be discriminated from these lesions based on the absence of terminal bars and/or cilia with carcinoid lesions. Clinical history (a radiographically detectable lesion) and physiological changes are essential elements in the establishment of carcinoid lesions. Immunocytochemical staining with chromogranin, neuron specific enolase, or serotonin, as well as histochemical detection of argentaffin or argyrophil, will help establish their neuroendocrine origin. Atypical carcinoid tumors, usually associated with the physiological carcinoid syndrome of right sided fibrosis of the heart, cyanotic flushing of the skin, and liver metastasis, generally have classical malignant features that may be difficult to distinguish from small cell carcinomas.

DeMay, A&S 2e. Carcinoid tumors (typical carcinoid), p1189-1191

39 **d** **small cell carcinoma**

Small cell carcinoma is a highly malignant neuroendocrine neoplasm that is ultrastructurally part of the amine precursor uptake and decarboxylation (APUD) tumors due to its cytoplasmic evidence of androgenic amines (membrane bound granules). These cells contain hyperchromatic, stippled chromatin, coarse clumping, nuclear molding, scanty cytoplasm, and micronucleoli. An important diagnostic feature of small cell carcinoma is the presence of paranuclear cytoplasmic inclusions–blue cytoplasmic globules found indenting the nuclei (best visualized with Diff-Quik staining). The cellular groupings characteristically have vertebral column formation, microbiopsy aggregates, and cords, nests, or ribbons. "Crush artifact," or degenerative nuclear material related to the mechanical crushing associated with the preparation of FNA specimens, is found in the background of most small cell carcinomas. This artifact presents as long clumpy streams of basophilic material. A variant of small cell carcinoma, intermediate cell small cell carcinoma, represents both fusiform and polygonal types, which are typically better preserved with open coarse chromatin patterns and enlarged cell areas. Immunocytochemical staining with chromogranin is helpful in establishing the neurosecretory nature of this tumor, but will not differentiate it from carcinoid lesions. Furthermore, the absence of lymphogranular bodies (best demonstrated with the Romanowsky or Diff-Quik stain) will help differentiate these lesions from malignant lymphoid processes.

DeMay, A&S 2e. Small cell carcinoma, p966-969

40 **a** **normal pulmonary constituents**

In addition to bronchial epithelial cells, cells not typically found with conventional exfoliative pulmonary cytology (sputum, bronchoscopy) but found in FNA specimens include sheets of mesothelial cells, fibroconnective tissue elements, fibroblasts, smooth muscle cells, adipose tissue, and hepatocytes.

DeMay, A&S 2e. The cells, p1159-1160

ISBN 978-089189-6357 ©ASCP 2015

41 a aspiration of necrotic center

Aspiration of the center of a lesion yields a specimen composed predominantly of diathesis and necrotic debris. When performing FNA, special attention needs to be given so that multiple sites of neoplasm are aspirated, especially along the peripheral margins (>10 planes).

DeMay, A&S 2e. Fine needle aspiration biopsy, p536-538; Complications associated with deep target biopsy, p541-542; Performing the biopsy, p543-544

42 c squamous carcinoma

Pleomorphic cells with caudate or spindle formations with refractile cytoplasm, anisonucleosis, and opaque ink dotlike nuclei are diagnostic of squamous cell carcinoma. A necrotic background is helpful in establishing this lesion.

DeMay, A&S 2e. Keratinizing (well differentiated) SCC, p562-566

43 d adenocarcinoma, prostate

Cells representing prostatic adenocarcinomas present in discohesive sheets, clusters, and microacinar formations with increased nuclear sizes, overlapping nuclei, and the important finding of macronucleoli.

DeMay, A&S 2e. Adenocarcinoma, p1409-1410

44 d metastatic melanoma

Melanoma typically presents in single cells, aggregates, or as spindle cells with bizarre malignant nuclear features, macronucleoli, intranuclear cytoplasmic invaginations, and possibly intracytoplasmic golden-brown pigment. Due to the fact that these diseases may be amelanotic, it may be helpful to confirm this disease process with S100, HMB45, melan A, or MITF (microphthalmia associated transcription factor)—all of which preferentially react with melanoma cells.

DeMay, A&S 2e. Metastasis, p1279

45 b neural sheath tumors

These lesions are typically paravertebral in origin and arise from the sympathetic or intercostal nerves. They include malignant schwannoma, neurilemoma, and neurofibroma.

DeMay, A&S 2e. Neurogenic tumors, p1235-1236

46 a Hashimoto thyroiditis

A predominantly rich heterogeneous population of lymphocytes and follicular center cells with associated Hürthle cells are diagnostic of Hashimoto thyroiditis. Colloid, if present, is scanty. Hürthle cells represent mitochondria rich follicular cells found singly and in clusters, containing abundant eosinophilic, granular cytoplasm. The nuclei are round to oval and often possess prominent nucleoli. Hürthle cells are found in Hashimoto thyroiditis, Hürthle cell neoplasms, and benign goiters.

DeMay, A&S 2e. Hashimoto thyroiditis, p874-877

47 c *Pneumocystis jiroveci*

Pneumocystis jiroveci is considered an opportunistic protozoan that may be seen in immunosuppressed individuals secondary to immunologic disorders, malignancies, or HIV infection, and in premature infants or patients receiving chemotherapy. Cytologic identification rests on the presence of frothy mats of eosinophilic material with interspersed "contact lens" shaped structures containing intranuclear trophozoites.

DeMay, A&S 2e. Pneumocystis jiroveci, p1472

48 b abscess

Abscesses of the lung typically present as cavitating lesions with the cytologic evidence described in the question. These inflammatory processes may be secondary to bacterial invasion, which may be apparent in the background or contained within the cytoplasm of histiocytes. Special stains may be required for differentiation of specific infectious process.

DeMay, A&S 2e. Abscess, p1161-1162

49 c gastroenteric cysts

These cystic lesions may arise from the foregut and are cytologically composed of gastric or intestinal epithelial cells.

DeMay, A&S 2e. Foregut cysts, p122

50 b malignant lymphoma

These monoclonal neoplasms cytologically present with a predominant population of small cleaved lymphocytes (80%), and a lesser population of small noncleaved/round lymphocytes and large lymphocytes. Their inability to express dual tumor cell marking as seen in small round cell lymphoma (noncleaved, well differentiated lymphocytic lymphoma) helps differentiate these 2 lesions.

DeMay, A&S 2e. Small lymphocytic lymphoma, p998-1000

51 c pneumothorax

Pneumothorax occurs in 5%–50% of the pulmonary aspirations performed. Although most resolve without further intervention, only a minority of the cases (10%) may require a chest tube or therapy. Decreasing the number of FNA passes to only those that are necessary will help decrease the chance of inducing this condition. In addition, there is a decreased chance of pneumothorax if both pleural surfaces are penetrated rapidly without crossing the fissures.

DeMay, A&S 2e. Complications associated with deep target biopsy, p541-542

52 b hamartoma

Hamartomas of the lung present with groups or sheets of benign epithelial cells, adipocytes, possible cartilage, and a background of fibromyxoid stroma. The cytologic diagnosis of this lesion is similar to that of pleomorphic adenoma of the salivary gland.

DeMay, A&S 2e. Hamartoma, p1167-1168

53 d malignant lymphoma

These monoclonal neoplasms cytologically present with a predominant population of small cleaved lymphocytes (80%), and a lesser population of small noncleaved/round lymphocytes and large lymphocytes. Their inability to express dual tumor cell marking as seen in small round cell lymphoma helps differentiate these 2 lesions.

DeMay, A&S 2e. Small lymphocytic lymphoma, p998-1000

54 d granuloma

Elongated, round, or oval cells presenting singly or in syncytial aggregates with oval/reniform nuclei containing finely granular, evenly distributed chromatin and micronucleoli are diagnostic of epithelioid histiocytes. These cells are part of the spectrum of granulomatous inflammation. Other cells associated with granulomatous inflammation include multinucleated histiocytes, fibroblasts, and acute or chronic inflammatory cells.

DeMay, A&S 2e. Granulomas, p1162

55 a Sjögren syndrome

This autoimmune disease, related to either Mikulicz disease or Sjögren syndrome, is a benign lymphoepithelial lesion involving the destruction of the salivary gland lymphoid tissue and the lacrimal glands (Mikulicz only). FNA cytology reveals the presence of reactive lymphoid hyperplasia and myoepithelial cell proliferation (benign lymphoepithelial lesion). Similar findings may be seen in human immunodeficiency virus infected patients or those suffering active acquired immunodeficiency disease.

DeMay, A&S 2e. Lymphoepithelial sialadenitis, p789-790

56 a bronchogenic adenocarcinoma

Bronchogenic adenocarcinomas cytologically present in 2D acinar clusters with smooth "community" borders and single cells and demonstrate hypochromatic/bland chromatin, or if less well differentiated, hyperchromasia. The presence of central macronucleoli is helpful in establishing this disease process. These true tissue fragments possess frothy cytoplasm, high N:C ratios, and uniform or lobulated nuclei.

DeMay, A&S 2e. Adenocarcinoma, p1176-1178

57 b sialadenitis

The cytology associated with acute sialadenitis reveals degenerated ductal cells, acinar groups, and adipocytes, as well as abundant necrotic debris, polymorphonuclear neutrophils, and macrophages.

DeMay, A&S 2e. Acute sialadenitis, p786

58 b negative

Nuclear molding or cohesion in small cells may be associated with neurosecretory tumors. In contrast, lymphocytic lesions will not demonstrate true cohesive properties–they may "kiss" but do not "hug." Chromogranin or neuron specific enolase will immunocytochemically identify small cell carcinomas, whereas common leukocyte antigen will positively identify lymphomas.

DeMay, A&S 2e. Small cell carcinoma, p1182-1185

59 c plasmacytoma

FNA of plasma cell myelomas reveals cells with "clock face" chromatin, immature cells with fine chromatin and prominent nucleoli, and occasionally binucleate and bizarre multinucleated giant cells. The cytoplasm is generally blue or amphophilic with perinuclear hofs and intranuclear or intracytoplasmic Russell bodies (representing immunoglobulin, usually IgG or IgA).

DeMay, A&S 2e. Plasmacytoma, p1000-1002

60 a invasive thymoma

Invasive thymomas cytologically present with bland morphologic appearance. Capsular invasion is required before rendering an invasive diagnosis. Paraneoplastic syndromes, such as myasthenia gravis, are commonly found in patients with thymoma.

DeMay, A&S 2e. Invasive thymoma, p1227

61 c pleomorphic adenoma

Sheets and clusters of cuboidal cells containing round to oval nuclei and micronucleoli represent the ductal epithelial component of pleomorphic adenoma (benign mixed tumor). Fibromyxoid and chondroid mesenchymal elements (staining bright magenta with Diff-Quik staining) and myoepithelial spindle cells, typically arranged in cords and as single cells, may predominate in the smears.

DeMay, A&S 2e. Pleomorphic adenoma (benign mixed tumor), p793-796

62 d pleomorphic adenoma

Sheets and clusters of cuboidal cells containing round to oval nuclei and micronucleoli represent the ductal epithelial component of pleomorphic adenoma (benign mixed tumor). Fibromyxoid and chondroid mesenchymal elements (staining bright magenta with Diff-Quik staining) and myoepithelial spindle cells, typically arranged in cords and as single cells, may predominate in the smears.

DeMay, A&S 2e. Pleomorphic adenoma (benign mixed tumor), p793-796

63 d treat with Carnoy fixative

Carnoy fixative may be utilized for bloody specimens, lysing the red blood cells that obscure the cellular detail. A 1:14 mixture of glacial acidic acid to 95% ethanol is appropriate.

64 c metastatic colonic adenocarcinoma

The presence of tall columnar or "cigar shaped" cells in aggregates with frankly malignant nuclear features, granular cytoplasm, or the presence of malignant signet ring cells may suggest a diagnosis of metastatic adenocarcinoma of the colon. Correlation with the primary lesion is critical.

DeMay, A&S 2e. Metastases, p1277-1278

65 a malignant schwannoma

Malignant schwannoma (neurofibrosarcoma), a nerve tissue tumor (of neural sheath) related to von Recklinghausen disease and generally arising within the posterior mediastinum, cytologically presents as monotonous synovial sarcoma. The presence of Verocay bodies, palisading nuclei with "flamelike" cytoplasm, and spindle cells with oval, curved, or twisted nuclei, is an essential component in establishing a primary schwannoma. Immunocytochemistry for S100 protein and Leu 7 may be positive. Thymoma, hemangioma, and parathyroid adenoma are all considered anterior mediastinal lesions.

DeMay, A&S 2e. Schwannoma (neurolemmoma), p1237

ISBN 978-089189-6357 ©ASCP 2015

66 c reactive bronchial cells

Radiation and chemotherapy induced changes characteristically produce macrocytic cells. These reactive cells may share "atypical" nuclear morphology with carcinoma, but the presence of benign products of functional differentiation, such as the presence of terminal bars and/or cilia, are often seen in these faux "abnormal" cells.

DeMay, A&S 2e. Radiation/chemotherapy, p1166

67 c peripheral lesions

Peripheral lesions, such as bronchioloalveolar carcinomas, generally do not exfoliate in sputum cytology as efficiently as central pulmonary neoplasms. Gaining access to these lesions via bronchoscopy may also prove inadequate. Therefore, the use of FNA in evaluating peripheral (especially small) lung lesions is considered a highly effective diagnostic procedure.

DeMay, A&S 2e. Fine needle aspiration biopsy, p1156-1159

68 c osteoblastoma

This vertebral column neoplasm typically presents in children and adolescents.

DeMay, A&S 2e. Osteoblastoma, p701-702

69 b aspiration pneumonia, plant material

Vegetable material may falsely give the interpretation of a squamous malignancy; however, their double refractile cell walls and smudged nuclear features help establish this process as plant material. Food particles may be secondary to aspiration pneumonia.

DeMay, A&S 2e. Aspiration pneumonia, p1166

70 c chondroblastoma

These benign lesions generally arise within the long bones in teenage boys and may involve the knee.

DeMay, A&S 2e. Chondroblastoma, p691

71 c cholangiocarcinoma, well differentiated

Cholangiocarcinoma of the liver presents in its well differentiated forms similar to benign ductal epithelium, except for its hypercellularity, minimal anisokaryosis, and nuclear crowding. Lesions may be differentiated from hepatocellular carcinoma by their immunocytochemical positivity with CEA and negativity for α-fetoprotein.

DeMay, A&S 2e. Cholangiocarcinoma, p1272-1273

72 d chondrosarcoma

Chondrosarcomas are malignant tumors often arising in the axial skeleton, pelvis, femur, or humerus. They typically affect older patients.

DeMay, A&S 2e. Chondrosarcoma (conventional), p692

73 b PAS+/Ewing sarcoma

These highly anaplastic lesions, of parasympathetic nerve origin, tend to affect the femur, fibula, or tibia in adolescent males. The malignant cells are glycogen+ (PAS+). In addition, a characteristic dimorphic pattern of large blastemic cells and lymphocytoid cells are seen with Diff-Quik staining.

DeMay, A&S 2e. Ewing sarcoma, p697-699

74 b fibroma

Fibromas are scirrhous ovarian lesions that yield hypocellular aspirates containing slender spindle fibroblasts. The differential diagnosis is a benign thecoma; however, thecomas cytologically present as pump spindle cells with vacuolated lipid+ cytoplasm, have an increased cytoplasmic mass, and have irregular nuclei.

DeMay, A&S 2e. Ovarian fibroma and fibrothecoma, p1412

75 b liposarcoma

Pleomorphic liposarcomas are often large in size and arise within the deep soft tissues of the retroperitoneal area or the extremities of middle aged to older patients.

DeMay, A&S 2e. Pleomorphic liposarcoma, p655-656

76 b luteal cyst

FNA of ovarian luteal cysts reveals sheets of luteal cells possessing granular and frothy cytoplasm, low N:C ratios, and predictable nuclei with prominent nucleoli. These cells resemble oncocytes as seen in the salivary glands, thyroid, and kidney. A bloody background may include the presence of normal follicular cells, stromal cells, and hemosiderin laden macrophages.

DeMay, A&S 2e. Corpus luteum cysts, p1421-1422

77 d oncocytic neoplasm

These renal cortical neoplasms represent 5% of all renal tumors. Differentiation between oncocytoma and oncocytic renal cell carcinoma should be reserved until a complete clinical, gross, and microscopic analysis is performed.

DeMay, A&S 2e. Oncocytoma, p1351-1352

78 b osteosarcoma

Osteosarcoma represents the most common primary bone malignancy and typically involves the long bones of adolescent males.

DeMay, A&S 2e. Osteosarcoma, p699-700

79 d angiosarcoma

These highly malignant vascular lesions often strike the elderly and predominantly arise within the liver, breast, bone, spleen, or the subcutaneous tissues. Immunocytochemical confirmation with factor VIII antigen may help in the differentiation of these lesions from other soft tissue sarcomas.

DeMay, A&S 2e. Angiosarcoma, p681-682

80 a seminoma

Seminomas cytologically present as large discohesive germ cells containing irregular chromatin and macronucleoli. The background contains a lymphocytic infiltrate, PAS positivity, and a "tigroid" pattern demonstrated with Diff-Quik. Granulomas are often seen and serve as a diagnostic clue for seminomas of the testes and dysgerminomas of the ovaries.

DeMay, A&S 2e. Germinoma (seminoma/dysgerminoma), p1415-1416

81 c mature cystic teratoma

The aspiration of a mature cystic teratoma or dermoid cyst yields squamous epithelial and adnexal components such as anucleate squames, superficial and intermediate cells, hair shafts, and sebaceous fluid. The background is generally granular, amorphous, or basophilic with a proteinaceous precipitate.

DeMay, A&S 2e. Mature cystic teratoma, p1232

82 b eosinophilic granuloma

Eosinophilic granulomas are a histiocytosis affecting the skull, ribs, or the spine of children and the ribs, mandible, or clavicle in adults. Cytologically, the presence of multinucleated and mononucleate histiocytes containing kidney bean shaped indented nuclei (Langerhans), which stain positive for S100, and an abundant population of normal eosinophils identify the lesion. Tingible body macrophages and Charcot-Leyden crystals may accompany these lesions.

DeMay, A&S 2e. Eosinophilic granuloma, p578

83 b aspiration may precipitate a hypertensive crisis

Pheochromocytomas, the most common adrenal medulla neoplasm, represent chromaffin paragangliomas. A urinary excretion of free catecholamines (norepinephrine & epinephrine) or catecholamine metabolites (vanillylmandelic acid and total metanephrines) or elevated plasma levels of metanephrines is typically the best mechanism for establishing this disease process. There is a possibility of initiating a hypertensive crisis as a result of aspiration biopsy. Nonfunctioning lesions cytologically present as loosely cohesive, pleomorphic, spindle appearing cells containing intranuclear inclusions, finely granular, regularly distributed chromatin, and prominent nucleoli. Single cells usually predominate in the aspiration of these types of lesions. Another variant of pheochromocytomas may be highly anaplastic. Overall, 3 diagnostic categories are usually seen: spindle, epithelioid, and ganglion.

DeMay, A&S 2e. Paragangliomas, p690

84 a dysgerminoma

Sheets and syncytia of cells possessing frothy, vacuolated basophilic cytoplasm, pleomorphic nuclei containing irregularly distributed chromatin, and prominent nucleoli are observed in ovarian dysgerminomas. The presence of a lymphocytic infiltrate is important in defining these lesions as germ cell tumors. Differential diagnoses include yolk sac tumors (YSTs) and embryonal carcinoma (EC); however, dysgerminomas are characteristically negative for α-fetoprotein, whereas YST and EC are typically positive and also lack a lymphoid infiltrate. Granulomas are often seen and serve as a diagnostic clue for germinomas.

DeMay, A&S 2e. Germinoma (seminoma/dysgerminoma), p1415-1416

85 d cytomegalovirus

Cytomegalovirus infections are herpetic infections found in immunocompromised patients, including those with HIV or cancer.

DeMay, A&S 2e. Viruses (cytomegalovirus), p54

86 c perform cultures for identification of possible inflammatory process

An inaccurate evaluation of inflammatory aspirates may account for false negative or false positive cytologic diagnoses. Although the Diff-Quik stain may be helpful in allowing for better cell recovery, a negative aspirate does not rule out the possibility of a bacterial process that must be cultured for microbiologic identification.

DeMay, A&S 2e. Abscess, p1161-1162

87 c benign fibrous histiocytoma

These lesions are composed of benign appearing fibroblasts arising from lesions contained within the extremities. The absence of nuclear pleomorphism helps discriminate these cells from malignant fibrous histiocytomas.

DeMay, A&S 2e. Benign fibrous histiocytoma, p1200

88 d follicular

Follicular cysts generally present in FNA cytology as hypocellular samples of granulosa and theca cells in clusters or sheets with high N:C ratios and folded bean shaped nuclei scattered among a proteinaceous or bloody background. If hypercellular samples are seen, the cellular morphology may be quite reactive and mimic malignant features–making differentiation from a malignant neoplasm difficult.

DeMay, A&S 2e. Functional cysts: follicular cysts, p1421

89 b serous cystadenoma

Monotonous sheets of epithelial columnar cells with regularly arranged nuclei containing micronucleoli (resembling mesothelial cells) found among a granular background are diagnostic of serous cystadenoma. Their lack of classic malignant nuclear morphology rules out the possibility of a serous cystadenocarcinoma. In addition, the absence of signet ring morphology helps differentiate these lesions from mucinous cystadenomas.

DeMay, A&S 2e. Serous cystadenoma, p1309-1310

90 b mucinous cystadenocarcinoma

Mucinous cystadenocarcinomas (MCAs) resemble colonic carcinomas but lack the extensive necrosis; furthermore, MCAs are generally unilateral while metastatic lesions are often bilateral.

DeMay, A&S 2e. Mucinous cystic neoplasms, p1310-1312

91 d mesenchymal repair

Mesenchymal repair, as well as epithelial repair, may be associated with wound healing, trauma, inflammation, chemotherapy or radiation, and ischemic tissue processes.

DeMay, A&S 2e. Fibrosis, p1166

92 c endometriotic cyst

Endometriotic cysts, related to ovarian endometriosis, are often termed "chocolate cysts" on gross examination due to their copious presence of old hemolyzed blood. FNA reveals typical endometrial glandular and stromal cells found among a background consisting of fresh and old blood as well as hemosiderin laden macrophages.

DeMay, A&S 2e. Endometriotic cyst and endometriosis, p1422

ISBN 978-089189-6357 ©ASCP 2015

93 d Brenner tumor

These solid tumors are composed of sheets of squamoid epithelial cells with regular nuclei containing prominent folds resembling "coffee bean" morphology. Hyalinized eosinophilic globules may be seen with concentrically arranged follicular cells. A differential diagnosis is granulosa cell tumor; however, the cells associated with Brenner tumor are larger with more abundant cytoplasm.

DeMay, A&S 2e. Brenner tumor, p1425

94 b benign lymphocytic population, seminoma

Seminomas cytologically present as large discohesive germ cells containing irregular chromatin and macronucleoli. The background contains a lymphocytic infiltrate, PAS positivity, and a "tigroid" pattern demonstrated with Diff-Quik. Granulomas are often seen and serve as a diagnostic clue for seminomas of the testes and dysgerminomas of the ovaries.

DeMay, A&S 2e. Seminoma/dysgerminoma, p1415-1416

95 a Leishmania

These intracellular parasites may be differentiated from *Pneumocystis jiroveci* by their negative reaction with GMS.

DeMay, A&S 2e. Sinus histiocytosis, p983-984

96 a follicular cyst

Follicular cysts may contain mature ova encircled by sheets and clusters of normal follicular cells. Follicular cysts generally present in FNA cytology as hypocellular samples of granulosa and theca cells in clusters or sheets of cells with high N:C ratios and folded bean shaped nuclei scattered among a proteinaceous or bloody background. If hypercellular samples are seen, the cellular morphology may be quite reactive and mimic malignant features—making differentiation from a malignant neoplasm difficult.

DeMay, A&S 2e. Functional cysts: follicular cysts, p1421

97 d colorectal/carcinoma

These faux "terminal bars" represent microvilli manifesting their glycocalyx and "rootlets" that extend into the body of the plasma membrane. Terminal barlike structures may be seen with gastrointestinal carcinomas, bronchioloalveolar adenocarcinomas, endocervical adenocarcinomas, and mucinous tumors (benign & malignant) of the ovary.

DeMay, A&S 2e. Glandular cells, p566-568

98 d granulosa cell tumor

Granulosa cell tumors are estrogen producing lesions that may be related to the subsequent development of endometrial adenocarcinomas. FNA cytology reveals cells in sheets with uniformly arranged nuclei containing nuclear grooves and micronucleoli. The presence of rosettes (although rare) provides proof of Call-Exner bodies that may contain intraluminar eosinophilic material.

DeMay, A&S 2e. Granulosa cell tumor, p1412-1413

99 c normal biliary duct

Ductal epithelium of the pancreas cytologically presents as monolayer or honeycombing sheets of cells with round, regular, predictable spatially arranged nuclei. These cells resemble endocervical cells.

DeMay, A&S 2e. Ductal cells, p1300-1301

100 c adenocarcinoma

Adenocarcinomas involving the gallbladder present with cytologic features that mirror pancreatobiliary carcinoma. Clinical history usually includes gallstones and is more often seen in Asians and Native Americans than Caucasians or African Americans.

DeMay, A&S 2e. Extrahepatic biliary tract and gallbladder, p1326

101 b the cells of the fibrolamellar variant of HCC are larger and more dispersed, with fewer trabeculae

The diagnosis of fibrolamellar hepatocellular carcinoma (HCC), although similar to well differentiated HCC, is based on the cytologic identification of cells with oncocytic cytoplasm, pale intracytoplasmic bodies, and an associated lamellar fibrosis (dense fibrous connective tissue with parallel rows of fibroblasts), which is rare in well differentiated HCC. As indicated in the question, the cells of fibrolamellar HCC are larger, more dispersed, not commonly arranged in trabeculae, and associated with bile ducts—all factors that contrast with the cytologic identification of well differentiated trabecular HCC. Clinically, the fibrolamellar variant of HCC is typically seen in younger patients (35 years of age), whereas ordinary HCC (>60 years of age) commonly affects more women than men and carries a better prognosis. Moreover, ordinary HCC is generally associated with an underlying cirrhosis or hepatitis, and fibrolamellar HCC is more likely associated with focal nodular hyperplasia.

DeMay, A&S 2e. Fibrolamellar variant of hepatocellular carcinoma, p1266-1267

102 d pancreatitis

A hypocellular sample of degenerated acinar cells in cohesive sheets containing abundant granular cytoplasm, numerous polymorphonuclear neutrophils, and lipid laden macrophages distributed amongst a background of necrosis is suggestive of acute pancreatitis. Necrotic fat, collagen, neutrophils, reactive mesothelial cells, and fibroconnective tissue may accompany these cellular findings.

DeMay, A&S 2e. Pancreatitis, p1303-1305

103 c mucinous cystic tumor/surgical resection

These lesions are considered borderline tumors, which, due to the inadequacy of cytomorphologic criteria to effectively predict their benign or malignant nature, must be resected. As indicated in answer 119, mucinous cystadenomas present with tall columnar morphology and mucus laden cytoplasm (mucicarmine +), and a fibrillar mucinous background.

DeMay, A&S 2e. Mucinous cystic neoplasms, p1310-1311

104 d prostatic hyperplasia

Cells arranged in monolayers and sheets with well defined honeycomb arrangement, basal cells (resembling myoepithelial cells), and spindle cells are helpful in establishing the diagnosis of benign prostatic hyperplasia.

DeMay, A&S 2e. Benign prostatic hyperplasia, p1409

105 a pancreatitis

Cytology includes the finding of inflammatory cells and histiocytes contained within a necrotic background. Although epithelial cells are rare to absent, reactive mesenchymal cells may be found demonstrating "atypical" morphology, which must be discriminated from malignancy.

DeMay, A&S 2e. Pancreatitic pseudocyst, p1306

106 b small round cells→small cleaved→large cleaved → small noncleaved→large noncleaved→immunoblastic→ plasma cell

Antigenic stimulation allows for differentiation of the lymphocytes within the lymphoid follicles as indicated.

DeMay, A&S 2e. Lymphocyte differentiation, p969-971, f13.1782-784

107 a lymphoid

The presence of lymphogranular bodies as seen with the Romanowsky stain (more difficult with the Papanicolaou stain) will only identify these cells as lymphoid in origin. They cannot be used to differentiate reactive hyperplasia from malignant lymphoma; however, their presence rules out the possibility of a poorly differentiated metastatic epithelial malignancy.

DeMay, A&S 2e. Lymphoglandular bodies, p975-976

108 d anaplastic carcinoma, pancreas

Aspirates containing hypercellular populations of single, discohesive, pleomorphic mononucleate cells with classic malignant criteria, multinucleated anaplastic giant cells, and abnormal mitotic figures are diagnostic of pleomorphic giant cell carcinoma of the pancreas.

DeMay, A&S 2e. Undifferentiated (anaplastic) carcinomas, p1316-1317

109 b well differentiated adenocarcinoma

Cells representing prostatic adenocarcinomas present in discohesive sheets, clusters, and microacinar formations with increased nuclear sizes, overlapping nuclei, and the important finding of macronucleoli. The absence of basaloid cells helps distinguish well differentiated lesions from dysplastic processes.

DeMay, A&S 2e. Adenocarcinoma, p1176-1180

110 c reactive condition

Lymphohistiocytic aggregates (not to be confused with lymphogranular bodies) are composed of reticular cells (stellate shaped with oval nuclei), germinal center cells, and tingible body macrophages. Their presence is usually indicative of a reactive lymphoid process.

DeMay, A&S 2e. Dendritic-lymphocytic aggregates, p973-974

111 b T cell and pan B cell surface antigens (Leu/CD5)

These neoplasms may be identified by their coexpression of pan B & T cell antigen using Leu1/CD5. Small cell noncleaved or round cell lymphoma (well differentiated lymphocytic lymphoma) cytologically presents as a monotonous population composed predominantly of small round cells. The absence of a polymorphic or heterogeneous pattern of mixed lymphocytes differentiates these malignancies from reactive lymphoid hyperplasia. Differentiation from undifferentiated B cell lymphoma/ Burkitt or non-Burkitt lymphoma is possible due to the clinical history associated with Burkitt and the presence of lipid+ cytoplasm associated with Burkitt lymphomas.

DeMay, A&S 2e. Small lymphocytic lymphoma, p998-999

112 a early reactive lymph node hyperplasia

Early phase lymph node reaction (immunoblastic hyperplasia) consists of a polymorphic population of large cleaved and noncleaved lymphocytes and immunoblasts, and a slightly greater population of small round and cleaved lymphocytes. Lymphohistiocytic aggregates (not to be confused with lymphogranular bodies) composed of reticular cells (stellate shaped with oval nuclei), germinal center cells, and tingible body macrophages are also identified. Early phase reactive lymphoid hyperplasia (EPRLH) may be differentiated from immunoblastic lymphomas (ILs) because EPRLH shows the presence of small round and small cleaved, large noncleaved, and cleaved lymphocytes, whereas ILs do not contain these key elements.

DeMay, A&S 2e. Immunoblastic lymphoma, p1008

113 d breast adenocarcinoma

Lobular carcinomas present as moderately cellular specimens composed of small monomorphic epithelial cells with minimal nuclear deviation or pleomorphism. The cells possess scanty cytoplasm, often with signet ring morphology or intracytoplasmic lumens. Nuclear overlapping and eccentric nuclei may be noted on high power. Rare vertebral column formation may be noted. Fibrocollagenous tissue may be interspersed amongst the groups of epithelial cells. Mucin positivity is usually noted.

DeMay, A&S 2e. Lobular carcinoma, p1090-1091

114 a small round lymphocytes, small cleaved lymphocytes, plasma cells

Late stage (end stage) reactive lymphoid hyperplasia is represented by the finding of a predominant population of small round and cleaved lymphocytes, and only scattered immunoblastic or plasmacytoid lymphocytes.

DeMay, A&S 2e. Chronic lymphadenitis (reactive hyperplasia), p977

115 a small round and small cleaved lymphocytes over large cleaved and noncleaved lymphocytes, lymphohistiocytic aggregates

The follicular hyperplasia variant of chronic lymphadenitis (reactive hyperplasia) presents as a heterogeneous or polymorphic population (in descending percentages) of small round and cleaved lymphocytes, large cleaved and noncleaved lymphocytes, immunoblasts, and plasma cells. This polymorphic pattern should preclude a diagnosis of lymphoma.

DeMay, A&S 2e. Follicular hyperplasia, p978-979

ISBN 978-089189-6357 ©ASCP 2015

116 c a benign cellular component

Cells originating from the seminal vesicles cytologically appear as single, often bizarre, "atypical" cells with intracytoplasmic yellow lipofuscin granules. The nuclei of these cells may appear quite abnormal; however, the cytoplasmic pigment should indicate the benignity of these cells.

DeMay, A&S 2e. The cells, p1406

117 c of monoclonal B cell origin

The immunocytochemical staining confirms the diagnosis of large cell noncleaved lymphoma (LCNL). LCNL may be differentiated from immunoblastic lymphomas (ILs) due to the lack of immunoblastic and plasmacytoid cells in LCNL–necessary components for establishing the diagnosis of IL. The FNA of large cell lymphomas typically exhibits with a predominant population (80%) of large cells with coarse irregular chromatin and prominent nucleoli. A smaller population of small round or cleaved lymphocytes completes the cytologic picture. The presence of lymphogranular bodies rules out the possibility of a true histiocytic (monocytic) lymphoma.

DeMay, A&S 2e. Diffuse large B cell lymphoma, p1006-1007

118 b benign lesions are more common than malignant tumors

The benign to malignant ratio of soft tissue lesions is 100:1.

DeMay, A&S 2e. Introduction, p630

119 b microcystic adenoma

These lesions commonly affect elderly patients, cytologically presenting as hypocellular specimens containing groups of cuboidal cells with PAS+, mucicarmine– cytoplasm. These lesions may be differentiated from mucinous cystadenomas, which present with tall columnar morphology and mucus laden cytoplasm (mucicarmine+).

DeMay, A&S 2e. Serous cystadenoma (microcystic adenoma), p1309-1310

120 c a polymorphic population of lymphoid cells

The follicular hyperplasia variant of chronic lymphadenitis (reactive hyperplasia) presents as a heterogeneous or polymorphic population (in descending percentages) of small round and cleaved lymphocytes, large cleaved and noncleaved lymphocytes, immunoblasts, and plasma cells. This polymorphic pattern should preclude a diagnosis of lymphoma.

DeMay, A&S 2e. Chronic lymphadenitis (reactive hyperplasia), p977

121 c nodular sclerosing type

The diagnosis of Hodgkin disease rests on the finding of the pathognomonic Reed-Sternberg (RS) cell, a cell with mirror image (binucleate) nuclei, as mononucleate cells ("Hodgkin cells"), lacunar cells (RS cells with clear surrounding cytoplasm), or merely as bare nuclei. The nuclei contain coarsely granular, irregularly distributed chromatin with irregular nuclear membranes and ill shaped macronucleoli. Associated cellular findings depend on which of the 4 Rye classification variants are represented: lymphocyte predominant (few RS cells [±polylobed RS cells], small round cells, and epithelioid histiocytes), nodular sclerosing (lower cellularity but increased number of mononuclear lacunar RS cells as well as "Hodgkin cells," fibrous connective tissue, small round lymphocytes, plasma cells, eosinophils), mixed cellularity (moderate population of RS cells, abundant eosinophils, neutrophils, plasma cells, small population of small round cells), or the lymphocyte depleted type (abundant polylobed RS, necrosis, and a scanty sample of small round cells and histiocytes).

DeMay, A&S 2e. Nodular lymphocyte predominant Hodgkin lymphoma, p1022

122 b bacterial infection

FNA of lymph nodes harboring acute lymphadenitis presents as a hypercellular population of neutrophils, rare lymphocytes, and tingible body macrophages in a necrotic background. The etiology is generally bacterial in origin and must be cultured for identification.

DeMay, A&S 2e. Acute lymphadenitis, p977

123 d Burkitt lymphoma

Burkitt lymphomas cytologically present as small noncleaved lymphomas with intermediate sized nuclei and frothy, vacuolated, lipid laden cytoplasm. These lesions mimic lymphocytic lymphomas (LLs), with the exception that LLs are T cell neoplasms that arise in the thymus.

DeMay, A&S 2e. Malignant lymphoma, p580

124 b islet cell tumor of the pancreas, β cell predominance

Chromogranin positivity indicates a neurosecretory (islet cell) pancreatic lesion, and the insulin production indicates the diagnosis of an insulinoma–a neoplasm composed predominantly of β cells.

DeMay, A&S 2e. Islet cell hyperplasia, p1323

125 d sarcoidosis

The finding of epithelioid macrophages (without intracytoplasmic inclusions), multinucleated histiocytes, and scattered lymphocytes indicates the diagnosis of granulomatous lymphadenitis. The presence of a necrotic background or neutrophilic infiltrate may help in determining whether the etiology is associated with caseous necrosis or suppurative inflammation. The diagnosis of sarcoidosis may only be suggested with the cytologic findings represented in granulomatous disease, generally presenting as a scanty sample and lacking a necrotic background. Schaumann and asteroid bodies may occasionally be seen.

DeMay, A&S 2e. Sarcoidosis, p987-988

126 b there is a lack of small round cells and immunoblasts in MCL; MCL is monoclonal for light chains

Further differentiation from reactive hyperplasia (RH) is possible due to the full range of heterogeneous cells that are seen in RH, including tingible body macrophages, lymphohistiocytic aggregates, and plasma cells. These elements are virtually absent in mixed lymphomas.

DeMay, A&S 2e. Follicular lymphoma, p1003-1005

127 d Hodgkin disease

The diagnosis of Hodgkin disease rests on the finding of the pathognomonic Reed-Sternberg (RS) cell, a cell with mirror image (binucleate) nuclei, as mononucleate cells ("Hodgkin cells"), lacunar cells (RS cells with clear surrounding cytoplasm), or merely as bare nuclei. The nuclei contain coarsely granular, irregularly distributed chromatin with irregular nuclear membranes and ill shaped macronucleoli. Associated cellular findings depend on which of the 4 Rye classification variants are represented: lymphocyte predominant (few RS cells [±polylobed RS cells], small round cells, and epithelioid histiocytes), nodular sclerosing (lower cellularity but increased number of mononuclear lacunar RS cells as well as "Hodgkin cells," fibrous connective tissue, small round lymphocytes, plasma cells, eosinophils), mixed cellularity (moderate population of RS cells, abundant eosinophils, neutrophils, plasma cells, small population of small round cells), or the lymphocyte depleted type (abundant polylobed RS, necrosis, and a scanty sample of small round cells and histiocytes).

DeMay, A&S 2e. Nodular lymphocyte predominant Hodgkin lymphoma), p1022

128 b drunken honeycombs and goblet cells

Secretory or mucinous ductal adenocarcinoma of the pancreas cytologically presents as "drunken honeycombs." Goblet cells (mucin positive) resemble benign muciphages. The cells are seen in sheets with increased cytoplasm (low N:C ratios), wobbly cell outlines, and loosely, unevenly spaced nuclei with folds and clefts. The nuclei may have irregular chromatin, and macronucleoli may be present. The differential diagnosis: cells in a monolayer formation containing overlapping bland nuclei, anisonucleosis, thick appearing nuclear membranes with prominent nucleoli, a loss of polarity, and crowded sheets represent a well differentiated nonsecretory pancreatic adenocarcinoma. An inconspicuous population of bizarre malignant tumor cells may accompany these otherwise deceptively malignant cellular findings.

DeMay, A&S 2e. Ductal adenocarcinoma, p1313-1316

129 a oncocytic neuroendocrine carcinoma of the pancreas

Oncocytic neuroendocrine carcinomas of the pancreas are confirmed as mentioned in answer 124. However, the neoplastic cells morphologically resemble oncocytes such as those found within the salivary glands, kidneys, and thyroid.

DeMay, A&S 2e. Neuroendocrine carcinomas, p1188-1192

130 d small round lymphocytes, small cleaved lymphocytes, large cleaved lymphocytes, large noncleaved lymphocytes, immunoblasts, plasma cells

Early phase lymph node reaction (immunoblastic hyperplasia) consists of a polymorphic population of large cleaved and noncleaved lymphocytes and immunoblasts, and a slightly greater population of small round and cleaved lymphocytes. Lymphohistiocytic aggregates (not to be confused with lymphogranular bodies) composed of reticular cells (stellate shaped with oval nuclei), germinal center cells, and tingible body macrophages are also identified. Immature plasmacytoid cells with prominent nucleoli help support a diagnosis of infectious mononucleosis. Early phase reactive lymphoid hyperplasia (EPRLH) may be differentiated from immunoblastic lymphomas (ILs) because EPRLH shows the presence of small round and small cleaved, large noncleaved and cleaved lymphocytes, whereas ILs do not contain these key elements.

DeMay, A&S 2e. Follicular hyperplasia, p1222-1223

131 c cat scratch disease

Cat scratch disease differs cytologically from toxoplasmosis due to a predominant population of epithelioid cells, the additional presence of neutrophils and eosinophils, and a possible microabscess related necrotic background. A Warthin-Starry silver stain will confirm the presence of Gram– bacterium. *Toxoplasma gondii,* on the other hand, may be found in patients who are exposed to feline feces (often from the dust of cat litter). Specimens may indicate the presence of small lymphocytes, immunoblasts, plasma cells, tingible body macrophages, lymphohistiocytic aggregates, and rare epithelioid histiocytes. These cells represent a diagnostic triad of marked follicular hyperplasia, small granulomas, and monocytoid B cells.

DeMay, A&S 2e. Cat scratch disease, p988

132 b Burkitt lymphoma

The starry sky pattern represents tingible body macrophages in the presence of undifferentiated small noncleaved lymphocytes.

DeMay, A&S 2e. Malignant lymphoma, p580

133 c clear cell renal cell carcinoma

The identification of lipid laden cytoplasm as demonstrated by special staining with oil red O in concert with the described cellular findings is important in establishing the diagnosis of clear cell renal cell carcinoma. These findings may also prove useful in differentiating these lesions from primary transitional cell carcinoma and oncocytoma.

DeMay, A&S 2e. Conventional (clear & granular) renal cell carcinoma, p1356-1359

ISBN 978-089189-6357 ©ASCP 2015

134 a metastatic breast carcinoma
Lobular carcinomas present as moderately cellular specimens composed of small monomorphic epithelial cells with minimal nuclear deviation or pleomorphism. The cells possess scanty cytoplasm, often with signet ring morphology or intracytoplasmic lumens giving the nucleus a targetoid appearance. Cells may be cohesive with vertebral column formation, contain hyperchromatic nuclei with nucleoli, and have frothy cytoplasm. The background is often thick and eosinophilic with interspersed fat vacuoles and small fibrous stromal elements. Nuclear overlapping and eccentric nuclei may be noted on high power. Rare vertebral column formation may be noted. Fibrocollagenous tissue may be interspersed amongst the groups of epithelial cells. Mucin positivity is usually noted.
DeMay, A&S 2e. Lobular carcinoma, p1090-1091

135 b 20s-40s
Papillary carcinoma (PTC) of the thyroid accounts for 75% of all thyroid carcinomas in the US and is 2-4× more common in women. This lesion, unlike follicular and anaplastic carcinomas of the thyroid, is etiologically related to iodized salt or radiation exposure. As indicated in the question, the peak incidence is between the ages of 20 and 40; however, PTC is the most common thyroid cancer in young children and may occur at any age. Strictly stated, the younger the patient and the smaller the lesion (4 cm), the better the prognosis. Despite being more common in women, men are more likely to have a poorer prognosis.
DeMay, A&S 2e. Papillary thyroid carcinoma, p892-893

136 b metastatic colonic carcinoma
Metastatic carcinomas represent 90% of the liver malignancies. The most common metastases are adenocarcinomas and gastrointestinal malignancies (colorectal, stomach, pancreatic). Other metastatic lesions include those from the lungs, breast, and kidney followed by gastrointestinal leiomyosarcomas, melanomas, lymphomas, and neuroendocrine tumors. The presence of tall columnar or "cigar shaped" cells in aggregates with frankly malignant nuclear features, granular cytoplasm, or the presence of malignant signet ring cells may suggest a diagnosis of metastatic adenocarcinoma of the colon. Correlation with the primary lesion is critical.
DeMay, A&S 2e. Metastases, p1277-1278

137 d hepatoblastoma
Hepatoblastoma (HB) is a rare primary liver lesion usually found in children <3 years of age. This embryonal tumor may be associated with congenital anomalies rather than cirrhosis. HB is third in incidence of the intra-abdominal childhood malignancies, just behind neuroblastoma and Wilms tumor. There are 3 distinct variants of HB, variants that are epithelial, epithelial and mesenchymal (mixed), or anaplastic; however, these epithelial cells may have anaplastic, embryonal, or fetal differentiation. In this question, the anaplastic variant of HB is described, a lesion that is similar to other "small blue cell tumors." Cells of embryonal differentiation are cytologically identified as more mature, arranged in cords or ribbons with typical malignant nuclear features. The fetal type cells are even larger than the anaplastic or embryonal types, possess granular or clear cytoplasm (often containing fat, glycogen, or bile), typical malignant nuclear features, and lower N:C ratios than the other cell types. These cells are loosely cohesive, and arranged in sheets, acini, or 3D structures (disorganized trabeculae). The fetal cells of HB may also be associated with extramedullary hematopoiesis (megakaryocytes and immature red and white blood cells). Lastly, the mesenchymal variant of HB has undifferentiated cells, osteoid, or metaplastic components such as squamous cells, skeletal tissue, muscle, or cartilage.
DeMay, A&S 2e. Hepatoblastoma, p1270-1272

138 c basal cell adenoma
Basal cell adenomas (BCAs) are cytologically composed of a pure population of epithelial cells. Small cohesive basaloid cells in cords, aggregates, or irregular clusters with high N:C ratios and predictable nuclear features (lacking atypia) in the presence of copious amounts of metachromatic basement membrane are diagnostic of BCA. However, the fibrous stroma component necessary for the diagnosis of pleomorphic adenoma is absent in these lesions. Clinically, the absence of neural symptoms may also help differentiate BCA from adenoid cystic carcinomas.
DeMay, A&S 2e. Basal cell adenoma, p796-797

139 a follicular cells
Follicular cells present as small cells with uniform nuclei found in clusters with or without associated colloid and as monolayer sheets with honeycombing (resembling endocervical cells). Single cells may be observed.
DeMay, A&S 2e. Follicular cells, p861-862

140 d papillary carcinoma
Papillary carcinoma generally presents in monolayer sheets or in papillary groupings with fibrovascular cores. The cells contain irregular nuclear membranes with bland chromatin features, nuclear grooves, and intranuclear intracytoplasmic inclusions representing cytoplasmic intranuclear invaginations or nuclear pseudoinclusions. Colloid, foreign body giant cells, and psammoma bodies may accompany these findings.
DeMay, A&S 2e. Cytology of papillary carcinoma, p895-897

141 a mucoepidermoid carcinoma

High grade mucoepidermoid carcinomas (MECs) of the salivary gland present with predominant populations of malignant squamous cells revealing typical nonkeratinizing or keratinizing features. Mucus producing columnar cells containing bland nuclei and foamy cytoplasm and a population of benign polygonal intermediate cells define low grade MEC. The differential diagnosis of a high grade MEC includes a pure keratinizing squamous cell carcinoma, a diagnosis that may be preferred in the presence of pearl formations.

DeMay, A&S 2e. Mucoepidermoid carcinoma, p804-807

142 c Hürthle cells

Hürthle cells represent mitochondria rich follicular cells found singly and in clusters, containing abundant, eosinophilic, granular cytoplasm. The nuclei are round to oval and often possess prominent nucleoli. Hürthle cells are found in Hashimoto thyroiditis, Hürthle cell neoplasms, and benign goiters.

DeMay, A&S 2e. Hürthle cells, p863-864

143 d Hodgkin disease

The diagnosis of Hodgkin disease rests on the finding of the pathognomonic Reed-Sternberg (RS) cell, a cell with mirror image (binucleate) nuclei, as mononucleate cells ("Hodgkin cells"), lacunar cells (RS cells with clear surrounding cytoplasm), or as bare nucleoli. The nuclei contain coarsely granular, irregularly distributed chromatin with irregular nuclear membranes and ill shaped macronucleoli. Associated cellular findings depend on which of the 4 Rye classification variants are represented: lymphocyte predominant (few RS cells [±polylobed RS cells], small round cells and epithelioid histiocytes), nodular sclerosing (lower cellularity but increased number of mononuclear lacunar RS cells as well as "Hodgkin cells," fibrous connective tissue, small round lymphocytes, plasma cells, eosinophils), mixed cellularity (moderate population of RS cells, abundant eosinophils, neutrophils, plasma cells, small population of small round cells), or the lymphocyte depleted type (abundant polylobed RS, necrosis, and a scanty sample of small round cells and histiocytes).

DeMay, A&S 2e. Nodular lymphocyte predominant Hodgkin lymphoma, p1022

144 b Hashimoto thyroiditis

A predominantly rich heterogeneous population of lymphocytes and follicular center cells with associated Hürthle cells are diagnostic of Hashimoto thyroiditis. Colloid, if present, is scanty.

DeMay, A&S 2e. FNA biopsy of Hashimoto thyroiditis, p874-875

145 b adenoid cystic carcinoma

Adenoid cystic carcinomas are cytologically identified by the presence of small round epithelial cells in clusters, acinar formations, and 3D tissue fragments in balls or cylinders containing central, eosinophilic, hyaline/homogeneous, fibrillar basement membrane material. Adenoid cystic carcinomas are frequent submaxillary and minor salivary gland neoplasms arising from the intercalated ducts. These lesions often present as painful lesions due to perineural invasion.

DeMay, A&S 2e. Adenoid cystic carcinoma, p802-804

146 d metastatic melanoma

Melanoma typically presents in single cells, in aggregates, or as spindle cells with bizarre malignant nuclear features, macronucleoli, intranuclear cytoplasmic invaginations, and possibly intracytoplasmic golden-brown pigment. Due to the fact that these diseases may be amelanotic, it may be helpful to confirm this disease process with S100, HMB45, melan A or MITF (microphthalmia associated transcription factor)–all of which preferentially react with melanoma cells.

DeMay, A&S 2e. Metastases, p1279

147 a follicular neoplasm

Follicular neoplasms cytologically present as a hypercellular population of overlapping follicular cells with cohesive microfollicular or trabecular groupings. Colloid is scanty to absent. The diagnosis of follicular neoplasm is given to those samples in which definitive atypical nuclear features are absent. Follicular adenoma should be reserved for histologic diagnosis only due to the possibility of capsular invasion by these benign appearing cells and the lack of distinguishable cytologic criteria necessary to differentiate these lesions from well differentiated carcinomas.

DeMay, A&S 2e. Follicular neoplasms, p882-885

148 a colloid goiter

Benign follicular cells in monolayer or honeycombing sheets in the presence of abundant colloid (appearing as ropy amorphous background material) and (as seen) associated hemosiderin laden macrophages and fibroblasts are typical findings associated with the FNA of benign colloid nodules.

DeMay, A&S 2e. Goiter, p881-882

149 a acinic cell carcinoma

Hypercellular specimens composed of acinic cells (without ducts) in sheets, acini, or tubules containing uniform to slightly enlarged central or eccentric nuclei, nucleoli, and clear or granular (PAS+) cytoplasm with intracytoplasmic granules are representative of acinic cell carcinoma. Fibrofatty stroma is absent while a lymphocytic infiltrate may be common. Acinic cell carcinomas are considered rare lesions predominantly arising within the parotid gland.

DeMay, A&S 2e. Acinic cell carcinoma, p807-808

150 d lipophagic granuloma

Lipid laden macrophages predominate in aspiration biopsy specimens in patients who have received lymphangiography. Special staining with oil red O may help elucidate the benign nature of these cells.

DeMay, A&S 2e. Foreign body granulomas, p989

151 c metastatic adenocarcinoma, breast

Metastatic carcinomas represent the most common lymph node malignancy, even more common than primary lymphoid neoplasms. FNA of this lymph node shows an infiltrating ductal carcinoma of the breast, a tumor that presents as hypercellular epithelial cells in well formed microacini with malignant nuclear characteristics. Cohesive clusters of "foreign" cells are helpful in establishing a diagnosis of metastatic carcinoma.

DeMay, A&S 2e. Metastatic malignancy, p930-932

ISBN 978-089189-6357 ©ASCP 2015

152 d lymphoma

Large cell or histiocytic lymphoma accounts for the most common primary lymphoma of the thyroid. These cells present as a predominant population of large lymphocytes with irregular nuclear membranes and coarse, irregular chromatin patterns with prominent nucleoli, as well as small cleaved lymphocytes with similar nuclear features. The presence of lymphogranular bodies as seen with the Romanowsky stain will help identify these cells as being of lymphoid origin, differentiating the process from poorly differentiated malignancies. Lymphomas involving the thyroid may be primary or represent metastatic neoplasms.

DeMay, A&S 2e. Hematologic neoplasms, p927-929

153 a immunoblastic hyperplasia

Early phase lymph node reaction (immunoblastic hyperplasia) consists of a polymorphic population of large cleaved and noncleaved lymphocytes and immunoblasts, and a slightly greater population of small round and cleaved lymphocytes. Lymphohistiocytic aggregates (not to be confused with lymphogranular bodies) composed of reticular cells (stellate shaped with oval nuclei), germinal center cells, and tingible body macrophages are also identified. Immature plasmacytoid cells with prominent nucleoli help support a diagnosis of infectious mononucleosis. Early phase reactive lymphoid hyperplasia (EPRLH) may be differentiated from immunoblastic lymphomas (ILs) because EPRLH shows the presence of small round and small cleaved, large noncleaved and cleaved lymphocytes, whereas ILs do not contain these key elements.

DeMay, A&S 2e. Paracortical, or diffuse immunoblastic, hyperplasia, p981-982

154 b papillary carcinoma

Papillary carcinoma generally presents in monolayer sheets or in papillary groupings with fibrovascular cores. The cells contain irregular nuclear membranes with bland chromatin features, nuclear grooves, and intranuclear intracytoplasmic inclusions representing cytoplasmic intranuclear invaginations or nuclear pseudoinclusions. Colloid, foreign body giant cells, and psammoma bodies may accompany these findings.

DeMay, A&S 2e. Cytology of papillary carcinoma, p895-898

155 b giant cell anaplastic carcinoma

These lesions generally affect elderly females and present cytologically as anaplastic giant pleomorphic tumor cells with classic nuclear morphology. Abundant diathesis and abnormal mitotic figures are common findings in these aspirations.

DeMay, A&S 2e. Giant cell (anaplastic) medullary carcinoma, p915

156 d adenoid cystic carcinoma

Aspirates of adenoid cystic carcinoma display sharply circumscribed "hyaline" globules associated with neoplastic basaloid cells.

DeMay, A&S 2e. Adenoid cystic carcinoma, p802-804

157 b granulomatous lymphadenitis

The finding of epithelioid macrophages (without intracytoplasmic inclusions), multinucleated histiocytes, and scattered lymphocytes indicates the diagnosis of granulomatous lymphadenitis. The presence of a necrotic background or neutrophilic infiltrate may help in determining whether the etiology is associated with caseous necrosis or suppurative inflammation.

DeMay, A&S 2e. Granulomatous hyperplasia, p986-987

158 a adenocarcinoma

Cells representing prostatic adenocarcinomas present in discohesive sheets, clusters, and microacinar formations with increased nuclear sizes, overlapping nuclei, and the important finding of macronucleoli. The absence of basaloid cells helps distinguish well differentiated lesions from dysplastic processes.

DeMay, A&S 2e. Adenocarcinoma, p1176-1182

159 c plasma cell myeloma

FNA of plasma cell myelomas reveal cells with "clock face" chromatin, immature cells with fine chromatin and prominent nucleoli, and occasionally binucleate and bizarre multinucleated giant cells. The cytoplasm is generally blue or amphophilic with perinuclear hofs and intranuclear or intracytoplasmic Russell bodies (representing immunoglobulin, usually IgG or IgA).

DeMay, A&S 2e. Plasmacytoma/plasma cell myeloma, p1000-1002

160 b large cell cleaved lymphoma

Large cell cleaved lymphomas typically present as a predominant population (80%) of large cleaved cells with coarse irregular chromatin and prominent nucleoli. A smaller population of small round or cleaved lymphocytes completes the cytologic picture. Differentiation from immunoblastic lymphomas is based on the absence of large immunoblasts and plasmacytoid cells as well as the absence of mature lymphocytes. The presence of lymphogranular bodies rules out the possibility of a true histiocytic (monocytic) lymphoma.

DeMay, A&S 2e. Diffuse large B cell lymphoma, p1006-1007

161 a follicular (reactive) hyperplasia

The follicular hyperplasia variant of chronic lymphadenitis (reactive hyperplasia) presents as a heterogeneous or polymorphic population (in descending percentages) of small round and cleaved lymphocytes, large cleaved and noncleaved lymphocytes, immunoblasts, and plasma cells. This polymorphic pattern should preclude a diagnosis of lymphoma.

DeMay, A&S 2e. Chronic lymphadenitis, p572

162 b cat scratch disease

Cat scratch disease is marked by a predominant population of epithelioid cells, the additional presence of neutrophils and eosinophils, and a possible microabscess related necrotic background. A Warthin-Starry silver stain will confirm the presence of Gram– bacteria. Alternatively, *Toxoplasma gondii* may be found in patients who are exposed to feline feces (often from the dust of cat litter). Specimens may indicate the presence of small lymphocytes, immunoblasts, plasma cells, tingible body macrophages, lymphohistiocytic aggregates, and rare epithelioid histiocytes. These cells represent a diagnostic triad of marked follicular hyperplasia, small granulomas, and monocytoid B cells.

DeMay, A&S 2e. Cat scratch disease, p988

163 a osteosarcoma

Osteosarcoma cytologically presents as round to polygonal cells with pleomorphic sarcomatous cytoplasm in the company of an eosinophilic (metachromatic with Romanowsky stain) osteoid matrix. Multinucleated giant tumor cells are common findings.

DeMay, A&S 2e. Osteosarcoma, p699-700

164 d Burkitt lymphoma

Burkitt lymphomas cytologically present as small noncleaved lymphomas with intermediate nuclei and frothy, vacuolated, lipid laden cytoplasm. These lesions mimic lymphocytic lymphomas (LLs) with the exception that LLs are T cell neoplasms that arise in the thymus.

DeMay, A&S 2e. Burkitt lymphoma, p1008-1010

165 a small cell noncleaved lymphoma

Small cell noncleaved or round cell lymphomas (well differentiated lymphocytic lymphoma) cytologically present as a monotonous population composed predominantly of small round cells. The absence of a polymorphic or heterogeneous pattern of mixed lymphocytes and the presence of a positive staining reaction with Leu1/CD5 differentiate these malignancies from reactive lymphoid hyperplasia. Differentiation from undifferentiated B cell lymphoma/Burkitt or non-Burkitt lymphoma is possible due to the clinical history associated with Burkitt and the presence of lipid+ cytoplasm associated with Burkitt lymphomas.

DeMay, A&S 2e. Small lymphocytic lymphoma, p998-999

166 c malignant fibrous histiocytoma

Soft tissue aspirations containing bizarre giant tumor cells with classic malignant nuclear morphology and spindle shaped and polygonal fibroblasts occurring singly and in overlapping fashion, seen in combination with a lymphocytic infiltrate, are diagnostic of malignant fibrous histiocytoma.

DeMay, A&S 2e. Undifferentiated pleomorphic sarcoma (so called malignant fibrous histiocytoma), p667-668

167 b seminoma

Seminomas cytologically present as large discohesive germ cells containing irregular chromatin and macronucleoli. The background contains a lymphocytic infiltrate, PAS positivity, and a "tigroid" pattern demonstrated with Diff-Quik. Granulomas are often seen and serve as a diagnostic clue for seminomas of the testes and dysgerminomas of the ovaries.

DeMay, A&S 2e. Germinoma (seminoma/dysgerminoma), p1415-1416

168 a lipoma

Lipomas are characterized in cytology by the presence of mature adipose tissue in sheets with "chicken wire" appearance. The cells have eccentrically located nuclei, single large lipid droplets within the cytoplasm, and anatomizing capillaries. Oily material may "bead up" on Diff-Quik preparations.

DeMay, A&S 2e. Lipoma, p649-652

169 d hepatocytes, suggest reaspiration

This inadequate or unsuccessful lung aspirate reveals normal hepatocytes that are identified as polygonal cells arranged in monolayer formations. The cytoplasm is described as granular with bile inclusions, while the nuclei are generally round to oval with prominent nucleoli. Many cells are binucleate, while others may contain intranuclear cytoplasmic invaginations. Care should be exercised to prevent confusion of these cells with indigenous pulmonary mucosa.

DeMay, A&S 2e. Miscellaneous cells, p1160

170 c faulty technique–aspiration of necrotic center

Represented is a necrotic center of a centrally detected squamous cell carcinoma of the lung. Aspiration of the center of this lesion yielded a specimen composed predominantly of diathesis and necrotic debris. When performing FNA, special attention needs to be given so that multiple sites of neoplasm are aspirated, especially along the peripheral margins (>10 planes).

DeMay, A&S 2e. Fine needle aspiration biopsy, p1156-1159

171 d coccidioidomycosis

Coccioidomycosis is endemic to the southwestern United States. Most patients are asymptomatic, but immunocompromised patients are more susceptible to infection. The organisms are large with thick walled spherules containing endospores. The spherules may be extracellular or engulfed by macrophages. Empty spherules may appear fractured or empty. Contaminants and pollen grains can simulate the organisms. *Cryptococcus* has a polysaccharide capsule with narrow, teardrop buds. *Histoplasma* are small, budding yeasts, usually present within macrophages.

DeMay, A&S 2e. Coccidioides immitis, p1471

172 d any of the above

Intranuclear cytoplasmic invaginations (INCIs), or pseudoinclusions, are often found within papillary carcinoma of the thyroid, melanomas, and hepatocellular carcinomas. The presence of INCIs are helpful in confirming these malignant diseases; however, they have been reported in benign lesions as well, such as benign liver conditions.

DeMay, A&S 2e. Glandular cells, p568

ISBN 978-089189-6357 ©ASCP 2015

173 c chromogranin

Islet cell tumors (pancreatic endocrine neoplasms) present as loosely cohesive clusters or rosettes and as single cells containing eccentrically located nuclei and sparsely fine, red granular cytoplasm demonstrated on Diff-Quik. The chromatin is described as salt & pepper. Immunocytochemical studies for chromogranin, neuron specific enolase, insulin, gastrin, or argyrophilic positivity may help identify these neuroendocrine tumors.

DeMay, A&S 2e. Islet cell, p1301-1302

174 b Echinococcus granulosus

Hydatid sand is composed of scoleces and hooklets derived from *Echinococcus granulosus*. Aspiration of cystic liver nodules is generally contraindicated due to the possibility of anaphylaxis.

DeMay, A&S 2e. Hydatid cysts, p1256

175 a ductal adenocarcinoma

Cells in a monolayer formation containing overlapping bland nuclei, anisonucleosis, thick appearing nuclear membranes with prominent nucleoli, a loss of polarity, and crowded sheets represent a well differentiated nonsecretory pancreatic adenocarcinoma. An inconspicuous population of bizarre malignant tumor cells may accompany these otherwise deceptively benign cellular findings.

DeMay, A&S 2e. Ductal adenocarcinoma, p1313-1316

176 a α-fetoprotein–, keratin+

Hepatocellular carcinoma (HCC) will stain positive for α-fetoprotein, whereas pancreatic carcinomas are negative. Both lesions are positive for low (CAM5.2) and high (AE1/AE3) molecular weight keratin. The morphologic presence of "tombstone cells" (tall columnar) helps support a diagnosis of pancreatic carcinoma rather than HCC.

DeMay, A&S 2e. Hepatocellular carcinomas, p1260-1266

177 b Kaposi sarcoma

The FNA of Kaposi sarcoma presents with bland, slender, spindle shaped cells arranged in sheets and bundles with hyperchromatic nuclei. A very important component of this diagnosis is the presence of hemorrhagic background and the finding of hemosiderin contained within the cytoplasm of the cells. PAS+ nonspecific hyaline globules may be identified. Kaposi sarcoma most likely does not represent a malignant process, but rather a proliferative or hyperplastic process (Gallo). Its natural history typically has a fatal outcome within 6 months.

DeMay, A&S 2e. Kaposi sarcoma, p679-680

178 b cholangiocarcinoma

Well differentiated cholangiocarcinomas present cytologically as hypercellular specimens containing sheets of cells with slightly enlarged, overlapping nuclei and micronucleoli. Their resemblance to normal ductal cells may cause difficulty in establishing a malignant diagnosis. Careful attention should be given to mild nuclear deviations in light of a radiographically identified neoplasm. Cholangiocarcinomas are negative for α-fetoprotein and positive for CEA, whereas hepatocellular carcinomas are positive and negative, respectively.

DeMay, A&S 2e. Cholangiocarcinoma, p1272-1273

179 a Aspergillus species, rule out secondary malignancy by re-aspirating from various areas of the mass

Mycotic infections (aspergillosis, blastomycosis, or others) secondary to malignant processes are often due to a cancer causing postobstructive pneumonitis. These coexisting secondary infections are often peripherally located to the malignancy; therefore, thorough sampling becomes an important aspect in the evaluation of lung masses. The presence of fungal elements may not preclude the possibility of a primary lesion that was missed due to improper sampling. *Aspergillus* species present as thick hyphae with dichotomous branching occurring at 45° angles.

DeMay, A&S 2e. Aspergillus species, p1470-1471

180 a chromogranin

Small cell carcinoma is a highly malignant neuroendocrine neoplasm that is ultrastructurally part of the amine precursor uptake and decarboxylation (APUD) tumors due to its cytoplasmic evidence of androgenic amines (membrane bound granules). These cells contain hyperchromatic, stippled chromatin, coarse clumping, nuclear molding, scanty cytoplasm, and micronucleoli. An important diagnostic feature of small cell carcinoma is the presence of paranuclear cytoplasmic inclusions–blue cytoplasmic globules found indenting the nuclei (best visualized with Diff-Quik staining). The cellular groupings have vertebral column formation, microbiopsy aggregates, and cords, nests, or ribbons. "Crush artifact," or degenerative nuclear material related to the mechanical crushing associated with the preparation of FNA specimens, is found in the background of most small cell carcinomas. This artifact presents as long clumpy streams of basophilic material. A variant of small cell carcinoma, intermediate cell small cell carcinoma, represents both fusiform and polygonal types, which are typically better preserved with open coarse chromatin patterns and enlarged cell areas. Immunocytochemical staining with chromogranin is helpful in establishing the neurosecretory nature of this tumor, but will not differentiate it from carcinoid lesions. Furthermore, the absence of lymphogranular bodies (best demonstrated with the Romanowsky or Diff-Quik stain) will help differentiate these lesions from malignant lymphoid processes.

DeMay, A&S 2e. Small cell carcinoma, p1182-1185

181 c acute lymphadenitis

FNA of lymph nodes harboring acute lymphadenitis presents as a hypercellular population of neutrophils, rare lymphocytes, and tingible body macrophages in a necrotic background. The etiology is generally bacterial in origin and must be cultured for identification.

DeMay, A&S 2e. Acute lymphadenitis, p977

182 d hepatocellular carcinoma

Trabecular (well differentiated) hepatocellular carcinomas present with confluent trabeculating structures on low power analysis. Hyperchromatic nuclei with overlapping features revealing high N:C ratios are unlike those found with poorly differentiated nontrabecular lesions. Hepatocytes arranged in cords and circumscribed by endothelium are typically found in well differentiated hepatocellular carcinoma. Poorly differentiated lesions present with pronounced nuclear abnormalities and lack the trabecular organization. Elevated α-fetoprotein may be demonstrated by serum analysis.

DeMay, A&S 2e. Hepatocellular carcinoma, p1026-1030

183 b mesothelial cells

Mesothelial cells representing nondiagnostic elements from the visceral or parietal pleura appear in sheets with regularly spaced, round to oval uniform nuclei, often containing intranuclear grooves.

DeMay, A&S 2e. Mesothelial cells, p1160

184 b *Pneumocystis jiroveci*

Pneumocystis jiroveci is considered an opportunistic protozoan which may be seen in immunosuppressed individuals secondary to immunologic disorders, malignancies, or HIV infection, and in premature infants or patients receiving chemotherapy. Cytologic identification rests on the presence of frothy mats of eosinophilic material with interspersed "contact lens" shaped structures containing intranuclear trophozoites.

DeMay, A&S 2e. Pneumocystis jiroveci, p1472

185 a reactive

Polygonal cells arranged in rows or trabeculae with dense, granular cytoplasm, enlarged centrally placed bi- or multinucleated cells with smooth nuclear membranes, prominent nucleoli, intranuclear cytoplasmic invaginations, and intracytoplasmic bile pigmentation are diagnostic of reactive hepatocytes. These changes are commonly associated with conditions such as alcoholic cirrhosis or viral hepatitis. Bile ductal cells, fibrous connective tissue, and numerous lymphocytes represent concomitant cytologic findings.

DeMay, A&S 2e. Diffuse liver diseases, p1253-1255

186 a Warthin tumor

Warthin tumor (papillary cystadenoma lymphomatosum) cytologically presents with reactive lymphoid populations and oxyphilic/oncocytic epithelial cells. Oncocytes, cytologically presenting as cuboidal cells with eosinophilic granular cytoplasm and central or eccentric nuclei with prominent nucleoli, are suspended within a watery, proteinaceous, or dirty background. The concomitant finding of a lymphocytic infiltrate (representing a germinal center) alongside the oncocytic population excludes the diagnosis of pure oncocytoma or oxyphilic adenoma. Atypical squamous metaplasia (elongated, caudate shaped cells) may be present if the lesion is infarcted or infected; therefore, exercise caution to prevent overinterpretation of these lesions as squamous cell carcinoma.

DeMay, A&S 2e. Warthin tumor, p798-800

187 d pleomorphic adenoma

Sheets and clusters of cuboidal cells containing round to oval nuclei and micronucleoli represent the ductal epithelial component of pleomorphic adenoma (benign mixed tumor). Fibromyxoid and chondroid mesenchymal elements (staining bright magenta with Diff-Quik staining) and myoepithelial spindle cells, typically arranged in cords and as single cells, may predominate in the smears.

DeMay, A&S 2e. Pleomorphic adenoma (benign mixed tumor), p793-796

188 a adenocarcinoma, poorly differentiated

Poorly differentiated adenocarcinomas may be difficult to separate from other poorly differentiated malignancies, including squamous cell carcinoma and large cell undifferentiated carcinoma. Aspirates yield hypercellular samples containing a heterogeneous population of single cells and slightly cohesive fragments. Anisokaryosis, fine to coarsely granular, irregularly distributed chromatin patterns, multiple macronucleoli, and elevated N:C ratios are common findings. The hallmark for identifying these lesions as glandular in origin is the identification of frothy, lacy, vacuolated to granular cytoplasmic textures.

DeMay, A&S 2e. Adenocarcinoma, p1176-1182

189 a metastatic squamous cell carcinoma

Squamous cell carcinoma cytologically resembles those neoplasms identified in their primary esophageal location. Pleomorphic, keratinizing cells with irregular chromatin, keratinizing pearls, and cellular cannibalism represent many of the features that are found amongst a necrotic background. Poorly differentiated lesions will display classic malignant nuclear features and homogeneous, dense cytoplasm.

DeMay, A&S 2e. Squamous cells, p563-566

190 a secretory ductal carcinoma, pancreas

Secretory or mucinous ductal adenocarcinoma of the pancreas cytologically presents as "drunken honeycombs." Goblet cells (mucin positive) resemble benign muciphages. The cells are seen in sheets with increased cytoplasm (low N:C ratios), wobbly cell outlines, and loosely, unevenly spaced nuclei with folds and clefts. The nuclei may have irregular chromatin and macronucleoli may be present.

DeMay, A&S 2e. Ductal adenocarcinomas, p1313-1316

191 d squamous carcinoma

Pleomorphic cells with caudate or spindle formations with refractile cytoplasm, anisonucleosis, opaque ink dotlike to vesicular nuclei, and coarsely granular, irregularly distributed chromatin are representative of squamous cell carcinoma. A necrotic background is helpful in establishing this lesion.

DeMay, A&S 2e. Squamous cells, p563-566

192 a granuloma

Liver granulomas may be cytologically identified by the presence of single and multinucleated giant cells, epithelioid histiocytes, lymphocytes, and plasma cells. Fibrous connective tissue may be interspersed amongst the inflammatory cellular findings.

DeMay, A&S 2e. Granuloma, p1256-1257

ISBN 978-089189-6357 ©ASCP 2015

193 d   normal parenchyma

Cells representing normal acinar structures composed of serous and mucous glandular fragments are seen in the photomicrograph. These cells are cuboidal in shape with granular (serous) or vacuolated (mucinous) cytoplasm and eccentrically located nuclei. Interspersed adipose tissue is also a common finding in normal salivary gland aspirates. Rarely, ductal cells and myoepithelial cells are seen.

DeMay, A&S 2e. Acinic cells, p779

194 b   acute pancreatitis

A hypocellular sample of degenerated acinar cells in cohesive sheets containing abundant granular cytoplasm, numerous polymorphonuclear neutrophils, and lipid laden macrophages distributed among a background of necrosis is suggestive of acute pancreatitis. Necrotic fat, collagen, neutrophils, reactive mesothelial cells, and fibroconnective tissue may accompany these cellular findings.

DeMay, A&S 2e. Pancreatitis, p1303-1305

195 c   chromogranin

Pheochromocytoma, the primary differential diagnosis of this image given the characteristic "salt & pepper" chromatin, stains positively with chromogranin and other neuroendocrine markers, which would be confirmatory in this case.

DeMay, A&S 2e. Pheochromocytomas, p1394-1395

196 c   inhibin

Adrenal cortical tumors stain positively for inhibin, calretinin, melan A/MART1, CD56, and synaptophysin. Characteristic features of stripped nuclei and frothy background material are seen, in keeping with the cytoplasmic fragility of benign and malignant adrenal cortical epithelium.

DeMay, A&S 2e. Inhibin, p1524

197 a   bronchioloalveolar carcinoma

This cellular aspiration shows bland cuboidal to columnar neoplastic cells in papillary clusters and flat sheets. The nuclei are enlarged with increased N:C ratio. The nuclear membrane is slightly irregular. Nuclear pseudoinclusions and psammoma bodies may be seen. No terminal bars or cilia are seen.

DeMay, A&S 2e. Bronchioloalveolar carcinoma, p1178-1179

198 d   calcitonin

Medullary carcinoma is derived from the c cells of the thyroid; the source of calcitonin, with serum levels often increased in these patients. Calcitonin can also be detected by immunostains on biopsy material and can serve as a tumor marker in these patients.

DeMay, A&S 2e. Calcitonin, p848

199 c   glomerulus structure

Intact glomeruli are infrequently aspirated. This aspirate yielded an intact glomerulus structure, characterized by a lobulated cluster of capillaries, mesangial and capsular cells.

DeMay, A&S 2e. Glomeruli, p1348

200 b   metastatic signet ring cell adenocarcinoma

The nuclear features of signet ring cell adenocarcinoma can be quite deceptively bland; however, in general, there is often some degree of anaplasia. The large cytoplasmic vacuole, with its characteristic displacement of the nuclei, is an important clue to the diagnosis. It should be recognized that signet ring cell adenocarcinoma can arise from many sources, including stomach, pancreas, breast, and others.

DeMay, A&S 2e. Signet ring cell carcinoma, p1182

201 c   CD10–, CK7–

Chromophobe renal cell carcinomas sometimes stain negative for both CK7 and CD10. Clear cell renal cell carcinomas are CD10+, CK7–. Papillary renal cell carcinomas are CK7+ and CD10+. Urothelial carcinomas are CK7+/CK20+ and CD10–. Note how the cells of a chromophobe carcinoma display distinct cell membrane, similar to cell "walls" of vegetable cells.

DeMay, A&S 2e. Chromophobe renal cell carcinoma, p1361-1362

202 a   parathyroid hormone

Elevated parathyroid hormone levels are seen in patients with functioning parathyroid adenomas.

DeMay, A&S 2e. Parathyroid, p1239

203 b   multiple myeloma

Plasmacytoma/multiple myeloma is characterized by discohesive cells with eccentric nuclei, coarse chromatin, and basophilic cytoplasm. Multinucleated forms may be present.

DeMay, A&S 2e. Plasmacytoma/plasma cell myeloma, p1000-1002

204 c   benign gastric tissue

Endoscopic ultrasound guided biopsy is a useful tool, but is often contaminated by tissue fragments from normal organs that the needle passes through en route to the actual target. Onsite identification and recognition of this tissue will aid the clinician in obtaining diagnostic material. The large, flat sheets of uniform cells with uniform, nonoverlapping nuclei, depicted here are most consistent with normal gastric tissue. There are no features of malignancy, neuroendocrine origin or acinar structures.

DeMay, A&S 2e. Gastrointestinal cells, p1302

205 a   metastatic squamous cell carcinoma

Pleomorphic cells with dense and focally keratinized cytoplasm with dense, coarse chromatin and pyknotic nuclei arranged singly and in small sheets characterize squamous cell carcinoma. Necrosis, debris and anucleate ghost cells may be present in the background.

DeMay, A&S 2e. Branchial cleft cyst, p755-756

206 b   nodular fasciitis

A mixed population of plump spindled or stellate cells with abundant cytoplasm, often mixed with loose myxoid or fibrillary stroma and inflammatory cells, is most consistent with nodular fasciitis. The nuclei show benign features including smooth nuclear membranes and lack of hyperchromasia.

DeMay, A&S 2e. Nodular fasciitis, p656-657

207 **d** **follicular neoplasm**

Aspirates from follicular neoplasms of the thyroid are usually quite cellular with minimally atypical follicular cells arranged in monotonous crowded microfollicles or in syncytial groups. Colloid is variable, but usually scanty. Cytoplasm is delicate, ill defined, and sometimes absent. Surgical excision is recommended to evaluate for vascular or capsular invasion seen with follicular carcinomas.

DeMay, A&S 2e. FNA biopsy: the gold standard, p849-853

208 **b** **thyroglossal duct cyst**

Thyroglossal duct cysts are usually located at or near the midline of the thyroid. The aspirate contains cystic debris, and varying numbers of benign appearing squamous cells, macrophages, inflammatory cells, or thyroid tissue.

DeMay, A&S 2e. Thyroglossal duct cysts, p754-755

209 **a** **squamous cell carcinoma**

Pleomorphic cells with dense and focally keratinized cytoplasm with dense, coarse chromatin arranged singly and in small sheets characterize squamous cell carcinoma.

DeMay, A&S 2e. Squamous cell carcinoma, p1173-1175

210 **c** **low grade chondrosarcoma**

This aspirate displays abundant cartilagenous matrix with a moderate number of minimally atypical cells. The findings are diagnostic of a cartilagenous neoplasm. Although the cellularity is suspicious for low grade chondrosarcoma, open biopsy would be recommended for confirmation. The abundant cartilagenous matrix and lack of anaplasia would rule out other considerations.

DeMay, A&S 2e. Chondrosarcoma, p692-694

211 **c** **ductal adenocarcinoma**

Note the irregular nuclear distribution and crowding, irregular nuclear membranes, and small nucleoli, consistent with well differentiated adenocarcinoma.

DeMay, A&S 2e. Ductal adenocarcinoma, p1313-1316

212 **b** **benign gastric mucosal cells**

Note the extremely uniform regularly spaced nuclei without significant membrane irregularity. The cytoplasm is mucinous, without goblet cells (which would suggest duodenal sampling). Gastric mucus producing (foveolar) cells may be abundant in EUS FNA samples of the pancreatic body or tail which are taken through the stomach. The duodenum is more commonly transgressed in sampling the pancreatic head.

DeMay, A&S 2e. Gastric mucous cells, p1302

213 **c** **metastatic small cell carcinoma**

The aspirate smear was highly cellular. The field demonstrates small but pleomorphic cells with little or no cytoplasm, smudgy appearing nuclei and evidence of nuclear molding. The nuclear edges are quite irregular. There are strands of DNA artifact across the cell group. These are the typical cytologic features of small cell undifferentiated carcinoma, in this case metastatic clinically from the lung. The primary was detected by bronchial washing cytology in this case.

DeMay, A&S 2e. Location, location, location, p621-625

214 **b** **pancreatic endocrine neoplasm**

Monotonous discohesive cells with eccentric nuclei "plasmacytoid" cells, typical of a pancreatic endocrine neoplasm.

DeMay, A&S 2e. Pancreatic endocrine neoplasms, p1321-1323

215 **c** **papillary thyroid carcinoma**

Small uniform "lymphocytelike" cells occur singly and in fragments. The background has a foamy quality and lacks colloid.

DeMay, A&S 2e. Papillary thyroid carcinoma, p892-893

216 **b** **flow cytometry**

A diffuse monotonous population of lymphoid cells. Cells have scant basophilic cytoplasm with numerous lymphoglandular bodies in the background. Flow cytometry would best confirm the diagnosis of lymphoma in this case.

DeMay, A&S 2e. Flow and image cytometry, p1528-1529

217 **c** **these cells are diagnostic, and adequacy of the FNA is complete**

Pancreas EUS FNA specimens typically have adequacy statements provided as part of the routine patient workup in many medical centers. Diff-Quik stains are utilized as a rapid staining technique in these situations where samples can be prescreened for adequacy. Features of malignancy are identified here (including increased N:C ratios, disorderly arrangement, and discohesion of the group). However, a statement of adequacy and the presence of diagnostic cells is routinely the primary information that should be rendered by a cytotechnologist.

DeMay, A&S 2e. FNA biopsy of the pancreas, p1298-1300

218 **b** **solid pseudopapillary tumor**

Note the high cellularity with cells loosely attached to fibrovascular cores and single cells. The individual cells are relatively bland and monomorphic with ovoid nuclei and occasional nuclear grooves. Cytoplasm may be tapered and cytoplasmic hyaline globules may be seen. This is a rare low grade neoplasm with an excellent prognosis usually affecting young women.

DeMay, A&S 2e. Solid pseudopapillary neoplasm, p1323-1324

219 **c** **cells consistent with peripheral ganglion sampling**

Ganglion cells are the cell bodies of sensory neurons, found outside of the CNS and typically associated with blood vessels and lymph nodes. Ganglion cells cluster near satellite nerve cells and have cytologic features including large polygonal cells with well defined cell borders, abundant granular cytoplasm with large, centrally or eccentrically located vesicular nuclei, and prominent nucleoli.

DeMay, A&S 2e. Peripheral nervous system tumors, p1236-1237

ISBN 978-089189-6357 ©ASCP 2015

220 c giant cell tumor of bone

There are 2 large multinucleated giant cells in the center of the image. They are surrounded by plump oval stromal cells. Cellularity is moderate to high in keeping with a neoplasm but with the stromal cells and giant cells appearing quite bland. These are the features of giant cell tumor of bone as seen in cytologic smears. While giant cell tumors are generally benign they can be unpredictable, producing recurrence, bland isolated metastasis usually in the lung, or undergoing frank malignant transformation. In the last situation they loose the features of giant cell tumor and cytologically appear as high grade spindle cell sarcomas sometimes producing osteoid (osteogenic sarcoma).

DeMay, A&S 2e. Giant cell tumor of bone, p696-697

221 c metastatic renal cell carcinoma

A large sheet of uniform epithelial appearing cells is seen. The cells have a finely granular and occasionally partly clear cytoplasm. The cells look like what one would expect to see from a touch preparation of a conventional renal cell carcinoma. The cells lack a perinuclear hof as would be expected with plasma cells, and they lack the very large nucleoli and abundant cytoplasm as well as pleomorphism seen with alveolar rhabdomyosarcoma, though some renal cell carcinomas may have all of those features. The cells are much too large and have too much cytoplasm for rhabdomyosarcoma. The cell sheets have a penetrating blood vessel, which is found in renal cell carcinoma and hepatocellular carcinoma.

DeMay, A&S 2e. Metastasis, p817

222 c pulmonary hamartoma

A biphasic admixture of benign appearing respiratory epithelium and fibromyxoid/chondroid elements is present, characteristic of a pulmonary hamartoma.

DeMay, A&S 2e. Hamartoma, p1167-1168

223 c metastatic melanoma

Although the large binucleate cells present with macronucleoli may be seen in each of the above entities, the finely granular cytoplasmic pigment distinguishes this tumor as metastatic melanoma.

DeMay, A&S 2e. Melanoma, p588-590

224 a metastatic Merkel cell carcinoma

A tight fragment of hyperchromatic small cells displaying nuclear molding, karyorrhexis, and extensive background necrosis. Although morphologically small cell carcinoma would be the primary differential diagnosis, given the patient's history, metastatic Merkel cell carcinoma is the appropriate choice of the given options.

DeMay, A&S 2e. Merkel cell carcinoma, p761

225 c antithyroid peroxidase antibodies

Antithyroid peroxidase antibodies are often elevated in patients with Hashimoto thyroiditis.

DeMay, A&S 2e. Antithyroid antibodies, p848

226 b colon

This aspirate of metastatic adenocarcinoma of the colon displays cell groups that are crowded and disorderly with some formation of microacinar glandular arrangements. The cells can vary from tall columnar with cigar shaped nuclei to round cells with irregular nuclei. The nuclei are pleomorphic with irregular nuclear membranes. The chromatin is coarse and dark with prominent nucleoli. The cytoplasm is granular with vacuolization. There is a tumor diathesis.

DeMay, A&S 2e. Metastases, p1277-1279

227 a obtain material for a core biopsy or cell block to perform immunohistochemical stains

Gastrointestinal stromal tumors (GISTs) are the most common spindle cell neoplasms of the stomach. EUS FNA usually demonstrates a cellular spindle cell lesion with usually low grade monomorphic nuclei. Definitive diagnosis requires a panel of immunochemical stains including c-kit (CD117), CD34, smooth muscle actin, desmin, and S100.

DeMay, A&S 2e. Gastrointestinal cells, p1302

228 a PLAP+, CK−

Germinoma, like other germ cell tumors, are characteristically PLAP+, CK−. CK positivity is usually seen in carcinoma, GFAP positivity in glial neoplasms, and HMB45 positivity in melanomas.

DeMay, A&S 2e. Germ cell tumors, p1414-1416

229 b anaplastic thyroid carcinoma, giant cell variant

Aspirates of anaplastic carcinoma of the thyroid are cellular with large pleomorphic tumors cells that lack evidence of keratinization.

DeMay, A&S 2e. Anaplastic (undifferentiated) thyroid carcinoma, p907-909

230 c inhibin

Adrenal cortical carcinoma stains positively for inhibin, calretinin, melan A/MART1, CD56, and synaptophysin.

DeMay, A&S 2e. Inhibin, p1524

231 c osteosarcoma

This aspirate displays the cytologic characteristics of osteosarcoma; bizarre, pleomorphic cells in a background of metachromatic staining osteoid.

DeMay, A&S 2e. Osteosarcoma, p699-701

232 c CAM5.2+

This aspirate displays large pleomorphic cells with granular cytoplasm consistent with hepatocellular carcinoma. No glandular differentiation is identified. Hepatocellular carcinoma is usually CAM5.2+. Cytokeratin AE1/AE3 is positive in most carcinomas, but not hepatocellular carcinoma. CDX2 positivity suggest GI origin. CEA positivity indicates adenocarcinoma such as cholangiocarcinoma.

DeMay, A&S 2e. Fine needle aspiration biopsy of hepatocellular carcinoma, p1262

233 a intraperitoneal hemorrhage

The image is from a hepatic adenoma, which displays hepatocytes with mildly increased N:C ratios and disorganization of the cellular architecture. Biliary epithelium is absent. These lesions are at risk for spontaneous rupture and abdominal (intraperitoneal) hemorrhage.

DeMay, A&S 2e. Liver cell adenoma, p1258-1259

234 a cholangiocarcinoma

Aspirates of cholangiocarcinoma display cytologic features of adenocarcinoma; 3D fragments of malignant appearing cells with increased N:C ratios and macronucleoli.

DeMay, A&S 2e. Cholangiocarcinoma, p1272-1273

235 a polymorphous low grade adenocarcinoma

Aspirates of polymorphous low grade adenocarcinoma are from a basaloid tumor with monotonous neoplastic cells with branching, cordlike or papillary fronds, well defined lumens and peripheral palisading of the nuclei.

DeMay, A&S 2e. Adenocarcinoma, p760-761

236 a flow cytometry

This image displays non-Hodgkin lymphoma characterized by a monotonous population of large lymphocytes. Abundant karyorrhectic nuclei and lymphoglandular bodies are evident in the background. Flow cytometry is useful for confirming clonality and subtyping of malignant lymphomas.

DeMay, A&S 2e. Malignant lymphoma, p572-574

ISBN 978-089189-6357 ©ASCP 2015

Chapter 9

Cytopreparatory Techniques/Lab Operations

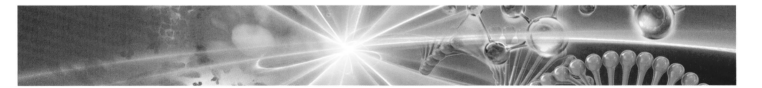

1   Which of the following is considered a hazardous chemical?
   a   ethanol
   b   saline
   c   Scott water
   d   lithium carbonate

2   What will allow for increased adherence of cerebrospinal fluids and urines to the glass slides?
   a   Hanks balanced salt solution
   b   polylysine coated slides
   c   nonalbuminized slides
   d   95% ethanol

3   What type of fire extinguisher is to be used for burning liquids?
   a   type A
   b   type C
   c   type B
   d   type D

4   Which statement regarding thionin blue is true?
   a   it must be dissolved in 100% ethanol
   b   it will not stain red blood cells
   c   the formula requires normal acetic acid
   d   it is a synonym for toluidine blue

5   All of the following are components of the material safety data sheets except:
   a   date material was prepared
   b   permissible exposure limits
   c   emergency first aid procedures
   d   type of gloves required for cleanup

6   If sputum specimens must be preserved before cytopreparation, which fixative is best?
   a   100% ethanol
   b   95% ethanol
   c   70% ethanol
   d   50% ethanol

7   What chemicals should not be stored together because of their incompatibility?
   a   acetic acid and acetone
   b   ammonia and acetic acid
   c   flammable liquids and nitric acid
   d   chlorine with any flammable liquids

8   What is considered an alternative processing method (in lieu of the centrifugation/sediment method) for preparing cell blocks?
   a   plasma thrombin method
   b   saponin method
   c   Hanks method
   d   thionin method

9   When handling chemicals:
   a   reuse all unlabeled vials to prevent wastefulness
   b   label all containers with common name only
   c   dispose of gloves at the end of each day to prevent contamination
   d   pour acid into water, never water into acid

10 The earliest action required in the event of a fire is:
   a   tell visitors to exit
   b   telephone the switchboard
   c   pull the fire alarm and rescue burning people
   d   contain the fire with a fire blanket

11 After performing FNA, a sound methodology for preparing the smears that will ensure adequate cytologic evaluation, is to:
   a   express a minimum of 10 mL, let air material air dry, then forcibly crush the aspirated material with a second slide to ensure material is adequately broken up; fix slides immediately (as needed)
   b   express 10 drops on the edge of the slide, then place a cover slip on top; proceed with staining
   c   spray the specimen through the air onto the slide; air dry all slides
   d   express a small drop near the frosted end of the slide, then place a second slide on top and quickly pull slides apart; fix a designated number of slides immediately, and purposely air dry others

12 Screening errors may be attributed to:
   a   inadequate sampling
   b   good sampling preparation
   c   well established quality control
   d   atrophy in postmenopausal females

13 The fire extinguisher that can be used for burning wood, paper, or refuse and is also considered general purpose is type:
   a B
   b D
   c A
   d C

14 Should a chemical come in contact with your skin, you should:
   a rinse the contaminated clothing with water
   b flush the area with 95% EtOH
   c clean the area with neutralizing agents or ointments
   d read material safety data sheets and wash the chemical off with soap and water if possible

15 When processing fine needle aspiration specimens, one should:
   a process all smears with the Papanicolaou stain; air dried smears should never be used unless necessary for possible lymphopoietic malignancies
   b process a few fixed smears with the Papanicolaou stain and a few air dried smears with a compatible stain (Romanowsky or Diff-Quik)
   c process a few air dried smears with the Papanicolaou stain and a few alcohol fixed smears with a compatible stain (Romanowsky or Diff-Quik)
   d process all smears with the Papanicolaou stain; batch FNA slides with the general processing of Pap tests—this will insure optimal staining for most pathologic processes

16 What is a sound procedure for a dealing with a small chemical spill?
   a evacuate the building
   b evacuate all people from the building
   c use the "spill up" kit available
   d solid spills must be diluted with water before cleaning up

17 The optimal thickness of the coverslip used for cytology is:
   a 0.5
   b 1.0
   c 1.5
   d 2

18 When handling hazardous materials, one must make sure to:
   a inform the laboratory workers by word of mouth
   b keep the material safety data sheet within the laboratory procedure manual
   c conduct weekly employee information training
   d maintain warning labels and common chemical names on all materials

19 Which of the following describes the advantages of using the Saccomanno technique over the "pick and smear" or direct spreading technique for processing sputum specimens?
   a Saccomanno technique is the method of choice for preparing fresh sputum specimens
   b using the Saccomanno technique allows the entire sputum specimen to be sampled; it yields slides with a uniform, even distribution of the cells, and eliminates the mucus within the specimen
   c when using the Saccomanno technique, it is not necessary to have cells prefixed in polyethylene glycol and alcohol solution, as is the case with the direct smear method
   d the Saccomanno technique allows for better cytologic identification of cellular groupings and clusters

20 One of the best methods for preventing the spread of infectious agents while working in the laboratory is:
   a wearing adhesive bandages
   b hand washing
   c washing all counters with Hanks balanced salt solution
   d wearing a cloth lab coat

21 When using the Cytospin centrifugation technique for preparing transudative fluids (such as urines and cerebrospinal fluids), which of the following processing methodologies will help ensure specimen adequacy?
   a add 1 mL of Saccomanno fixative if preparing for the Pap stain, place 10-15 drops of specimen into the chamber, and centrifuge at 100 rpm for 10-15 minutes
   b add a few drops of Saccomanno fixative if preparing for the Pap stain, place 2-5 drops of specimen into the chamber, and centrifuge at 500-600 rpm for 4-5 minutes
   c add 10 mL of Saccomanno fixative if preparing for the Pap stain, place 10 mL (equal volumes) of specimen into the chamber, and centrifuge at 1,500-2,000 rpm for 10 minutes
   d do not add Saccomanno fixative (regardless of the staining technique to be used), place 5 mL of specimen into the chamber, and centrifuge at 1,000-1,500 rpm for 4-5 minutes

22 For a cancer screening program to become successful, which of the following is considered a prerequisite?
   a the disease must affect a small percentage of the population
   b a suitable test must be at no cost to be effective
   c the physical and psychological harm of the test and treatment should outweigh the benefit
   d the cost benefit analysis should show the screening is economically beneficial

23 What is considered a universal precaution?
   a pregnant or nursing mothers should never be allowed to process cytologic specimens
   b make sure to recap all needles prior to discarding
   c use biological safety hoods for processing gynecologic specimens
   d decontaminate the work area at least once per shift with an appropriate germicide

ISBN 978-089189-6357 ©ASCP 2015

24 The primary reason for using a liquid based monolayer specimen preparation system for Papanicolaou smears is it:
a provides a cleaner background and helps prevent overlapping and crowding of cells
b allows an identical number of cells to be aliquoted every time for each slide prepared
c uses fixatives that enlarge the cells, making it easier to visualize small cell lesions and diagnose abnormal conditions
d spreads a monolayer of cells over the entire glass slide, increasing the surface area of the slide utilized and the number of cells that can be diagnosed

25 The fixative of choice for preparing cell blocks is:
a 30% formalin
b 10% formalin
c 25% glacial acetic acid
d 1:1 diethyl ether in 95% ethyl alcohol

26 A slide should be "fixed" for:
a 15-30 minutes
b 45-60 minutes
c 5-10 minutes
d a minimum of 1 hour

27 Fresh body fluids, those without added fixatives, are suggested for cytopreparation because:
a alcohol acts as a tissue culture medium, cultivating bacterial growth, which may interfere with cytopreparation
b prefixed specimens cannot be destained if needed
c fresh specimens stain more readily with eosin Y
d alcohol coagulates proteins, rendering processing of the specimen difficult

28 Which applies regarding the Papanicolaou staining process?
a filter stains weekly
b check the percent of lithium blue each day when using the regressive staining procedure
c maintain the alkalinity of the bluing solution when using the progressive staining procedure
d store all stains in clear bottles to minimize oxidation

29 The cytologic evaluation of urine specimens is most optimal when the urine is:
a preserved with alcohol
b refrigerated
c fresh
d preserved with carbowax

30 Regarding cytologic fixatives, which of the following is true?
a 100% ethanol has many advantages over 95% ethanol
b 95% ethanol is suitable only for gynecological smears
c 100% methanol produces less cell shrinkage
d 80% isopropanol is unacceptable for cytologic fixation

31 What is a suitable lysing agent for excessively bloody specimens?
a 1:14 glacial acetic acid in 95% ethanol
b 10 mol urea
c 1:1 hydrochloride in 95% ethanol
d 1:50 glacial acetic acid in 95% ethanol

32 Which EA stain is most useful in helping to distinguish endometrial adenocarcinomas from endocervical adenocarcinomas?
a EA35
b EA36
c EA50
d EA65

33 To achieve the best results, the pH of the EA solution should be:
a 1.5-2.0
b 2.5-3.0
c 3.0-4.0
d 4.5-5.0

34 If nuclear overstaining occurs:
a HCl concentration is too dilute; increase the concentration
b ammonium hydroxide concentration is too weak; increase the concentration
c air dry the slide completely before staining
d decrease the fixation time before staining

35 If the oven temperature is excessively high during the preparation of a cell block slide, what effect may occur?
a slides are too blue
b darker nuclei
c slides are yellow
d lighter nuclei

36 What coating fixative is best for specimens that must be transported?
a commercial hair spray
b 95% ethanol
c polyethylene glycol
d 2% glacial acetic acid

37 With regard to centrifugation, cells sediment best at what centrifugal force and for how long?
a 300 g, 15 minutes
b 500 g, 5 minutes
c 600 g, 10 minutes
d 1,200 g, 10 minutes

38 The total surface area covered by the pores of nucleopore filters is roughly:
a 2%
b 10%
c 20%
d 50%

39 Which is true regarding the progressive Papanicolaou staining process?
a hydrochloric acid (HCl) removes excess hematoxylin
b nuclei are overstained then destained
c lithium carbonate is used to blue or set the hematoxylin
d nuclei are understained then blued with HCl

40 If the nuclei appear too pale after staining:
a decrease the alkalinity of the tap water rinse
b increase the alkalinity of the tap water rinse
c decrease time in hematoxylin
d change the stains daily

41 Water in the xylene will cause:
   a excessive basophilia
   b excessive eosinophilia
   c a milky haze on the slide
   d dark nuclear features

42 Which EA stain contains half the original amount of light green?
   a EA65
   b EA50
   c EA36
   d EA35

43 In order to minimize the possibility of "floaters" found in cerebrospinal fluid specimens, one should:
   a delete the OG
   b separate equipment and staining dishes
   c use polycarbonate filters only
   d use cellulosic filters only

44 What is an effective fire safety precaution?
   a make sure to store incompatible chemicals together
   b have your evacuation plan memorized
   c store flammable liquids in glass bottles
   d keep all chemicals on the workbench

45 What solvent has a detrimental effect on both polycarbonate and cellulosic filters?
   a 1-propanol
   b 100% ethanol
   c chloroform
   d 3N ammonium hydroxide

46 A stain useful for rapid examination of nonfixed fluids is:
   a EA65
   b Papanicolaou
   c toluidine blue
   d Hanks

47 What produces the "hill and valley" effect on cellulosic filters?
   a expanding in 100% EtOH
   b expanding in 100% acetone
   c expanding in methyl alcohol
   d not expanding in 95% EtOH

48 If the cytoplasm appears too green, one should:
   a increase eosin or decrease the staining time in the EA
   b increase the light green concentration in the EA
   c increase the staining time in EA
   d change the EA more often

49 In regressive Papanicolaou staining, the nuclei are:
   a understained
   b overstained
   c stained to desired intensity
   d stained after the cytoplasmic stains

50 When staining a bronchial washing specimen, the slides are most commonly overstained with nuclear stain and then passed through a weak acidic solution. This process is known as:
   a progressive staining
   b regressive staining
   c counterstaining
   d Papanicolaou staining

51 A liter of pleural fluid is received from a patient with a smoking history, a lung mass and a history of lymphoma. What is the best way to process the specimen?
   a submit the fluid to microbiology for culture and sensitivity
   b prepare a single Diff-Quik cytospin
   c prepare slides for cytologic evaluation and submit material for flow cytometry
   d prepare a cell block and perform an immunohistochemical panel to include S100, leukocyte common antigen (CD45), calretinin and vimentin

52 To achieve proper Köhler illumination, you must:
   a routinely have the microscope professionally adjusted twice a year
   b focus the microscope, close the field diaphragm and focus the edges, center the light beam, and open the field diaphragm until its edges just clear the field of view
   c close the field diaphragm, center the light beam, and clean the microscope stage
   d clean off the microscope eyepieces and clean the microscope objective lenses with xylene

53 One advantage of the Romanowsky stain over the Papanicolaou stain is:
   a it provides better nuclear detail
   b it more clearly demonstrates the presence of keratinization
   c it is more similar to the stain typically used in histology
   d it is easier to discern cytoplasmic features

54 Which of the following cytology preparations is classified as "selective cellular enhancement" technique?
   a Millipore filter preparation
   b direct smear
   c liquid based preparations
   d cytospin

55 In the daily routine quality control process, the Papanicolaou stained slides were noted to have a hazy film that reduced the clarity of the cytoplasmic and nuclear outlines. What may be the reason for this?
   a the absolute alcohol is contaminated
   b the eosin needs to be changed
   c the hematoxylin needs to be changed
   d the OG-6 needs to be replaced

56 Volatile and flammable chemicals such as xylene need to be stored in:
   a a microbiologic safety hood
   b a cool, well ventilated metal cabinet
   c a drying oven
   d a cabinet under a sink

ISBN 978-089189-6357 ©ASCP 2015

57 The appropriate sequence of events for destaining cytology slides is to:

  a soak in xylene, remove coverslip, proceed backwards through the staining process, and then soak in a dilute hydrochloric acid
  b soak in a dilute hydrochloric acid, remove coverslip, pass through xylene, and then proceed backwards through the staining process
  c remove coverslip, remove excess mounting media with xylene, and then soak in a dilute hydrochloric acid
  d soak in xylene, remove coverslip, proceed forwards through the staining process, and then soak in a dilute hydrochloric acid

58 Modified Carnoy fixative is particularly useful:

  a concentration of cellular material into pellets
  b bluing of the nuclear stain
  c fixation of cell blocks
  d the lysing of red blood cells in bloody samples

59 Droplets noted under the coverslip are indicative of:

  a expired mounting media
  b Scott tap water not adequately rinsed off slide
  c water contamination in the xylene
  d pH of the water was too alkaline

60 Brilliant cresyl blue, toluidine blue, and new methylene blue are examples of what type of staining?

  a supravital staining
  b regressive staining
  c counterstaining
  d passive staining

61 Which of the following serves as a blueing agent in the progressive Papanicolaou staining method?

  a absolute alcohol
  b tap water if pH is consistently higher than 8
  c dilute hydrochloric acid
  d EA polychrome

62 Which Papanicolaou stain component targets and stains nucleolar material?

  a modified OG-6
  b Harris hematoxylin
  c modified EA
  d Gill 2 hematoxylin

63 When preparing cytologic specimens, which of the following statements is true?

  a stains should be checked and documented for quality on a daily basis
  b stains and solutions should be filtered monthly
  c stains should be labeled on the cover of the staining dish
  d stains should be checked and documented for quality on a weekly basis

64 When preparing a batch of Pap counterstain, what is the proper formula for calculating how much dye is required if the dye content is <100%?

  a percent of dye content divided by amount of dye required
  b percent of dye content multiplied by percent aqueous solution
  c amount of dye required multiplied by percent dye content
  d amount of dye required divided by percent dye content

65 Of the options listed, the most practical method for making cells blocks from fine needle aspirations is by placing the specimen material into:

  a 10% buffered formalin and centrifuging
  b normal saline and centrifuging
  c polyethylene glycol and leaving sit for 1 hour
  d hemacyte agent and centrifuging

66 The preparation/stain that best demonstrates amyloid and colloid in thyroid aspirates is?

  a ethanol fixed/Pap
  b air dried/Diff-Quik
  c thin layer prep/Pap
  d cytospins/Pap

67 The Papanicolaou stain array contains the following stains:

  a nuclear stain methylene blue and cytoplasmic stains orange G, eosin Y, and light green
  b nuclear stain hematoxylin and cytoplasmic stains orange G, eosin Y, and light green
  c nuclear stain methylene blue and cytoplasmic stains acridine orange and bismarck brown
  d nuclear stain hematoxylin and cytoplasmic stains acridine orange and bismarck brown

68 Why is methanol fixation not recommended for use on ThinPrep specimens when suspecting a lymphoid lesion?

  a methanol causes excessive swelling of the lymphoid elements
  b cells do not adhere to the ThinPrep specimens
  c methanol does not preserve antigens necessary for lymphoid antigen markers
  d methanol induces false positive reactions with lymphoid antigen markers

69 Which of the following fixatives crosslinks proteins?

  a 95% ethanol with air dried smears
  b 10% buffered formalin
  c Saccomanno fixative
  d 95% ethanol with wet smears

70 In the Papanicolaou staining array, the dye orange G:

  a stains cytokeratin intermediate filaments orange
  b is a component of the polychromatic mixture EA
  c stains cytoplasm containing a large component of the protein keratin
  d is a plant extract

71 A staining format that utilizes overstaining of a specimen with an unacidified hematoxylin followed by hydrochloric (HCl) acid rinses describes:
a progressive staining
b supravital staining
c special staining
d regressive staining

72 Universal precautions, including the use of gloves and protective eyewear, are advisable in the preparation of fresh specimens:
a only when the patient has a history of a dangerous infection
b only when the person handling the specimen has broken skin with specimens from all patients and at all times
c only when cytopreparation takes place outside a biosafety hood
d one cannot rely on clinical history to flag a specimen as potentially infectious

73 Which of the following specimens presents the LEAST actual risk of transmission of the patient's known infection to laboratory workers handling the fresh specimen?
a a fine needle aspiration from a known AIDS patient
b urine containing large numbers of *Schistosoma haematobium* ova
c pleural fluid from a patient with chronic hepatitis B
d bronchial washings from a patient with active pulmonary tuberculosis

74 What is the single most effective way to prevent the spread of infections?
a frequent changing of gloves
b use of personal protective equipment
c hand washing
d washing gloves when contaminated

75 At the conclusion of a fine needle aspiration procedure, used 25 gauge needles should be:
a sterilized and reused
b placed in a red biohazard bag
c recapped and placed in the regular trash can
d placed in a puncture resistant container for disposal

76 What does this safety symbol represent?

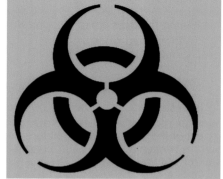

a radiation danger
b flammable material
c biohazard material
d carcinogen

77 When removing a chemical from its original container and placing it in a smaller container for short term use, what information needs to be on the smaller container?
a nothing if it will be used up within a few days
b name of the chemical and the date of transfer
c name of the chemical and name and address of manufacturer
d name of the chemical, the hazard, and the date of transfer

78 On the hazard communication label found on chemical containers, the red diamond indicates:
a health hazard
b fire hazard
c reactivity/instability
d electrical hazard

79 All flammable chemicals should be kept:
a in a cool, dry closet
b in a closed fire cabinet
c under the sink
d in a sealed plastic bin

80 What is the appropriate way to dispose of chemical wastes?
a flush down the sink with running cold water
b pour into single waste container for disposal and pick up
c pour into labeled containers and place in regular trash
d comply with local, state, and federal regulations

81 Which of the following chemicals is considered a carcinogen?
a ethyl alcohol
b xylene
c Scott tap water
d hematoxylin

82 MSDS sheets for chemicals must contain:
a fire and exposure hazard data
b the expiration date for the chemical
c the lot number of manufacture
d applications in laboratory procedures

83 What is the correct laboratory procedure for the manipulation of hazardous chemicals?
a pour concentrated solutions into less concentrated solutions
b pour water into acid
c fill reagent bottles to full capacity
d pour less concentrated solutions into concentrated solutions

84 MSDS is an acronym for:
a microchip safety data system
b multilevel skills development system
c management safety data sheet
d material safety data sheet

ISBN 978-089189-6357 ©ASCP 2015

85 The purpose of an MSDS is:
   a to advise as to how to proceed in the event of a chemical exposure
   b to alert hospital administration that a chemical exposure has occurred
   c to provide information as to how the chemical is manufactured
   d to provide a procedure for the use of a particular chemical

86 When a chemical is spilled on the skin, what is the most appropriate course of action?
   a wipe the affected are with a clean cloth
   b flush affected area with water continuously for 15 minutes
   c use a neutralizing agent on the skin before washing with soap and water
   d report incident to supervisor if a rash occurs

87 A material safety data sheet is developed for each chemical by:
   a the manufacturer
   b the laboratory manager
   c the hospital administrator
   d OSHA

88 On the hazard communication label found on chemical containers, the blue diamond indicates:
   a health hazard
   b fire hazard
   c reactivity/instability
   d electrical hazard

89 What would be considered appropriate storage for a bottle of glacial acetic acid?
   a under the sink next to the bleach
   b on an upper level wall shelf, out of the way
   c in the flammables cabinet
   d in a separate cabinet

90 According to the College of American Pathologists checklist for laboratory accreditation, how often must employees participate in fire drills?
   a at least once per month
   b at least once per year
   c at least once every 6 months
   d at least once every 2 years

91 Portable fire extinguishers are classified by their ability to handle specific classes and sizes of fires. An extinguisher with a green triangle containing the letter A is used for:
   a electrical fires
   b burning liquids
   c burning combustible materials
   d all types of fires

92 In the event of a fire, what is generally the first response in the fire plan?
   a close all windows and doors to contain the fire
   b attempt to extinguish the fire if it is small enough and staff are trained
   c be sure that all people are out of immediate danger
   d pull the fire alarm

93 Review of laboratory safety policies and procedures must be completed:
   a only when changes occur
   b every 6 months
   c at least annually
   d every 2 years

94 OSHA stands for:
   a On Site Health Administration
   b Occupational Safety and Health Administration
   c Operations Safety Hospital Administration
   d Online Safety Hospital Administration

95 Which activities are allowed in laboratory technical work areas?
   a mouth pipetting
   b manipulation of contact lenses
   c computer data access
   d eating and drinking

96 Eyewash plumbing should be flushed for ~3 minutes:
   a every day
   b every week
   c every month
   d every 6 months

Cytopreparatory Techniques/ Lab Operations *Answer Key*

1 **a** ethanol
Examples of other hazardous chemicals include chloroform, ammonium hydroxide, and bleach.
Carson, Histotechnology 4e. Ethyl alcohol (ethanol), p33

2 **b** polylysine coated slides
The coating on these slides will increase the cellular yield in normally hypocellular specimens.
Carson, Histotechnology 4e. Poly-L-lysine coated slides, p73

3 **c** type B
Type B extinguishers are for burning liquids, and type C extinguishers should be used in the event of an electrical fire.
Carson, Histotechnology 4e. Fire & explosive hazards, p91

4 **b** it will not stain red blood cells
Thionin blue, methylene blue, and toluidine blue are all stains that allow for rapid examination of wet specimens. Toluidine blue may be used on centrifuged or other specimens for quick examination of the cellularity/ diagnosis. One drop of this stain on the unfixed specimen allows for excellent cell examination. This technique may be used for quick diagnosis or to decrease the possibility of unidentified "floaters."
Carson, Histotechnology 4e. Toluidine blue wet film, p328

5 **d** type of gloves required for cleanup
Material safety data sheets (MSDSs) must be kept for all laboratory chemicals. The date the MSDS was prepared, chemical identity, hazard emergency information, physical hazards, first aid protocols, disposal methods, and the common chemical name are some of the important informative data found for each chemical.
Carson, Histotechnology 4e. Hazard identification, p93-95

6 **c** 70% ethanol
70% ethanol is preferred for collecting sputum specimens over 95% ethanol due to its possibility for mucoprotein coagulation.
Carson, Histotechnology 4e. Fixation, p317-318

7 **c** flammable liquids and nitric acid
A list of chemicals that may and may not be stored together should be posted in clear sight of the storage area for the benefit of all laboratory personnel.
Carson, Histotechnology 4e. p92-93

8 **a** plasma thrombin method
The plasma thrombin clot (PTC) method may be used as an alternative to the conventional fixed sediment (FS) methodology for cell block preparation. In the PTC method, equal drops of plasma and thrombin are added to the centrifugate to allow for a clot to form. The clot is placed onto lens paper and processed using conventional histologic processing techniques. Another alternative to the FS method is the bacterial agar methodology. This method uses Bouin fluid as a fixative (centrifugate is allowed to sit in fixative for 2 hours). The supernatant is poured off, and the sediment is removed and placed on tissue paper, cut in half, and placed into a petri dish with melted agar. After the agar hardens, the specimen is placed onto tissue paper, loaded into a cassette, and processed using conventional histologic processing.
Carson, Histotechnology 4e. Cell blocks, p324-325

9 **d** pour acid into water, never water into acid
This information is key in the proper disposal of acid.
Carson, Histotechnology 4e. Hazardous chemical disposal, p92-93

10 **c** pull the fire alarm and rescue burning people
Pull the alarm to notify others in danger, remove visitors, and if possible, contain the fire with an appropriate extinguisher.
Carson, Histotechnology 4e. Fire & explosive hazards, p91-92

11 **d** express a small drop near the frosted end of the slide, then place a second slide on top and quickly pull slides apart; fix a designated number of slides immediately, and purposely air dry others
In preparing FNA smears for cytologic interpretation, it is important to express a tiny drop of the harvest onto the slide, being careful not to spray the specimen through the air, which may create aerosols that are potentially infectious. The spreader slide must be gently lowered onto the diagnostic slide in a crosswise fashion over the droplet and pulled down over the length (taking care not to spread to the edges) of the diagnostic slide with a smooth motion.
Carson, Histotechnology 4e. Smear preparation, p316-320

12 **a** inadequate sampling
It is estimated that 2/3-1/2 of the screening errors that occur in gynecologic cytopathology are related to inadequate samples or poor specimen preparation of the smear taker, and up to 1/2 of the false negative cases are related to the laboratory (inadequate screening, poor quality control, inadequate interpretation). Errors in each area are in the range of 5%-10%.
DeMay, A&S 2e. Historical perspectives, p2-4

ISBN 978-089189-6357 ©ASCP 2015

13 c A

Type B extinguishers are for burning liquids, and type C extinguishers should be used in the event of an electrical fire.

Carson, Histotechnology 4e. Fire & explosive hazards, p91-92

14 d read material safety data sheets and wash the chemical off with soap and water if possible

Removing the contaminated clothing and flushing the affected area with water, when appropriate as determined by MSDS instructions, followed by cleaning with soap and water is important. Always immediately seek medical care.

Carson, Histotechnology 4e. Chemical hazards, p88-91

15 b process a few fixed smears with the Papanicolaou stain and a few air dried smears with a compatible stain (Romanowsky or Diff-Quik)

Preparing a few air dried slides allows for staining with a compatible stain such as Romanowsky or Diff-Quik. Air drying the cells has many advantages and, contrary to popular belief, provides essential information that often cannot be appreciated with the conventional fixed based Papanicolaou stain. In addition to increasing cell adherence to the slide, staining air dried slides allows for the cytologic visualization of extracellular substances (mucin, ground substance, colloid) and enhances the ability to appreciate cytoplasmic pleomorphism, gland and lymphoreticular differentiation, and microbiologic agents.

DeMay, A&S 2e. Routine stains, p1504-1505

16 c use the "spill up" kit available

After seeking information from the MSDS, spill pillows and silicone absorbent may be used to cleanup the spill. Proper disposal is imperative.

Carson, Histotechnology 4e. Chemical hazards, p88-91

17 b 1.0

The refractive index of the mounting media together with a maximum coverslip thickness of 0.96-1.06 mm will allow for the most effective microscopy in cytology (based on the corrective figure of 0.17 mm-0.18 mm objectives). Cytologic specimens are generally thicker than tissue sections; therefore, a 1.5 mm coverslip may be used.

DeMay, A&S 2e. Diffraction, p1596-1597

18 d maintain warning labels and common chemical names on all materials

Warning labels must describe the common chemical name, potential health hazards, and manufacturer's address. The warning diamond, designed by the National Fire Protection Association), is divided into 4 sections and graded from 0-4. The left side of the diamond (blue in color) is the health hazard section:

0 normal material
1 slightly hazardous
2 hazardous
3 extreme danger
4 deadly

The top section of the diamond (red in color) is fire hazard (flash points):

0 will not burn
1 not exceeding 200°F
2 >100°F
3 <100°F
4 <73°F

The far right side of the diamond (yellow) is reactivity/instability:

0 stable
1 unstable as heated
2 violent chemical change
3 shock and heat
4 may detonate

The bottom section of the diamond (white) refers to specific hazards:

ACID acid
ALK alkali
COR corrosive
OXY oxidizer
P polymerization
☢ radioactive
W use no water

Carson, Histotechnology 4e. Chemical hazards, p88-94

19 b using the Saccomanno technique allows the entire sputum specimen to be sampled; it yields slides with a uniform, even distribution of the cells and eliminates the mucus within the specimen

The Saccomanno technique is the methodology of choice for prefixed sputum specimens (polyethylene glycol and 70% ethanol). The advantages are as listed in the answer; however, the disadvantage of this technique (when compared to the direct or "pick and smear" technique) is that cellular groupings are often disassociated in the blending process. For instance, the cytologic diagnosis of small cell neuroendocrine carcinoma (which possesses cells in molding groups or in streaks) may be more difficult, as well as adenocarcinomas that present in tight cohesive clusters. If either are suspected, one should blend the specimen at lower speeds or prepare the sputum by gently crushing an aliquot of the specimen between 2 slides, separate the slides, and equally distribute the smeared material over both slides with an applicator slick (direct smear method). Excessively mucoid or bloody specimens prepared by the direct smear technique may be treated with bromhexin, the saponin method, or dithiothreitol.

Carson, Histotechnology 4e. Mucoid specimens, p320-322

20 b hand washing

Proficient and efficient hand washing will reduce the possibility of contracting disease or contaminating the workplace.

Carson, Histotechnology 4e. Biological or infectious hazards, p86-87

21 b add a few drops of Saccomanno fixative if preparing for the Pap stain, place 2-5 drops of specimen into the chamber, and centrifuge at 500-600 rpm for 4-5 minutes

When preparing specimens for cytocentrifugation with the Cytospin, Saccomanno fixative should be added for slides that are to be stained with the Pap stain. Only a few drops of the specimen need to be added (using a disposable pipette) to the cytofunnel chamber to achieve optimal results. 4 drops are usually sufficient for body fluids and bronchial or gastrointestinal washings, 2 drops for urines, and 4-6 drops for patients with known infectious disease. Centrifugation should be performed at 500 rpm for 5 minutes (cerebrospinal fluid) or 600 rpm for 4 minutes (all others); if performed any faster or longer, the specimens are at risk for air drying or cell lysis.

Carson, Histotechnology 4e. t14.2 Cytocentrifuge preparations, p321

22 d the cost benefit analysis should show the screening is economically beneficial

In order to help ensure a successful screening program, the disease has to represent an important health problem with a known natural history and recognizable early stage, be of moderate cost, and be effectively managed if treated at an early stage.

DeMay, A&S 2e. Screening, p1571-1573

23 d decontaminate the work area at least once per shift with an appropriate germicide

Taking universal precautions, such as wearing barrier protection, masks, gloves, face shield, disposable fluid resistant gowns, and the practice of safe cytopreparatory techniques under biological fume hoods will help decrease the possibility of exposure of yourself or others to infectious diseases, especially hepatitis B or the human immunodeficiency virus.

Carson, Histotechnology 4e. Biological or infectious hazards, p86-88

24 a provides a cleaner background and helps prevent overlapping and crowding of cells

Additional advantages of liquid based monolayer systems for cytopreparation are that they help to minimize the amount of blood and inflammatory cells present in the specimen, as well as decrease any protein or mucus that may interfere with the ability of the diagnostician to render a satisfactory or adequate diagnosis.

DeMay, A&S 2e. Liquid based preparations, p1547-1548

25 b 10% formalin

Alcohol shrinks and hardens tissue, making microtomy quite difficult. Fixation with a 1:9 solution of 40% formaldehyde and water creates a 10% formalin solution. Formalin should be neutral (pH 7.0) and be stored in the dark to prevent the formation of formic acid.

Carson, Histotechnology 4e. Cell blocks, p324-325

26 a 15-30 minutes

Fixing cells <15 minutes may create undesirable effects such as lack of crisp nuclear detail or pale nuclei. A minimum of 15 minutes is required to remove the wax cellular coating (2% carbowax) used to preserve the cells for transport. Fixation longer than 30 minutes has not been shown to provide additional benefit.

Carson, Histotechnology 4e. Fixation, p317-318

27 d alcohol coagulates proteins, rendering processing of the specimen difficult

Fresh body fluids are preserved in their own culture medium, which helps to prevent cellular degeneration. Performing membrane filtration is easier with unfixed fluids due to the ease with which soluble proteins pass through the filter. Alcohol denatures these proteins, often clogging the membrane and creating difficulty in filtration.

Carson, Histotechnology 4e. Fixation, p317-318

28 c maintain the alkalinity of the bluing solution when using the progressive staining procedure

The color change will not occur at a pH <8.0. If the laboratory is using running tap water to blue its nuclei, the pH should be tested to ensure its feasibility. Chlorine may also cause cellular fading; therefore, these levels should also be tested if using tap water as a blueing agent.

DeMay, A&S 2e. Bluing hematoxylin, p1556-1557

29 c fresh

For related information, see question 4.

30 c 100% methanol produces less cell shrinkage

This effect allows for better cell preservation. Hospitals that do not have a license to buy ethanol may choose to use this fixative in place of ethanol.

DeMay, A&S 2e. Fixation, p1548-1551

31 a 1:14 glacial acetic acid in 95% ethanol

Glacial acetic acid diluted 1:14 (modified Carnoy) is an excellent lysing agent for hemolyzing red blood cells and allowing for the enhancement of the cellular foreground.

Carson, Histotechnology 4e. Prefixatives, p318

ISBN 978-089189-6357 ©ASCP 2015

32 d EA65

EA65 will often stain endocervical adenocarcinomas (granular cytoplasm), and eosinophilic and endometrial adenocarcinomas (frothy, vacuolated cytoplasm) basophilic or cyanophilic.

Carson, Histotechnology 4e. EA, p326-328

33 d 4.5-5.0

Maintaining a consistent pH between 4.5 and 5.0 will allow for optimal color consistency.

Carson, Histotechnology 4e. EA, p326-328

34 a HCl concentration is too dilute; increase the concentration

If the HCl is too dilute, the hematoxylin removal may be inadequate, resulting in overstained nuclei.

Carson, Histotechnology 4e. The nuclear dyes, p112-116

35 c slides are yellow

Once the slides are yellow (due to a much higher temperature than necessary to bake the tissue section onto the slide[s] before staining), the condition is irreversible.

Carson, Histotechnology 4e. Cell blocks, p324-325

36 c polyethylene glycol

2% polyethylene glycol (carbowax) and 95% ethanol is a cellular fixative that coats the cells with a waxy substance that helps to prevent air drying during transport of the specimen.

Carson, Histotechnology 4e. Fixation, p317-318

37 c 600 g, 10 minutes

Whole cells sediment most efficiently at 600 g for 10 minutes. The centrifugal speed may be determined by measuring (in centimeters) the center of the centrifuge head to the bottom of the specimen holder. This number can then be applied to a centrifugal force chart that will read the optimal number of rpm necessary to spin the sample.

Carson, Histotechnology 4e. t14.2 Cytocentrifuge preparations, p321

38 a 2%

These pores are visible when viewing polycarbonate (nucleopore) filters under the microscope unless the pores are dissolved with chloroform. Nucleopore filters may also be used to make imprint smears.

DeMay, A&S 2e. Membrane filtration, p1546-1547

39 c lithium carbonate is used to blue or set the hematoxylin

Blueing is necessary to change the nuclear stain color from red to blue using an alkaline solution such as lithium carbonate, ammonium hydroxide, or Scott tap water. Running water may also be used as long as the pH is >8.0.

DeMay, A&S 2e. Bluing hematoxylin, p1556-1557

40 b increase the alkalinity of the tap water rinse

A deep blue can be attained if the alkalinity of the blueing agent (progressive staining) is >8.0.

DeMay, A&S 2e. Bluing hematoxylin, p1556-1557

41 c a milky haze on the slide

Care should be exercised to drain the slides properly between steps, thus preventing the possibility of water contamination in the clearing solution. The addition of silicic acid pellets to the previous 100% ethanol may alleviate this problem.

DeMay, A&S 2e. Xylene, p1566-1567

42 a EA65

EA65 may be preferred for nonglycogenated preparations. EA36 was the original Papanicolaou stain, and EA50 uses a different solvent.

Carson, Histotechnology 4e. EA, p326-328

43 b separate equipment and staining dishes

"Floaters" are considered cross contaminated cells from one specimen to the glass slide of another specimen. Their presence on a different focal plane or field when viewing the slide, as well as the morphologic recognition of like cells in another specimen, will help determine their origin as a contaminant. Cytopreparatory steps that may help reduce the possibility of "floaters" include gentle agitation during the staining process, performing toluidine blue wet preparations before processing cells to determine the possibility of malignant cells, and daily filtering of all stains.

Carson, Histotechnology 4e. Cross contamination, p328

44 b have your evacuation plan memorized

In the event of a fire, there may be no time to consider a possible evacuation plan. An evacuation plan should be placed in clear view, and all employees should familiarize themselves with the escape route.

Carson, Histotechnology 4e. General safety practices, p95

45 b 100% ethanol

Absolute ethanol will dissolve both polycarbonate and cellulose membrane filters. Expanding cellulose filters in 95% ethanol before using them will reduce the "hill and valley" effect often encountered when microscopically viewing membrane filters. Additionally, flattening the filter onto the slide and mounting media by rolling a wooden applicator stick over the surface of the freshly stained filter helps to keep the cells on the filter in the same focal plane.

DeMay, A&S 2e. Membrane filtration, p1546-1547

46 c toluidine blue

This stain may be used on centrifuged or other specimens for quick examination of the cellularity/diagnosis. One drop of toluidine blue on the unfixed specimen allows for excellent cell examination. This technique may be used for quick diagnosis or to decrease the possibility of unidentified "floaters."

Carson, Histotechnology 4e. Cross contamination, p328

47 d not expanding in 95% EtOH

Expanding cellulose filters in 95% ethanol before using them will reduce the "hill and valley" effect often encountered when microscopically viewing membrane filters. Additionally, flattening the filter onto the slide and mounting media by rolling a wooden applicator stick over the surface of the freshly stained filter helps to keep the cells on the filter in the same focal plane.

DeMay, A&S 2e. Membrane filtration, p1546-1547

48 a increase eosin or decrease the staining time in the EA

The desired amount of green cytoplasm may be determined based on these principles. Conversely, when all green disappears, the stain is exhausted and should be replaced.

Carson, Histotechnology 4e. EA, p326-328

49 b overstained

Regressive staining requires overstaining with an unacidified hematoxylin followed by the removal of the excess hematoxylin with hydrochloric acid. Next, a running bath is necessary to stop the action of the hydrochloric acid. This may be a contraindication when staining nongynecologic slides due to the possibility of decreased cellular adhesion when the slides are soaking in a running water bath.

DeMay, A&S 2e. Papanicolaou stain, p1552-1562

50 b regressive staining

An aqueous hydrochloric acid solution (0.25%) is used to remove the excess hematoxylin from the nucleus. This technique is typically used for nongynecologic specimens and is referred to as regressive staining.

DeMay, A&S 2e. Rinses, p1559-1560

51 c prepare slides for cytologic evaluation and submit material for flow cytometry

Flow cytometry may be useful to evaluate for the presence of lymphoma in cytologic fluids. The fluid needs to be submitted fresh or in RPMI. In patients with known diagnoses of lymphoma, the cell marker profile of the fluid can be compared to the cell marker profile of the original lymphoma.

DeMay, A&S 2e. Flow & image cytometry, p1528

52 b focus the microscope, close the field diaphragm and focus the edges, center the light beam, and open the field diaphragm until its edges just clear the field of view

The common method of coordinating the components of a microscope is to perform Köhler illumination. Köhler illumination images the light condenser in the plane of the object, thereby coordinating it with where the visualizing system is focused.

DeMay, A&S 2e. Köhler illumination, p1603-1604

53 d it is easier to discern cytoplasmic features

The Papanicolaou stain and the Romanowsky stain are both used in cytologic preparations. Each has its own advantages. The advantages of the Papanicolaou stain include better nuclear detail, cellular transparency, better demonstration of keratinization and squamous differentiation, and similarity to histologic stains. The Romanowsky stain gives more cytoplasmic detail and detail of background substances present in cytologic smears.

DeMay, A&S 2e. Routine stains, p1504-1505

54 c liquid based preparations

Selective cellular enhancement techniques according to the AMA Current Procedural Terminology 2008 Professional Edition include liquid based slide preparation methods.

DeMay, A&S 2e. Liquid based preparations, p1547-1548

55 a the absolute alcohol is contaminated

In order to achieve proper slide dehydration, the Papanicolaou stained slide is exposed to 95% alcohol followed by absolute (100%) alcohol.

DeMay, A&S 2e. Papanicolaou stain, p1552-1556

56 b a cool, well ventilated metal cabinet

A cool, well ventilated metal cabinet should be used to store volatile, flammable, and explosive materials such as xylene.

Carson, Histotechnology 4e. Chemical hazards, p88-90

ISBN 978-089189-6357 ©ASCP 2015

57   **a**   soak in xylene, remove coverslip, proceed backwards through the staining process and then soak in a dilute hydrochloric acid

Destaining of a cytology slide is done by following these steps: First you must remove the coverslip by soaking in xylene or a xylene substitute. Once the coverslip is removed, continue to soak the slide until all evidence of residual mounting media is removed. Next, begin moving the slide backwards through the staining process to remove the counterstain. The final step is the removal of the nuclear stain by soaking the slide in a dilute solution of hydrochloric acid for 5-10 minutes.

DeMay, A&S 2e. Destaining, p1561-1562

58   **d**   the lysing of red blood cells in bloody samples

Modified Carnoy solution, in addition to urea, 1% saponin, and glacial acetic acid, is useful in the lysing of red blood cells in bloody cell samples.

Carson, Histotechnology 4e. Bloody specimens, p322

59   **c**   water contamination in the xylene

Water droplets under the coverslip are indicative of inadequate dehydration of the slide and/or water being present in the xylene bath of the stainer.

DeMay, A&S 2e. Xylene, p1566-1567

60   **a**   supravital staining

Supravital staining is defined as any mechanism used to demonstrate a process(es) or structure(s) within living cells. In the cytopreparation arena, supravital staining with toluidine blue assists in the detection of a bloody fluid specimen prior to contaminating the staining solutions with "floaters." It can also be utilized for the detection of crystals and casts in urine, as well as the evaluation of overall cellularity and amount of fresh blood within a specimen.

Carson, Histotechnology 4e. Toluidine blue wet film, p328

61   **b**   tap water if pH is consistently higher than 8

Ammonium hydroxide, lithium carbonate, and Scott tap water are the most commonly used blueing reagents; however, tap water with a pH higher than 8 also serves as a blueing agent. In contrast, absolute alcohol dehydrates, dilute hydrochloric acid removes excess nuclear stain (regressive staining), and EA polychrome stains the cytoplasm and the nucleolar material (RNA).

DeMay, A&S 2e. Scott tap water substitute, p1554-1555

62   **c**   modified EA

Modified EA is a polychrome stain that consists of light green, SF yellowish, and eosin Y. The eosin Y component is an acidic dye that not only stains the nucleolar material (RNA), but also the cytoplasm of superficial cells, red blood cells, and cilia.

Carson, Histotechnology 4e. EA, p326-327

63   **a**   stains should be checked and documented for quality on a daily basis

Stains should be checked and documented for quality on a daily basis. In the staining setup, staining dishes should be labeled for content as the covers can be removed and misplaced.

DeMay, A&S 2e. Quality control and quality assessment, p1541-1542

64   **d**   amount of dye required divided by percent dye content

The amount of dye needed for preparing a batch of Papanicolaou counterstain such as modified OG or modified EA is determined by utilizing the following formula: amount of dye required divided by the percent of dye content indicated on the vial.

DeMay, A&S 2e. Papanicolaou stain, p1552-1553

65   **a**   10% buffered formalin and centrifuging

Cell blocks from aspirations oftentimes provide crucial information. Cells blocks can be created by placing an aspirate in a liquid fixative such as Bouin solution or 10% neutral buffered formalin. The specimen material is then centrifuged and the supernatant decanted, leaving a small pellet for embedding and sectioning.

Carson, Histotechnology 4e. Cell blocks, p324-325

66   **b**   air dried/Diff-Quik

In addition to being simple to prepare and permitting immediate evaluation, air dried/Diff-Quik preparations highlight amyloid and colloid although Pap stained preparations provide superior nuclear detail.

DeMay, A&S 2e. Routine stains, p1504-1505

67   **b**   nuclear stain hematoxylin and cytoplasmic stains orange G, eosin Y, and light green

Choice b correctly describes the modern Papanicolaou stain array. The original Papanicolaou array included bismarck brown, but this inactive dye has not been included for many years. Methylene blue is a nuclear dye used in Romanowsky type stains, not in the Papanicolaou array. Acridine orange combines with RNA and DNA, is fluorescent in ultraviolet light and is used mainly in research.

DeMay, A&S 2e, Papanicolaou stain, p1552-1553

68   **c**   methanol does not preserve antigens necessary for lymphoid antigen markers

Methanol tends to lead to overall cellular shrinkage and does not preserve the antigen necessary for lymphoid antigen markers.

Carson, Histotechnology 4e. Actions of fixatives, p245

69 **b** **10% buffered formalin**

Aldehyde fixatives like formalin (formaldehyde) achieve fixation by the mechanism of crosslinking proteins. Alcohol fixatives like ethanol (ethyl alcohol) denature or coagulate proteins. Saccomanno fixative is a prefixative that contains 50% ethanol and 2% carbowax.

Carson, Histotechnology 4e. Prefixatives, p318

70 **c** **stains cytoplasm containing a large component of the protein keratin**

Orange G is a synthetic dye of relatively small size, and it rapidly penetrates and stains cytoplasm rich in the structural protein keratin, for example the cells of keratinizing squamous cell carcinoma. EA is a mixture of the synthetic dyes eosin Y and light green, and does not include orange G. Cytokeratin is an intermediate filament, a component of the cytoskeleton, and it is labeled with immunostaining, not with orange G.

DeMay, A&S 2e. Papanicolaou stain, p1552-1553

71 **d** **regressive staining**

The regressive staining format requires intentional overstaining of cellular elements, followed by extraction of the excess hematoxylin with hydrochloric acid.

DeMay, A&S 2e. Hematoxylin, p1556-1557

72 **c** **with specimens from all patients and at all times**

One cannot rely on clinical history to flag a specimen as potentially infectious. The patient could harbor an undiscovered infection or the history accompanying the specimen may be incomplete. All fresh specimens should be treated as potential biohazards that require universal precautions.

Carson, Histotechnology 4e. Biological infectious hazards, p86-88

73 **b** **urine containing large numbers of *Schistosoma haematobium* ova**

Schistosoma ova are not the infectious stage in the life cycle of these parasites. The cercarial stage must be produced in order for the parasite to infect humans. In contrast, HIV, hepatitis B, and the tubercle bacillus are all highly infectious in the described specimens.

DeMay, A&S 2e. Schistosomiasis, p451-452

74 **c** **hand washing**

Hands come into contact with many organisms and can transmit infections. Therefore, frequent hand washing is the most important factor in the preventing of the spread of infections among hospital personnel and patients.

Carson, Histotechnology 4e. General safety practices, p95

75 **d** **placed in a puncture resistant container for disposal**

All disposable sharps should be placed into a puncture resistant container for transport or disposal.

Carson, Histotechnology 4e. Handling tissue waste, p87-88

76 **c** **biohazard material**

The 4 interlocking circles are the universal symbol for biohazard materials.

Carson, Histotechnology 4e. Hazard identification, p93-94

77 **d** **name of the chemical, the hazard, and the date of transfer**

All hazardous chemicals must have warning labels on them, which must include the chemical and common name, warnings about health and physical hazards, and the name and address of the manufacturer the product is purchased from. If the chemical is taken from the original container and put into a smaller container for ongoing use, the smaller container must be labeled properly with the name of the chemical, the hazards, and the date of the transfer.

Carson, Histotechnology 4e. Hazard identification, p93-94

78 **b** **fire hazard**

All chemical containers are required to indicate hazard levels in specific categories. The red diamond indicates the fire hazard, the blue diamond indicates the health hazard, the yellow diamond indicates reactivity/instability, and the white diamond indicates other specific hazards.

Carson, Histotechnology 4e. Hazard identification, p93-94

79 **b** **in a closed fire cabinet**

Flammables must be stored in explosion proof fire cabinets, refrigerators, or freezers, which should always be closed when not in direct use.

Carson, Histotechnology 4e. Fire & explosive hazards, p91-92

80 **d** **comply with local, state, and federal regulations**

The College of American Pathologists checklist for laboratory accreditation requires that chemical waste disposal comply with all local, state, and federal regulations. Certain hazardous chemicals cannot be disposed of in the sewer system. Some chemicals cannot be mixed together for disposal, nor can they be placed in landfills.

Carson, Histotechnology 4e. Chemical hazards, p88-91

81 **b** **xylene**

Xylene is on the list of chemicals found in the cytology laboratory that are considered carcinogenic.

Carson, Histotechnology 4e. Chemical hazards, p88-91

82 **a** **fire and exposure hazard data**

OSHA requires that employees working with chemicals have access to up to date material safety data sheets. Each sheet must contain information about the hazards of the chemical, the name of the manufacturer with contact information, requirements for handling the chemical, and cleanup information.

DeMay, A&S 2e. Compliance resources, p1591

ISBN 978-089189-6357 ©ASCP 2015

83 a pour concentrated solutions into less concentrated solutions

All chemicals should be treated as potential hazards. Proper handling of chemicals can reduce risks. Reagents should be added slowly, by pouring concentrated solutions into less concentrated solutions while stirring. Always pour acid into water; never pour water into acid. Reagent bottles should be filled to within 1/4 of their capacity to allow for heat expansion.

Carson, Histotechnology 4e. Chemical hazards, p88-91

84 d material safety data sheet

Material safety data sheet (MSDS) means written or printed material concerning a hazardous chemical prepared to comply with OSHA Hazard Communication standards. Manufacturers of chemicals must ensure that the hazards of all chemicals are evaluated, and that information concerning their hazards is transmitted to employers and employees. This transmittal of information is to be accomplished by means of comprehensive hazard communication programs, which include container labeling and other forms of warning, MSDS, and employee training.

Carson, Histotechnology 4e. Hazard identification, p93-94

85 a to advise as to how to proceed in the event of a chemical exposure

Employers shall provide employees with information (MSDS or other written communication) and training to the extent necessary to protect them from the hazards of handling or working with chemical substances. An MSDS contains general information about a chemical product: its name and manufacturer, its properties and hazards, handling and storage, first aid measures in event of exposure, and accidental release measures.

Carson, Histotechnology 4e. Hazard identification, p93-94

86 b flush affected area with water continuously for 15 minutes

General instructions for chemical spills on the skin include 1) removal of all contaminated clothing as quickly as possible; 2) flushing the area continuously for 15 minutes under a safety shower, faucet or eye wash; 3) washing off chemical with soap and water; and 4) obtaining immediate medical attention. Do NOT use neutralizing agents, creams, lotions, or salves on the affected skin.

Carson, Histotechnology 4e. Hazardous chemical spills, p92

87 a the manufacturer

Manufacturers are required by OSHA to develop and provide material safety data sheets for each chemical they produce, and include the sheet with each shipment of the chemical.

Carson, Histotechnology 4e. Hazard identification, p93-94

88 a health hazard

All chemical containers are required to indicate hazard levels in specific categories. The red diamond indicates the fire hazard, the blue diamond indicates the health hazard, the yellow diamond indicates reactivity/instability, and the white diamond indicates other specific hazards.

Carson, Histotechnology 4e. Hazard identification, p93-94

89 d in a separate cabinet

Chemicals should be stored in groups of similar reactivities and compatibilities. Incompatible chemicals should never be stored together. No dangerous chemicals should be placed on a high shelf because they could fall on someone. Refer to MSDS for specific information about the storage and handling of each chemical.

Carson, Histotechnology 4e. Chemical storage, p92

90 b at least once per year

Fire drills prepare employees to respond quickly & safely in the event of a fire. Every employee must participate in a fire drill at least once per year. Participation must be documented.

Carson, Histotechnology 4e. Fire & explosive hazards, p91-92

91 c burning combustible materials

A fire extinguisher identified with a green triangle containing the letter A is used for burning combustible materials such as wood, paper, clothing, or trash. It employs water or an all purpose dry chemical.

Carson, Histotechnology 4e. Fire & explosive hazards, p91-92

92 c be sure that all people are out of immediate danger

The acronym RACE provides the general plan for dealing with a fire. R stands for **rescue**–be sure that all persons are out of immediate danger. A stands for **alarm**–pull the fire alarm then notify authorities (if there is time). C stands for **contain**–close all doors and windows to contain the fire. E stands for **extinguish/evacuate**–attempt to put out the fire if it is small and staff are properly trained in the use of the fire extinguisher; evacuate the area.

Davis, Laboratory Safety—A Self Assessment Workbook, p29 [ISBN 978-089189-5701]

93 c at least annually

Individual laboratory safety policies and procedures are revised as needed, but a full review of all policies and procedures must be completed and documented at least annually.

CAP Laboratory Accreditation General Checklist. GEN.00016. 2007

94 b Occupational Safety and Health Administration

The Occupational Safety and Health Administration is a division of the US Department of Labor and is the main federal agency charged with the enforcement of safety and health legislation in the workplace.

United States Department of Labor. Occupational Health and Safety Administration. http://www.OSHA.gov

95 c computer data access

Smoking, eating and drinking, application of cosmetics and lip balm, manipulation of contact lenses, and mouth pipetting are all prohibited in laboratory technical work areas.

Clinical and Laboratory Standards Institute (formerly NCCLS). Clinical Laboratory Safety; Approved Guideline 2e. GP17-A2, 2004

96 b every week

Eyewash plumbing should be flushed weekly for ~3 minutes to decrease bacterial growth in the water lines and minimize the possibility of infections resulting from use of the eyewash station.

Davis, Laboratory Safety—A Self Assessment Workbook, p148 [ISBN 978-089189-5701]

ISBN 978-089189-6357 ©ASCP 2015

Chapter 10

Laboratory Management & Administration

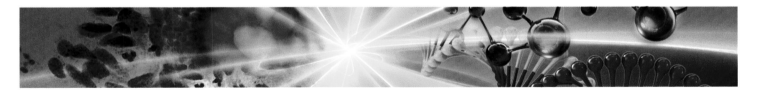

1 **What individual is qualified as General Supervisor under CLIA '88?**
 a PhD degree with 1 year of experience in cytopathology
 b MS degree with 5 years of experience, 1 in cytopathology
 c BS degree with 5 years of experience, 2 in cytopathology
 d BS degree with 3 years of experience, 2 in cytopathology

2 **What is considered a necessary component of an annual report?**
 a cytology-histology correlation
 b number of patients requesting information
 c needs assessment of the personnel benefits
 d the square footage of the cytotechnologist's workspace

3 **Cytopreparatory technicians, those individuals responsible for the preparation of cytologic material, are required to meet what CLIA regulation?**
 a cytology degree, certification by the American Society for Clinical Pathology
 b cytology degree, certification by the American Society for Cytotechnologists
 c high school degree, supervision by the General Supervisor
 d no degree required, only supervision by General Supervisor

4 **CLIA '88 regulations require that original requisitions be kept for a minimum of:**
 a 2 years
 b 5 years
 c 10 years
 d 20 years

5 **All of the following are considered important managerial responsibilities, except:**
 a adhering to the laboratory procedure manual
 b planning a weekly budget
 c organization of staff
 d development of internal and external quality control and quality assurance

6 **Optimally, each cytotechnologist participates in continuing education:**
 a at least 1 hour per year
 b in house as well as through professional societies
 c through all of the professional agencies at least 5× per month
 d a minimum of 10 hours per week

7 **Under CLIA '88, the Technical Supervisor is defined as:**
 a the cytotechnologist supervisor
 b the cytotechnologist in charge of the laboratory
 c the pathologist in charge of cytology
 d both the cytotechnologist supervisor and the pathologist in charge of cytology

8 **Under CLIA '88, copies of final reports must be kept for a minimum of:**
 a 2 years
 b 5 years
 c 10 years
 d 20 years

9 **Which statement is correct regarding specimen preparation?**
 a gynecologic specimens must be stained separately from nongynecologic specimens
 b staining quality should be checked weekly
 c all stains and solutions must be dated by the laboratory supervisor
 d all solutions must be filtered a minimum of once per month

10 **When ordering laboratory supplies, one may:**
 a jointly purchase supplies with the histology laboratory
 b make sure to accumulate inventory
 c order 3 years in advance
 d order supplies after the solution runs out to avoid oversupplying

11 **Accreditation of a cytotechnology program in the United States is determined by:**
 a American Society for Clinical Pathology
 b Commission for Allied Health Educational Programs
 c American Society for Cytotechnology
 d American Pathology Association

12 The CLIA regulations stipulate that glass slides must be kept for a minimum of:
a 2 years
b 5 years
c 10 years
d 20 years

13 Should a cytotechnology laboratory vacancy occur, the best mechanism to compensate until the position if filled is to:
a maximize the total number of specimens each cytotechnologist can review
b increase productivity
c stagger work hours/split shifts to cover the laboratory operations
d train individuals on the job until it can be filled by a qualified individual

14 A primary cytotechnologist diagnostic error is defined as:
a missing by 1 grade, ASCUS to LGSIL
b failing to determine specimen type
c incorrect judgment of specimen adequacy
d missing an obvious malignancy

15 The purpose of quality control and quality assurance protocols is:
a to ensure that the job gets done right the first time
b to ensure that the job eventually gets done correctly
c to increase revenues for the laboratory
d to identify strengths so that administration can see that the laboratory is doing a good job

16 A uniform, strict set of guidelines that apply to all laboratories reimbursable by Medicare/Medicaid are referred to as:
a Clinical Laboratory Improvement Amendments of 1988 (CLIA '88)
b Occupational Safety and Health regulations
c Bethesda System terminology
d interlaboratory comparison regulations

17 CLIA '88 requires:
a 10% review of focused or high risk cases as well as random review
b 10% random review only
c 10% focused or high risk only
d 10% of abnormal diagnoses

18 Quality assurance is defined as:
a collecting the data to determine efficacy of the individual and/or laboratory
b determining patterns or trends in test accuracy with the collected data
c reexamination of the negative material
d performing a 10% review on all gynecologic cases

19 Which are considered important budgetary considerations for laboratory operations?
a calculating the direct and indirect costs associated with laboratory operations
b cost of equipment maintenance on a 5 year basis
c deflation of supplies
d enforcing the 100 slide limit on each cytotechnologist to maximize profit

20 Regarding laboratory procedure manuals, which of the following statements are correct?
a laboratory manual must be kept, reviewed periodically, and signed by the Technical Supervisor
b laboratory manual must be kept, reviewed periodically, and signed by the General Supervisor
c laboratory manuals are not required under CLIA '88
d laboratory manuals must be updated each week as required by CLIA '88

21 What is an important employee record to maintain for each of the laboratory personnel?
a employee's future job plans
b employee's education
c accidents occurring at home
d outside income

22 On the average, (1) how many women are diagnosed with cervical cancer annually, (2) how many die of the disease, and (3) how does this compare with the incidence and mortality data from 50 years ago?
a 2,500; 1,300; decrease of 90%
b 5,000; 2,500; decrease of 30%
c 13,000; 5,000; decrease of 70%
d 26,000; 13,000; decrease of 25%

23 When conducting appraisal of new employees, one should consider:
a not performing an interview to rule out possible biases
b emphasizing their negative attributes only to increase their productivity
c measuring specific variables
d emphasizing their positive attributes to keep the laboratory from any possible employee litigation

24 A process by which a nongovernmental agency recognizes a program or laboratory as competent is termed:
a accreditation
b licensure
c OSHA
d Clinical Laboratory Improvement Act of 1988

25 What is considered methodology to ensure productivity?
a review of the individual's workload every 6 months by the Technical Supervisor
b maximizing the governmental slide limits
c performing 20% rescreen on all focused cases
d identifying the number of malignancies missed per week

26 When conducting quality control on gynecologic cases:
a the laboratory supervisor should pick a number, and each cytotechnologist should re-evaluate his/her own specimens
b the Technical Supervisor must review 10% of each cytotechnologist's workload for that particular day
c a blind or random sampling method should be conducted independently of each cytotechnologist's work
d 10% of the cytotechnologist's abnormal diagnoses should be reviewed by the Technical Supervisor

ISBN 978-089189-6357 ©ASCP 2015

27. The governing agency responsible for overseeing safety is referred to as:
   a CLIA
   b JCAHO
   c OSHA
   d ASCP

28. In the workload log record each cytotechnologist should include all of the following, EXCEPT:
   a number of cases/slides reviewed
   b number of discrepancies
   c workload limit
   d number of well preserved slides

29. The process by which a public authority grants permission to an individual or organization to engage in professional practice is called:
   a accreditation
   b certification
   c licensure
   d articulation

30. The Clinical Laboratory Improvement Amendments of 1988 (CLIA '88) require all of the following conditions, EXCEPT:
   a all cases of atypical squamous cells of undetermined significance (ASCUS) are considered part of the 5 year retrospective review process
   b a diagnosis of a high grade squamous intraepithelial lesion mandates follow-up of the patient
   c daily record of the number of slides reviewed as well as the amount of time spent reviewing the slides must be kept for each cytotechnologist
   d board certified pathologists may not perform primary review of >100 cytology slides in any 24 hour period

31. According to most organizational theorists, the administrative process includes:
   a planning and organizing
   b clerical work and proofreading
   c specimen processing and bench work
   d buying and selling

32. In forecasting inventory needs, which method is more responsive to change?
   a moving average
   b regression analysis
   c exponential smoothing
   d base index

33. Which rate setting technique is best suited to departments in which the cost of supplies is high in relation to the cost of labor?
   a hourly rate
   b surcharge
   c weighted value
   d per diem

34. What budgeting process identifies resources for budget items such as buildings and major equipment purchases?
   a physical plant
   b revenue
   c operational
   d capital

35. Which measure of CAP Workload productivity will reflect a potential personnel shortage?
   a paid productivity
   b worked productivity
   c specified productivity
   d unspecified productivity

36. In the CAP Workload Recording Method of determining labor costs, what calculation represents the mean number of workload units required to perform a procedure once?
   a unit volume per procedure
   b raw count
   c item for count
   d unit for count

37. Which coding system provides the reasoning and justification for ordering and performing laboratory procedures?
   a Current Procedural Terminology
   b HCFA Common Procedural Coding System
   c International Classification of Diseases 9
   d International Classification of Functioning, Disability and Health

38. Practices that result in failure to comply with governmental regulations involving intentional deception for personal gain are considered:
   a fraud
   b abuse
   c misdemeanor
   d battery

39. The ratio of the average annual investment return for a capital purchase to the initial investment cost defines its:
   a present value
   b time adjusted return
   c payback
   d average rate of return

40. Which method of cost accounting examines only those additional costs required to perform potential increases in test volume?
   a macro
   b micro
   c mini
   d incremental

41. What element of negligence requires that damages be shown to be the direct result of a negligent act?
   a duty
   b breach of duty
   c standard of care
   d proximate cause

42. What type of budget allows periodic negotiation and adjustment without requiring sanctions from external authorities?
   a appropriation
   b fixed forecast
   c variable
   d limited term

43 In a quality systems design, what documents whether a procedure performs at preset specifications?
   a proficiency testing
   b process validation
   c calibration
   d process control

44 What are the basic output units for analyzing productivity in the CAP Laboratory Management Index Program (LMIP)?
   a billable and total test
   b labor and FTE
   c consumable and equipment
   d discharges and outpatient visits

45 What type of budget report plots budgeted revenue and collections against expenses?
   a departmental trend summary
   b fund-balance statement
   c profit and loss statement
   d cost reports

46 What type of witness to a legal proceeding is permitted to offer an opinion based on "reasonable scientific certainty"?
   a ordinary
   b expert
   c fact
   d reasonable

47 Which LMIP measure represents the ratio of onsite testing to outsourced testing?
   a onsite billable per technical FTE
   b onsite billable per total billable tests
   c onsite billable per total FTE
   d worked to paid hours

48 In examining LMIP data to manage cost effectiveness, which ratio can be expected to increase as the total number of billable tests increases?
   a total laboratory expenses per discharge
   b total labor expense per onsite billable test
   c labor and direct expense per onsite billable test
   d consumable and direct expense per onsite billable test

49 Besides OSHA, which of the following federal agencies regulates laboratory operations?
   a Federal Bureau of Investigation
   b Central Intelligence Agency
   c Department of Transportation
   d Social Security Administration

50 A cytology supervisor is experiencing significant difficulty recently with a piece of laboratory equipment. The equipment service vendor arrives to investigate and requests copies of the laboratory orders and reports pertaining to 400 patients who had testing done on the suspect equipment. How should the supervisor respond?
   a deny the request because this would be a HIPAA violation
   b allow the vendor to take the records since they will be used for business purposes
   c provide the requested copies if the vendor has signed a business associate agreement with the laboratory
   d provide the requested copies if the orders and reports are hand delivered to the vendor by a laboratory employee

51 The Clinical Laboratory Improvement Amendments of 1988 (CLIA '88) mandate a 5 year retrospective review of all negative Pap tests diagnosed on all patients with a current cytologic diagnosis of:
   a invasive cancer only
   b atypical squamous cells of undetermined significance (ASCUS) or higher
   c low grade squamous intraepithelial lesion (LSIL) or higher
   d high grade squamous intraepithelial lesion (HSIL) or higher

52 Workload screening limits of 100 cytologic smears (or 200 liquid based preparations) in a 24 hour period are intended as:
   a a screening limit for pathologists only
   b the absolute daily maximum number of slides allowed by law
   c a screening limit for cytotechnologists only
   d a daily performance target established to measure competency

53 Photographed patient records that need to be discarded should be:
   a placed in a nonbiohazard trash can
   b shredded
   c placed in an open recycle bin
   d torn at least twice; shredding is not required

54 Annual statistics of the cytology laboratory must document which of the following:
   a number of Pap tests reported without an endocervical component
   b number of negative Pap tests reclassified as abnormal
   c number of Pap tests reviewed for 5 year retrospective rescreen
   d number of Pap tests reported as satisfactory for evaluation

55 According to CLIA '88, in the case of a Pap test referred to the Technical Supervisor for review, which of the following is not required in the report?
   a the specific test performed
   b the address of the laboratory
   c the pathologist's signature
   d the name of the screening cytotechnologist

ISBN 978-089189-6357 ©ASCP 2015

56 Random and focused 10% quality control (QC) presignout rescreen of negative Pap tests may be performed by:
a solely the technical supervisor of the laboratory
b cytotechnologists who excel in their competency review
c cytotechnologists with at least 5 years' experience
d cytotechnologists qualifying for general supervisor status under CLIA '88

57 In evaluating cytotechnologist competency, tracking an individual's abnormal rate is useful when compared to:
a the number of positive cases referred to the pathologist
b the number of false negative cases referred on routine QC
c the number of individual cases with histologic correlation
d the laboratory's abnormal rate

58 Which of the following Pap tests should not be billed?
a sample contains inadequate cellularity
b sample is extensively obscured by blood
c sample is received without proper patient identifier
d sample demonstrates obscuring foreign material

59 A cytotechnologist must have how many years of full time experience before he/she is eligible to perform quality control presignout rescreening of Pap tests?
a 1
b 3
c 5
d 10

60 Your laboratory monitors the rate of HPV DNA+ ASCUS Pap tests as a QC measure. 25% of your ASCUS Pap tests are high risk HPV+. As medical director you conclude that:
a your laboratory screens a low risk patient population
b the sensitivity of your HPV test needs to be adjusted
c your laboratory is overcalling ASCUS
d similar results were noted in the ALTS trial

61 How frequently must every CLIA licensed laboratory ensure that each cytotechnologist and pathologist is enrolled, takes, and passes a CMS approved gynecologic cytology proficiency test?
a annually
b depends on state licensure requirements
c biannually
d upon renewal of laboratory certification

62 Which of the following is not required on the cytology specimen requisition?
a patient age/date of birth
b patient gender and ethnic designation
c date of specimen collection
d specimen source

63 As defined by Medicare, which of the following represents a "screening" high risk Pap test?
a early onset of sexual activity (under the age of 20)
b previous abnormal Pap test in a postmenopausal patient
c history of sexually transmitted disease (excluding HIV)
d <3 negative Pap tests in the previous 7 years

64 Which of the following statements regarding the cytology laboratory procedure manual is correct:
a a hard copy of the procedure manual must be kept in every work area
b copies of discontinued procedures must be kept for 5 years
c product inserts may substitute for written procedures
d review of the manual must be performed by the Technical Supervisor

65 An effective benchmark for measuring diagnostic performance by cytotechnologists and pathologists in gynecologic cytology is:
a 5 year retrospective review of current abnormal cases
b individual competency review every 6 months
c random and focused rescreening of quality control (QC) cases
d determining individual ASC:SIL ratios

66 For each pathologist, what percentage of Pap tests interpreted as NILM must be subjected to quality control (QC) rescreen?
a none
b 10%
c 20%
d 100%

67 According to CLIA '88, every cytology professional (cytotechnologist or pathologist) engaged in screening or review of Pap tests (gynecologic cytology) must:
a show evidence of 10 hours of continuing education in gynecologic cytology biennially
b participate in unknown gynecologic cytology case review at least 4× annually
c participate in an annual CMS approved proficiency testing program with a laboratory pass rate of at least 90%
d participate in an annual CMS approved proficiency testing program with an individual passing score of at least 90%

68 The Medicare definition of a "diagnostic" high risk Pap test is:
a any sign of symptom related to a gynecologic disorder
b <3 negative Pap tests in the previous 7 years
c history of an abnormal Pap within the last 3 years
d history of exposure to diethylstilbestrol

69 6 Sigma is:
a a concept of using well defined statistical tools and measures to improve processes
b related to CLIA '88 mandated gynecologic cytology proficiency testing compliance
c a measure of the image resolving power of a microscope objective
d a measure of stability of alternating current stability for high sensitivity medical instruments

70 A cytotechnologist notices that a specimen currently being processed belongs to a famous athlete who is in the Baseball Hall of Fame. Is it acceptable for the cytotechnologist to share this discovery with her family and/or her coworkers?
  a yes, but only with her coworkers, not with her family
  b yes, this is public information
  c no, since the diagnosis has not yet been reported to the patient's physician
  d no, sharing this information violates HIPAA

71 A cytology supervisor is experiencing significant difficulty recently with a piece of laboratory equipment. The equipment service vendor arrives to investigate and requests copies of the laboratory orders and reports pertaining to 400 patients who had testing done on the suspect equipment. How should the supervisor respond?
  a deny the request because this would be a HIPAA violation
  b allow the vendor to take the records since they will be used for business purposes
  c provide the requested copies if the vendor has signed a business associate agreement with the laboratory
  d provide the requested copies if the orders and reports are hand delivered to the vendor by a laboratory employee

72 Which of the following must be included in the cytology laboratory's annual statistical report?
  a ratio of liquid based to conventional Pap tests
  b percentage of Pap tests screened on an imaging device
  c data from cytologic histologic correlation
  d number of cases rescreened for 5 year retrospective review

73 When a physician of healthcare worker is reviewing a patient's records, HIPAA clearly states that:
  a the records should be reviewed with as many colleagues as possible
  b it is OK to leave the patient's records out to review later
  c the patient's information can be emailed to colleagues for opinions
  d the patient's records should be reviewed in private, and consults should be done privately and only as needed

74 When preparing cytologic specimens, which of the following statements is true?
  a changing solutions and stains weekly is sufficient
  b the Technical Supervisor is responsible for checking and labeling solutions and stains
  c cross contamination is best avoided by staining gynecologic and nongynecologic cases in separate staining setups
  d the decision to filter stains is based only on stain quality

75 In reference to Pap test classification by Medicare as "screening" vs "diagnostic," which statement is true?
  a only the referring physician or reviewing pathologist may determine the risk classification
  b the screening cytotechnologist or referring clinician may determine the risk classification
  c only the referring clinician may determine the risk classification
  d the risk classification is determined by the patient's insurance and history of prior abnormal Pap(s)

76 Which of the following risk factors indicates the need for a focused presignout quality control (QC) rescreen of a patient's Pap test?
  a family history of cervical cancer
  b previous abnormal Pap test result
  c previous unsatisfactory Pap test result
  d no transformation zone component

77 Who needs to worry about protecting patient privacy and confidentiality?
  a physicians
  b employees who need access to patient records
  c nurses
  d all employees

78 A patient comes into the emergency room for treatment and refuses to sign an authorization form. The patient may:
  a be refused treatment
  b be forced to sign the authorization
  c be treated without further discussion
  d be talked about among colleagues

79 A 30-year-old female who has had 3 prior NILM Pap tests in the last 5 years has a current Pap test interpreted as ASC-H. Her high risk HPV DNA test is negative. Which of the following statements is true?
  a this patient does not need colposcopy
  b this patient should have colposcopy
  c if colposcopy, biopsy and ECC are all normal, the ASC-H diagnosis was an overcall
  d HPV testing is the recommended triage for ASC-H in women 30 and older

80 Which of the following is not required in the cytopathology laboratory procedure manual?
  a criteria for specimen rejection
  b cytopreparatory techniques
  c manufacturer's procedure manuals for all laboratory instrumentation
  d requirements for specimen collection and processing

81 The 4 Pap tests listed below are submitted to a pathologist for review. The pathologist's review of which case would not count towards the laboratory's 10% quality control (QC) presignout rescreening requirement?
  a NILM–reactive changes
  b NILM–Candida
  c NILM–herpes
  d ASCUS

ISBN 978-089189-6357 ©ASCP 2015

82 Quality control (QC) rescreening of negative Pap tests must be completed when?
- a within 30 days of reporting the negative result
- b within 72 hours of reporting the negative result
- c within 1 year of reporting the negative result
- d prior to reporting the negative result

83 The acceptable deviation of a determined laboratory analysis from its true value is its:
- a standard deviation
- b allowable error
- c predictive value
- d coefficient of variance

84 According to Maslow's hierarchy of needs, which of the following is a primary need and thus serves as a prime motivator in the workplace?
- a acceptance by peers
- b recognition for accomplishments
- c job security
- d job satisfaction

85 In a criterion based job description, what factor is important to task completion but has little impact on outcomes if the task is performed incorrectly?
- a critical task
- b essential task
- c outcome metrics
- d key job area

86 What common term is defined as the official acknowledgment of technical or professional competence?
- a peer assurance
- b credentialing
- c registration
- d regulation

87 Analysis of what type of costs enables the measurement of productivity in terms of fluctuations in the cost to produce a given service?
- a unit
- b direct
- c indirect
- d mixed

88 Which of the following measures of group effectiveness is defined by the ratio of outputs to inputs?
- a production
- b adaptiveness
- c development
- d efficiency

89 Which federal agency regulates market entry of medical devices, laboratory instruments, reagents, and systems?
- a Centers for Disease Control
- b Health Care Financing Administration
- c Food and Drug Administration
- d Department of Defense

90 Which of the following facilities would be subject to the regulations of the National Labor Relations Act?
- a a VA hospital with annual receipts of $1,000,000
- b a nursing home with annual receipts of $90,000
- c a for profit adult day care center with annual receipts of $125,000
- d a not for profit hospital with annual receipts of $300,000

91 When negligence appears so obvious that the court shifts the burden of proof to the defendant, the concept is referred to as:
- a negligence ipso facto
- b res ipsa loquitor
- c negligence per se
- d respondeat superior

92 A manager following McGregor theory Y leadership style would do which of the following?
- a require employees to set their own goals and objectives
- b closely supervise and control staff work responsibilities
- c motivate staff with financial reward for good performance
- d structure workflow according to published standards

93 Costs that are sensitive to changes in test volume are called:
- a fixed
- b variable
- c direct
- d indirect

94 Which agency investigates alleged discrimination cases under Title VII?
- a National Labor Relations Board
- b Equal Employment Opportunity Commission
- c US Department of Labor
- d Affirmative Action

95 Which method of costing (cost accumulation) attempts to allocate indirect costs to the hospital laboratory?
- a direct
- b standard
- c variance
- d full

96 According to Herzberg 2 factor motivation theory, what 2 factors contribute to strong motivation of employees?
- a hygiene factors and satisfiers
- b interpersonal factors and motivators
- c good feelings and personal factors
- d recognition and expectation

97 A technologist commits a major error in laboratory testing that results directly in the death of a patient. The family of the patient brings suit against the technologist, the pathologist, and the hospital administrators. What is the legal premise that gives them the right to sue the hospital administrators?
- a res ipsa loquitor
- b respondeat superior
- c procedenti ab utroque
- d locum tenens

98 Which one of the following questions can be legally asked on an employment application?
 a Have you ever been arrested?
 b Do you have any relatives employed by this company?
 c Do you have a disability?
 d Do you prefer to be addressed as Ms, Mrs, or Mr?

99 What set of laws and regulations pertains to labor relations in the private sector?
 a Civil Service Reform Act
 b National Labor Relations Act
 c state labor laws
 d local jurisdiction laws

100 In plotting statistical tests of method comparison data, what calculation is a measure of proportional bias?
 a slope of the line
 b intercept of the line
 c standard error
 d correlation coefficient

101 What is the most commonly cited reason for conducting a performance appraisal?
 a documentation of disciplinary action
 b behavior modification
 c salary and promotion decisions
 d competency assessment

102 In the context of employee performance appraisal, a standard may be defined as a:
 a reference for the formation of judgments
 b clear definition of what constitutes good or bad performance
 c mutual consent to specified goals
 d measure to which like objects are expected to conform

103 The Age Discrimination in Employment Act (ADEA) protects employees against discrimination in terms of paid benefits and continued employment to workers over what age?
 a 18
 b 21
 c 40
 d 70

104 What agency is responsible for oversight of labor relations in the federal sector?
 a National Labor Relations Board
 b Equal Employment Opportunity Commission
 c Merit Systems Protection Board
 d Federal Labor Relations Authority

105 According to Herzberg's 2 factor motivation theory, a marginal employee will be more likely to perform at unacceptable levels when what factors are absent?
 a motivators
 b hygiene
 c interpersonal
 d expectation

106 Which of the following quality improvement tools is best for determining the significance of data?
 a Pareto diagram
 b fishbone diagram
 c scatter diagram
 d affinity diagram

107 Which legal doctrine holds an employer liable for the actions of an employee?
 a res ipsa loquitor
 b respondeat superior
 c negligence per se
 d compar sit laudatio

108 What method of process control can be used to assess the repeatability and accuracy of test results?
 a reference sample
 b control sample
 c gold standard
 d predictable standard

109 According to French and Raven's bases of power model, a manager who is able to lead by the charisma of her personality demonstrates what type of power of influence?
 a reward
 b expert
 c referent
 d legitimate

110 What factor is the most common reason for CLIA proficiency testing failure?
 a imprecision
 b inaccuracy
 c bias
 d internal coefficient of variation

111 What is the most important management decision in the implementation of a Westgard process control system?
 a number of controls analyzed
 b desirable error detection rate
 c acceptable rejection rate
 d acceptable standard deviation

112 A member of the laboratory team likes to work alone, prefers to solve new problems, likes analysis and putting things into logical order, and works best following a predetermined plan. What Myers-Briggs type is this person most likely to be?
 a introvert, intuiting, thinking, judging
 b extrovert, sensing, feeling, perceiving
 c introvert, sensing, thinking, judging
 d extrovert, intuiting, feeling, judging

113 The ability of a laboratory analysis to measure or detect a given test outcome consistently over time refers to the test's:
 a sensitivity
 b specificity
 c precision
 d accuracy

ISBN 978-089189-6357 ©ASCP 2015

114 The ability of a laboratory analysis to detect the smallest amount of an element or analyte is a measure of its:

a specificity
b sensitivity
c precision
d accuracy

115 In examining Levy-Jennings process control charts, a change in the precision of a test would be reflected as a:

a dispersion
b trend
c shift
d cluster

116 Which term refers to governmental control over an economic market?

a accreditation
b certification
c licensure
d regulation

117 Laboratories in which of the following settings are exempt from CLIA '88 regulation?

a physician office
b Pap test laboratories
c skilled nursing facilities
d Department of Defense drug surveillance facilities

Laboratory Management & Administration *Answer Key*

1 d BS degree with 3 years of experience, 2 in cytopathology

The cytotechnology supervisor is regarded as the General Supervisor. This individual must possess at least 3 years of experience. In addition, only cytotechnologists who qualify for General Supervisor status under CLIA '88 are permitted to perform intralaboratory quality control or 10% rescreen.

DeMay, A&S 2e. CLIA '88, p1583-1588

2 a cytology-histology correlation

Some of the annual statistics required by cytopathology laboratories include the cytotechnologist worklogs, workload statistics, quality control data and quality assurance guidelines, total number of specimens processed, and a breakdown of number of specimens by diagnosis.

Keebler CM, Somrak TM, The Manual of Cytotechnology. Recordkeeping practices, p338

3 d no degree required, only supervision by General Supervisor

Cytopreparatory technicians must meet no minimal education requirements. On the job training is acceptable.

Keebler CM, Somrak TM, The Manual of Cytotechnology. Support personnel, p337

4 a 2 years

These requisitions may be kept in hard files or on microfilm with accompanying biopsy or autopsy reports if applicable.

Keebler CM, Somrak TM, The Manual of Cytotechnology. Recordkeeping practices, p338-340

5 b planning a weekly budget

A yearly or biannual long range budget should be developed based on the patterns or trends from past budgets and predictions for the upcoming year. Before developing a budget, a complete cost analysis for performing the laboratory tests (eg, supplies, equipment/ instrument or capital purchases, continuing education costs) should be developed to include direct and indirect costs, and personnel costs need to be determined (including possible increases in salary or differential pay). Periodic reassessment throughout the year is necessary to establish the baseline necessary to determine requirements for future budgetary processes.

Keebler CM, Somrak TM, The Manual of Cytotechnology. Budget process, p358-362

6 b in house as well as through professional societies

Continuing education is essential for each cytotechnologist to keep abreast of the evolving nature of diagnostic cytopathology. Key considerations include developing in house workshops; attending regional, state, or national meetings; subscribing to the American Society of Cytopathology teleconferencing series; purchasing the numerous ASCP educational programs (eg, *Check Sample*, Chapter 12: Laboratory management and administration answer key); subscribing to the ASCP nongynecologic PTTM slide program; or participating in the College of American Pathologists Interlaboratory Comparison program.

Keebler CM, Somrak TM, The Manual of Cytotechnology. Continuing Education, p362

7 c the pathologist in charge of cytology

The Technical Supervisor of the laboratory must be a board certified pathologist. Subspecialization in cytopathology is not mandated by CLIA '88. The cytotechnology supervisor is regarded as the General Supervisor. This individual must possess at least 3 years of experience. In addition, only cytotechnologists who qualify for General Supervisor status under CLIA '88 are permitted to perform intralaboratory quality control or 10% rescreen

DeMay, A&S 2e. CLIA '88, p1583-1588

8 c 10 years

These reports must be available as hard copies for a minimum of 10 years.

Keebler CM, Somrak TM, The Manual of Cytotechnology. Recordkeeping practices, p338-340

9 a gynecologic specimens must be stained separately from nongynecologic specimens

Gynecologic processing must be performed independently of nongynecologic specimens due to the possibility of "floaters."

Keebler CM, Somrak TM, The Manual of Cytotechnology. Specimen preparation, p340

10 a jointly purchase supplies with the histology laboratory

Bulk discounts may be realized if the laboratory has the potential to jointly purchase supplies with the histology laboratory.

Keebler CM, Somrak TM, The Manual of Cytotechnology. Laboratory supplies, p361

11 b Commission for Allied Health Educational Programs

The Commission for Allied Health Educational Programs (CAHEP) is responsible for accrediting all Cytotechnology programs as recommended by the American Society for Cytopathology (Cytotechnology Program Review Committee).

12 b 5 years

All glass slides must be kept for a minimum of 5 years, regardless of whether they are normal or abnormal, gynecologic or nongynecologic.

Keebler CM, Somrak TM, The Manual of Cytotechnology. Recordkeeping practices, p338-340

13 c stagger work hours/split shifts to cover the laboratory operations

Overtime scheduling may be needed to maintain productivity and ensure timely patient diagnoses. Flexible time shifts may provide some support when recruiting for vacant positions.

Keebler CM, Somrak TM, The Manual of Cytotechnology. Position vacancy, p361

14 d missing an obvious malignancy

A primary error is a misdiagnosis that would have changed the clinical management of the patient. This error must be originally made by the cytotechnologist who screened the specimen. The error should be noted in the personnel file for determination of a possible plan of action.

Keebler CM, Somrak TM, The Manual of Cytotechnology. Primary error, p363

ISBN 978-089189-6357 ©ASCP 2015

15 a to ensure that the job gets done right the first time

Eliminating mistakes begins by establishing a stringent set of guidelines that each cytotechnologist must follow. Updated and current procedure manuals that reflect the current practice of the laboratory and identify the expected role of the cytotechnologist will help ensure quality and performance within the workplace. Timely appraisal of individual performance standards ensures that if mistakes do occur, they are eliminated with the utmost efficiency.

Keebler CM, Somrak TM, The Manual of Cytotechnology. Quality management, p365

16 a Clinical Laboratory Improvement Amendments of 1988 (CLIA '88)

The CLIA '88 regulations attempt to regulate all laboratories to ensure quality patient care.

DeMay, A&S 2e. CLIA '88, p1583-1588

17 a 10% review of focused or high risk cases as well as random review

CLIA '88 regulations require that a 10% random and focused review be performed blindly without the knowledge of which case will be re-reviewed by a General Supervisor level cytotechnologist.

DeMay, A&S 2e. CLIA '88, p1583-1588

18 b determining patterns or trends in test accuracy with the collected data

Quality control is the collection of the data necessary to establish statistical information needed to evaluate the efficacy of the laboratory. Quality assurance is using the collected data to establish patterns or trends that the laboratory can use to improve its operation.

Keebler CM, Somrak TM, The Manual of Cytotechnology. Quality assurance/quality control measures and practices, p353-355

19 a calculating the direct and indirect costs associated with laboratory operations

A yearly or biannual long range budget should be developed based on the patterns or trends from past budgets and predictions for the upcoming year. Before developing a budget, a complete cost analysis for performing the laboratory tests (eg, supplies, equipment/instrument or capital purchases, continuing education costs) should be developed to include direct and indirect costs, and personnel costs need to be determined (including possible increases in salary or differential pay). Periodic reassessment throughout the year is necessary to establish the baseline necessary to determine requirements for future budgetary processes.

Keebler CM, Somrak TM, The Manual of Cytotechnology. Budget process, p358-362

20 a laboratory manual must be kept, reviewed periodically, and signed by the Technical Supervisor

The Technical Supervisor of the laboratory must be a board certified pathologist. Subspecialization in cytopathology is not mandated by CLIA '88. The cytotechnology supervisor is regarded as the General Supervisor. This individual must possess at least 3 years of experience. In addition, only cytotechnologists who qualify for General Supervisor status under CLIA '88 are permitted to perform intralaboratory quality control or 10% rescreen.

DeMay, A&S 2e. CLIA '88, p1583-1588

21 b employee's education

An employee's education and experience are 2 important records that should be maintained for each cytotechnologist. Other records include his or her attendance, productivity, reliability, professionalism, and diagnostic accuracy.

Keebler CM, Somrak TM, The Manual of Cytotechnology. Personnel issues, p362-365

22 c 13,000; 5,000; decrease of 70%

The incidence of cervical cancer has decreased overall 70% since the test was implemented (1950s). It stands today as the most successful cancer screening test in medicine.

American Cancer Society Facts and Figures; 2002: http://cancer.org.

23 c measuring specific variables

Measuring specific variables allows the interviewer to evaluate each of the candidates fairly with relatively unbiased interpretations. Collected data can be kept on file should the future necessitate.

Keebler CM, Somrak TM, The Manual of Cytotechnology. Performance standards, p365

24 a accreditation

Accreditation is awarded to institutions, whereas licensure is awarded to individuals.

Keebler CM, Somrak TM, The Manual of Cytotechnology. Laboratory accreditation, p334

25 a review of the individual's workload every 6 months by the Technical Supervisor

The Technical Supervisor, a cytopathologist who is the typically the director of the cytology laboratory, must review the productivity of each cytotechnologist within the laboratory to determine his or her competency and productivity levels.

Keebler CM, Somrak TM, The Manual of Cytotechnology. Productivity issues, p363

26 c a blind or random sampling method should be conducted independently of each cytotechnologist's work

CLIA '88 regulations require that a 10% random and focused review be performed blindly without the knowledge of which case will be re-reviewed by a General Supervisor level cytotechnologist.

DeMay, A&S 2e. CLIA '88, p1583-1588

27 c OSHA

The Occupational Safety and Health Administration establishes guidelines and monitors compliance with chemical and biohazardous regulations.

Keebler CM, Somrak TM, The Manual of Cytotechnology. Chemical safety, p372

28 d number of well preserved slides

Each cytotechnologist must strictly comply with the CLIA '88 guidelines to ensure quality of patient care.

DeMay, A&S 2e. CLIA '88, p1583-1588

29 c licensure

Licensure is the legal process governing the right to professional practice. Certification is the process by which a peer group or governmental agency recognizes that an organization or individual has met certain requirements. Articulation refers to terms of agreement between educational institutions relating to student placement.

Snyder JR, Wilkinson DS, eds. Management in Laboratory Medicine. Laboratory regulation, certification and accreditation, p371

30 a all cases of atypical squamous cells of undetermined significance (ASCUS) are considered part of the 5 year retrospective review process

The only cases warranting a 5 year retrospective review are those currently diagnosed as high grade intraepithelial lesions or above.

Keebler CM, Somrak TM, The Manual of Cytotechnology. Quality control practices, p340-342

31 a planning and organizing

The administrative process includes planning, organizing, directing, and controlling.

Snyder JR, Wilkinson DS, eds. Management in Laboratory Medicine. The nature of management in laboratory medicine, p10

32 c exponential smoothing

Exponential smoothing responds to trends better than the moving average approach because its weights are based on historical data.

Snyder JR, Wilkinson DS, eds. Management in Laboratory Medicine. Inventory management and cost containment, p557-559

33 b surcharge

The surcharge or cost plus technique is useful for departments in which supply costs exceed labor costs to provide a service. The hourly rate method is better suited to departments in which there is a good association between the service provided and the time required to provide the service. In the weighted value approach, relative value of a procedure is assigned depending upon the direct cost of performing it.

Snyder JR, Wilkinson DS, eds. Management in Laboratory Medicine. Budgeting laboratory resources, p490

34 d capital

The capital budget identifies resources for the acquisition and maintenance of physical resources such as buildings and major equipment.

Snyder JR, Wilkinson DS, eds. Management in Laboratory Medicine. Budgeting laboratory resources, p480

35 c specified productivity

Specified productivity reflects activities not included in calculations of CAP Workload unit time and therefore may better reflect the need for additional personnel.

Snyder JR, Wilkinson DS, eds. Management in Laboratory Medicine. Laboratory cost accounting, p502-504

36 a unit volume per procedure

Unit volume per procedure is the mean number of workload units required to perform a procedure 1 time. Raw count is a total of the items to be counted and item for count specifies what is to be counted.

Snyder JR, Wilkinson DS, eds. Management in Laboratory Medicine. Laboratory cost accounting, p494

37 c International Classification of Diseases—9

The International Classification of Disease–9 provides the coding framework for justifying laboratory testing. Current Procedural Terminology codes identify services for Medicare, Medicaid, and many third party reimbursement payers.

Snyder JR, Wilkinson DS, eds. Management in Laboratory Medicine. Coding, billing, and reimbursement management, p509-514

38 a fraud

Fraud is a felony offense involving intentional misrepresentation to knowingly gain personal benefit. Abuse is considered a misdemeanor offense and involves practices that fail to follow standard practice and result in improper reimbursement. Battery is the infliction of nonconsensual touching.

Snyder JR, Wilkinson DS, eds. Management in Laboratory Medicine. Coding, billing, and reimbursement management, p509-515

39 d average rate of return

The average rate of return for a capital purchase is the average annual investment return divided by the initial investment cost. Payback analysis determines the time in the life of the instrument when cash flows can recover the original investment. The present value of an item is what it would cost at some future point if the present cost were invested and earned returns equal to a specific amount. The time adjusted return method is a calculation of the rate at which the net present value totals 0.

Snyder JR, Wilkinson DS, eds. Management in Laboratory Medicine. Budgeting laboratory resources, p483-485

40 d incremental

The incremental method examines the additional costs associated with increases in test volume. The macro method assigns direct cost to the appropriate cost center, whereas the micro method examines the cost per test of direct and indirect labor, materials, instrumentation, and overhead.

Snyder JR, Wilkinson DS, eds. Management in Laboratory Medicine. Laboratory cost accounting, p494-500

41 d proximate cause

The plaintiff must show proximate cause, or that the injury or damage resulted directly from the negligent act.

Snyder JR, Wilkinson DS, eds. Management in Laboratory Medicine. Medicolegal concerns in laboratory medicine, p412

42 b fixed forecast

Fixed forecast budgets permit renegotiation of budget elements without external sanctioning. Appropriation budgets from governmental agencies are apportioned periodically from central agencies and cannot be renegotiated during a given budget period.

Snyder JR, Wilkinson DS, eds. Management in Laboratory Medicine. Budgeting laboratory resources, p475

43 b process validation

Process validation ensures that a new procedure will perform according to preset specifications. Process control enables identification of opportunities to reduce error and decrease variation.

Snyder JR, Wilkinson DS, eds. Management in Laboratory Medicine. Quality management in the laboratory, p400

ISBN 978-089189-6357 ©ASCP 2015

44　a　billable and total test

The billable and total tests are the basic output units of productivity, while labor, FTE, and financial costs represent basic input units.

Snyder JR, Wilkinson DS, eds. Management in Laboratory Medicine. Assessing laboratory operating performance: the laboratory management index program, p452

45　c　profit and loss statement

Profit and loss statements reflect budgeted revenue and actual collections vs actual expenses.

Snyder JR, Wilkinson DS, eds. Management in Laboratory Medicine. Budgeting laboratory resources, p479-480

46　b　expert

Only an expert witness may offer an opinion based on reasonable scientific certainty. An ordinary or fact witness may offer only an opinion based on his or her own experience.

Snyder JR, Wilkinson DS, eds. Management in Laboratory Medicine. Medico legal concerns in laboratory medicine, p417

47　b　onsite billable per total billable tests

Onsite billable per total billable tests measures the percentage of tests performed in-house vs that sent to reference laboratories.

Snyder JR, Wilkinson DS, eds. Management in Laboratory Medicine. Assessing laboratory operating performance: the laboratory management index program, p456

48　a　total laboratory expenses per discharge

The total laboratory expense per discharge can be expected to increase as the total number of billable tests increases. The other 3 measures listed can be expected to decrease as the total number of billable tests increases.

Snyder JR, Wilkinson DS, eds. Management in Laboratory Medicine. Assessing laboratory operating performance: the laboratory management index program, p456-457

49　c　Department of Transportation

The Department of Transportation regulates laboratory operations related to safe practices in packaging, transporting, and handling biologic materials.

Snyder JR, Wilkinson DS, eds. Management in Laboratory Medicine. Laboratory regulation, certification, and accreditation, p389

50　c　provide the requested copies if the vendor has signed a business associate agreement with the laboratory

Generally, whenever a third party such as a service vendor accesses or uses protected health information provided by a covered entity for purposes other that the diagnosis and treatment of the patient, a business associate agreement is required.

HIPAA. United States Public Law 104-191. Health Insurance Portability and Accountability Act of 1996 (HIPAA, Title II)

51　d　high grade squamous intraepithelial lesion (HSIL) or higher

CLIA '88 requires that previous negative Pap tests over the last 5 years must be reviewed on all patients with a current diagnosis of HSIL or higher.

DeMay, A&S 2e. CLIA '88, p1583-1588

52　b　the absolute daily maximum number of slides allowed by law

The 100 smear (or 200 liquid based preparations) workload limit over 24 hours was established as the daily screening maximum allowed by law. It applies to anyone who screens and evaluates cytologic slides and includes gynecologic and nongynecologic slides, and slides evaluated for quality control (QC).

Cibas ES, Ducatman BS. Cytology: Diagnostic Principles and Clinical Correlates. 3rd ed. Philadelphia: Saunders; 2009

53　b　shredded

Paper records with personal patient identifiers (PPIs) must be either shredded or placed in a closed receptacle for delivery to a company contracted to destroy records for the facility.

HIPAA. United States Public Law 104-191. Health Insurance Portability and Accountability Act of 1996 (HIPAA, Title II)

54　b　number of negative Pap tests reclassified as abnormal

Laboratories must keep a record of any negative case that was reclassified as abnormal. Only unsatisfactory cases must be reported in annual statistics. Pap tests lacking an endocervical component are not considered unsatisfactory.

Cibas ES, Ducatman BS. Cytology: Diagnostic Principles and Clinical Correlates. 3rd ed. Philadelphia: Saunders; 2009

55　d　the name of the screening cytotechnologist

According to CLIA '88, all pathologist reviewed cases must include the name and address of the laboratory, the test performed the test result, and the pathologist's signature (which may be electronic). The name of the screening cytotechnologist is this subset of cases is not required.

DeMay, A&S 2e. CLIA '88, p1583-1588

56　d　cytotechnologists qualifying for General Supervisor status under CLIA '88

Quality control presignout rescreening must be performed by either the Technical Supervisor (board certified pathologist) or by a cytotechnologist qualified as a Cytology General Supervisor under CLIA '88.

Cibas ES, Ducatman BS. Cytology: Diagnostic Principles and Clinical Correlates. 3rd ed. Philadelphia: Saunders; 2009:510

57　d　the laboratory's abnormal rate

A cytotechnologist's abnormal rate is most useful when compared to the overall abnormal rate in the laboratory. The laboratory should establish an unacceptable deviation from the laboratory abnormal rate to determine if remedial action is required.

Cibas ES, Ducatman BS. Cytology: Diagnostic Principles and Clinical Correlates. 3rd ed. Philadelphia: Saunders; 2009:515-516

58　c　sample is received without proper patient identifier

Samples considered unsatisfactory for processing (eg, irresolvable lack of patient identifier, or glass slide(s) broken beyond repair) should not be billed.

Cibas ES, Ducatman BS. Cytology: Diagnostic Principles and Clinical Correlates. 3rd ed. Philadelphia: Saunders; 2009:507

59 **b** 3

Quality control presignout rescreening must be performed by a cytotechnologist qualified as a Cytology General Supervisor. This means the individual must be qualified as a cytotechnologist under CFR 493.1483, and have at least 3 years of full time experience (at least 2,080 hours per year) working as a cytotechnologist within the preceding 10 years (CFR 493.1469).

DeMay, A&S 2e. CLIA '88, p1583-1588

60 **c** your laboratory is overcalling ASCUS

The NCI-ALTS trial was demographically representative of the US population. The target rate of ASCUS is ~50% high risk HPV+.

Stoler MH. Testing for human papillomavirus: data driven implications for cervical neoplasia management. Clin Lab Med. Sep 2003;23(3):569-583

61 **a** annually

Every CLIA licensed laboratory must enroll each of its cytotechnologists and pathologists performing gynecologic testing in a CMS approved cytology proficiency testing program. Each cytotechnologist and pathologist must take and pass proficiency testing each year.

DeMay, A&S 2e. CLIA '88, p1583-1588

62 **b** patient gender and ethnic designation

Although the patient gender is required, the ethnic designation is not.

Cibas ES, Ducatman BS. Cytology: Diagnostic Principles and Clinical Correlates. 3rd ed. Philadelphia: Saunders; 2009:500

63 **d** <3 negative Pap tests in the previous 7 years

According to Medicare, a screening (high risk) Pap test includes the following: early onset of sexual activity (<16 years of age); multiple sexual partners (25 in lifetime); history of STD (including HIV); DES exposure or abnormal Pap within past 3 years (women of child bearing age only).

Cibas ES, Ducatman BS. Cytology: Diagnostic Principles and Clinical Correlates. 3rd ed. Philadelphia: Saunders; 2009:505

64 **d** review of the manual must be performed by the Technical Supervisor

The cytology procedure manual must be reviewed by the Technical Supervisor who is the pathologist in charge of the cytology laboratory. Frequency of review is determined by the regulatory body that surveys and accredits the laboratory. Annual review of the laboratory procedure manual is good practice and is required by some regulatory agencies.

Keebler, CM Somrak, TM. The Manual of Cytotechnology. Recordkeeping practices, p338-340

65 **d** determining individual ASC:SIL ratios

Tracking ASC:SIL ratios alone does not address accuracy but can be useful in identifying individuals who may need additional training. A cytotechnologist's ASC:SIL ratio should be calculated based on the diagnosis they submit to the pathologist. The pathologists' ASC:SIL ratio should be calculated based on their final diagnosis.

Cibas, ES Ducatman, BS. Cytology: Diagnostic Principles and Clinical Correlates Second Edition. 2003. Saunders, p474

66 **a** none

Pap tests signed out by MDs or DOs who are certified in Anatomic Pathology by the American Board of Pathology or the American Osteopathic Board of Pathology, or who possess qualifications that are equivalent to those required for the above certifications, are not subject to rescreening requirements.

DeMay, A&S 2e. CLIA '88, p1583-1588

67 **d** participate in an annual CMS approved proficiency testing program with an individual passing score of at least 90%

CLIA '88 requires individuals to be tested annually if they evaluate gynecologic cytology samples. CMS approved proficiency testing currently consists of a 10 glass slide test and constitutes a recertification of the individual rather than the composite laboratory performance.

DeMay, A&S 2e. CLIA '88, p1583-1588

68 **a** any sign of symptom related to a gynecologic disorder

A Pap test on a patient presenting with a gynecologic disorder is defined by Medicare as a "diagnostic" high risk Pap test. The other choices represent examples of high risk "screening" Pap tests.

Cibas ES, Ducatman BS. Cytology: Diagnostic Principles and Clinical Correlates. 3rd ed. Philadelphia: Saunders; 2009:505

69 **a** a concept of using well defined statistical tools and measures to improve processes

6 Sigma is a well defined concept employing a host of statistical tools, such as control charts, to measure baseline performance of a process and develop methods for its subsequent improvement.

Chowdhury S. The Power of Six Sigma: An Inspiring Tale of How Six Sigma is Transforming the Way we Work.

70 **d** no, sharing this information violates HIPAA

All individuals are entitled under HIPAA to the privacy and confidentiality of their protected health information (PHI). Disclosure of the athlete's PHI to anyone without a need to know represents a HIPAA violation.

HIPAA. United States Public Law 104-191. Health Insurance Portability and Accountability Act of 1996 (HIPAA, Title II)

71 **c** provide the requested copies if the vendor has signed a business associate agreement with the laboratory

Generally, whenever a third party such as a service vendor accesses or uses protected health information provided by a covered entity for purposes other that the diagnosis and treatment of the patient, a business associate agreement is required.

HIPAA. United States Public Law 104-191. Health Insurance Portability and Accountability Act of 1996 (HIPAA, Title II)

72 **c** data from cytologic-histologic correlation

Cytology/histology correlation is required data in the annual cytology statistical report. Other requirements include: workload statistics, quality control records, number of specimens processed, and a breakdown of the number of specimens by diagnosis.

Keebler, CM Somrak, TM. The Manual of Cytotechnology 7e. Recordkeeping practices, p338

ISBN 978-089189-6357 ©ASCP 2015

73   **d**   the patient's records should be reviewed in private and consults should be done privately and only as needed

All patient's records should be kept confidential and released on a need to know basis only.

Perney S. HIPAA Training Handbook for the Healthcare Staff; An Introduction to Confidentiality and Privacy Under HIPAA. USA: Opus Communications Inc.; 2002:12

74   **c**   cross contamination is best avoided by staining gynecologic and nongynecologic cases in separate staining setups

Cross contamination of one specimen by another is best prevented during staining, when separate gynecologic and nongynecologic staining setups are in place. If separate staining for these specimens cannot be performed, all stains and solutions should be changed and filtered between gynecologic and nongynecologic staining runs.

Keebler, CM Somrak, TM. The Manual of Cytotechnology 7e. Specimen preparation, p340

75   **c**   only the referring clinician may determine the risk classification

A Pap test on a patient presenting with a gynecologic disorder is defined by Medicare as a "diagnostic" high risk Pap test. The other choices represent examples of high risk "screening" Pap tests.

Cibas ES, Ducatman BS. Cytology: Diagnostic Principles and Clinical Correlates. 3rd ed. Philadelphia: Saunders; 2009:505

76   **b**   previous abnormal Pap test result

Quality control presignout rescreening should include a mix of randomly selected routine Pap tests and focused rescreening of high risk cases. Patients with a previous abnormal Pap test should be considered high risk and be targeted for focused quality control rescreening.

Keebler, CM Somrak, TM. The Manual of Cytotechnology. Record keeping practices, p342.

77   **d**   all employees

It is the responsibility of all employees of an organization to help keep the privacy of patients as they receive care. Also, they need to help protect the confidentiality of information that is given to them to provide for those patients.

Perney S. HIPAA Training Handbook for the Healthcare Staff; An Introduction to Confidentiality and Privacy Under HIPAA. USA: Opus Communications Inc.; 2002:30-31

78   **c**   be treated without further discussion

A patient cannot be denied treatment if they choose not to sign an authorization form for any reason.

Perney S. HIPAA Training Handbook for the Healthcare Staff; An Introduction to Confidentiality and Privacy Under HIPAA. USA: Opus Communications Inc.; 2002:18-19

79   **b**   this patient should have colposcopy

Since ASC-H identifies a patient population at high risk for CIN2/3, colposcopy is mandatory and not based on HPV triage. Initial colposcopy, biopsies and endocervical sampling may be falsely negative, though, and these patients should be followed with repeat Pap tests at 6 & 12 months or HPV testing at 12 months.

Stoler MH. Testing for human papillomavirus: data driven implications for cervical neoplasia management. Clin Lab Med 2003;23(3):569-583

80   **c**   manufacturer's procedure manuals for all laboratory instrumentation

While manufacturer's procedure manuals may be used as references or supplements to the laboratory's written procedures, they are not required in the procedure manual, nor can they serve as a replacement for specific procedures.

Cibas ES, Ducatman BS. Cytology: Diagnostic Principles and Clinical Correlates. 3rd ed. Philadelphia: Saunders; 2009:499

81   **d**   ASCUS

10% of negative cases must be rescreened prior to signout. Any case falling into a category of Epithelial Cell Abnormalities, including ASCUS, should not be counted towards the 10% QC rescreening requirement. This case could however be included in a laboratory's hierarchical review process for other reasons.

DeMay, A&S 2e. CLIA '88, p1583-1588

82   **d**   prior to reporting the negative result

Cases must be prospectively (presignout) quality control rescreened.

DeMay, A&S 2e. CLIA '88, p1583-1588

83   **b**   allowable error

Allowable error defines how far from the true value a test result can be and remain acceptable.

Snyder JR, Wilkinson DS, eds. Management in Laboratory Medicine. Process control and method evaluation, p302

84   **c**   job security

Primary needs are physiologic (food, clothing, shelter) and safety (from harm, disease, disaster). In the workplace, money is a motivator to satisfy physiologic needs, and such things as insurance benefits and job security satisfy safety needs. Acceptance, recognition, and job satisfaction are motivators to satisfy secondary needs in Maslow's Hierarchy.

Snyder JR, Wilkinson DS, eds. Management in Laboratory Medicine. Motivation—managerial assumptions and effects, p97-98

85   **a**   critical task

Critical tasks are those that are significant in the completion of a task but have little impact on outcomes when performed poorly. Essential tasks are those involving the utmost attention to detail and accuracy. Outcome metrics evaluate the performance, cost effectiveness, quality, and quantity of a task. Key job areas define major job roles and responsibilities.

Snyder JR, Wilkinson DS, eds. Management in Laboratory Medicine. Staffing and scheduling of laboratory personnel, p232

86   **b**   credentialing

Credentialing is the common term applied to the official acknowledgment of professional or technical competence. Peer assurance defines a voluntary process of subjecting to oversight by an external professional constituent organization; registration usually occurs at the state level and involves filing name and qualifications of a professional to practice; regulation refers to governmental control of an economic market.

Snyder JR, Wilkinson DS, eds. Management in Laboratory Medicine. Laboratory regulation, certification, and accreditation, p375

87 **a** unit

Examining unit costs identifies changes in the cost to produce a unit of service and enables monitoring of productivity.

Snyder JR, Wilkinson DS, eds. Management in Laboratory Medicine. Introduction to laboratory financial management, p465

88 **d** efficiency

Efficiency is the ratio of outputs to inputs. Production refers to a laboratory's ability to meet the organization's needs in terms of quality and quantity of laboratory testing. Adaptiveness relates to a laboratory's response to internal and external change forces. Development refers to operations investment over the long term.

Snyder JR, Wilkinson DS, eds. Management in Laboratory Medicine. Leadership styles and group effectiveness, p127

89 **c** Food and Drug Administration

The Food and Drug Administration regulates market entry of medical devices, laboratory instruments, and reagents and supplies under the Food, Drug and Cosmetic Act.

Snyder JR, Wilkinson DS, eds. Management in Laboratory Medicine. Laboratory regulation, certification, and accreditation, p385

90 **d** a not for profit hospital with annual receipts of $300,000

Amendments to the National Labor Relations Act apply to hospitals with annual receipts exceeding $250,000, nursing homes with receipts over $100,000 per year, and to voluntary not for profit health care institutions with receipts of $300,000 or more annually to NLRA regulation.

Snyder JR, Wilkinson DS, eds. Management in Laboratory Medicine. Labor relations and the clinical laboratory, p271

91 **b** res ipsa loquitor

Res ipsa loquitor, or "the thing speaks for itself," refers to negligence so apparent that the court shifts the burden of proof from the plaintiff to the defendant. Negligence per se exists when a practice is in direct violation of a state law or federal regulation that establishes a standard of care. Respondeat superior, or "look to the one higher up," is the legal doctrine by which plaintiffs can sue an employer for the negligent actions of an employee. Negligence ipso facto is nonsense.

Snyder JR, Wilkinson DS, eds. Management in Laboratory Medicine. Medicolegal concerns in laboratory medicine, p412

92 **a** require employees to set their own goals and objectives

Theory Y managers motivate staff by allowing them to direct and control themselves. Theory X managers structure, control, and closely supervise their staff under the assumption that they are incapable of doing it for themselves.

Snyder JR, Wilkinson DS, eds. Management in Laboratory Medicine. Managerial assumptions and effects, p101

93 **b** variable

Fixed costs remain unchanged over time, while variable costs fluctuate in proportion to volume. Direct costs include all those that can be specifically associated with a test, while indirect costs, or overhead, are the costs included in the expense of operating a laboratory.

Snyder JR, Wilkinson DS, eds. Management in Laboratory Medicine. Introduction to laboratory financial management, p463-465

94 **b** Equal Employment Opportunity Commission

Title VII of the Civil Rights Act guarantees equality to all people and is enforced by the Equal Employment Opportunity Commission. Affirmative Action refers to programs designed to reverse the effects of discrimination.

Snyder JR, Wilkinson DS, eds. Management in Laboratory Medicine. Interviewing and employee selection, p198

95 **d** full

As methods for accumulating direct and indirect costs of operation, direct costing allocates all direct costs to the laboratory while full costing assigns indirect costs to the laboratory. Standard costs indicate the total cost of efficient operation.

Snyder JR, Wilkinson DS, eds. Management in Laboratory Medicine. Introduction to laboratory financial management, p465

96 **a** hygiene factors and satisfiers

The combination of hygiene factors and satisfiers tends to produce strong employee motivation.

Snyder JR, Wilkinson DS, eds. Management in Laboratory Medicine. Motivation—managerial assumptions and effects, p99-100

97 **b** respondeat superior

Respondeat superior is the legal doctrine by which employers are responsible for the actions of employees. Res ipsa loquitor addresses negligence that is so obvious that the court shifts the burden of proof away from the plaintiff and toward the defendant. Locum tenens is a temporary substitute for a doctor or clergy member. Procedenti ab utroque is a phrase from a Latin hymn.

Snyder JR, Wilkinson DS, eds. Management in Laboratory Medicine. Medicolegal concerns in laboratory medicine, p413

98 **b** Do you have any relatives employed by this company?

It is legal to inquire about relatives who may work for the same company in order to abide by requirements of nepotism policies. It is not legal to ask for the names of family members specifically, except to ask whom to notify in case of emergency. It is legal to inquire about convictions, but not arrests. Employers may ask about impairments that would interfere with ability to perform the job, but not about disabilities in general. Questions as to form of address can be construed as attempts to identify marital status or gender, both of which are unlawful questions.

Snyder JR, Wilkinson DS, eds. Management in Laboratory Medicine. Interviewing and employee selection, p201

99 **b** National Labor Relations Act

Labor relations are regulated through the National Labor Relations Act for the private sector and through the Civil Service Reform Act for the federal sector.

Snyder JR, Wilkinson DS, eds. Management in Laboratory Medicine. Labor relations and the clinical laboratory, p269

ISBN 978-089189-6357 ©ASCP 2015

100 a   slope of the line

The slope of the regression line reflects proportional bias. The Y intercept of the line detects constant bias, and the standard error determines the scatter of plots about the line. The correlation coefficient is not well suited for method comparison studies in the clinical lab, owing to its variability with the distribution of data.

Snyder JR, Wilkinson DS, eds. Management in Laboratory Medicine. Process control and method evaluation, p317

101 c   salary and promotion decisions

The most commonly cited reason for conducting employee performance evaluation is as a means to make decisions related to salary and promotion.

Snyder JR, Wilkinson DS, eds. Management in Laboratory Medicine. Standards and appraisals of laboratory performance, p246

102 d   measure to which like objects are expected to conform

A standard is a measure to which like objects are expected to conform. A criterion is a reference used in forming judgments.

Snyder JR, Wilkinson DS, eds. Management in Laboratory Medicine. Interviewing and employee selection, p195-219

103 c   40

The ADEA provides protection against age discrimination to workers over 70 years of age and eliminates mandatory retirement. Amendments also protect workers over age 40 from discriminatory practices related to paid benefits or continued employment.

Snyder JR, Wilkinson DS, eds. Management in Laboratory Medicine. Interviewing and employee selection, p199

104 d   Federal Labor Relations Authority

Collective bargaining in the federal sector is overseen by the Federal Labor Relations Authority.

Snyder JR, Wilkinson DS, eds. Management in Laboratory Medicine. Labor relations and the clinical laboratory, p270

105 b   hygiene

Hygiene or environmental factors are related to dissatisfaction, the absence of which encourages unacceptable performance. Motivators are related to job satisfaction and encourage performance above accepted levels.

Snyder JR, Wilkinson DS, eds. Management in Laboratory Medicine. Motivation—managerial assumptions and effects, p99-100

106 a   Pareto diagram

A Pareto diagram is best suited for use in determining the significance of data. Fishbone, or cause and effect, diagrams are useful in distinguishing the true cause of an observed effect from randomly associated causes. Scatter diagrams plot 2 characteristics on an X&Y axis to determine the existence of relationship between the characteristics. Affinity diagrams are useful in defining groups of items from among large quantities of descriptive or verbal data.

Snyder JR, Wilkinson DS, eds. Management in Laboratory Medicine. Problem solving—the decision making process, p69

107 b   respondeat superior

Respondeat superior, or "look to the one higher up," is the legal doctrine by which plaintiffs can sue an employer for the negligent actions of an employee. Res ipsa loquitor, or "the thing speaks for itself," refers to negligence so apparent that the court shifts the burden of proof from the plaintiff to the defendant. Negligence per se exists when a practice is in direct violation of a state law or federal regulation that establishes a standard of care. Compar sit laudatio is a phrase from a Latin hymn.

Snyder JR, Wilkinson DS, eds. Management in Laboratory Medicine. Medico legal concerns in laboratory medicine, p413

108 a   reference sample

The reference sample method assesses laboratory performance by examining the results of tests repeated on same and different days for the ability to repeat identical and accurate results consistently.

Snyder JR, Wilkinson DS, eds. Management in Laboratory Medicine. Process control and method evaluation, p293

109 c   referent

Referent power arises solely from a leader's personality. Reward power uses the expectation of gaining substantial gain. Expert power results from the use of specialized cognitive knowledge or technical skill. Legitimate power is the authority arising from the formal organizational structure.

Snyder JR, Wilkinson DS, eds. Management in Laboratory Medicine. Leadership styles and group effectiveness, p130

110 c   bias

Failure to control for bias is the most common reason for CLIA PT failure.

Snyder JR, Wilkinson DS, eds. Management in Laboratory Medicine. Process control and method evaluation, p310

111 d   acceptable standard deviation

In the development of a Westgard process control system, managers must decide on a number of factors, including error rate, false rejection rate, and number of controls, but the most important decision is setting the standard deviation for the analysis, as it determines acceptance or rejection of data.

Snyder JR, Wilkinson DS, eds. Management in Laboratory Medicine. Process control and method evaluation, p300

112 a   introvert, intuiting, thinking, judging

The personality described is that of an intuiting, thinking, judging introvert.

Snyder JR, Wilkinson DS, eds. Management in Laboratory Medicine. Leadership styles and group effectiveness, p138-141

113 c   precision

The ability of a laboratory test to detect minute amounts of an analyte is a measure of the test's sensitivity. Specificity refers to the ability of an analysis to reliably detect a specific element in the presence of possible confounding factors. Accuracy refers to how close to the true value of an analyte a test can measure. Precision relates to the ability of a test to consistently measure at the same value with repeated performance over time.

Snyder JR, Wilkinson DS, eds. Management in Laboratory Medicine. Process control and method evaluation, p319

114 b   sensitivity

The ability of a laboratory test to detect minute amounts of an analyte is a measure of the test's sensitivity. Specificity refers to the ability of an analysis to reliably detect a specific element in the presence of possible confounding factors. Accuracy refers to how close to the true value of an analyte a test can measure. Precision relates to the ability of a test to consistently measure at the same value with repeated performance over time.

Snyder JR, Wilkinson DS, eds. Management in Laboratory Medicine. Process control and method evaluation, p319

115 a   dispersion

Data points tend to be either dispersed or contracted with a change in precision. Trends are seen when the testing conditions worsen over time, and shifts may be caused by changes in method or reagents.

Snyder JR, Wilkinson DS, eds. Management in Laboratory Medicine. Process control and method evaluation, p298

116 d   regulation

Regulation is the term applied to the governmental control of an economic market for the purpose of public protection.

Snyder JR, Wilkinson DS, eds. Management in Laboratory Medicine. Laboratory regulation, certification, and accreditation, p371

117 d   Department of Defense drug surveillance facilities

Facilities subject to regulation by the Substance and Mental Health Services Administration are exempt from CLIA '88, including drug surveillance facilities in the Department of Defense.

DeMay, A&S 2e. CLIA '88, p1583-1588

ISBN 978-089189-6357 ©ASCP 2015

Chapter 11

Molecular Techniques & Special Stains

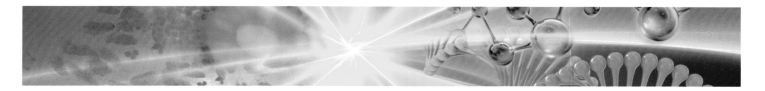

1   One of the principal preparation differences between the Romanowsky and Papanicolaou stains is:
   a   air drying artifact is associated with the Romanowsky stain
   b   increased cell adherence to the slide is associated with the Romanowsky stain
   c   alcohol fixation is mandatory for Romanowsky staining
   d   an increased propensity for "floaters" within the Romanowsky stain due to cells falling off the prepared slides

2   Which of the following cellular elements are best visualized with the Romanowsky stain when compared with the Papanicolaou stain?
   a   mucin
   b   keratin
   c   viral changes
   d   euchromatin

3   What morphologic enhancements does the Romanowsky stain have over the Papanicolaou stain?
   a   the Romanowsky stain enables better differentiation of nuclear chromasia
   b   the Romanowsky stain is more helpful when analyzing 3D tissue fragments
   c   the cellular morphology demonstrated with the Romanowsky stain is akin to that seen with H&E
   d   the Romanowsky stain is a metachromatic stain enabling better visualization of various mucins, neurosecretory granules, and stromal elements

4   Which of the following special stains may prove useful when differentiating plasmacytomas from small cell cleaved lymphomas?
   a   rhodanine
   b   Congo red
   c   PAS
   d   methyl green pyronine

5   A 63-year-old male with a 50 year history of moderate alcohol intake now presents with multiple liver nodules. Cellular morphology reveals cells that suggest a diagnosis of cholangiocarcinoma over hepatocellular carcinoma. Which of the following enzyme reactions would help confirm this suspicion?
   a   aminopeptidase
   b   acid phosphatase
   c   aryl sulfatase
   d   lysozyme

6   A 55-year-old female with a prior history of partial colectomy for rectal cancer now presents with a 1.5 cm solitary lung mass. Cellular morphology reveals cells that more closely resemble bronchogenic adenocarcinoma rather than metastatic colonic adenocarcinoma. Which of the following enzyme reactions will confirm lung primary over a metastatic colonic carcinoma?
   a   alcian blue
   b   Congo red
   c   alkaline phosphatase
   d   lysosyme

7   The periodic acid-Schiff (PAS) stain verifies the presence of:
   a   keratohyalin granules
   b   hyaluronic acid
   c   carbohydrate moieties
   d   neutral mucin

8   Which of the following special stains is useful when determining muscle fibers?
   a   argentaffin silver stain
   b   oil red O
   c   methyl green pyronine
   d   Masson trichrome

9   Epithelial lesions are immunocytochemically positive for which of the following intermediate filaments?
   a   keratin
   b   vimentin
   c   desmin
   d   actin

10 Immunocytochemical markers are helpful because:
   a they are specific for specific tumor types
   b the FDA must approve them for use before testing begins
   c they often aid in the diagnosis of lesions that are difficult to classify
   d they do not require confirmation by additional diagnostic studies

11 Melanomas may react to all of the following immunocytochemical markers, except:
   a S100
   b epithelial membrane antigen
   c vimentin
   d factor VIII

12 Which of the following special stains may be helpful in differentiating spindle cell neoplasms?
   a melanin
   b phosphotungstic acid-hematoxylin
   c orcein stain
   d Congo red

13 Which of the following intermediate filament immunocytochemical markers will help identify the possibility of a rhabdomyosarcoma?
   a desmin
   b vimentin
   c glial fibrillary acidic protein (GFIP)
   d neurofilament

14 Carcinoid tumors may be confirmed with which of the special stains?
   a PAS
   b argentaffin
   c rubeanic acid
   d alcian blue

15 High molecular weight keratin is expressed in which of the following lesions?
   a dysgerminoma
   b endodermal sinus tumor
   c squamous cell carcinoma
   d malignant lymphoma

16 Electron microscopy was performed due to the unknown histogenesis of a liver lesion thought to be metastatic. Features revealed intracellular lumens forming flocculent filled acini lined by microvilli. Which of the following lesions is likely?
   a squamous cell carcinoma
   b adenocarcinoma
   c sarcoma
   d lymphoma

17 The distinction of hemosiderin laden macrophages from malignant melanoma may be aided by:
   a Nile blue sulfate
   b iron stain
   c GMS
   d alcian blue

18 The identification of lipid is best achieved with what special stain?
   a Nile blue sulfate
   b Sudan black
   c Giemsa
   d Feulgen

19 When differentiating metastatic hepatocellular carcinoma (HCC) from melanoma, α-fetoprotein would stain:
   a positive for HCC, negative for melanoma
   b negative for HCC, positive for melanoma
   c positive for both
   d negative for both

20 Which special stain may aid in the diagnosis of metastatic melanoma?
   a keratin
   b neuron specific enolase
   c S100
   d LCA

21 What special stain is most helpful in identifying *Pneumocystis jiroveci*?
   a iron
   b Feulgen
   c GMS
   d mucicarmine

22 Well differentiated mucus producing adenocarcinomas may be distinguished from poorly differentiated squamous cell carcinomas by using:
   a mucicarmine
   b Giemsa
   c Gram-Weigert
   d Feulgen

23 The identification of fungi may be determined best with what special stain?
   a GMS
   b oil red O
   c Biebrich-Scarlet
   d iron

24 The Feulgen reaction is used for the identification of:
   a DNA
   b melanin
   c fat
   d glycogen

25 Which special stain may aid in differentiating histiocytes from mesothelial cells?
   a Feulgen
   b Prussian blue
   c Rakoff
   d neutral red-Janus green

ISBN 978-089189-6357 ©ASCP 2015

26 What immunocytochemical stain will help differentiate malignant lymphoma from a neuroendocrine tumor?
   a keratin; lymphoma is positive, neuroendocrine tumors are negative
   b HMB45; lymphoma is positive, neuroendocrine tumors are negative
   c leukocyte common antigen; lymphoma is positive, neuroendocrine tumors are negative
   d PAS; lymphomas are negative, neuroendocrine tumors are positive

27 Immunocytochemistry might be helpful in differentiating pancreatic adenocarcinoma (PAC) from hepatocellular carcinoma (HCC) by staining with:
   a keratin; HCC is positive, PAC is negative
   b α-fetoprotein; HCC is positive, PAC is negative
   c keratin; HCC is negative, PAC is positive
   d immunocytochemistry is not helpful in distinguishing these tumors

28 What immunocytochemical stain will have a positive staining reaction and help in the confirmation of a metastatic sarcoma?
   a keratin
   b vimentin
   c α-fetoprotein
   d neuron specific enolase

29 Metastatic colonic adenocarcinoma to the liver could be differentiated from primary hepatocellular carcinoma (HCC) by using what immunocytochemical stain?
   a keratin–low molecular weight (CAM5.2); HCC is strongly positive, colonic adenocarcinoma is negative
   b keratin–high molecular weight (AE1/AE3); HCC is negative to weakly positive, colonic adenocarcinoma is strongly positive
   c HMB45; HCC is positive, colonic adenocarcinoma is negative
   d S100; HCC is negative, colonic adenocarcinoma is positive

30 Most fungi will stain positive with which of the following special stains?
   a PAS
   b Nile blue sulfate
   c Shorr
   d Rakoff

31 Immunocytochemical staining for chromogranin is helpful for the identification of:
   a lymphoma
   b adenocarcinoma
   c squamous carcinoma
   d carcinoid tumors

32 Small cell carcinoma may be differentiated from malignant lymphoma by using what special stain?
   a chromogranin
   b S100
   c HMB45
   d α-fetoprotein

33 If staining for glycogen, which special stain is required?
   a mucicarmine
   b PAS
   c Nile blue sulfate
   d neutral red

34 What immunocytochemical stain might help in differentiating metastatic pleomorphic carcinoma of the pancreas from metastatic fibrous histiocytoma (MFH) in liver aspirations?
   a keratin; positive for carcinoma, negative for MFH
   b keratin; negative for carcinoma, positive for MFH
   c HMB45; positive for carcinoma, negative for MFH
   d HMB45; negative for carcinoma, positive for MFH

35 *Cryptococcus* may be identified best with what special stain?
   a mucicarmine
   b Gram
   c PAS-D
   d Janus green

36 HMB45 may be a useful marker for determining the presence of:
   a undifferentiated squamous carcinoma
   b hepatocellular carcinoma
   c poorly differentiated adenocarcinoma
   d metastatic melanoma

37 A helpful stain for the identification of hematopoietic and lymphoid cells is:
   a Gram
   b PAS
   c Romanowsky
   d mucicarmine

38 A false positive immunohistochemical result may be due to:
   a destruction of antigens in the specimen by air drying
   b use of outdated reagents
   c antibody crossreactivity with antigens other than the one evaluated for by the test
   d overheating of cell block material

39 A false negative immunocytochemical result may be due to:
   a ineffective blocking of endogenous enzymes
   b use of outdated reagents
   c antibody crossreactivity with antigens other than the one evaluated for by the test
   d interpretation of background melanin pigment

40 Diff-Quik stained, air dried preparations from a thyroid aspiration as best utilized for:
   a accentuating nuclear detail
   b highlighting colloid and amyloid
   c optimizing cellularity
   d eliminating obscuring colloid

41 The main advantage of in situ hybridization (ISH) for pathology is:
    a ISH amplifies DNA and/or RNA
    b ISH detects and localizes specific DNA or RNA sequences within morphologically preserved cells and tissue
    c ISH is a commercially prepared technique, that requires no validation
    d ISH detects and localizes specific DNA or RNA sequences, which have been amplified

42 A 69-year-old male had a nephrectomy 2 years prior for conventional renal cell carcinoma. He recently noted a nonpainful mass in the subcutaneous tissue around his left elbow, which had been slowly enlarging over several weeks. Which of the following panels of immunohistochemical markers would best support your interpretation?
    a CK20+, PSA–, uroplakin+
    b CK7–, CD10+, renal cell carcinoma antigen (RCA+)
    c CK7–, CK20–, RCA–
    d WT1+, CK–, EMA+

43 An aspirate is performed of a lower back soft tissue mass of a 38-year-old male. A differential consideration of schwannoma would stain positive with which of the following immunostains?
    a CD34
    b c-kit (CD117)
    c S100
    d CD68

ISBN 978-089189-6357 ©ASCP 2015

44 A bronchoalveolar lavage is performed on a 40-year-old male with fever, cough and patchy radiologic opacities of his lungs, bilaterally. Which of the stains listed below would yield a more definitive diagnosis of the process shown in the image above?

a iron stain
b Gomori methenamine silver stain
c Congo red stain
d trichrome stain

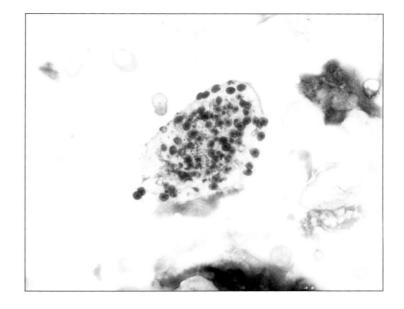

45 In the pleural fluid cell block preparation shown in the image, the differential diagnosis is metastatic adenocarcinoma vs mesothelioma. Which panel will be most helpful?

a B72.3, carcinoembryonic antigen (CEA), vimentin, leukocyte common antigen
b B72.3, MOC31, BerEP4, calretinin
c calretinin, vimentin, leukocyte common antigen, chromogranin
d calretinin, S100, thyroid transcription factor, CEA

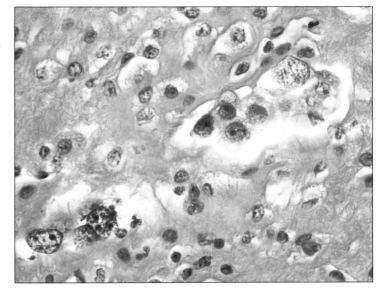

46 Which immunostain would help confirm the morphologic impression depicted in this image from an aspirate of a 4 cm mass in the liver of a 68-year-old female?

a TTF1
b inhibin
c HepPar 1
d CD10

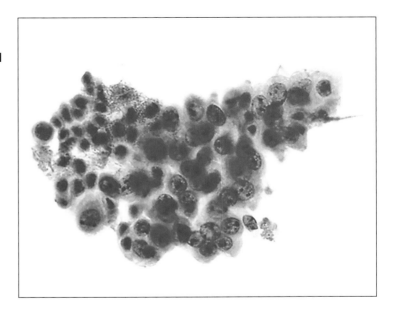

47 Which positive immunostain from the aspirate of a
    3 cm liver mass in a 73-year-old male would help
    confirm the morphologic impression?
    a HepPar1
    b CDX2
    c chromogranin
    d PSA

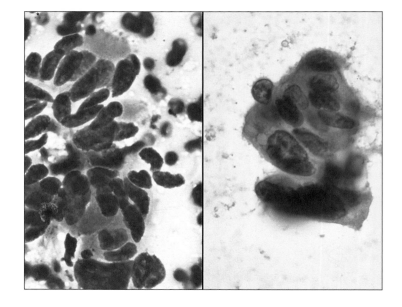

48 Which immunostain from this aspirate of a 4 cm mass
    in the right kidney of a 64-year-old female would
    confirm the morphologic impression?
    a CD10
    b CK7/CK20
    c CDX2
    d EMA

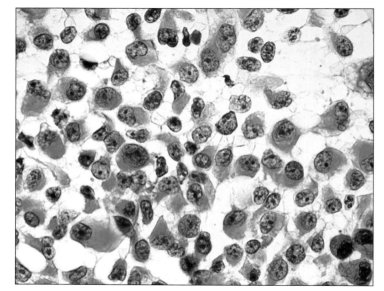

49 A supraclavicular lymph node FNA from a
    24-year-old male is suspicious for Hodgkin disease.
    Reed-Sternberg cells are diagnostic for Hodgkin
    lymphoma and are identified with the following cell
    marker:
    a α fetoprotein
    b CD15/LeuM1
    c B-72.3
    d Leu7

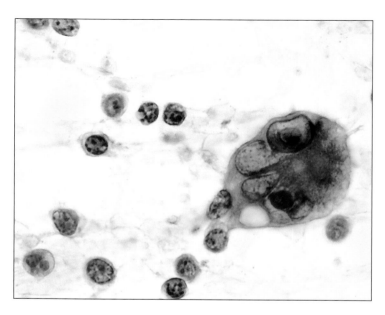

ISBN 978-089189-6357 ©ASCP 2015

Molecular Techniques & Special Stains
Answer Key

1 **b** **increased cell adherence to the slide is associated with the Romanowsky stain**

Air drying is generally the first step in the Romanowsky or Diff-Quik stains, allowing for better cellular adhesion to the slide and decreasing the likelihood that cells will "fall off" the slide, as will often occur when immersing fresh specimens into the alcoholic medium for fixation for compatibility with the Papanicolaou stain. It should be noted, though, that Romanowsky staining is compatible with alcohol fixed material, yields excellent cytoplasmic detail, and helps with visualization of stromal components.

DeMay, A&S 2e. Romanowsky stain, p1505

2 **a** **mucin**

Air drying is generally the first step in the Romanowsky or Diff-Quik stains, allowing for better cellular adhesion to the slide and decreasing the likelihood that cells will "fall off" the slide, as will often occur when immersing fresh specimens into the alcoholic medium for fixation for compatibility with the Papanicolaou stain. It should be noted, though, that Romanowsky staining is compatible with alcohol fixed material, yields excellent cytoplasmic detail, and helps with visualization of stromal components.

DeMay, A&S 2e. Romanowsky stain, p1505

3 **d** **the Romanowsky stain is a metachromatic stain enabling better visualization of various mucins, neurosecretory granules, and stromal elements**

Air drying is generally the first step in the Romanowsky or Diff-Quik stains, allowing for better cellular adhesion to the slide and decreasing the likelihood that cells will "fall off" the slide, as will often occur when immersing fresh specimens into the alcoholic medium for fixation for compatibility with the Papanicolaou stain. It should be noted, though, that Romanowsky staining is compatible with alcohol fixed material, yields excellent cytoplasmic detail, and helps with visualization of stromal components.

DeMay, A&S 2e. Romanowsky stain, p1505

4 **d** **methyl green pyronine**

Methyl green pyronine (MGP) binds to the cytoplasm and/or nucleus of cells with abundant RNA (endoplasmic reticulum or pronounced nucleoli). Cell markers such as leukocyte common antigen (LCA) are usually negative with plasma cells and therefore may also be helpful in differentiating these 2 malignancies.

DeMay, A&S 2e. Methyl green pyronine (MSP) stain, p1506

5 **a** **aminopeptidase**

Aminopeptidase positivity suggests bile duct, kidney, bladder, or stomach origin rather than hepatocellular carcinoma. Negative staining with α-fetoprotein, an oncofetal glycoprotein, may be helpful in this case but does not necessarily exclude hepatocellular carcinoma. Antinuclear staining for bile canaliculi may also have utility.

DeMay, A&S 2e. Aminopeptidase, p1507

6 **c** **alkaline phosphatase**

Alkaline phosphatase, although nonspecific, reacts with adenocarcinomas including those from the lung, ovary, endometrium, or kidneys but does not react with lesions of gastrointestinal tract origin. In this case, a positive reaction would exclude the probability that the patient has a metastatic colonic adenocarcinoma and may verify a new primary malignancy. Aryl sulfatase, on the other hand, would react just the opposite, failing to react with the suspected bronchogenic tumor. If it were suspected that the cells were metastatic from the colon, a positive reaction would be seen.

DeMay, A&S 2e. Alkaline phosphatase, p1507

7 **c** **carbohydrate moieties**

Periodic acid-Schiff stain will color fungi, carbohydrates, and glycogen as magenta red.

DeMay, A&S 2e. Periodic acid-Schiff (PAS) stain, p1506

8 **d** **Masson trichrome**

Masson trichrome stains will help identify skeletal or smooth muscle differentiation vs nonmuscle fibers.

DeMay, A&S 2e. Masson trichrome, p1506

9 **c** **desmin**

Epithelial tumors are generally positive for keratin and soft tissue tumors are positive for vimentin, but not exclusively. Certain tumors of both categories such as renal cell carcinoma and synovial sarcoma as well as Wilms tumor and mesotheliomas are some of the lesions that crossreact with both immunocytochemical stains.

DeMay, A&S 2e. Desmin, p1517

10 **c** **they often aid in the diagnosis of lesions that are difficult to classify**

Immunocytochemical stains are useful but are often not specific. It is reasonable that other diagnostic procedures be performed to rule on the sensitivity of immunocytochemical markers. They can often be as misleading as they are useful.

DeMay, A&S 2e. Immunocytochemistry, p1507

11 **d** **factor VIII**

Factor VIII marks endothelial components only.

DeMay, A&S 2e. Factor VIII related antigen, p17

12 **a** **melanin**

Spindle cell melanomas and clear cell sarcoma can be differentiated from other spindle cell or pleomorphic sarcomas owing to their melanin positivity.

DeMay, A&S 2e. Melanin stains, melanocytic proteins, p1517

13 **c** **glial fibrillary acidic protein (GFIP)**

Vimentin is found in mesenchymal cells and sarcomas, desmin is found in all kinds of muscle tissue but is more sensitive to skeletal muscle, neurofilaments are found in neuronal tumors, and glial acidic proteins mark glial supportive cells of the central nervous system.

DeMay, A&S 2e. Glial fibrillary acidic protein (GFAP), p1517

14 b argentaffin

Silver stains may be useful when demonstrating neurosecretory granules from neuroendocrine lesions such as carcinoid tumors, small cell carcinomas, islet cell tumors, medullary carcinomas, paragangliomas, and neuroblastomas. However, immunocytochemical staining with neuron specific enolase or chromogranin may prove more useful.

DeMay, A&S 2e. Chromaffin, argentaffin & argyrophil staining, p1506

15 c squamous cell carcinoma

High molecular weight keratin is expressed in squamous cell carcinomas and mesotheliomas, whereas low molecular weight keratins are expressed in all cell lines with epithelial differentiation, such as endodermal, neuroectodermal, mesenchymal, or germ cell tumors.

DeMay, A&S 2e. Cytokeratin, p1515

16 b adenocarcinoma

In contrast to adenocarcinomas and lymphomas, squamous cell carcinomas would reveal tonofilaments such as intercellular bridges (desmosomes) and microvilli attached at their tips by desmosomes.

DeMay, A&S 2e. Uranyl acetate and lead citrate stain (electron microscopy), p1524

17 b iron stain

PAS stains for hemosiderin and may prove useful in discriminating hemosiderin laden macrophages from melanoma. These benign cells are also immunocytochemically negative for S100, HMB45, melan A and MITF (microphthalmia associated transcription factor)—all which are positive in a high percentage of melanomas.

DeMay, A&S 2e. The cytoplasm, p1487

18 b Sudan black

Sudan black will stain phospholipids black.

DeMay, A&S 2e. Lipid, p1506

19 a positive for HCC, negative for melanoma

α-fetoprotein will positively distinguish hepatocellular carcinoma from melanoma but will not differentiate liver cell dysplasias and germ cell neoplasms.

DeMay, A&S 2e. α-fetoprotein, p1522

20 c S100

S100, HMB45, melan A or MITF (microphthalmia associated transcription factor) all preferentially react with melanoma cells.

DeMay, A&S 2e. S100 protein, p1510

21 c GMS

Gomori methenamine silver stains for fungi and *Pneumocystis jiroveci*. These infectious agents will stain characteristically gray to black.

DeMay, A&S 2e. Pneumocystis jiroveci, p1472

22 a mucicarmine

Mucicarmine stains for intracellular mucin, found within mucus producing glandular lesions. Mucin will stain rose to red in color.

DeMay, A&S 2e. Mucicarmine, p1506

23 a GMS

Gomori methenamine silver stains for fungi and *Pneumocystis jiroveci*. These infectious agents will stain characteristically gray to black.

DeMay, A&S 2e. Fungus, p1470

24 a DNA

The Feulgen reaction will positively stain double stranded nucleic acid deep red to purple in color. RNA does not stain with Feulgen.

Koss LG. Diagnostic cytology. Cytologic techniques/principles of operation of a laboratory of cytology, p1492-1505

25 d neutral red-Janus green

Neutral red-Janus green, a supravital stain that must be performed on nonfixed specimens, will positively identify white blood cells and histiocytes from mesothelial cells.

Koss LG. Diagnostic cytology. Cytologic techniques/principles of operation of a laboratory of cytology, p1492-1505

26 c leukocyte common antigen; lymphoma is positive, neuroendocrine tumors are negative

Neuroendocrine tumors such as carcinoid tumors, small cell carcinomas, neuroblastomas, medullary tumors of the thyroid, and pituitary tumors may stain positive with chromogranin or neuron specific enolase. Lymphomas are positive for common leukocytic antigen.

DeMay, A&S 2e. Other cell markers, p18

27 b α-fetoprotein; HCC is positive, PAC is negative

α-fetoprotein will positively distinguish hepatocellular carcinoma from melanoma but will not differentiate liver cell dysplasias and germ cell neoplasms.

DeMay, A&S 2e. α-fetoprotein, p1522

28 b vimentin

Vimentin will strongly express positivity in cells of mesenchymal origin.

DeMay, A&S 2e. Vimentin, p1516

29 b keratin—high molecular weight (AE1/AE3); HCC is negative to weakly positive, colonic adenocarcinoma is strongly positive

Only high molecular weight (MW) keratin is effective in discriminating these lesions. Low MW keratin will positively identify both neoplasms with equal intensity.

DeMay, A&S 2e. Cytokeratin, p1514

30 a PAS

Periodic acid-Schiff stain will color fungi, carbohydrates, and glycogen as magenta red.

DeMay, A&S 2e. Periodic acid-Schiff (PAS) stain, p1506

ISBN 978-089189-6357 ©ASCP 2015

31 **d** **carcinoid tumors**

Neuroendocrine tumors such as carcinoid tumors, small cell carcinomas, neuroblastomas, medullary tumors of the thyroid, and pituitary tumors may stain positive with chromogranin or neuron specific enolase.

DeMay, A&S 2e. Chromogranin, p1519

32 **a** **chromogranin**

Lymphomas are positive for common leukocytic antigen.

DeMay, A&S 2e. Chromogranin, p1519

33 **b** **PAS**

Neuroendocrine tumors such as carcinoid tumors, small cell carcinomas, neuroblastomas, medullary tumors of the thyroid, and pituitary tumors may stain positive with chromogranin or neuron specific enolase.

DeMay, A&S 2e. Periodic acid-Schiff (PAS) stain, p1506

34 **a** **keratin; positive for carcinoma, negative for MFH**

Keratin intermediate filaments will identify pancreatic carcinomas as epithelial lesions but will not stain malignant fibrous histiocytoma. However, keratin may be co-expressed in muscle sarcomas, synovial sarcomas, epithelioid sarcomas, and Wilms tumors.

DeMay, A&S 2e. Filaments, p1514

35 **a** **mucicarmine**

The mucinous capsule of *Cryptococcus neoformans* will stain rose to red.

DeMay, A&S 2e. Cryptococcus neoformans, p1471

36 **d** **metastatic melanoma**

HMB45 preferentially reacts with melanoma cells.

DeMay, A&S 2e. HMB45, 1517

37 **c** **Romanowsky**

The Romanowsky stains may be used to analyze lymphoreticular and hematopoietic specimens that are air dried. This stain may prove particularly useful when differentiating lymphopoietic malignancies.

DeMay, A&S 2e. HMB45, p1505

38 **c** **antibody crossreactivity with antigens other than the one evaluated for by the test**

False positive immunohistochemical results may be due to antibody crossreactivity with antigens, drying of the cells during the collection, fixation or staining procedures, inappropriate fixation, ineffective blocking of endogenous enzymes, binding to endogenous biotin, nonspecific binding of the antibody to Fc receptors or binding of the biotinylated label to avidin in the tissues. Choices a, b & d may cause false negative results.

Koss LG, Melamed KR. Koss' Diagbostic Cytology and Its Histopathologic Bases 4e, p1540

39 **b** **use of outdated reagents**

False negative immunocytochemical results may be due to use of outdated reagents. The problems in choices a, c & d are at particular risk for a false positive interpretation.

Koss LG, Melamed KR. Koss' Diagbostic Cytology and Its Histopathologic Bases 4e, p1540

40 **b** **highlighting colloid and amyloid**

As Diff-Quik stained air dried smears nicely illustrate extracellular matrix/material, they assist in highlighting colloid and amyloid in thyroid FNAs.

DeMay, A&S 2e. Diff-Quik staining, 1505

41 **b** **ISH detects and localizes specific DNA or RNA sequences within morphologically preserved cells and tissue**

The benefit of in situ hybridization (ISH) to pathology is that the context of the morphologically preserved cells and tissue remains, while DNA and/or RNA sequences are detected and localized. The ISH techniques routinely used in pathology include fluorescence in situ hybridization and chromogenic in situ hybridization.

DeMay, A&S 2e. In situ hybridization (ISH) techniques, p1529-1530

42 **b** **CK7–, CD10+, Renal cell carcinoma antigen (RCA+)**

Renal cell carcinoma, conventional type, should be CK7–, CD10+ and RCA +. Chromophobe renal cell carcinoma will stain positively for CK7 in contrast to conventional renal cell carcinoma. Chromophobe renal cell carcinoma will not stain for CD10. Conventional clear cell carcinoma with eosinophilia will not stain for parvalbumin, c-kit, or Ksp cadherin. Any panel to detect renal cell carcinoma should contain both positive and negative staining antibody reagents.

DeMay, A&S 2e. Renal cell carcinoma, p1523

43 **c** **S100**

Schwanomas can be found in aspirates from many anatomic sites, especially soft tissue. The cytologically benign, but sometimes mildly atypical wavy or serpentine spindled cells may be admixed with a fibrillary or myxoid stroma and stain positively for S100.

DeMay, A&S 2e. Peripheral nervous system tumors, p1236-1237

44 **b** **Gomori methenamine silver stain**

Pneumocystis is an opportunistic infection that appears as amphophilic foamy casts on Papanicolaou stain. The 4-8 μm cup shaped cysts stain with Grocott modification of Gomori methenamine silver stain.

DeMay, A&S 2e. Pneumocystis jiroveci, p1172

45　b　B72.3, MOC31, BerEP4, calretinin

Immunohistochemical markers can be used to distinguish mesothelioma from metastatic adenocarcinoma. Markers that typically stain mesothelioma include calretinin, HBME1, CK5/6 and vimentin. Markers that typically stain metastatic carcinoma include MOC31, BerEP4, LeuM1 (CD15), B72.3, and CEA.

DeMay, A&S 2e. Other markers, p1523-1524

46　c　HepPar1

This aspirate displays the classic features of hepatocelluar carcinoma; large cells resembling hepatocytes with enlarged, atypical nuclei displaying prominent nucleoli and intranuclear inclusions. The cells may be present singly and in thickened trabeculae. Naked nuclei and necrosis may be present in the background. Hepatocellular carcinomas stain positively with HepPar1 and AFP. Inhibin stains adrenal cortical carcinoma. CD10 stains renal cell carcinomas. TTF1 is positive in many pulmonary primaries, primarily adenocarcinoma, small cell carcinoma and other nonsquamous cell carcinomas. All of these are in the differential diagnosis.

DeMay, A&S 2e. Transcription factors, p1520-1521

47　b　CDX2

This aspirate of metastatic colonic adenocarcinoma shows the characteristic cytologic features of hyperchromatic columnar cells in a necrotic or dirty background. CDX2 is positive in typical adenocarcinomas of the colon.

DeMay, A&S 2e. CDX2, p1521

48　b　CK7/CK20

Urothelial carcinoma from any site, including the renal pelvis stains positively for CK7/CK20. The morphology of urothelial carcinoma may include cercariform cells, cells with eccentric nuclei, and tapered cytoplasmic processes with blunt ends.

DeMay, A&S 2e. CK7 & CK20, p1521

49　b　CD15/LeuM1

While there are several immunocytochemical stains which can identify Reed-Sternberg cells to verify a diagnosis of Hodgkin lymphoma, CD15 (LeuM1) is the most viable. Abnormal cells in Hodgkin lymphoma routinely stain with CD15 and CD30.

DeMay, A&S 2e. Transmembrane glycoproteins, p1521-1522

ISBN 978-089189-6357　©ASCP 2015

Chapter 12

Molecular Diagnostics & Theranostics

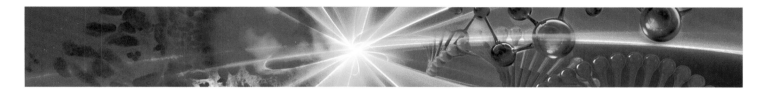

1 Which of the following describes the role of molecular diagnostics as it relates to the practice of cytopathology?
   a no value as an adjunctive testing modality for establishing the diagnosis of precancerous disease
   b increasing number of molecular techniques are available for infectious diseases and tumor diagnostics
   c a poor reflex for equivocal morphology
   d often difficult to standardize procedures and an overall lack of automation

2 Which statements regarding the utility of cotesting cytopathology with molecular diagnostics are considered true?
   a cotesting may impede service/patient care due to decreased turn around time
   b cotesting is often cost prohibitive due to poor reimbursement
   c cytology professionals are not educated to perform molecular testing
   d integrating reporting enhances the overall standard of care

3 Rare abnormal cells with atypical features suggesting a high grade intraepithelial lesion were found in a liquid based cytology preparation. DNA analysis for low and high risk HPV DNA was inconclusive. Polymerase chain reaction (PCR), using a universal consensus oligonucleotide primer for high risk HPV DNA types 16, 18, 31, 33, 35, 41, and 45, was used to test the residual cellular material from the vial. The PCR reaction was positive. Which of the following statements apply?
   a colposcopy is likely to reveal a high grade squamous intraepithelial lesion
   b PCR is not useful in confirming HPV DNA
   c high risk primers comprise HPV types 6 and 11
   d PCR is the most useful tool for evaluating gynecologic material

4 Which of the following molecular assays are least commonly used as adjunctive tests in cytopathology?
   a fluorescence in situ hybridization (FISH)
   b Hybrid Capture 2
   c polymerase chain reaction
   d strand displacement amplification

5 A consensus universal primer is designed to show cross reactivity for common nucleic acid sequences. For purposes of testing HPV in vitro, these primers are grouped into low and high risk genotype sequences in order to separate those patients with low potential for developing cervical intraepithelial neoplasia from those at high risk who need to be triaged into colposcopy or biopsy. Which of the following statements is true regarding these universal primers?
   a low risk types include 16, 18, 31, 33, 35, 45, 51, 52, 56, 58, 59, and 68
   b high risk types include 6, 11, 42, 43, and 44
   c a quantitative index of viral load is provided when using consensus primers
   d specimens are considered positive if any of the low risk or high risk viral infections are found within each respective probe cocktail

6 One of the advantages of using in situ hybridization testing for HPV DNA is:
   a it can be performed on archival tissue specimens
   b it can be performed on circulating peripheral blood
   c it is more sensitive than a Pap test
   d it is more sensitive than polymerase chain reaction

7 Which of the following statements represents the molecular function of Hybrid Capture 2 testing?
   a antibodies attach to captured hybrids reacting with a substrate to emit an amplified chemiluminescent signal
   b specimens are morphologically analyzed with fluorescence in situ hybridization (FISH)
   c specimens are morphologically analyzed with bright field microscopy using chromogenic detection
   d cleavage based amplification is utilized for the reaction

8 Flow cytometry of Pap tests with suspected cytologic changes of cervical intraepithelial neoplasia will help the pathologist determine that:
   a DNA aneuploidy confirms high grade lesions
   b DNA aneuploidy confirms low grade lesions
   c DNA aneuploidy is strongly associated with nononcogenic, nontransforming episomal HPV infections
   d flow cytometry cannot be used to analyze cervical samples owing to its inability to distinguish polyploidy from aneuploidy in any cervical intraepithelial lesion

9 An advantage of coupling in situ hybridization with cytopathology in the interpretation of precancerous or equivocal cytopathology specimens is that:
   a true replication/cloning of oligonucleotide targeted endogenous genetic aberrations allows for amplification of a single genetic copy
   b conventional microscopy (bright field) can be used to interpret genetic signals
   c genetic signals are measured by a luminometer
   d restriction fragment length polymorphisms (RFLPs) may provide confirmation of equivocal morphologic interpretations

10 The molecular assay which utilizes/amplifies specific targets by adding dideoxynucleotides (ddATP, ddCTP, ddGTP, and ddTTP) to 4 separate DNA synthesis reactions containing oligonucleotides, template and DNA polymerase is referred to as:
   a signal amplification for Hybrid Capture 2
   b in situ hybridization
   c polymerase chain reaction (PCR)
   d branched DNA amplification

11 Which of the following applications describes a signal amplification system that targets nucleic acids using a series of probes binding to a target, producing an overlap that is cut by an enzyme, where the addition of a complementary FRET probe with a reporter molecule located in the proximity of a quencher molecule subsequently binds to a signal probe producing a flap (which is cut by the earlier enzyme) releasing the reporter molecule from the quencher molecule ultimately producing a quantifiable signal?
   a Qβ replicase assay
   b ligase chain reaction
   c strand displacement amplification
   d invader (cleavage based) amplification

12 Which of the following molecular assays can be used for determining oncogenic HPV from liquid based specimens?
   a western blots
   b invader (cleavage based) amplification
   c mitochondrial DNA polymorphisms
   d cycling probe assays

13 A ThinPrep Pap test from a 44-year-old female with no previous history of abnormal cytology reveals few rare immature metaplastic cells with high N:C ratios, hyperchromasia, and irregular nuclear membranes. Based on these findings, which of the following may be recommended?
   a PCR testing for low risk HPV
   b loop electrosurgical excision procedure (LEEP)
   c Hybrid Capture 2 testing for high risk HPV
   d repeat Pap test in 1 year

14 The most important aspect of Hybrid Capture 2 testing is the:
   a negative predictive value
   b positive predictive value
   c specificity
   d sensitivity in CIN1

15 Hybrid Capture 2, the only commercially available HPV test approved by the Food and Drug Administration for use with liquid based Pap tests, is a nucleic acid signal amplification based assay that hybridizes a RNA probe with the target HPV DNA gene in vitro. How does the system allow for visualization of a positive product?
   a captured RNA-DNA hybrids with alkaline phosphatase conjugated antibodies are detected with a chemiluminescent substrate and signaled by a luminometer
   b it is a quantitative assay that uses type specific primers that hybridize with RNA-DNA hybrids and are detected with ethidium bromide
   c it uses a Southern blot analysis of DNA hybrids that are visualized with radioactive 32P via autoradiography
   d it uses tissue in situ hybridization of cellular and viral nucleic acid sequences visualized by biotinylated probes

16 An advantage of Hybrid Capture 2 assays, as compared to other molecular assays, is its:
   a ability to differentiate integrated from episomal viral infections
   b ability to provide specific virus genotyping
   c specificity for high risk viral types
   d sensitivity for HSIL and cancer

17 Cervical squamous intraepithelial lesions have a progressive dysfunction of proliferative ability where proliferating cells and mitotic figures increase as a factor of increasing CIN grades. Which of the following immunocytochemical markers may be useful markers of proliferation?
   a HPV E6/E7
   b p53
   c Rb
   d Ki67

18 An advantage of in situ hybridization, as compared to other molecular assays for diagnosing precancerous cervical lesions, is its:
   a excellent tissue or cytology localization of HPV infected cells
   b labeling as an analyte specific reagent
   c increased sensitivity over Hybrid Capture 2
   d use of a thermal cycler to clone low signal viral copies to help the gynecologist predict the likelihood for a clinically visible lesion in the future

19 Flow cytology was performed on a bronchial washing specimen from a 66-year-old male with a history of smoking but nondiagnostic cytology. A high S phase fraction was determined, which may indicate:
   a reactive bronchial alveolar cells
   b idiopathic pulmonary hemosiderosis
   c hamartoma
   d bronchogenic carcinoma

ISBN 978-089189-6357 ©ASCP 2015

20 Which molecular assay has increased sensitivity and specificity over immunohistochemistry for determining overexpression of the *HER2*/neu gene (chromosome 17 (17q11.2-q12) in breast cancer?
   a fluorescence in situ hybridization (FISH)
   b RFLP typing
   c bisulfite DNA sequencing
   d single strand conformation polymorphism (SSCP)

21 Which assay will allow for increased sensitivity (as compared to cytology) for establishing the diagnosis of low grade malignant tumors from benign urothelial cells?
   a Hybrid Capture 2
   b pyrosequencing
   c fluorescence in situ hybridization (FISH)
   d cleavage based amplification

22 For purposes of CLIA '88, HPV testing is considered:
   a low complexity
   b moderate complexity
   c high complexity
   d CLIA '88 does not rule on the complexity of HPV testing in the laboratory

23 Which FDA approved urologic assay uses a multicolor test that detects aneuploidy for chromosomes 3,7, 9p21, and 17?
   a Urovysion (Abbott Molecular)
   b BTA TRAK test (Polymedco)
   c APTIMA (Gen-Probe)
   d NMP22 (Matritech)

24 Which disease/genetic mutation/adjunctive molecular assay can assist fine needle aspiration cytology to classify genetic mutations that can aid in stratifying aggressive vs less aggressive tumors?
   a retinoblastoma/p53/PCR
   b pancreatic cancer/RET tyrosine kinase domain (RETTK)/PCR
   c thyroid (papillary) cancer/*KRAS* mutations/PCR
   d neuroblastoma/*NMYC*/fluorescence in situ hybridization (FISH)

25 Which of the following oncogenes is considered a tumor suppressor protein (which normally functions to prevent cells from dividing in the absence of an appropriate signal) where its deletion or inactivation can be used as a biomarker for tumor progression in many types of cancer, including esophagus, head and neck, bladder, colon, lung, melanoma, and cervix?
   a p16
   b *KRAS*
   c *BRCA1* and *BRCA2*
   d *NMYC*

26 Which of the following cancers are associated with translocations resulting in the chromosomal abnormality t(14;18), t(8;14)?
   a follicular lymphoma
   b acute lymphocytic leukemia
   c multiple myeloma
   d Waldenström macroglobulinemia

27 Which of the following statements regarding molecular diagnostics is false?
   a over 5,000 diseases have direct genetic causes
   b it provides a high sensitivity and increased specificity for most tests and adds diagnostic utility
   c it may provide a viable reflex for equivocal morphology
   d turnaround time of FDA approved tests may prohibit use in gynecologic cytopathology

28 The p16 immunohistochemical stain can be used in the differential diagnosis of cervical precancer vs a reactive process. In the cell, p16 functions as:
   a a cell cycle inhibitor; therefore, strong overexpression implies the lesion of interest is most likely benign
   b a cell cycle inhibitor; therefore, absence of expression means the lesion of interest is most likely to be precancer
   c a cell cycle inhibitor that is paradoxically overexpressed in precancer
   d a cell cycle promoter; therefore, overexpression means the lesion of interest is most likely precancer

29 Why is p16 immunohistochemistry a useful tool for cervical neoplasia identification?
   a p16 overexpression is a surrogate for high risk HPV oncogene activity
   b p16 overexpression is a good marker for the presence of any type of HPV
   c p16 is only expressed in high grade lesions
   d if p16 is negative, the lesion is most likely also HPV−

30 When evaluating breast carcinoma in a cytologic preparation for HER2/neu overexpression by immunocytochemistry, one looks for:
   a nuclear staining
   b punctate staining
   c plasma membrane staining
   d cytoplasmic staining

31 What is the most useful feature of clinically validated high risk HPV DNA testing?
   a it is very specific and therefore has a high positive predictive value
   b it is very sensitive and therefore has a high negative predictive value
   c it is very sensitive and therefore has a high positive predictive value
   d it is very specific and therefore has a high negative predictive value

32 A nuclear counterstain utilized in the preparation and analysis of fluorescent in situ hybridization (FISH) specimens is:
   a PAS (periodic acid-Schiff)
   b Feulgen
   c DAPI (4'-6-diamidino-2-phenylindole)
   d GMS (Gomori methenamine silver)

33 A 62-year-old female presents with a 3 cm mass in the anterior rectum. Cytologic analysis reveals a poorly differentiated adenocarcinoma. Which of the following immunohistochemical markers might be recommended to assist the clinician in determining the appropriate therapeutic regimen if they are concerned the patient might be resistant to cisplatin and would like to measure oxaliplatin response?

a excision repair cross complementing polypeptide (ERCC1)
b minichromosome maintenance and topoisomerase IIα (ProEx C)
c BRAF to determine EGFR inhibitor response
d microsatellite instability MLH1

34 A 12-year-old female with a previous diagnosis of Ewing sarcoma presents with multiple lung nodules in the hilar area of the right lung. Which of the following FISH assays is necessary to confirm a diagnosis of metastatic sarcoma?

a ALK 2p23 gene rearrangement
b EWSR 10q23,3 deletion
c EWSR 18q11 and 18q11.2 rearrangement
d EWSR1 22q12 rearrangement

35 Which of the following molecular biomarkers when overexpressed may assist the clinician with determining cervical intraepithelial disease progression caused by aberrant S phase induction?

a epithelial growth factor receptor (EGFR; ErbB1; HER1 in humans)
b minichromosome maintenance and topoisomerase IIα (ProEx C)
c estrogen receptor
d excision repair cross complementing polypeptide (ERCC1)

36 Identification of which mutation has been known to occur in classic Cowden syndrome, a heritable hamartoma syndrome with a high risk of breast tumor development?

a epithelial growth factor receptor (EGFR; ErbB1; HER1 in humans)
b ALK 2p23 gene rearrangement
c PTEN del(10)q23.3
d HER2/neu

37 A deep soft tissue aspiration reveals dispersed cells, stripped nuclei, acinar structures, and small to medium size cells with rounded and fusiform bland nuclei with inconspicuous nucleoli. FISH analysis of the cells reveals a cytogenetic anomaly t(X;18) (p11.2;q11.2). The diagnosis is consistent with:

a synovial sarcoma
b Ewing sarcoma
c pleomorphic sarcoma
d tuberculosis granuloma

38 Which of the following genetic aberrations, when identified in non-small cell lung cancer, would suggest a therapeutic regimen using Xalkori (crizotinib)?

a BCR/ABL fusion
b EML4/ALK fusions
c BRAF mutations
d EGFR mutations

39 A 30-year-old female presents with an acetic white lesion on the left quadrant of the cervix. The cytologic diagnosis rendered is HSIL (severe dysplasia) and is confirmed as CIN2 by histopathologic analysis. The patient is 6 months pregnant and the clinician is concerned that a LEEP may compromise the patient's pregnancy. After discussing the options with the patient, the pathologist recommends a marker to determine the likelihood that the disease will progress. Which of the following makers may assist the clinician in determining the likelihood of more rapid progression and help the patient decide whether she could wait for treatment post pregnancy vs immediate therapeutic intervention?

a FISH analysis of PTEN to determine a lipid phosphatase signal of phosphoinositol-3-kinase/AGT pathway
b chromogenic in situ hybridization for high risk HPV
c polymerase chain reaction to determine overexpression of E1 oncoprotein
d analysis of minichromosome maintenance and topoisomerase II α proteins with ProEx C

40 The following represents a cytologic sample from a 43-year-old female. A differential diagnosis of hairy cell leukemia is being considered. Which of the following immunohistochemical markers would be used to assist in your confirmation?

a CD20 pan B cell
b ANXA1: annexin A1; CBA44
c CD23
d PAX5

41 Which of the following markers would be helpful in differentiating mantle cell lymphoma?

a ANXA1
b BCL2 and BCL6
c cyclin D1/PRAD1
d CBA44/ZAP70

42 The following cells represent a fine needle aspiration of a 1 cm mass from the neck of a 35-year-old male with night sweats of 4 months duration. Which of the following immunohistochemical markers would help confirm the diagnosis?

a BCL2
b cyclin D1/PRAD1
c ZAP70
d fascin

ISBN 978-089189-6357 ©ASCP 2015

43 All of the following are considered hematopoietic markers for the confirmation of Hodgkin lymphoma, EXCEPT:
    a ALK
    b CD15
    c CD30
    d ANXA1

44 Which of the following immunohistochemical markers would be helpful in confirming a diagnosis of T cell/NK cell lymphoma?
    a CD1a/CD2/CD3/CD4/CD5/CD7/CD8/CD43/CD56/CD57/GRANB
    b CD10/CD20/CD23/CD79a/PAX5/BCL2/BCL6
    c ALK/CD15/CD30/fascin/PAX
    d CYCLIN/MUM1/CBA44/ZAP70

45 A 46-year-old female with a history of hereditary nonpolyposis colon cancer presents with recent weight loss, abdominal pain and tenderness in the lower abdomen presents with blood in the stool has a positive fecal occult test. Cytology of rectal brushings from a 4 cm mass reveals a grade 4 adenocarcinoma. Which of the following molecular assays will assist the clinician with responsiveness to EGFR inhibitor therapy and to assist with the differentiation of microsatellite instability?
    a CMYC 8q24 rearrangement
    b CEBPA mutational analysis
    c BRAF mutation analysis
    d BCR/ABL mutation analysis

46 A 58-year-old female with stage IV ductal carcinoma of the breast is being tested for the presence of circulating tumor cells. Results show that 8 cells/7.5 mL of blood. Based on the results, what are the clinical implications?
    a predictive of shorter progression free survival and shorter overall survival
    b predictive of longer progression free survival and greater overall survival
    c indeterminate of determination of progression
    d circulating tumor cells cannot be determined for breast cancer

47 What test would you recommend for screening of patients with chronic myelogenous leukemia (CML) who fail to achieve hematologic response at 3 months?
    a ALK 2p23 gene rearrangement
    b BCR/ABL kinase gene mutation analysis
    c CMYC 8q24 rearrangement
    d BRAF mutation analysis

48 Which of the following molecular assays identifies the fusion gene transcript and determination of baseline level expression in newly diagnosed CML patients?
    a BRAF mutation analysis
    b ALK 2p23 gene rearrangement
    c BCR/ABL quantitative PCR major and/or minor
    d CMYC 8q24 rearrangement

49 A 52-year-old male with a previously established diagnosis of melanoma presents with multiple nodules in the left lower lobe of the lung. Anaplastic cells are identified after needle aspiration. Which of the following positive mutations would assist the clinician in choosing vemurafenib therapy over other forms of chemotherapy?
    a BRAF V600
    b EGFR
    c KRAS
    d BCR/ABL mutation positive

50 A 62-year-old male presents with a 3 cm hilar mass in the upper lobe of the right lung. Subsequent CT scans reveal multiple masses in the liver. Fine needle aspiration biopsy reveals pleomorphic cells in loose aggregates with anisonucleosis and anisocytosis. Which of the following positive mutations would be helpful in triaging the patient for gefitinib and erlotinib therapy?
    a BRAF V600
    b HER2/neu
    c EGFR
    d KRAS

51 Which marker can assist the clinician with patient responsiveness to EGFR (tyrosine kinase inhibitor) therapy for colorectal cancer?
    a JAK2
    b PML RARA
    c KRAS
    d UGT1A1

52 Positivity by which of the following tests places a patient at a higher risk for Burkitt lymphoma?
    a HER2/neu by immunocytochemistry
    b epidermal growth factor (HER1) by immunocytochemistry
    c BCR/ABL by in situ hybridization
    d EBV by in situ hybridization

53 A 43-year-old female presents with pelvic ascites and lower back pain. Peritoneal aspiration reveals cells with large vacuolated cytoplasm, anisokaryosis in loose 3D groupings. Which of the following biomarkers may be useful in differentiating epithelioid mesothelioma vs serous papillary carcinoma of the ovary?
    a anticaldesmon
    b DOG1 K9
    c microsatellite PMS2
    d microsatellite MSH6

54 Which of the following markers confirm the presence of a gastrointestinal stromal tumor (GIST)?
    a microsatellite instability MLH1
    b DOG1 (K9)
    c HER2
    d p16

55 Which of the following markers would aid in the diagnosis of a metastatic anaplastic squamous cell carcinoma in a lung aspirate from a primary esophageal carcinoma?
   a ALK1
   b p16
   c KRAS
   d HER1

56 A 33-year-old female presents with a 2 cm lesion in the upper right quadrant of the right breast. FNA reveals poorly differentiated anaplastic cells. FISH analysis with HER2 was positive for aneuploidy. The patient was treated with Herceptin and Lapatinib but had metastatic recurrence 6 months later. Which of the following therapeutic regimens would be recommended?
   a second course of trastuzumab/lapatinib
   b doxorubicin/Adriamycin
   c trastuzumab emtansine (T-DM1)
   d 5FU

57 A 66-year-old male with a history of grade IV colorectal cancer presents with multiple lesions in the liver. Immunohistochemical and molecular analysis reveals the cells are IHC3+ and FISH+ for HER2. Which of the following therapeutic regimens may increase/stabilize overall survival rate?
   a dual therapy with trastuzumab and Lapatinib
   b monotherapy with FOLFIRI
   c FOLFOX
   d triple therapy with FOLFIRI, FOLFOX and Avastin

58 Which of the following biomarkers may aid in assisting individuals with Lynch syndrome determine whether they are at an increased risk for hereditary nonpolyposis colon cancer?
   a p16
   b p21
   c p27^{Kip}
   d microsatellite instability marker 2

59 Which gene expression marker is consistently expressed in Reed-Sternberg cells from classic Hodgkin disease?
   a pERK1/2
   b human herpesvirus 8
   c multiple myeloma oncogene 1 (*MUM1*)
   d pRb (phosphorylated retinoblastoma suppressor protein)

60 Which of the following biomarkers may aid in determining cell progression of atypical cells of undetermined significance from a cervical sample and thus may prompt the clinical for increased surveillance?
   a p21
   b p16^{INK4a}
   c p27^{Kip}
   d pRb

61 Loss of which protein has been linked to tamoxifen resistant breast cancers?
   a p21
   b pRb
   c p16^{INK4a}
   d p27^{Kip}

62 A 28-year-old female with undifferentiated ductal carcinoma of the breast was estrogen receptor negative and progesterone receptor negative. Analysis with p27^{Kip} revealed strong reactivity. Based on the following, which of the following statements is true?
   a more likely to have a high tumor and a higher propensity for metastasis
   b more likely to have a lower tumor grade and greater prognosis
   c no information can be discerned from the molecular panel

63 A 53-year-old male with a 6 cm solitary nodule in the liver presents with hepatocellular carcinoma. The surgeon was unable to resect the entire tumor. Positivity by which of the following markers might suggest the patient is a candidate for sorafenib therapy?
   a p21^{Waf1}
   b p16^{INK4a}
   c p27^{Kip}
   d pERK

64 A FNA of a soft tissue lesion reveals pleomorphic spindle cells with malignant nuclear features. The cells were positive for intermediate filament, desmin, and to muscle specific actin and confirmed as leiomyosarcoma. Measurement of the overexpression of which protein may lead to a disruption of apoptosis and short term survival/poor prognosis?
   a SRV (survivin)
   b microsatellite instability MLH1
   c DOG1 (K9)
   d p16

ISBN 978-089189-6357   ©ASCP 2015

65 A ThinPrep Pap specimen taken from a 44-year-old female immunologically stained for the p16^{INK4a} protein. Which of the following represents the most appropriate clinical management?

   a recommend follow-up Pap test every 6 months to determine if progression to adenocarcinoma in situ occurs

   b immediate colposcopy

   c hysterectomy

   d HPV testing in 12 months

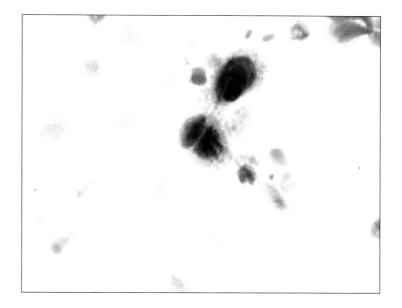

66 A 66-year-old former Hall of Fame pitcher for the Chicago Cubs, with a history of oropharyngeal cancer presents with a 2 cm cervical neck mass of unknown etiology. The cells illustrated were extracted from the mass and fixed in ethanol and processed for the Papanicolaou stain and in situ hybridization (ISH) using Inform HPV III Family 16 probe (Ventana Medical Systems). ISH stains revealed dark blue to black nuclear dots. The diagnosis is consistent with:

   a reactive lymphoid hyperplasia

   b branchial cleft cyst

   c metastatic squamous cell carcinoma

   d sialadenitis

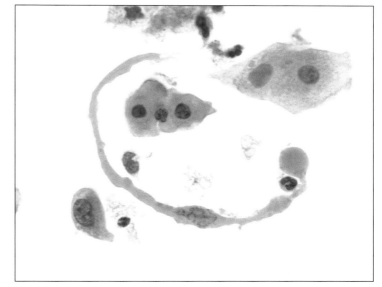

67 A 58-year-old female with a previous history of a breast malignancy presents with difficulty in breathing and a blood streaked sputum. A liquid based sputum sample was processed with a modified Pap stain and a fresh sample was submitted for FISH analysis. A multitarget FISH probe to the centromeric region of chromosome 6 and to the 5p15, 8q24 (site of the *MYC* gene) and 7p12 (site of the *EGFR* gene) loci revealed 5 cells with multiple gains. These cells represent the Pap stained cytology. The diagnosis is:

   a metastatic breast cancer (ductal)

   b metastatic colon cancer

   c primary lung cancer (squamous cell carcinoma)

   d benign respiratory epithelium

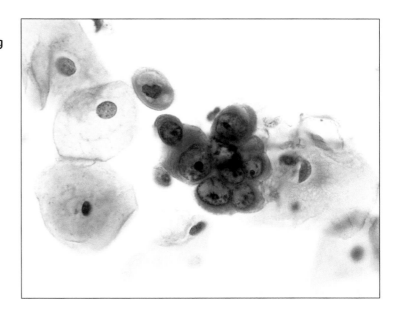

68 The abnormal urothelial cells shown have been treated with a UroVysion FISH probe set and were visualized with a fluorescent microscope. This FISH probe pattern is most consistent with:

a tetrasomy
b polysomy
c trisomy
d 9p21 homozygous deletion

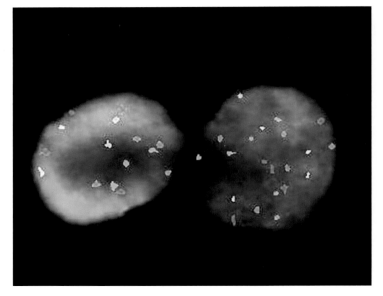

69 A 69-year-old patient has "smudge cells" in her peripheral smear and generalized lymphadenopathy. Fine needle aspiration of a cervical lymph node has been performed as shown in the image and needle rinses are submitted in RPMI for flow cytometry analysis. Which of the limited flow cytometry panel shown below would be most useful?

a CD3, CD20, CD79a, CD10
b CD3, CD4, CD8, CD45
c CD20, CD3, κ, λ
d CD56, CD3, κ, λ

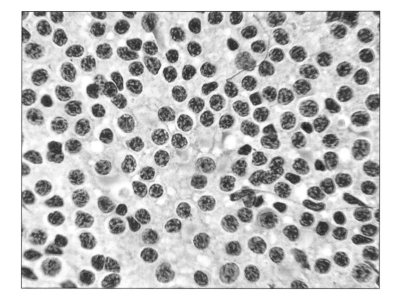

70 Positive results from which ancillary test would help confirm the morphologic impression in this aspirate of a 3 cm left supraclavicular mass from a 72-year-old male?

a flow cytometry
b S100 stain
c TTF1 stain
d PLAP stain

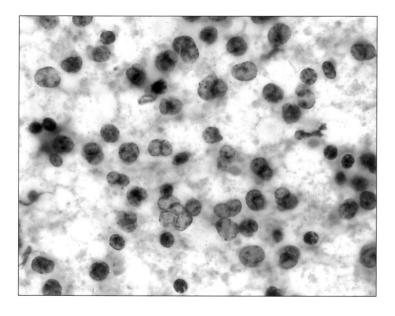

ISBN 978-089189-6357 ©ASCP 2015

71 FNA was performed on a 65-year-old male with a hypervascular 4 cm right kidney mass. What is the genetic abnormality seen in >90% of cases of this tumor?

a chromosome 11 translocations
b no genetic aberrations
c trisomy 7 and 17
d chromosome 3 aberrations, especially deletions

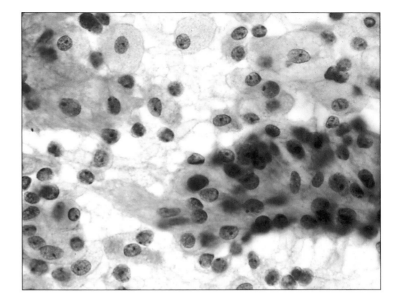

72 Which cytogenetic abnormality is associated with the entity depicted in this aspirate of a 3 cm subcutaneous mass from the ankle of a 34-year-old female?

a t(X;18)
b t(11;22)
c t(9;22)
d WT1

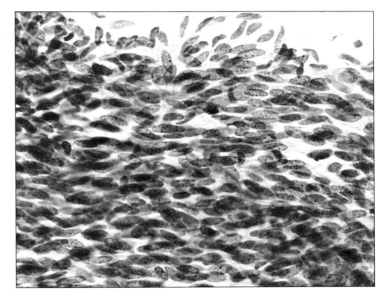

73 A 44-year-old female presents with a 2 cm lesion in the upper outer quadrant of the left breast. FNA reveals the following cells. The patient is confirmed with Stage 2 node negative disease. Which of the following tests would allow the oncologist to choose between a combination cyclophosphamide, doxorubicin (Adriamycin), fluorouracil (5FU) (CAF) chemotherapy vs Herceptin?

a microsatellite instability (ML1)
b HER2/neu
c KRAS
d BCR/ABL

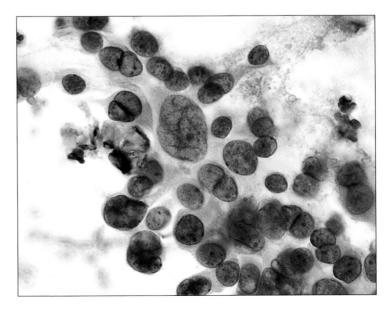

Molecular Diagnostics & Theranostics
Answer Key

1 **b** **increasing number of techniques for infectious diseases and tumor diagnostics**

The use of molecular tests has become invaluable, as adjunctive assays for establishing the diagnosis of precancerous cervical disease are now considered an important reflex for equivocal cellular morphology (ASCUS). Within the past 5 years, myriad platforms have been developed that have helped standardize the reliability of companion molecular diagnostics using semiautomation—increasing the overall sensitivity of testing.

Schmitt FC, Longatto-Filho A, Valent A, Vielh P. Molecular techniques in cytopathology practice. J Clin Pathol 2008 61(3):258-67 [PMID18037664]

2 **d** **integrating reporting enhances the overall standard of care**

Cotest results are now the standard of care for reporting atypical gynecologic Pap tests (ASCUS) under the 2006 ASCCP Guidelines for the management of abnormal cervical lesions. In addition, the efficiency of testing (turn around time of results) is not compromised using the latest generation of molecular assays.

Schmitt FC, et al. Molecular techniques in cytopathology practice. Clinic Pathol 2008;61(3):258-67 [PMID18037664]

3 **a** **colposcopy is likely to reveal a high grade squamous intraepithelial lesion**

Confirmation of high risk HPV DNA is possible with PCR. Quantitative RT-PCR may be even more useful in determining RNA transcripts in cervical infections with low viral copy number. However, PCR is not without its inherent limitations, including the relatively costly nature of performing the tests and the possibility of false positive results due to laboratory contamination or procedural errors.

DeMay, A&S 2e. PCR reaction based techniques, p1531

4 **d** **strand displacement amplification**

Common molecular tests in cytopathology include Hybrid Capture 2, in situ hybridization (cotesting for the cytologic diagnosis of ASCUS) and fluorescence in situ hybridization (useful for determining recurrent bladder cancer and prognostic markers for breast cancer).

Schmitt FC, et al. Molecular techniques in cytopathology practice. Clinic Pathol 2008;61(3):258-267 [PMID18037664]

5 **d** **specimens are considered positive if any of the low risk or high risk viral infections are found within each respective probe cocktail**

The probe cocktails simply indicate which patients are at low risk (probes that can hybridize to any of HPV types 6, 11, 42, 43, and 44) or high risk (types 16, 18, 31, 33, 35, 45, 51, 52, and 56).

Manos MM, et al. Identifying women with cervical neoplasia: using human papillomavirus DNA testing for equivocal Papincolaou results. JAMA 1999;281(17):1605-1610 [PMID10235153]

6 **a** **it can be performed on archival tissue specimens**

In situ hybridization can be performed on fresh unstained or archival (paraffin embedded) formalin fixed tissues as well as archived cervical smears or samples.

DeMay, A&S 2e. In situ hybridization (ISH) techniques, p1529-1530

7 **a** **antibodies attach to captured hybrids reacting with a substrate to emit an amplified chemiluminescent signal**

The specimen is initially hybridized with RNA probe (assume target sequence is present), captured by an RNA probe to detect hybrids, followed by conjugation with antibodies that attach to the captured hybrids ultimately reacting with a substrate to emit an amplified chemiluminescent signal.

Dehn D, Torkko KC, Shroyer KR. Human papillomavirus testing and molecular markers of cervical dysplasia and carcinoma. Cancer. 2007; 111(1):1-14 [PMID71219448]

8 **a** **DNA aneuploidy confirms high grade lesions**

DNA aneuploidy in cervical lesions is regarded as a true precursor for cervical cancer. Aneuploidy is absent in low grade lesions and thereby may help clinicians determine which patients need treatment. In addition, DNA aneuploidy in postirradiation cervicovaginal smears after cervical carcinoma may indicate recurrence.

DeMay, A&S 2e. Nonhematologic solid tumors, p1528-1529

9 **b** **conventional microscopy (bright field) can be used to interpret genetic signals**

In addition to the specificity of in situ hybridization, an added advantage is that the molecular signal can be compared with the cytomorphology such that the interpreter can view a microscopic signal in situ for comparative purposes.

Guo M, et al. A human papillomavirus testing system in women with abnormal Pap results: a comparison study with follow-up biopsies. Acta Cytol 2007;51(5):749-54 [PMID17910345]

10 **c** **polymerase chain reaction (PCR)**

PCR is the prototypical method for cloning and amplifying target nucleic acid in a rapid fashion (hours) such that the gene of interest can be detected in vitro.

DeMay, A&S 2e. PCR based techniques, p1531

11 **d** **invader (cleavage based) amplification**

Targets for this application include cystic fibrosis, factor V Leiden, and high risk human papillomavirus.

DeMay, A&S 2e. PCR reaction based techniques, p1531

12 **b** **invader (cleavage based) amplification**

Targets for this application include cystic fibrosis, factor V Leiden, and high risk human papillomavirus.

Wong AK, et al. Human papillomavirus (HPV) in atypical squamous cervical cytology: the Invader HPV test as a new screening assay. Clinic Microbiol 2008;46(3):869-875 [PMID18174309]

13 **c** **Hybrid Capture 2 testing for high risk HPV**

It may be appropriate to perform HPV testing for high risk (transforming) virotypes to determine if atypical cells of undetermined significance (ASCUS) or (ASC-H) are significant cytologic findings. If the HPV test is positive, colposcopy and biopsy are recommended (ALTS trial data, Shiffman and Solomon, National Cancer Institute). If the HPV high risk test is negative, the patient will be asked for

ISBN 978-089189-6357 ©ASCP 2015

a repeat Pap in 6 months or return to routine surveillance. Triage of atypical cells may help reduce unnecessary colposcopy on patients with equivocal Pap tests by determining which patients are truly at risk for progressive cervical intraepithelial disease. Between 10% and 20% of equivocal Pap tests confirmed positive for high risk HPV may prove to be high grade disease at colposcopy.

Dehn D, Torkko KC, Shroyer KR. Human papillomavirus testing and molecular markers of cervical dysplasia and carcinoma. Cancer 2007;111(1):1-14 [PMID17219448]

14   a   negative predictive value

Hybrid Capture 2 represents an FDA approved assay for the detection of high risk HPV. The sensitivity for detecting CIN2 or higher is 83%-96%, and the negative predictive value is 98%.

Dehn D, Torkko KC, Shroyer KR. Human papillomavirus testing and molecular markers of cervical dysplasia and carcinoma. Cancer 2007;111(1):1-14 [PMID17219448]

15   a   captured RNA-DNA hybrids with alkaline phosphatase conjugated antibodies are detected with a chemiluminescent substrate and signaled by a luminometer

Hybrid Capture 2 is the only commercially approved in vitro HPV test for determining low or high risk infections. The test uses microplates for capturing RNA hybrids and has an analytical sensitivity of 1.0 pg/mL (5,000 HPV genomes per test). The test is approved direct to vial or can be tested off liquid based medium.

Manos MM, et al. Identifying women with cervical neoplasia: Using human papillomavirus DNA testing for equivocal Papincolaou results. JAMA 1999;281(17):1605-1610 [PMID10235153]

16   d   sensitivity for HSIL and cancer

Hybrid Capture 2 represents an FDA approved assay for the detection of high risk HPV. The sensitivity for detecting CIN2 or higher is 83%-96%, and the negative predictive value is 98%.

Dehn D, Torkko KC, Shroyer KR. Human papillomavirus testing and molecular markers of cervical dysplasia and carcinoma. Cancer 2007;111(1):1-14 [PMID17219448]

17   d   Ki67

Studies have shown that expression of the proliferation marker Ki67 in normal, metaplastic, and dysplastic changes. The MIB1 monoclonal antibody shows progressively increased Ki67+ cells as CIN grades increase. Other studies have used Ki67 to discriminate HSIL from atypical atrophy

Bulten J, de Wilde PC, Schijf C et al. Decreased expression of Ki67 in atrophic cervical epithelium of postmenopausal women. J Pathol 2000;190(5):545–553 [PMID10727980].

18   a   excellent tissue or cytology localization of HPV infected cells

In addition to the specificity of in situ hybridization, an added advantage is that the molecular signal can be compared with the cytomorphology such that the interpreter can view a microscopic signal in situ for comparative purposes.

DeMay, A&S 2e. In situ hybridization (ISH) techniques, p1529-1530

19   d   bronchogenic carcinoma

Aneuploidy or high S phase fraction may assist in the confirmation of a malignant neoplastic disease. Flow cytometry may also prove useful in the diagnosis of high grade dysplasia from ulcerative colitis, carcinoma in situ in urothelial tumors, metastatic carcinomatous in cerebral spinal fluid specimens, and carcinoma of the breast via fine needle aspiration. It also has prognostic utility with hematopoietic lesions, neuroblastoma, medulloblastoma, and acute lymphoblastic leukemia.

DeMay, A&S 2e. Flow and image cytometry, p1528-1529

20   a   fluorescence in situ hybridization (FISH)

HER2 overexpression is associated with clinically aggressive breast tumors which have a higher recurrence rate and poorer prognosis. The use of a quantifiable FISH technique is considered more sensitive and specific when compared to the subjective interpretation of an immunohistochemical stain.

Sińczak-Kuta A, Tomaszewska R, Rudnicka-Sosin L, et al. Evaluation of HER2/neu gene amplification in patients with invasive breast carcinoma; Comparison of in situ hybridization methods. Pol J Pathol. 2007;58(1):41-50 [PMID17585541]

21   c   fluorescence in situ hybridization (FISH)

Although the sensitivity of cytology is good for establishing the diagnosis of high grade urothelial tumors, low grade tumors are difficult and often impossible to distinguish from benign urothelial cells. In addition, bladder cancer commonly recurs, and early recurrence is often difficult to detect cytologically with cystoscopic specimens. Utilization of FISH can help identify both low grade neoplasms and recurrent transitional cell carcinoma of the bladder.

Daniely M, Rona R, Kaplan T, et al. Combined morphologic and fluorescence in situ hybridization analysis of voided urine samples for the detection and follow-up of bladder cancer in patients with benign urine cytology. Urol Oncol 2008;26(3):332 [PMID17963263]

22   c   high complexity

The CLIA laboratory and staff must be approved for high complexity testing.

DeMay, A&S 2e. Compliance resources, p1591

23 a Urovysion (Abbott Molecular)

Although the sensitivity of cytology is good for establishing the diagnosis of high grade urothelial tumors, low grade tumors are difficult and often impossible to distinguish from benign urothelial cells. In addition, bladder cancer commonly recurs, and early recurrence is often difficult to detect cytologically with cystoscopic specimens. Utilization of FISH can help identify both low grade neoplasms and recurrent transitional cell carcinoma of the bladder.

Daniely M, Rona R, Kaplan T, et al. Combined morphologic and fluorescence in situ hybridization analysis of voided urine samples for the detection and follow-up of bladder cancer in patients with benign urine cytology. Urol Oncol 2008;26(3):332 [PMID17963263]

24 d neuroblastoma/ *NMYC*/fluorescence in situ hybridization (FISH)

In addition to overexpression of *NMYC* in the PI3K mediated VEGF regulation of neuroblastoma cells, p53 oncoproteins have been identified in up to 50% of all cancers, *KRAS* mutations have been found in pancreatic cancer, and the RET tyrosine kinase domain (RETTK) is overexpressed in papillary carcinoma of the thyroid.

Kang J, Rychahou PG, Ishola TA, Mourot JM, Evers BM, Chung DH. NMYC is a novel regulator of PI3K-mediated VEGF expression in neuroblastoma. Oncogene 2008;27(28):3999-4007 [PMID18278068]

25 a p16

Overexpression of p16^{INK4a} protein indicates infection and genomic integration of high risk human papillomavirus (high risk HPV) and may be useful for determining the progression of abnormal cervical lesions to carcinoma.

Holladay EB, Logan S, Arnold J, Knessel B, Smith GD. A comparison of the clinical utility of p16^{INK4a} immunolocalization to the presence of human papillomavirus by hybrid capture 2 for the detection of cervical dysplasia/neoplasia. Cancer Cytopathol 2006;108(6):451-461 [PMID17078096]

26 a follicular lymphoma

Translocations often given rise to the development of hematological malignancies, such as chronic myelogenous leukemia and follicular lymphoma.

DeMay, A&S 2e. Diagnostic, prognostic, and theranostic applications, p1532-1534

27 d turnaround time of FDA approved tests may prohibit use in gynecologic cytopathology

The efficiency of testing (turnaround time of results) is not compromised using the latest generation of molecular assays. In addition, cotesting cytology and high risk HPV molecular results are now considered the standard of care for reporting atypical gynecologic Pap tests (ASCUS).

Schmitt FC, Longatto-Filho A, Valent A, Vielh P. Molecular techniques in cytopathology practice. J Clin Pathol 2008 Mar;61(3):258-67 [PMID18037664]

28 c a cell cycle inhibitor that is paradoxically overexpressed in precancer

p16 is a cyclin dependent kinase inhibitor. High levels of p16 normally block the cell cycle. The E7 oncogene of high risk HPVs causes p16 to be overexpressed, but the site of p16's inhibition is also bypassed by HPV oncogene activation.

Thomison J 3rd, Thomas LK, Shroyer KR. Human papillomavirus: molecular and cytologic/histologic aspects related to cervical intraepithelial neoplasia and carcinoma. Hum Pathol 2008;39(2):154-166 [PMID08206494]

29 a p16 overexpression is a surrogate for high risk HPV oncogene activity

The E7 oncogene of virtually all high risk HPVs interacts with the retinoblastoma cell cycle control protein to turn on p16; therefore, p16 can act as a surrogate for the harder problem of detecting multiple high risk HPVs.

Thomison J 3rd, Thomas LK, Shroyer KR. Human papillomavirus: molecular and cytologic/histologic aspects related to cervical intraepithelial neoplasia and carcinoma. Hum Pathol 2008;39(2):154-166 [PMID08206494]

30 c plasma membrane staining

A membranous staining pattern is the hallmark of *HER2*/neu immunocytochemistry profile.

DeMay, A&S 2e. Growth factors and growth factor receptors, p1513-1514

31 b it is very sensitive and therefore has a high negative predictive value

Negative predictive value drives the value of HPV testing which is highly sensitive for CIN3.

Stoler MH, Castle PE, Solomon D, Schiffman M. The expanded use of HPV testing in gynecologic practice per ASCCP-guided management requires the use of well validated assays. Am J Clin Pathol 2007;127(3):335-337 [PMID17276947]

32 c DAPI (4'-6-diamidino-2-phenylindole)

DAPI is 4',6-diamidino-2-pheylindole, a commonly utilized fluorescent nuclear chromatin counterstain.

Halling KC. Kipp BR. Fluorescence in situ hybridization in diagnostic cytology. Hum Pathol 2007;38(8):1137-4114 [PMID17640552]

33 a excision repair cross complementing polypeptide (ERCC1)

ERCC1 polypeptide is required for nucleotide excision repair of damaged DNA. Increased levels are found in cisplatin resistant cells.

Jérôme Viguier et al. ERCC1 Codon 118 polymorphism is a predictive factor for the tumor response to oxaliplatin/5-fluorouracil combination chemotherapy in patients with advanced colorectal cancer. Clin Cancer Res 2005;11:6212 [PMID16144923]

ISBN 978-089189-6357 ©ASCP 2015

34   d   EWSR1 22q12 rearrangement

The chromosomal abnormality t(11;22)(q23;q12) has been detected in 90%-95% of primary and metastatic Ewing sarcoma, the second most common bone tumor in children. Detection of the rearrangement is evident in interphase cells.

Yamaguchi U et al. A practical approach to the clinical diagnosis of Ewing sarcoma/primitive neuroectodermal tumour and other small round cell tumours sharing EWS rearrangement using new fluorescence in situ hybridisation probes for EWSR1 on formalin fixed, paraffin wax embedded tissue. J Clin Pathol 2005;58(10):1051-1056 [PMID16189150]

35   b   minichromosome maintenance and topoisomerase II α (ProEx C)

ProEx C targets the minichromosome maintenance (MCM2) and topoisomerase II α (TOP2A) proteins, which when overexpressed allow for disease progression due to aberrant S phase induction. HPV oncoproteins E6 and E7 create aberrant S phase, and the levels of MCM2 and TOP2A proteins increase in proliferating cells. Specimens with p16+/ProEx C+ results showed the highest specificity for CIN2 and CIN3.

Ming Guo et al. Efficacy of p16 and ProExC immunostaining in the detection of high grade cervical intraepithelial neoplasia and cervical carcinoma. Am J Clin Pathol 2011;135(2):212-220 [PMID21228361]

36   c   *PTEN* del(10q23.3)

PTEN, a tumor suppressor gene located on 10q23.3, encodes a lipid phosphatase that regulates the G1, thus interfering with cell cycle arrest and subsequent apoptosis. *PTEN* mutations have been identified in 80% of Cowden syndrome, a heritable multiple hamartoma syndrome that increases the risk for breast, endometrial and thyroid cancer.

Iqbal UA et al. Mutational spectra of PTEN/MMAC1 gene: a tumor suppressor with lipid phosphatase activity. J Natl Cancer Inst 1999;91(22):1922-1932 [PMID10564676]

37   a   synovial sarcoma

SYT 18q11.*2* gene rearrangement translocation is highly specific for synovial sarcoma. Detection is in interphase cells.

Fisher C, de Brujin DRH, Guerts van Kessel A. Chapter IX: Synovial sarcoma. In Fletcher CDM, Unni KK, Mertens F, eds. World Health Organization Classification of Tumors: Pathology and Genetics of Tumours of Soft Tissue and Bone. Lyon, IARC Press, 2002, p200-204 [ISBN 9283224132]

38   b   *EML4/ALK* fusions

Rearrangements of the ALK locus are found in non-small cell lung cancers. *EML4/ALK* fusions are due to paracentric inversions on the short arm of chromosome 2. Late stage or metastatic non-small cell lung cancer can be treated with Xalkori (crizotinib).

Soda M, Choi YL, Enomoto M, et al: Identification of the transforming EML4-ALK fusion gene in non-small cell lung cancer. Nature 2007;448:561-566 [PMID1765570]

39   d   analysis of minichromosome maintenance and topoisomerase II α proteins with ProEx C

ProEx C targets the minichromosome maintenance (MCM2) and topoisomerase II α (TOP2A) proteins, which when overexpressed allow for disease progression due to aberrant S phase induction. HPV oncoproteins E6 and E7 created aberrant S phase and the levels of MCM2, and TOP2A proteins increase in proliferating cells. Specimens with p16+/ProEx C+ results showed the highest specificity for CIN2 and CIN3.

Ming Guo et al. Efficacy of p16 and ProExC immunostaining in the detection of high grade cervical intraepithelial neoplasia and cervical carcinoma. Am J Clin Pathol 2011;135(2):212-220 [PMID21228361]

40   b   *ANXA1*: annexin A1; CBA44

Annexin A1 (*ANXA1*) has been identified as a gene that is upregulated in hairy cell leukemia. The marker is important in differentiating from other B cell diseases, including splenic lymphoma with villous lymphocytes and variant hairy cell leukemia, which do not respond well to treatments effective with hairy cell leukemia.

Falini B et al. Simple diagnostic assay for hairy cell leukemia by immunocytochemical detection of annexin A1 (ANXA1). Lancet 2004;5:363(9427):1869-70 [PMID15183626]

41   c   cyclin D1/PRAD1

Cyclin D1 is a G1 cyclin that helps control the cell cycle progression by interacting with the retinoblastoma gene product (pRb), which when inactivated, is associated with mantle cell lymphoma. Mantle cell lymphomas are characterized by bcl1 rearrangement and cyclin D1 (PRAD1/CCND1) overexpression.

Jares P et al. Expression of retinoblastoma gene product (pRb) in mantle cell lymphomas: correlation with cyclin D1 (PRAD1/CCND1) mRNA levels and proliferative activity. Am J Pathol 1996;148(5):1591-1600 [PMID8623927]

42   d   fascin

Fascin is a sensitive marker for Reed-Sternberg cells and strongly positive in classic Hodgkin disease but cannot be used to rule out anaplastic large cell lymphoma.

Fan G et al. Comparison of fascin expression in anaplastic large cell lymphoma and Hodgkin disease. Am J Clin Pathol 2003;119(2):199-204 [PMID12579989]

43   d   *ANXA1*

Annexin A1 (*ANXA1*) has been identified as a gene that is upregulated in hairy cell leukemia. The marker is important in differentiating from other B cell diseases, including splenic lymphoma with villous lymphocytes and variant hairy cell leukemia, which do not respond well to treatments effective with hairy cell leukemia.

Falini B et al. Simple diagnostic assay for hairy cell leukemia by immunocytochemical detection of annexin A1 (ANXA1). Lancet 2004;5:363(9427):1869-70 [PMID15183626]

44 a CD1a/CD2/CD3/CD4/CD5/CD7/CD8/CD43/CD56/CD57/GRANB

Aggressive NK cell leukemia composed of immature NK cells. The disease is extremely rare. Cells are medium sized with irregular hyperchromatic nuclei and abundant cytoplasm containing azurophilic granules. Cells are positive for CD56, TIA1 and granzyme B, and some T cell specific antigens (CD2, CD3).

Medeiros LJ, Elenitoba-Johnson KS. Anaplastic large cell lymphoma. Am J Clin Pathol 2007;127(5):707-722 [PMID17511113]

45 c *BRAF* mutation analysis

Patients with primary or metastatic colorectal cancer with *BRAF* mutations are eligible for EGFR inhibitor therapy.

Tol J et al. (2009). BRAF mutation in metastatic colorectal cancer. NEJM 361:98-99 [PMID19571295]

46 a predictive of shorter progression-free survival and shorter overall survival

The Veridex, LLC CellSearch Circulating Tumor Cells Kit (Raritan, NJ) detects circulating epithelial tumor cells in peripheral blood. A count of 5 cells/7.5 mL or greater is predictive of a shorter progression free survival rate in patients with breast cancer.

Lucci A et al. Circulating tumour cells in nonmetastatic breast cancer: a prospective study. Lancet Oncol 2012;13(7):688-695 [PMID22677156]

47 b *BCR/ABL* kinase gene mutation analysis

The most common mechanism of resistance to Gleevec is due to mutations in the ABL kinase domain which prevents Gleevec from binding to the active site. Patients with a log increase in quantitative BCR/ABL levels should be assayed for the presence of Gleevec-resistance by quantitative RT-PCR. Increasing the dosage of Gleevec or adding another kinase inhibitor may help control the levels of BCR/ABL. Alternative therapies may be recommended if testing reveals a T315I mutation, indicating resistance to multiple targeted tyrosine kinase inhibitors.

Jones D et al. Laboratory practice guidelines for detecting and reporting BCR/ABL drug resistance mutations in chronic myelogenous leukemia and acute lymphoblastic leukemia. J Molec Diagn 2009;11:4-11 [PMID19095773]

48 c BCR/ABL quantitative PCR major and/or minor

Identification of a gene fusion transcript and baseline level of BCR/ABL (e13a2, e14a2, e1a2) expression confirms CML. The translocation is found in 99% of CML patients. The assay is also used to monitor the minimal resistance disease or remission in response to tyrosine kinase inhibitor therapy or stem cell transplantation.

Branford S et al. Real-time quantitative PCR analysis can be used as a primary screen to identify patients with CML treated with imatinib who have BCR/ABL kinase domain mutations. Blood 2004;104(9) [PMID15256429]

49 a *BRAF* V600

60% of melanomas have a mutation in the *BRAF* gene. Vemurafenib (Zelboraf) has been proven to improve survival in patients with untreated *BRAF* V600 mutation+ melanoma. Patients with *BRAF* V600E mutations can also be treated with dabrafenib (Tafinlar) and patients with V600K mutations with trametinib (Mekinist).

Bollag G et al. Clinical efficacy of a RAF inhibitor needs broad target blockade in BRAF-mutant melanoma. Nature 2010;467(7315):596-599 [PMID20823850]

50 c *EGFR*

EGFR mutations increase affinity to tyrosine kinase inhibitors. Gefitinib and erlotinib therapy, a tyrosine kinase inhibitor, has been proven to increase survival rates in patients with non-small cell lung cancer (NSCLC). In addition, detection of exon 19 deletions and exon 21 (L858R) substitution mutations of *EGFR* can be used to treat patients with NSCLC with Gilotrif (afatinib), an EGFR tyrosine kinase inhibitor.

Cataldo VD et al. Treatment of non-small cell lung cancer with erlotinib or gefitinib. N Engl J Med 2011;364:947-955 [PMID21388312]

51 c *KRAS*

30%-50% of colorectal tumors have mutated *KRAS* gene and these patients respond to anti-epidermal growth factor (EGFR) antibody therapy. Identification of 7 somatic mutations in KRAS oncogene qualifies patients for treatment with Erbitux (cetuximab) and Vectibix (panitumumab).

Wilson PM, Labonte MJ, Lenz HJ. Molecular markers in the treatment of metastatic colorectal cancer. Cancer J 2010;16(3):262-272 [PMID20526105]

52 d EBV by in situ hybridization

The Epstein-Barr virus has been associated with Burkitt lymphoma (an aggressive B cell lymphoma), Hodgkin disease and nasopharyngeal carcinoma.

Brady G et al. Epstein-Barr and Burkitt lymphoma. J Clin Pathol 2007;60(12):1397-1402 [PMID18042696]

53 a anticaldesmon

Anticaldesmon (regulatory protein found in smooth muscle) stains smooth muscle and myoepithelial cells. Although mesothelioma can be difficult to differentiate based on cytomorphology from adenocarcinoma, anticaldesmon may assist in differentiating epithelioid mesothelioma from serous papillary carcinoma of the ovary.

Comin CE et al. h-caldesmon, calretinin, estrogen receptor, and Ber-EP4: a useful combination of immunohistochemical markers for differentiating epithelioid peritoneal mesothelioma from serous papillary carcinoma of the ovary. Am J Surg Pathol 2007;3198:1139-1148 [PMID17667535]

54 b DOG1 (K9)

The calcium dependent chloride channel DOG1 (ANO1/TMEM16A) is expressed in 98% of gastrointestinal stromal tumors but is not expressed other sarcomas. Gastrointestinal stromal tumors (GIST) activate mutations of KIT or platelet derived growth factor receptor α (PDGFRA). Patients with GIST can be therapeutically treated with Gleevec/Glivec (imatinib) (tyrosine kinase inhibitors).

Simon S et al. DOG1 regulates growth and IGFBP5 in gastrointestinal stromal tumors. Cancer Res 2013;73(12):3661-3670 [PMID23576565]

55 d HER1

HER1, or EGFR, is expressed in epithelial tissues and overexpressed in squamous cell carcinoma. Identification of EGFR mutations is crucial when triaging patients with an established diagnosis of non-small cell lung cancer for gefitinib and erlotinib therapy.

Ciardello F, Tortora G. Epidermal growth factor receptor (EGFR) as a target in cancer therapy: understanding the role of receptor expression and the other molecular determinants that could influence the response to anti-EGFR drugs. Eur J Cancer 2003;39:1348-1354 [PMID12826036]

ISBN 978-089189-6357 ©ASCP 2015

56 c trastuzumab emtansine (T-DM1)

T-DM1 is a combination of human epidermal growth factor receptor 2 (HER2) antimicrotubule agent DM1 with trastuzumab. This antibody-drug conjugate has proven as effective therapy for patients presenting with recurrent or metastatic breast cancer who were previously treated with trastuzumab, lapatinib, an anthracycline, a taxane, and capecitabine.

Krop IE et al. A phase II study of trastuzumab emtansine in patients with humanepidermal growth factor receptor 2-positive metastatic breast cancer whowere previously treated with trastuzumab, lapatinib, an anthracycline, ataxane, and capecitabine. J Clin Oncol 2012;30(26):3234-3234 [PMID22649126]

57 a dual therapy with trastuzumab and lapatinib

Trastuzumab therapy, in combination with cisplatin and capecitabine or 5FU with HER2+ tumors, is an effective therapeutic regimen. Recently, lapatinib (an ATP competitive inhibitor that simultaneously inhibits both EGFR and HER2) has proven to be synergistic in inhibiting cell growth of HER2+ gastric cancers.

Wainberg ZA et al. Lapatinib, a dual EGFR and HER2 kinase inhibitor, selectively inhibits HER2-amplified human gastric cancer cells and is synergistic with trastuzumab in vitro and in vivo. Clin Cancer Res 2010;16(5):1509-1519 [PMID20179222]

58 d microsatellite instability marker 2

Patients diagnosed with hereditary nonpolyposis colon cancer are predisposed to cancer as a result of germ line mutation in the DNA mismatch repair (MMR) genes. Identification of the mutation is helpful for familial predictive testing. Lynch syndrome is defined as a mutation in MMR genes *MLH1, MSH2, MSH6* or *PMS2*. Screening with microsatellite instability analysis to determine loss of MMR proteins will aid in guiding disease surveillance. Recently, large 3' deletions of the *EPCAM* gene have also been associated with Lynch Syndrome. Mutation carriers have 25%-70% risk for colorectal cancer and a 30%-70% risk for endometrial cancer.

Vasen et al. Revised guidelines for the clinical management of Lynch syndrome (HNPCC): recommendations by a group of European experts. Gut 2013;62(6):812-823 [PMID23408351]

59 c multiple myeloma oncogene 1 (*MUM1*)

A t(6;14) translocation occurs with multiple myeloma that is specific to the *MUM1/FR4/ACSAT/Pip* gene. MUM is expressed in myeloma cells, Reed-Sternberg cells and normal and neoplastic T cells.

Kempf W et al. MUM1 expression in cutaneous CD30+ lymphoproliferative disorders: a valuable tool for the distinction between lymphomatoid papulosis and primary cutaneous anaplastic large cell lymphoma. Br J Dermatol 2008;158:1280-1287 [PMID18410414]

60 b p16^INK4a

p16 is involved in regulating the cell cycle. Mutations in p16—determined by p16^INK4a immunostaining—correlate with the severity of cytological/histologic abnormalities. p16^INK4a may be used as a biomarker to identify HR-HPV transformed cells originally interpreted as atypical cells of undetermined significance (ASCUS) or ASC-H (small cells that favor a high grade SIL) in Pap test samples.

Wentzensen N1, Bergeron C, Cas F, Vinokurova S, von Knebel Doeberitz M. Triage of women with ASCUS and LSIL cytology: use of qualitative assessment of p16^INK4a positive cells to identify patients with high grade cervical intraepithelial neoplasia. Cancer 2007;111(1):58-66 [PMID17186505]

61 a p21

p21 is transcriptionally regulated by the tumor suppressor gene p53. Overexpression of p16 (a result of p16 binding to cyclin/CDK complexes) inhibits retinoblastoma (Rb) protein phosphorylation. Loss of p21 has been associated with a tamoxifen growth inducing phenotype due to hyperphosphorylation of estrogen receptor α, thereby inducing gene expression of estrogen receptor regulated genes. Identification of a loss of p16 may assist the clinician with determining alternative therapeutic management in patients with tamoxifen resistant breast cancers.

Abukhdeir AM et al. Tamoxifen-stimulated growth of breast cancer due to p21 loss. Proc Natl Acad Sci USA 2008;105(1):288-293 [PMID18162533]

62 a more likely to have a high tumor and a higher propensity for metastasis

p27, a tumor suppressor gene that serves as a regulator of the cell cycle, is often inactivated in cancer. Inactivation of p27 occurs by the oncogenic activation of receptor tyrosine kinases (RTKs), phosphatidylinositol 3-kinase (PI3K), proto-oncogene c-Src, or Ras-mitogen activated protein kinase (MAPK), thus accelerating the proteolysis of the p27 protein and allowing cells to undergo uncontrolled proliferation leading to oncogenesis.

Chu I, Sun J, Arnaout A, Kahn H, Hanna W, Narod S, Sun P, Tan CK, Hengst L, Slingerland J. p27 phosphorylation by Src regulates inhibition of cyclin E-Cdk2. Cell 2007;128(2):281-294 [PMID17254967]

63 d pERK

pERK is a biomarker used in determining which patients should receive sorafenib/Nexavar (Bayer HealthCare Pharmaceuticals) therapy for hepatocellular carcinoma. Phosphorylated ERK (pERK) is a downstream component of the RAF/MEK/ERK signaling pathway. Sorafenib inhibits the serine-threonine kinases RAF1 and B-Raf, the receptor tyrosine kinase activity of vascular endothelial growth factor (VEGF) receptors 1, 2, and 3, and platelet derived growth factor receptor β. Sorafenib therapy has been proven to increase survival rates in patients with advanced hepatocellular carcinoma (HCC).

Zhang Z et al. Phosphorylated ERK is a potential predictor of sensitivity to sorafenib when treating hepatocellular carcinoma: evidence from an in vitro study. BMC Medicine 2009;7:41 [PMID19698189]

64 a SRV (survivin)

Survivin inhibits of apoptosis, regulates cell division, and is overexpressed in the most cancers. Patients with tumors that immunohistochemically reveal strong expression of survivin in the cytoplasm and the nucleus are at a significant increased risk of tumor related death compared to weaker staining tumors.

Taubert et al. Expression of survivin detected by immunohistochemistry in the cytoplasm and in the nucleus is associated with prognosis of leiomyosarcoma and synovial sarcoma patients. BMC Cancer 2010;10:65 [PMID20181247]

65 b immediate colposcopy

Overexpression of p16^INK4a protein indicates infection and genomic integration of high risk human papillomavirus (high risk HPV) and may be useful for determining the progression of abnormal cervical lesions to carcinoma.

Holladay EB, Logan S, Arnold J, Knessel B, Smith DG. A comparison of the clinical utility of p16^INK4a immunolocalization to the presence of human papillomavirus by Digene Hybrid Capture 2 for the detection of cervical dysplasia/neoplasia. Cancer Cytopathol 2006;108(6) [PMID17078096]

66 c metastatic squamous cell carcinoma

These cells represent a metastasis from a primary oropharyngeal carcinoma. A necrotic background lacking lymphoproliferative elements with keratinizing debris with scattered pleomorphic squamous cells possessing smudged opaque nuclei are represented. Intranuclear signals as confirmed via molecular confirmation with ISH assists with the diagnosis. Even in the absence of malignant morphology, the presence of true squamous elements and confirmation with ISH may help establish the diagnosis of metastatic carcinoma.

DeMay, A&S 2e. In situ hybridization (ISH) techniques, p1529-1530

67 a metastatic breast cancer (ductal)

FISH allows for the differentiation of true neoplastic glandular cells from reactive atypia. These cells, representing ductal carcinoma of the breast, present as hypercellular epithelial cells arranged in well formed microacini with pleomorphic nuclei, nuclear crowding and overlapping, hyperchromasia, irregular nuclear membranes, irregular chromatin, and prominent nucleoli.

DeMay, A&S 2e. Infiltrating ductal carcinoma, p1087-1090

68 b polysomy

Polysomy is defined as a cell nucleus that has an extra copy of 1 or more chromosomes, as represented by this image.

DeMay, A&S 2e. In situ hybridization (ISH) techniques, p1529-1530

69 c CD20, CD3, κ, λ

Flow cytometry can be used to demonstrate the presence of clonality in specimens of possible lymphoma/leukemia by testing for κ & λ. Additional B & T cell markers are also useful.

DeMay, A&S 2e. Lymphoreticular malignancies, p303-305

70 a flow cytometry

This aspirate shows the cytologic features of large cell lymphoma. The lymphoid cells are large and discohesive with nucleoli and convoluted nuclear membranes. Lymphoglandular bodies are present. Flow cytometry was positive for CD20, CD10, and monoclonal λ expression consistent with large cell lymphoma, B cell type. Although melanoma, seminoma, and poorly differentiated pulmonary carcinoma may be in the differential, the morphology is much more consistent with lymphoma.

DeMay, A&S 2e. Biology of non-Hodgkin lymphoma, p994-995

71 d chromosome 3 aberrations, especially deletions

The vast majority of clear cell renal cell carcinoma, including those related to the von Hippel-Lindau (VHL) disease, show 3p deletions. Trisomy 7 and 17 abnormalities are seen in papillary renal cell carcinoma.

DeMay, A&S 2e. Conventional (clear & granular) renal cell carcinoma, p1356-1360

72 a t(X;18)

Virtually all synovial sarcomas exhibit the cytogenetic abnormality of t(X;18). This specific abnormality is rarely seen in other sarcomas. t(11;22) is seen in Ewing or PNET. t(9;22) is relatively specific for extraskeletal myxoid chondrosarcoma. WT1 is typically seen in Wilms tumor.

DeMay, A&S 2e. t27.9 Recurrent diagnostic chromosomal abnormalities in adult and childhood sarcomas, p1534

73 b *HER2*/neu

HER2/neu (or erbB2) regulates cell growth and is overexpressed in 25% of breast cancers. Amplification is a predictor of tumor recurrence. Herceptin therapy has been shown to dramatically reduce the recurrence.

Wolff AC et al. Recommendations for human epidermal growth factor receptor 2 testing in breast cancer: American Society of Clinical Oncology/College of American Pathologists clinical practice guideline update. J Clin Oncol 2013;31(31):3997-4013 [PMID24101045]

Index

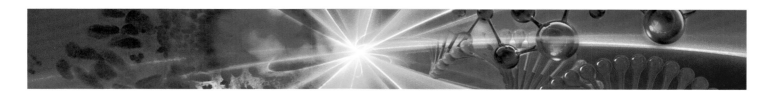

B

Bacterial vaginosis, 15
Barrett esophagus, 180
Basophilic watery diathesis, 82
BCR/ABL kinase gene mutation analysis, 382
BCR/ABL quantitative polymerase chain reaction (PCR), 382
Benign bile duct epithelium, 182
Benign chronic inflammation, 159
Benign collagen balls, 159
Benign diagnosis, 111
Benign fibrous histiocytoma, 310
Benign gastric mucosal cells, 322
Benign gastric tissue, 321
Benign lymphoepithelial cyst, 303
Benign mesothelial cells, 159
Benign radiation cellular changes, 10, 104
Bethesda System of classification, 33, 118
    criteria for, 115
    specimen adequacy clause of, 112
Bias, 357
Bicornuate uterus, 81
Bile duct brushings, 174, 176
Bilharzia, 237
Billable & total test, 352
Biohazard material, 338
Biopsy, 120
    cone artifact, 11
    fine needle aspiration, 373
Bipolar spindle cells, 162
Birth control pills, 97
Bladder dome, 255
Bladder washing, 256
Blastomyces dermatitidis, 208, 213
Bone marrow, 214
Bowen disease, 80
Bowenoid papulosis, 93
BRAF mutation analysis, 382
BRAF V600, 382
Brain metastasis, 125
Brain tissue, 159
Brenner tumor, 311
Bronchial aspiration, 200
Bronchial brushings, 183, 184, 185, 188, 189, 190, 191, 195, 201, 202, 203, 207
Bronchial hyperplasia, 211, 212
Bronchial metaplastic cells, 210
Bronchial obstruction, 186, 203
Bronchial washings, 184, 187, 202, 205, 206, 328
Bronchiectasis, 187
Bronchoalveolar lavage, 184, 204, 205, 363

Bronchopulmonary washing, 192
Brown artifact, 98
Brunn nests, 239
Budget, 343
Budget report, 344
Bullous dermatitis, 3

C

Caesarian section, 96
Calcium carbonate crystals, 255
Calcium dependent chloride channel (DOG1), 382
Cancer. See Carcinoma
Cancer screening program, 327
Candida, 213, 254
    albicans, 2, 181
    glabrata, 77
Cannonballs, 151
Capital budget, 352
Carbohydrate moieties, 365
Carbon histiocyte, 211
Carcinoembryonic antigen (CEA), 177
Carcinoid tumors, 177, 178, 208, 213, 306, 360
    of intestinal tract, 162
Carcinoma
    acinic cell, 304, 316
    adenoid cystic, 231, 304, 316, 317
    adenosquamous, 209
    adrenal cortical, 323
    alcian blue/colloid, 234
    anaplastic, 305
        pancreas, 312
        thyroid, giant cell variant, 323
    bladder, 238, 256
    breast, 159
    bronchioloalveolar, 309, 321
    bronchogenic, 379
    cervical, 72, 123
    chromophobe renal cell, 321
    clear cell renal cell, 314
    colloid, 230, 231, 236
    colonic, 161
    colorectal, 311, 373
    ductal of breast, 374
    exophageal, 163
    fibrolamellar hepatocellular, 311
    follicular, 258, 303
    giant cell anaplastic, 317
    hepatocellular, 320, 323, 360, 361, 366, 374
    hereditary nonpolyposis colon, 373
    infiltrating ductal, 235
    inflammatory, 230
    invasive, 208
    keratinizing, 9
    keratinizing squamous, 103
    large cell, 208, 306

    large cell nonkeratinizing, 9
    large cell squamous, 13
    lobular, 230, 233, 235
    lung, 149, 183
    medullary, 230, 234, 304, 305, 321
    meningeal, 136
    metastatic, 304
        anaplastic squamous cell, 374
        breast, 151, 158, 159, 315, 384
        colon, 82, 96
        colonic, 315
        lung, 151, 232
        Merkel cell, 323
        pancreatic, 282
        renal cell, 323
        small cell, 322
        squamous cell, 320, 321, 384
    microinvasive squamous, 11
    mucinous (colloid), 236, 365
    mucoepidermoid, 316
        well differentiated, 303
    nonkeratinizing squamous cell, 3, 88, 104
    nontrabecular hepatocellular, 305
    oat cell, 211
    oncocytic neuroendocrine, of pancreas, 314
    orpharyngeal, 375
    ovarian, 94
    pancreaticobiliary, 157
    papillary, 304, 315, 317
        of thyroid, 154, 269, 322
    papillary urothelial, 256
    renal cell, 154, 237, 252, 362, 367
    secretory ductal, of pancreas, 320
    small bowel, 161
    small cell, 90, 109, 152, 157, 159, 212, 216, 252, 306, 319, 361
        of the lung, 156
        neuroendocrine, 89, 104
        oat cell variety, 208
        squamous cell, 10, 95
    squamous cell, 3, 8, 11, 14, 182, 212, 254, 307, 320, 322, 365
        of bladder, 251
        differentiated urothelial, 253
        of esophagus, 209
        keratinizing, 88, 91, 99, 178, 181
            well differentiated, 209
        of lung, 200, 318
        nonkeratinizing, 95, 104, 179
        poorly differentiated, 208, 216
        of uterine cervix, 5, 33
    tamoxifen resistant breast, 374
    tubulal, 234, 236
    urothelial, 240, 249, 255, 256, 368
        grade III, 252
        low grade, 251
    uterine cervix
        squamous cell, 5
    vulva, 12
Carcinoma in situ, 9, 99, 101, 252

ductal, 231
small cell, 103
squamous, 11
urothelial, 255
of vulva, 4
Carnoy fixative, 308
Cat scratch disease, 314, 318
Cauda equina syndrome, 147
CD15/LeuM1, 368
CD20, 384
CDX2, 367
Cell blocks, 337
Cell cycle inhibitor, 380
Cell tumor of pancreas, 313
Cellular maturation, 77
Cellular morphology, 359
Cellulosic filters, 328
Centers for Medicare & Medicaid Services (CMS) approved proficiency testing program, 354
Centrifugal force, 328
Centrifugation/sediment method, 325
Cervical/endocervical smear, 7
Cervical smears, 5
Cervical squamous intraepithelial lesions, 370
Cervicitis, 105
chronic follicular, 105
chronic lymphocytic, 99
follicular, 7, 78, 104
granulomatous, 11, 90
Cervicography, 4
Charcot-Leyden crystals, 186, 211, 214
Chemical wastes, disposal of, 330
Chlamydial infection, 127
Chlamydia trachomatis, 14, 87
Cholangiocarcinoma, 303, 319, 324
well differentiated, 309
Cholecystectomy, 176
Chondroblastoma, 309
Chondrocalcinosis, 149, 155
Chondrosarcoma, 309
low grade, 322
Choriocarcinoma, 149
Chorioretinitis, 193
Choroid/ependymal cells, 156
Choroid plexus, 125
Chromatin degeneration, 4
Chromogranin, 319, 366
Chromosome 3 aberrations, 384
Chronic follicular gastritis, 177
Chylous effusion, 129
Ciliocytophthoria, 211
Cirrhosis, 2, 305
Civil Service Reform Act, 356
CK7/CK20, 368

Clinical information system (CIS), 90
Clinical Laboratory Improvement Amendments (1988) (CLIA '88), 4, 341, 342, 343, 344, 345, 351, 354
proficiency testing, 348
regulation, 349
Coating fixative, 328
Coccidioides, 215
Coccidioides immitis, 209, 213
coccidioidomycosis, 318
Cockleburs, 94
Coin lesion, 189
Collagen ball, 158
Collective bargaining, 357
College of American Pathologists (CAP) Laboratory Management Index Program (LMIP), 344
College of American Pathologists (CAP) Workload
productivity, 343
Recording Method, 343
Colloid goiter, 303, 316
Colonic brushings, 161, 165, 168, 173, 174
Colposcopy, 112, 119, 120, 121, 122, 124, 355, 378, 383
Commission for Allied Health Educational Programs, 350
Common leukocyte antigen, 157
Community borders, 152
Computer data access, 340
Computerized (axial) tomography (CAT or CT) scan, 40
Condyloma, 4
Condyloma acuminata, 106, 107
Condyloma infection, 9
Conjunctivitis, 151
Consensus universal primer, 369
Conventional microscopy, 378
Corn flaking, 98
Corpora amylacea, 211, 213, 252, 255
Corpus albicans, 2
Corpus luteum, 76
Corticosteroid therapy, 172
Cost accounting, 343
Cost benefit analysis, 334
Cost-plus technique, 352
Cotesting, 119, 120, 124, 378
Coverslip, 326, 329
Cowden syndrome, 372
Craniopharyngioma, 151
Credentialing, 355
Creola bodies, 211
Cresyl blue, 329
Criterion based job description, 347
Critical task, 355
Crohn disease, 171

Cross contamination, 355
Cryptococcus, 159, 361
Cryptococcus neoformans, 150, 152, 155, 209
Curschmann spirals, 186, 210, 211, 214
Cushing syndrome, 105
Cyclin D1, 381
Cystadenocarcinoma
mucinous, 99, 310
ovarian, 154
mucinous, 84
serous, 91, 158
papillary serous, 108
Cystadenoma, serous, 310
Cystic hyperplasia, 83
Cystic teratoma, 79
Cystitis, 251
granulomatous, 256
Cystitis cystica, 254
Cystitis glandularis, 253
Cytogenetic abnormality, 377
Cytologic analysis, 372
Cytologic-histologic correlation, 354
Cytologic specimens, 346
Cytology laboratory procedure, 345
Cytology laboratory's annual statistical report, 346
Cytology specimen requisition, 345
Cytology supervisor, 344, 346
Cytomegalovirus, 15, 94, 97, 209, 213, 215, 253, 256, 310
Cytopathology, 369
Cytopathology laboratory procedure manual, 346
Cytoplasmic streaming, 3
Cytoplasmic vacuolization, 85
Cytopreparation, 327
Cytopreparatory technicians, 341
Cytospin centrifugation technique, 326
Cytotechnologists, 341, 345, 346, 353
competency of, 345
worklogs of, 350
Cytotechnology laboratory vacancy, 342
Cytotechnology program, accreditation of, 341

D

DAPI, 380
Data points, 358
Defense, U.S. Department of, drug surveillance facilities of, 358
Del Castillo syndrome, 85, 106
Deoxyribonucleic acid (DNA) analysis, 369
Deoxyribonucleic acid (DNA) aneuploidy, 378
Desmin, 365

Diabetes mellitus (DM), 80, 98
Diagnostic performance, 345
Diathesis, 87, 96
Diff-Quik stain, 7, 333, 361, 365, 367
Direct costing, 356
Dispersion, 358
Disposable sharps, 338
Donovan bodies, 85
D-PAS+, 152
Ductal dilatation, 232
Ductal epithelium of pancreas, 311
Duodenal brushing, 166
Dysgerminoma, 310
Dyskeratocytes, 87
Dyskeratosis, 9, 78, 83
Dysphagia, 175
Dysplasia, 9, 10, 13, 187

E
EA65, 335
Early reactive lymph node hyperplasia, 312
Echinococcus granulosus, 153, 305, 319
Economic market, 349
Ectocervical scraping, 35
Ectocervical squamous lesions, 4
Effusion related disease, 149
Electron microscopy, 360
Elephantiasis, 128
Embryonal rhabdomyosarcoma, 152
EML4/ALK fusions, 381
Emphysema, 183
Endobronchial brushing, 192
Endocarditis, 193
Endocervical curettage (ECC), 6, 112, 120
Endocervical sampling, 121
Endocervical transformational zone component, 111, 118
Endocervical type glandular epithelium, 4
Endometrial cells, 111, 118
Endometrial curettings, 17
Endometrial hyperplasia, 79, 100, 102, 118
Endometrial polyps, 84
Endometrial sampling, 121
Endometriotic cyst, 310
Environmental factors, 357
Eosinophilic inclusions, 183
Ependymoma, 150
Epidermal growth factor receptor (EGFR), 382
Epidermoid cysts, 305
Epithelial lesions, 359
Epithelioid histiocytes, 212
Epstein-Barr virus, 382
Equal Employment Opportunity Commission (EEOC), 356

Esophageal brushings, 162, 163, 167, 169, 170, 171, 173, 174
Esophageal reflux, 181
Esophageal scraping, 162
Esophageal ulcers, 175
Esophageal washing, 175
Esophagitis, 181
Estrogen, 1
    ratio of, to follicle stimulating hormone, 1, 76
Ethanol, 332, 336
Ethanol (ethyl) alcohol (EA) stain, 328
Evacuation plan, 336
Excision repair cross complementing polypeptide (ERCC1), 380
Exophytic lesions, 86
Expert witness, 353
Exponential smoothing, 352
Extramedullary hematopoiesis, 129
Extrauterine tumors, 11
Eyewash plumbing, 331, 340

F
Factor VIII, 365
False negative immunocytochemical results, 361, 367
False positive immunohistochemical results, 361
Fascin, 381
Fat necrosis, 233, 235
Federal Labor Relations Authority, 357
Feminizing testicular syndrome, 58, 106
Ferruginous bodies, 211, 216
Fetal death in utero, 105
α-fetoprotein, 360, 366
Feulgen reaction, 360, 366
Fibroadenoma, 232, 235
Fibroblasts, 90
Fibrocystic diseases, 233, 235
Fibroma, 309
Fine needle aspiration (FNA), 40, 364, 373, 377
Fire drills, 339
Fire extinguishers, 325, 326, 331, 339
Fire plan, 331
Fire safety precaution, 328
Fixed costs, 356
Fixed forecast, 352
Flammable chemicals, storage of, 330
Floaters, 328, 335
Flow cytology, 370
Flow cytometry, 159, 324, 384
Fluorescent in situ hybridization (FISH) analysis, 372, 374, 375, 379, 380.71
Folic acid deficiency, 78, 85, 88
Follicular cells, 315

Follicular cysts, 310, 311
Follicular cytosis, 106
Follicular hyperplasia, 317
Food & Drug Administration (FDA), 356
Food contamination, 181
Formalin, 334, 338
Fraud, 352
French & Raven's bases of power model, 348
Full costing, 356
Fungating, 179
Fungi, 360

G
Ganglion cells, 322
Gartner cysts, 80
Gastric adenomatous polyps, 163
Gastric brushings, 161, 162, 164, 165, 166, 175
Gastric cytology, 163
Gastric lavage, 167
Gastric ulcer disease, 162
Gastric washings, 70, 163, 164, 172
Gastritis, 167
Gastroenteric cysts, 307
Gastrointestinal epithelium, 81
Gastrointestinal stromal tumor (GIST), 182, 323, 373
General Supervisor, 341, 353
Geotrichum candidum, 97
Germinoma, 323
Giant cell tumor of bone, 323
Giardia lamblia, 178
Glacial acetic acid, 331, 334
Glial fibrillary acidic protein (GFIP), 365
Glioblastoma multiforme, 151, 155
Glycogen, 81, 361
Glycogenated navicular cells, 81
Gomori methenamine silver (GMS) staining, 198, 366, 367
Goodpasture syndrome, 185
Gout/monosodium urate monohydrate, 155
Gouty arthritis, 125, 149
Granular cell tumors, 85, 215, 236
Granular intracytoplasmic inclusions, 94
Granuloma, 308, 320
    eosinophilic, 310
    lipophagic, 316
Granulosa cell tumor, 311
Granulosa-theca cell tumor, 82, 106
GYN cytology slides, 111
Gynecologic specimens, 350
Gynecomastia, 231, 236

H

I

J

K

L

Lumbar puncture, 133, 134
Luteal cyst, 309
Luteinizing hormone (LH), 1, 76
Lymphadenitis
  acute, 319
  chronic, 312
  granulomatous, 317
Lymph node hyperplasia, 267, 268
Lymphohistiocytic aggregates, 312
Lymphoid, 312
Lymphoid granulomatous disease, 268
Lymphoid lesion, 330
Lymphoma, 317, 366
  Burkitt, 158, 313, 314, 318, 373
  follicular, 380
  Hodgkin, 373
  immunoblastic, 267
  large cell, 180
    cleaved, 317
    noncleaved, 313
  malignant, 83, 307, 361
  Mantle cell, 372
  mixed cell, 268
  non-Burkitt, 158
  non-Hodgkin, 212, 304
  primary, 179
  small cell
    cleaved, 359
    noncleaved, 158, 318
    round, 266
  T cell/NK cell, 373
Lynch syndrome, 374

M

Macrocytosis, 87
Macronucleoli bodies, 8
Macrophages, 152
Malakoplakia, 253
Malignant fibrous histiocytoma, 318
Malignant melanoma, 152, 360
Malignant mesothelioma, 187
Malignant mixed tumor, 303
Malignant schwannoma, 308
Mallory bodies, 305
Malnutrition, 162
Mammogram, 159
Masculinizing tumor of the ovary, 1
Maslow's hierarchy of needs, 347
Masson trichrome, 365
Mastitis, 233
  granulomatous, 235
Material Safety Data Sheets (MSDSs), 325, 331, 332, 333, 339
Maturation index, 28
Mature cystic teratoma, 310
McGregor theory-Y leadership style, 347
Medulloblastoma, 150, 151, 156, 159
Megakaryocyte, 154
Melanin, 365

Melanoma
  metastatic, 307, 316, 323, 360, 367
Melanomas, 92, 154, 208, 360, 366
Meningioma, 150, 156
Meningiosarcoma, 150
Meningitis
  acute bacterial, 151, 156
  viral, 156
Meningoencephalitis, 127
Menometrorrhagia, 3
Menses, 1, 76
Menstrual cycle
  proliferative phase of, 99
  secretory phase of, 1, 76
Mesenchymal repair, 310
Mesonephric system, 4
Mesothelial cells, 152, 155, 156, 158, 320, 360
Mesothelioma, 128, 153, 157, 215, 363
  carcinomatous, 152, 154
Metaplastic dysplasia, 10, 102
Metastasis, 383
Metastatic malignant process, 153
Methanol, 337
Methylene blue, 329
Methyl green pyronine (MGP), 365
Michaelis-Gutmann bodies, 239
Microbacteria, 208
Microglandular hyperplasia, 2, 105
Microglandular pseudoparakeratosis, 76
Microhematuria, 249
Micronucleoli, diathesis, 90
Microphthalmia associated transcription factor (MITF), 272
Microsatellite instability marker 2, 383
Minichromosome maintenance & topoisomerase II α, 381
Mitotic figures, 1, 76
Mixed mesodermal tumor, homologous, 108
Mixed Müllerian tumor, 6, 100
  uterine, 11
Modified Carnoy fixative, 329
Modified ethanol (ethyl) alcohol (EA), 337
Molecular assays, 369, 370
Molecular diagnostics, 369, 371
Molluscum contagiosum, 98
Monosodium urate crystals, 149
Mott cell, 157
Mucicarmine, 126, 158, 214, 234, 366, 367
Mucinous cystic tumor/surgical resection, 311
Müllerian ducts, 5
Müllerian tumor, 4
Multinucleated bronchial, 214
Multinucleated giant histiocyte, 91

Multinucleation, 8
Multiple myeloma, 321
Multiple myeloma oncogene 1 (MUM1), 383
Multiple sclerosis, 149
Mycobacterium tuberculosis infection, 186
Myeloid metaplasia, 129
Myers-Briggs type, 348
Myocarditis, 127
Myoepithelial cells, 236
Myofibroblasts, 90
Myospherulosis, 236

N

National Labor Relations Act (NLRA), 347, 356
Navicular cells, 100
N:C ratios, 3, 87, 89, 106
Negative for intraepithelial lesion or malignancy (NILM), 96, 111, 118
Negative predictive value, 379
Negligence, 343, 347
Neoplasia
  cervical intraepithelial, 43, 87, 122
  vulvar epithelial, 82
  vulvar intraepithelial, grade 3 (VIN III), 6
Neoplasms
  alimentary tract, 169
  follicular, 304, 305, 316, 322
  hematopoietic, 306
  Hürthle cell, 305
  oncocytic, 309
  pancreatic endocrine, 322
  papillary, 187, 231
  papillary urothelial, of low malignant potential (PUNLMP), 252
  spindle cell, 360
Nephrolithiasis, 256
Neural sheath tumors, 307
Neuroblastoma, 151, 154, 156, 158
Neuroendocrine differentiation (ND), 10
Neuroendocrine tumors, 11, 212, 366
Neutral red-Janus green, 366
Nocardia asteroides, 209
Nodular fasciitis, 321
Nongonococcal urethritis, 151
Nonkeratinizing dysplasias, 80, 88, 102, 103, 106
Nonkeratinizing squamous lesion, 48
Nonkeratinizing stratified squamous, 210
Nonproductive cough, 201
Normal biliary duct, 311
Nose inhalant abuse, 214
Not for profit hospital, 356
Nuclear feathering, 109
Nuclear overstaining, 327
Nuclear pyknosis, 88, 104
Nucleopore filters, 328, 335